Discarded
University of Cincinnati
Blue Ash College Library

Magnetic Resonance Imaging: Atlas of the Head, Neck, and Spine

Magnetic Resonance Imaging: Atlas of the Head, Neck, and Spine

CATHERINE M. MILLS, M.D.
*Vice President and Medical Director
NMR of America, Inc.;
Assistant Clinical Professor of Radiology
University of California, San Francisco*

JACK de GROOT, M.D., Ph.D.
*Professor of Anatomy and Radiology
University of California, San Francisco*

JONATHAN P. POSIN, M.D.
*Director, North Bay MRI Center;
Assistant Clinical Professor of Radiology
University of California, San Francisco*

LEA & FEBIGER · PHILADELPHIA
1988

Lea & Febiger
600 South Washington Square
Philadelphia, Pa. 19106-4198
U.S.A.
(215) 922-1330

Library of Congress Cataloging-in-Publication Data

Mills, Catherine M.
  Magnetic resonance imaging: atlas of the head, neck, and spine / Catherine M. Mills, Jack de Groot, Jonathan P. Posin.
    p. cm.
  Includes index.
  ISBN 0-8121-1031-5
  1. Head—Imaging—Atlases. 2. Neck—Imaging—Atlases. 3. Spine—Imaging—Atlases. 4. Magnetic resonance imaging—Atlases. I. De Groot, J. (Jacob) II. Posin, Jonathan P. III. Title.
  [DNLM: 1. Head—anatomy & histology—atlases. 2. Neck—anatomy & histology—atlases. 3. Nuclear Magnetic Resonance—atlases. 4. Spine—anatomy & histology—atlases. WE 17 M657m]
QM535.M54 1988
617'.510757—dc19
DNLM/DLC
for Library of Congress   87-29344
                                              CIP

Copyright © 1988 by Lea & Febiger. Copyright under the International Copyright Union. All Rights Reserved. This book is protected by copyright. No part of it may be reproduced in any manner or by any means without written permission of the Publisher.

PRINTED IN THE UNITED STATES OF AMERICA

Print Number: 5 4 3 2 1

Foreword

MRI has dazzled the radiologic profession, the medical community at large, the financial community, and the public. Its workings seem both magical and a technologic tour de force. Radio waves weaker than those reaching us from commercial radio stations thousands of miles away are used to make life-like images of the inside of the body. Superconducting magnets that not too long ago were considered the stuff of accelerator laboratories and fusion research centers can now be found in hospitals, clinics, and shopping centers. Quantum mechanical principles are invoked to explain the workings of these magnets and the theory of the imaging process. Intimate molecular motions are reflected in images.

Intoxicated by the sheer weight of the technology and its access to information from deep in the molecule, many forget that an image is not a diagnosis. The quality of MRI as a diagnostic tool is no better than the interpretative ability of the physician conducting the study. Therefore, MRI, this youngest and most complex imaging technology, cannot be sundered from the oldest and most direct: anatomy. To understand MRI, we must first know how it maps the body onto an electronic image. This is why an atlas of this kind is a welcome and needed addition to the diagnostic library. This book has been prepared by three authors who mirror the disciplines they bring together so fruitfully. One is an anatomist who has been dedicated for many years to bringing to the physician pictures of the human body as it is. The others are young radiologists whose careers started when MRI began to realize its clinical potential and who contribute greatly to this realization. The reader can infer his own parable.

Much has been written about MRI. In addition to journals, the reader can find books that range from disorganized collections of "everyone's" work to tight compendiums written by one or two authors. The basic physics chapters and reviews are starting to assume a reassuring uniformity, including sometimes those written by physicians. Chapters on instrumentation range from the banal to the reasonable; none does justice to this rich and subtle subject. Literature regarding imaging techniques still ranges from the enlightened to the medieval. When MRI penetrated the consciousness of the radiologic community, much was written and said about future clinical applications. Not surprisingly, as working units became available, more was disproved than proved. Happily, we are now at a stage where the most grandiose expectations for MRI have been left behind. The papers that prove new clinical applications now appear more frequently than do those that disprove a previously "proven" application. Fantasy has left MRI and has settled on spectroscopy.

Five years from now, the practicing clinician will be as interested in the physics and instrumentation of MRI as he is today in the same aspects of x-ray CT or nuclear medicine. This is not necessarily bad: a great car driver does not need a Ph.D. in thermodynamics to win a race, nor does a jockey need to know the metabolic pathways of ATP and glucose to push his horse to the front. While a radiologist may not need to know the physics and instrumentation of MRI to serve his patients, knowledge of the way that the technique represents the human body is essential. This atlas speaks for the reality of MRI.

LEON KAUFMAN, PH.D.
*University of California,
San Francisco
Radiologic Imaging Laboratory*

Acknowledgments

We owe our thanks to many contributors who labored with us to bring this book to fruition. First, our deepest appreciation to Leon Kaufman, Ph.D., Director of the Radiologic Imaging Laboratory at the University of California, San Francisco, for his support, encouragement, and generous use of imagers and laboratory personnel. In particular, among the many helpful individuals at the R.I.L., we wish to thank Lawrence Crooks, Ph.D., and David Feinberg, Ph.D., for their sequencing software support, Mitsuaki Arakawa and John Hoenninger for their imaging hardware support, and Jeff Watts for his system software support. These individuals were responsible for the ongoing improvements in imager performance, ensuring that the Diasonics head images shown here were always state-of-the-art (and often compelling us to repeat images as we proceeded with this work). Equally valuable was the assistance provided by David Kramer, Ph.D., of the Technicare Corporation. Many individuals at both Diasonics (MRI), Incorporated and the Technicare Corporation provided technical and moral support, and both organizations also provided financial support to help to defray the costs of photographic reproduction. In that regard, we are indebted to the expert photographic work provided by John Sheldon, Deborah Kelly, and David Akers, who spent countless hours producing the highest-quality negatives and prints, doing justice to the spectacular images seen on the monitors after a rewarding imaging session. Such images are the result not only of well-tuned hardware and software, but of cooperative, motivated volunteers who spent many of their free hours lying immobile within a magnet. Two volunteers who deserve special mention are Anne Merrill Sandoval and Frank Gonzalez, who not only are excellent subjects, but are also excellent MRI technologists, responsible in their own right for the superlative spine images shown here. They received technical assistance from Carlos Sandoval, whose expertise ensured optimal performance of the Technicare system and its surface coils. Finally, thanks to those individuals who helped to bring order out of chaos. To Barbara diJeannene and Jill Lyon, who patiently typed and retyped this manuscript, and who endured the tedium of endless revisions and proofreading sessions, we owe our heartfelt thanks. So too, we thank our spouses for their patience and understanding, in particular the secretarial and technical support provided by Paula DeGroot, whose help certainly fell under the heading of "above and beyond the call of duty." We apologize to those not named here; they know that we appreciate their efforts in our behalf.

CATHERINE M. MILLS, M.D.
San Francisco, California
JACK DEGROOT, M.D., PH.D.
San Francisco, California
JONATHAN P. POSIN, M.D.
San Francisco, California

Contents

CHAPTER 1	Introduction	1
CHAPTER 2	Head, Axial Plane	3
CHAPTER 3	Head, Coronal Plane	61
CHAPTER 4	Head, Sagittal Plane	87
CHAPTER 5	Orbit	109
CHAPTER 6	Functional Systems	133
CHAPTER 7	Face, Neck and Cervical Spine, Axial Plane	161
CHAPTER 8	Face, Neck and Cervical Spine, Coronal Plane	183
CHAPTER 9	Face, Neck and Cervical Spine, Sagittal Plane	203
CHAPTER 10	Thoracic Spine	217

    a. Axial Series

    b. Coronal Series

    c. Sagittal Series

CHAPTER 11 Lumbar Spine   247

    a. Axial Series

    b. Coronal Series

    c. Sagittal Series

INDEX   283

1

Introduction

Few developments in the field of diagnostic imaging have generated as much excitement within the medical community as has magnetic resonance imaging (MRI). Though still in its infancy, when measured against the developmental time line of its predecessor, x-ray computed tomography, MRI has already proved its clear superiority in the area of central nervous system imaging.

At present, magnetic resonance imaging provides superlative sensitivity to pathologic change, increased contrast resolution, and comparable spatial resolution and clinical throughput when compared to computed tomography. These accomplishments are achieved without the limitations of ionizing radiation, beam-hardening artifacts, administration of intravascular or intrathecal contrast media, or lengthy computer reconstruction to obtain images in multiple orthogonal planes. It is not surprising that this diagnostic technique, with its clear advantages, has been so rapidly embraced by the medical community. As has been shown in the literature, however, the multiparametric nature of MRI yields a complexity and concomitant wealth of information that far exceed those characteristic of other techniques. MRI also requires new skills in the performance and interpretation of these examinations. This book provides the reader with a means to complement existing sources of information and to correlate the superb soft tissue contrast realized in magnetic resonance images with the appropriate anatomic and functional structures.

The MR images that follow were obtained in three orthogonal planes and appear in the variety of imaging sequences likely to be encountered on a routine clinical basis. These images were acquired on state-of-the-art superconducting magnetic resonance imagers operating at 0.35 and 0.6 T.

Given the state of flux of the MRI field, a wide variety of imagers will find their way into clinical practice, operating within a broad range of magnetic field strengths and with many different imaging sequences. This potential confusion has resulted in some consensus regarding the particular types of images that should be obtained to highlight certain of the better-understood tissue characteristics. With this in mind, signal acquisition techniques were selected that appropriately emphasized the T1 and T2 relaxation time differences known to be critical for neurodiagnosis. These images were obtained with the use of the spin echo technique of signal acquisition. The signal realized in magnetic resonance images is multiparametric and depends on hydrogen density, T1 and T2 relaxation times, and blood flow. Alterations in the parameters of the instrument, however, will emphasize particular contributors to the image intensity. Relatively short repetition and echo times provide images that highlight the T1 relaxation time characteristics, whereas long repetition and echo times highlight the T2 relaxation time characteristics.

The anatomic sections were obtained by serial sections in axial, coronal, or sagittal planes. The cadaver specimens were frozen prior to section; this procedure sometimes produces tissue swelling that effaces the normal cerebrospinal fluid spaces. Precautions were taken, however, to avoid artifact secondary to freezing; namely, most specimens were embalmed prior to being quickly frozen in dry ice. Sections approximately 4 mm thick then were made with use of a fine-tooth band saw (22 teeth/inch), were cleaned with running water, and were photographed within only a few hours of preparation to prevent desiccation. The anatomic sections were subsequently matched as closely as possible with the magnetic resonance images obtained from a volunteer subject. Although the magnetic resonance images were obtained from several different volunteers, an attempt was made to use images that not only were normal, but were anatomically similar. Note that several anatomic specimens were obtained from older individuals, who typically show large cerebrospinal fluid spaces due to atrophy of nervous tissue.

Where appropriate, pathologic examples have been included to complement normal images. In addition, because MRI clearly separates gray from white matter, and thus accurately visualizes the position of functional tracts as they extend from cortex to spinal cord, a separate section on functional neuroanatomy has been provided. Likewise, the improved visualization of vascular structures and associated pathologic processes has led to the inclusion of vascular anatomy and associated perfusion territories. Hopefully, both of these additions will be of particular use in clinical practice, as precise identification and localization of lesions can now be correlated to specific clinical symptoms.

Significant effort went into acquiring the best possible images for this atlas at the time it was sent to press. Unlike x-ray computed tomography, however, for which improvements in image quality usually coincided with each new generation of hardware, improvements in MRI are based for the most part on software improvement, and thus can occur at more frequent and less predictable intervals. In our experience, the time between new "generations" of magnetic resonance images has been measured in months, even in weeks; thus, our best efforts may be tempered somewhat by the inherent delay between the time this manuscript went to press and the time the reader is first able to obtain the finished product. In fact, we finally submitted this manuscript with a mixture of reluctance and pleasure, knowing that the true value of basic MRI anatomy, with careful correlation to specimens, function, vascular territories and pathology, would persist even in the face of further improvements in the technology.

2
Head, Axial Plane

Anatomic Level	Figures
Vertex	2.1–2.15
Centrum semiovale	2.16–2.23
Body of lateral ventricle	2.24–2.34
Internal capsule and thalamus	2.35–2.42
Midbrain	2.43–2.57
Pons	2.58–2.73
Medulla	2.74–2.88
Foramen magnum	2.89–2.95
Odontoid process of C2	2.96–2.100

A series of axial sections obtained from cadavers are matched with magnetic resonance images of a volunteer. Vascular territories are indicated by overlays on a companion image. Additional anatomic sections and magnetic resonance images that have slightly different angulation are displayed at each level. These images were generated on a second volunteer with the use of a different signal acquisition sequence. This chapter, therefore, reveals the variations seen as a result of changes in both patient position and imaging technique.

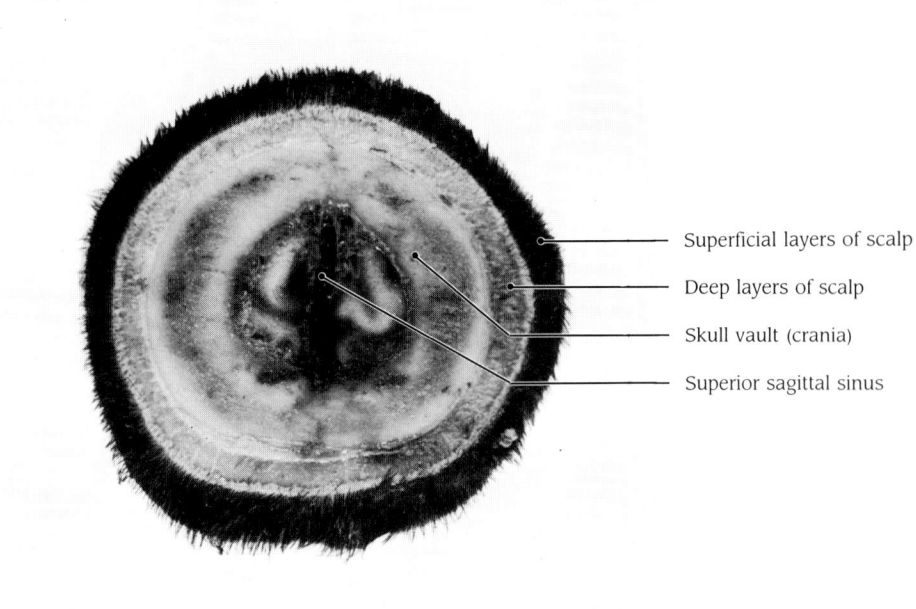
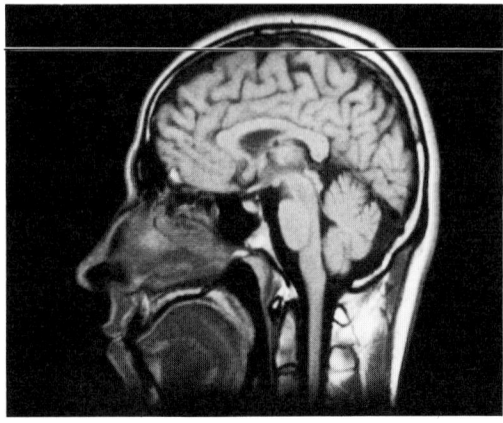

FIG. 2.1.

- Superficial layers of scalp
- Deep layers of scalp
- Skull vault (crania)
- Superior sagittal sinus

- The falx cerebri is formed by two layers of dura mater, which fuse with the endocranium and continue into the tentorium cerebelli. The superior sagittal sinus is enclosed by the layers of the falx cerebri and the endocranium, whereas the inferior sagittal sinus is solely contained within the falx.

- Although arachnoid granulations are most numerous in the superior sagittal sinus, they may occur in all dural venous sinuses, as well as in large cerebral veins.

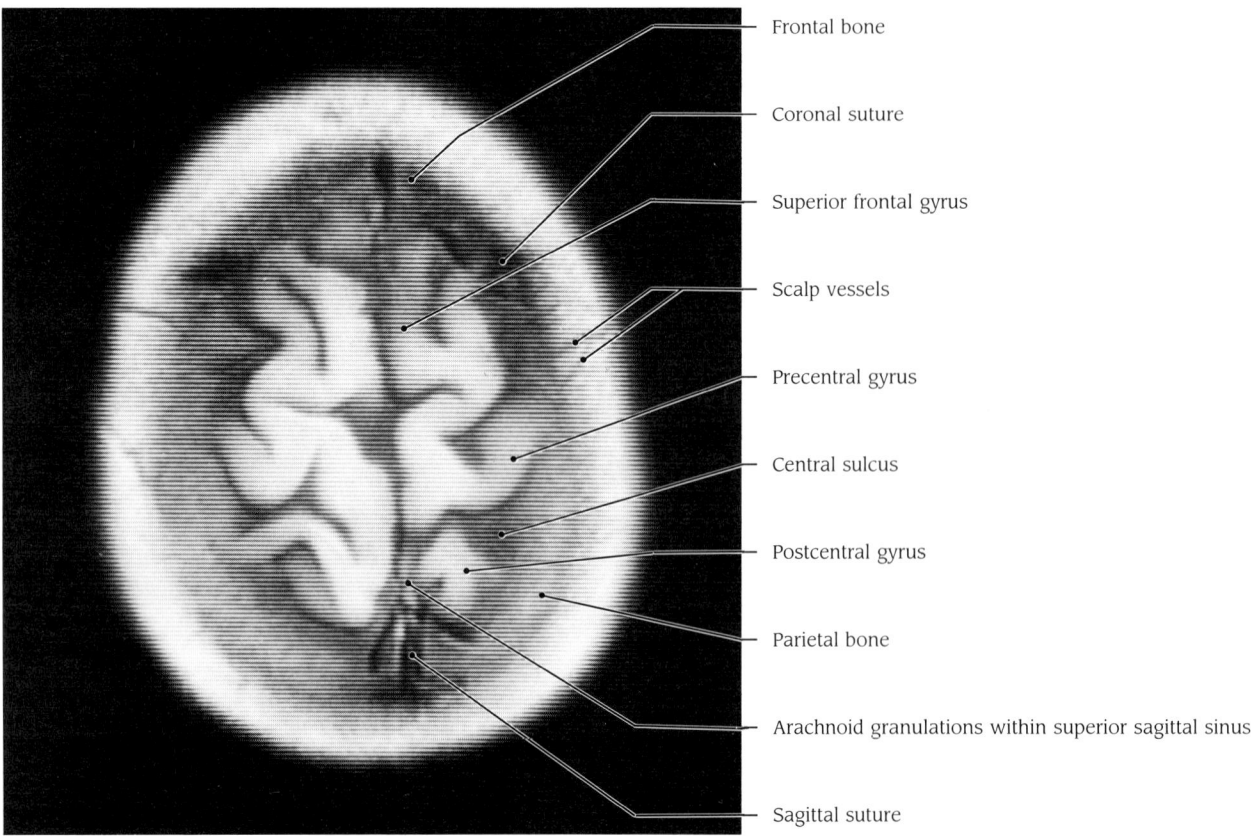

- Frontal bone
- Coronal suture
- Superior frontal gyrus
- Scalp vessels
- Precentral gyrus
- Central sulcus
- Postcentral gyrus
- Parietal bone
- Arachnoid granulations within superior sagittal sinus
- Sagittal suture

FIG. 2.2. TR = 500 msec, TE = 28 msec.

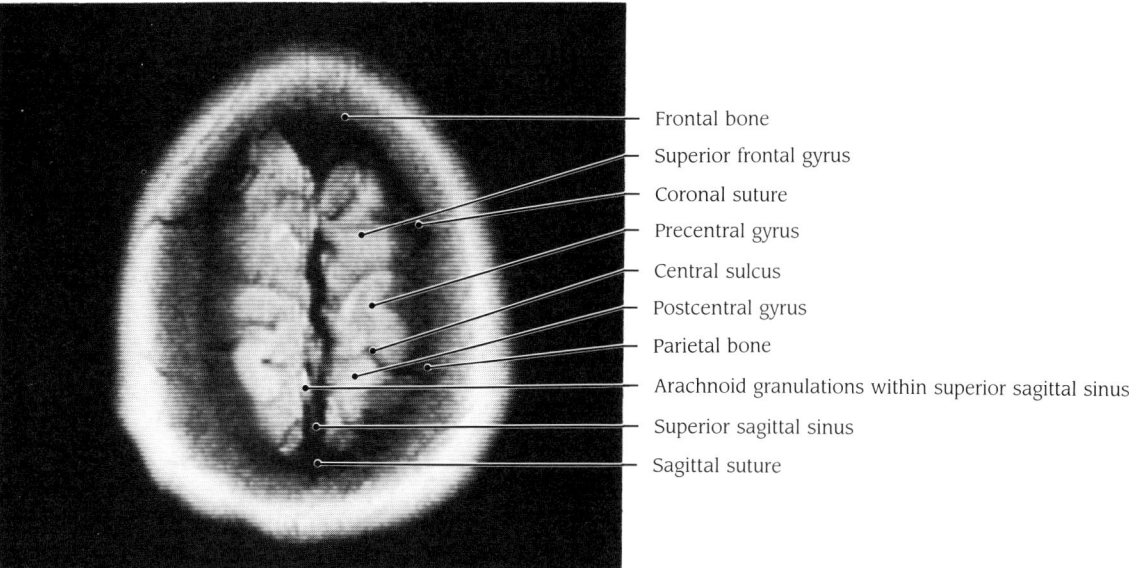

FIG. 2.3. TR = 2000 msec, TE = 28 msec.

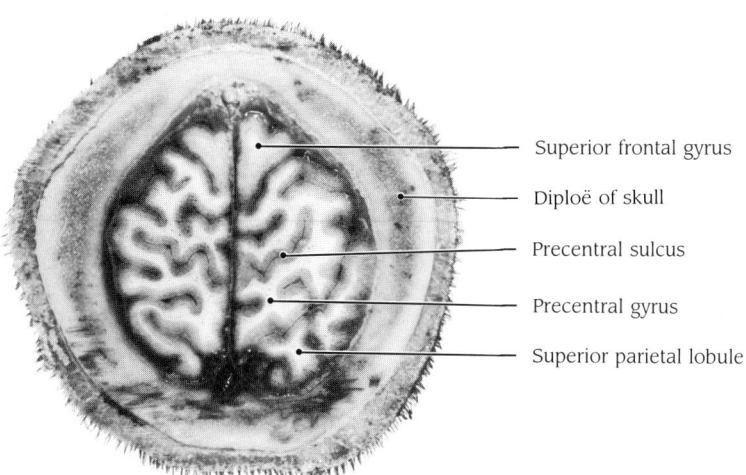

FIG. 2.4.

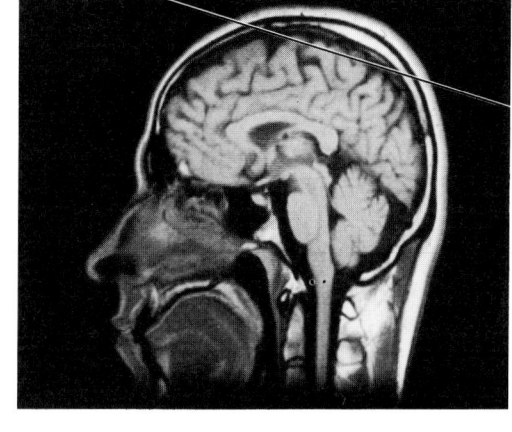

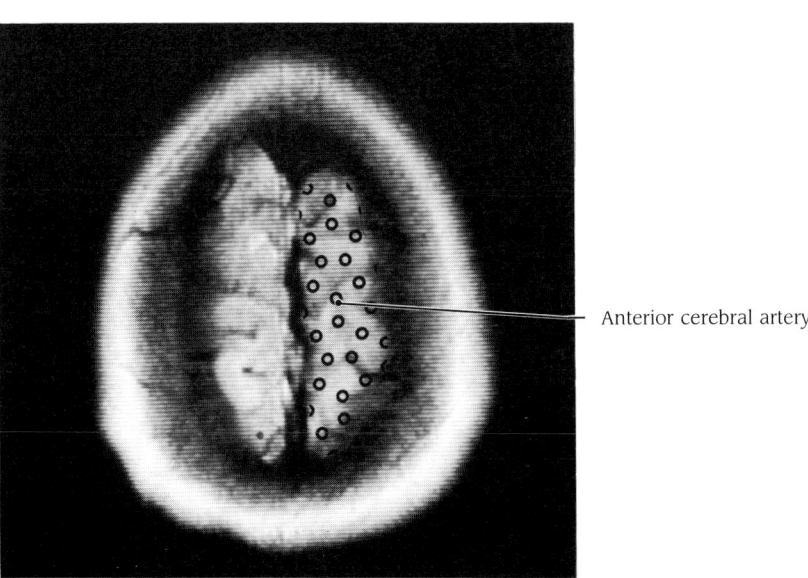

FIG. 2.5. TR = 2000 msec, TE = 28 msec.

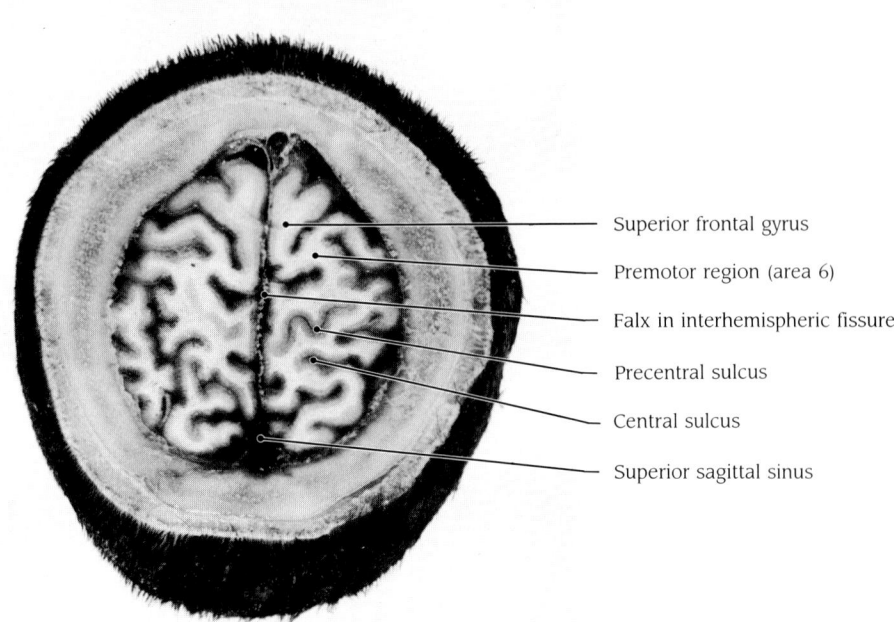

FIG. 2.6.

- Superior frontal gyrus
- Premotor region (area 6)
- Falx in interhemispheric fissure
- Precentral sulcus
- Central sulcus
- Superior sagittal sinus

- The precentral and postcentral gyri may be differentiated by the increased thickness of the gray matter of the precentral gyrus compared to that of the postcentral gyrus.
- The average thickness of the cranium varies considerably among individuals. Typically, the anterolateral aspects of the calvaria are thinner than the anterior and posterior portions.
- Variations in angulation produce differences in the apparent position of the central sulcus; with upward angulation, the central sulcus is shown more anteriorly placed than with downward angulation. Similarly, with differences in patient positioning, the superior and inferior parietal lobules appear differently, as these images show.

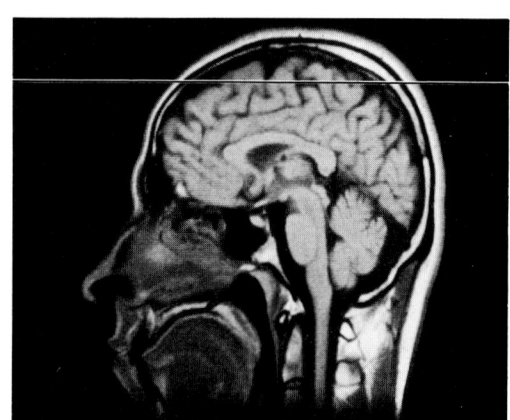

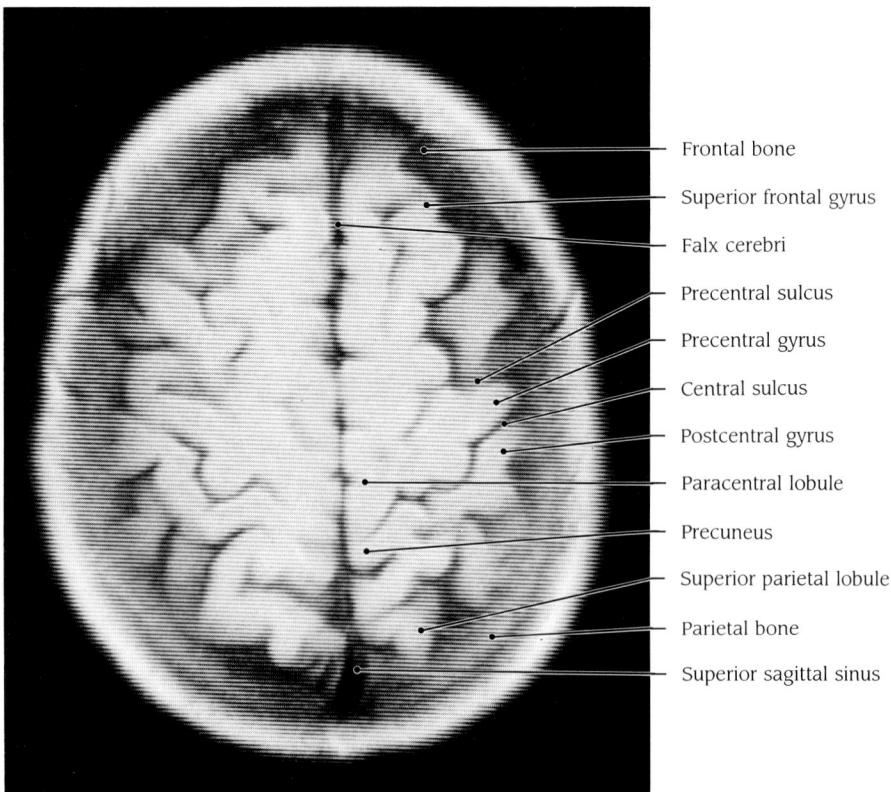

- Frontal bone
- Superior frontal gyrus
- Falx cerebri
- Precentral sulcus
- Precentral gyrus
- Central sulcus
- Postcentral gyrus
- Paracentral lobule
- Precuneus
- Superior parietal lobule
- Parietal bone
- Superior sagittal sinus

FIG. 2.7. TR = 500 msec, TE = 28 msec.

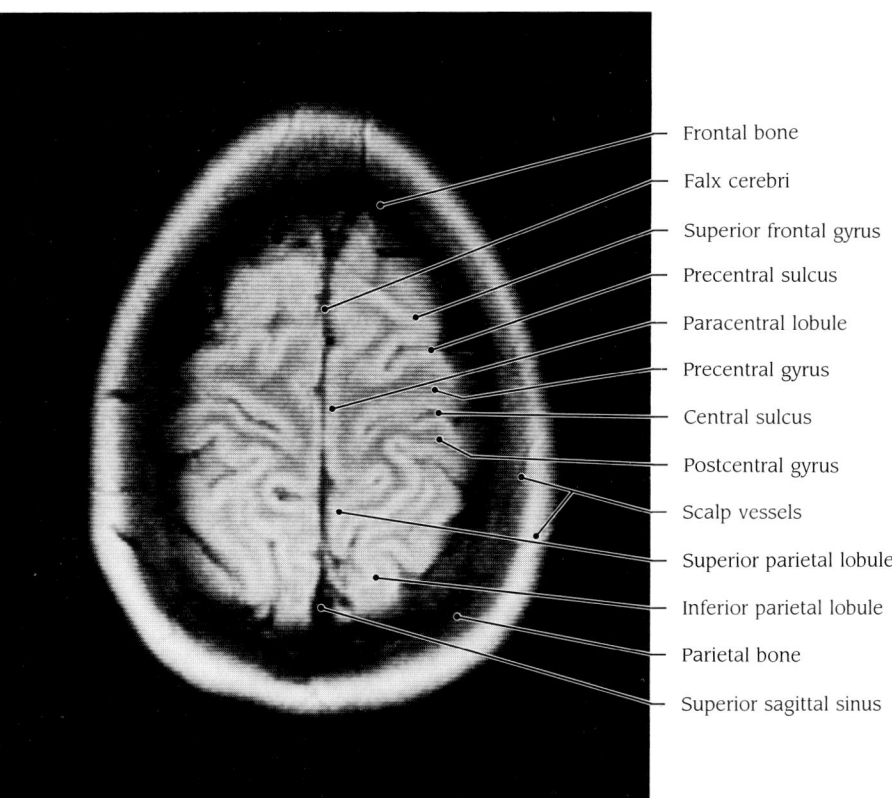

FIG. 2.8. TR = 2000 msec, TE = 28 msec.

- Frontal bone
- Falx cerebri
- Superior frontal gyrus
- Precentral sulcus
- Paracentral lobule
- Precentral gyrus
- Central sulcus
- Postcentral gyrus
- Scalp vessels
- Superior parietal lobule
- Inferior parietal lobule
- Parietal bone
- Superior sagittal sinus

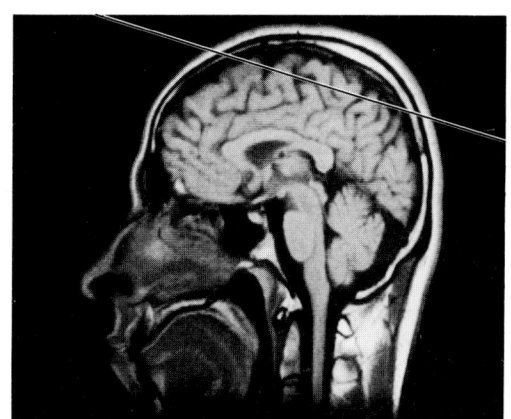

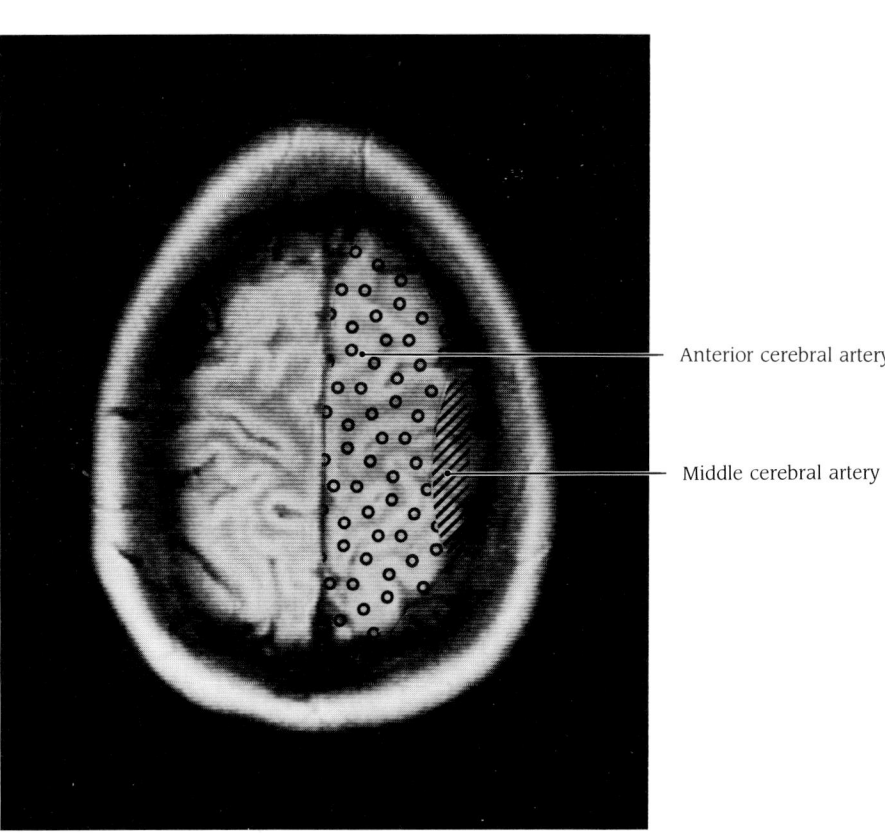

FIG. 2.9. TR = 2000 msec, TE = 28 msec.

- Anterior cerebral artery
- Middle cerebral artery

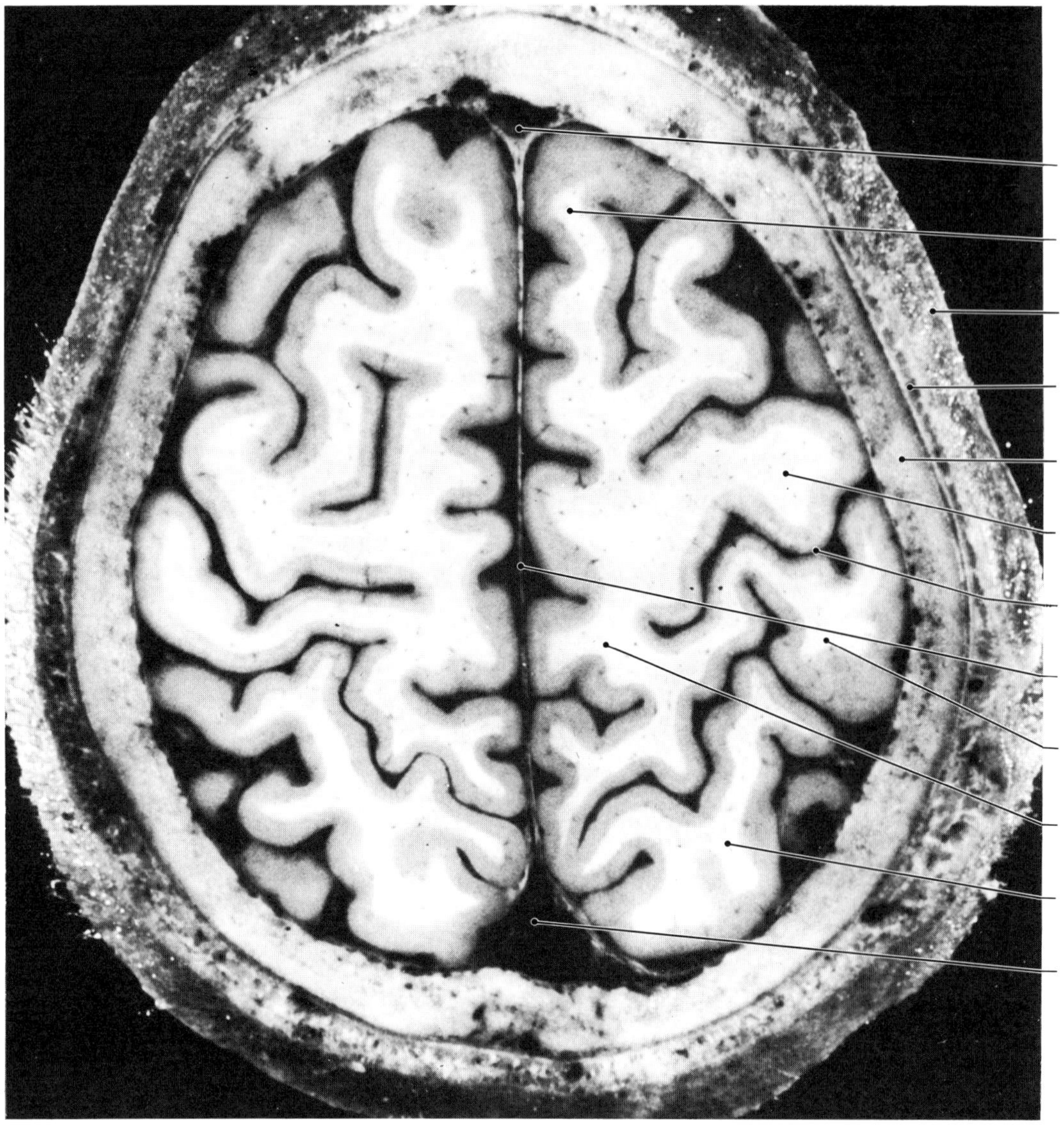

FIG. 2.10.

- Excellent contrast between gray and white matter permits identification of individual gyri.
- The falx usually is present in its entirety from anterior to posterior at this level.

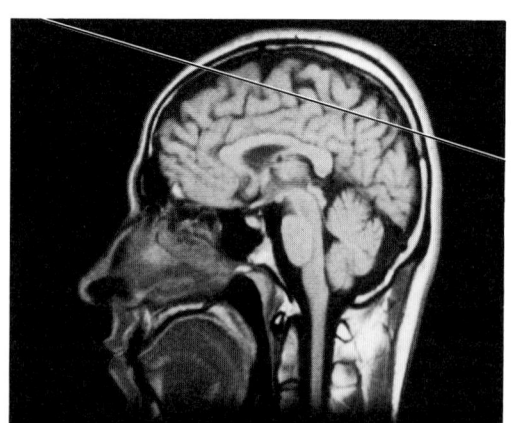

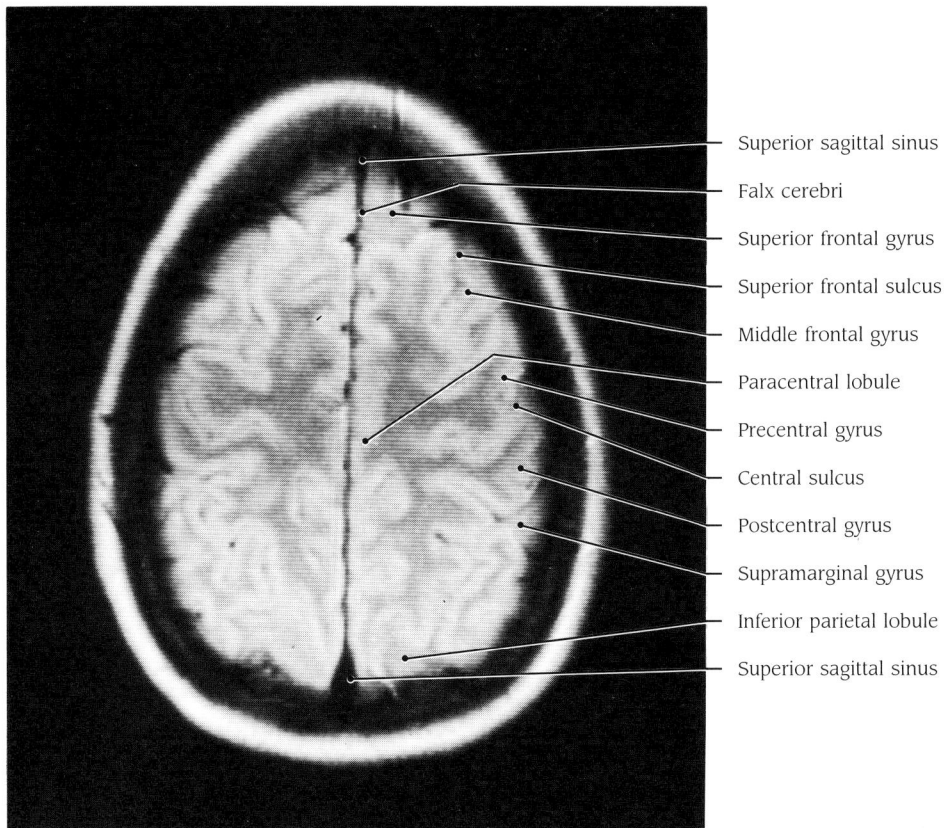

FIG. 2.11. TR = 2000 msec, TE = 28 msec.

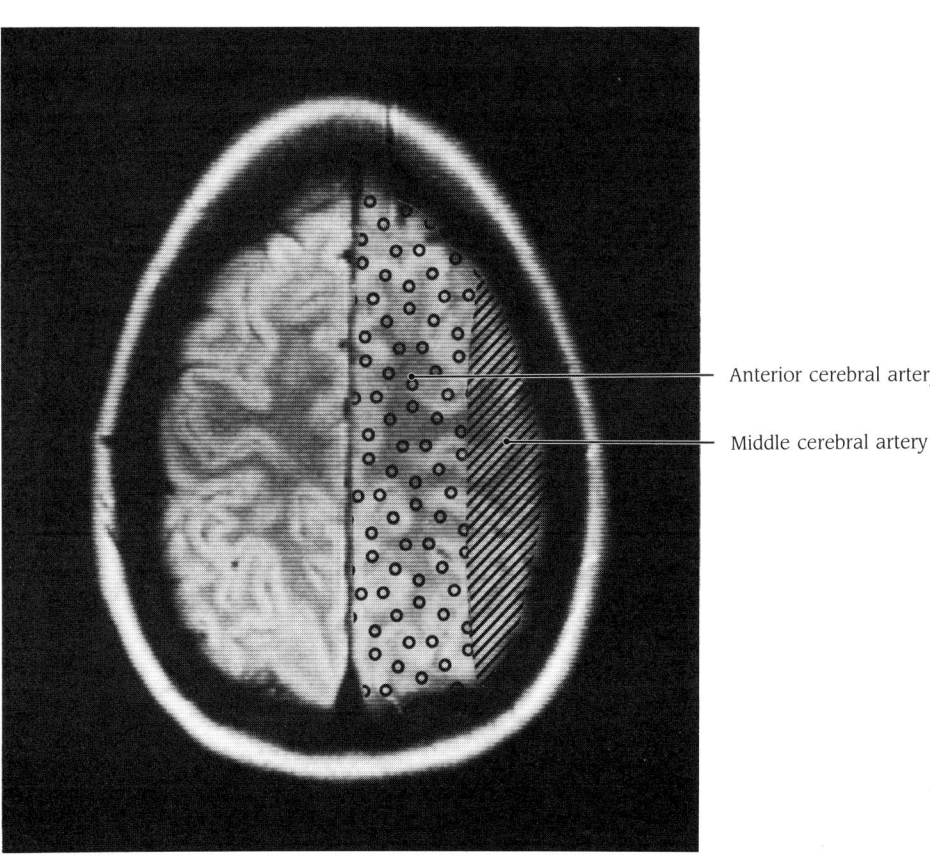

FIG. 2.12. TR = 2000 msec, TE = 28 msec.

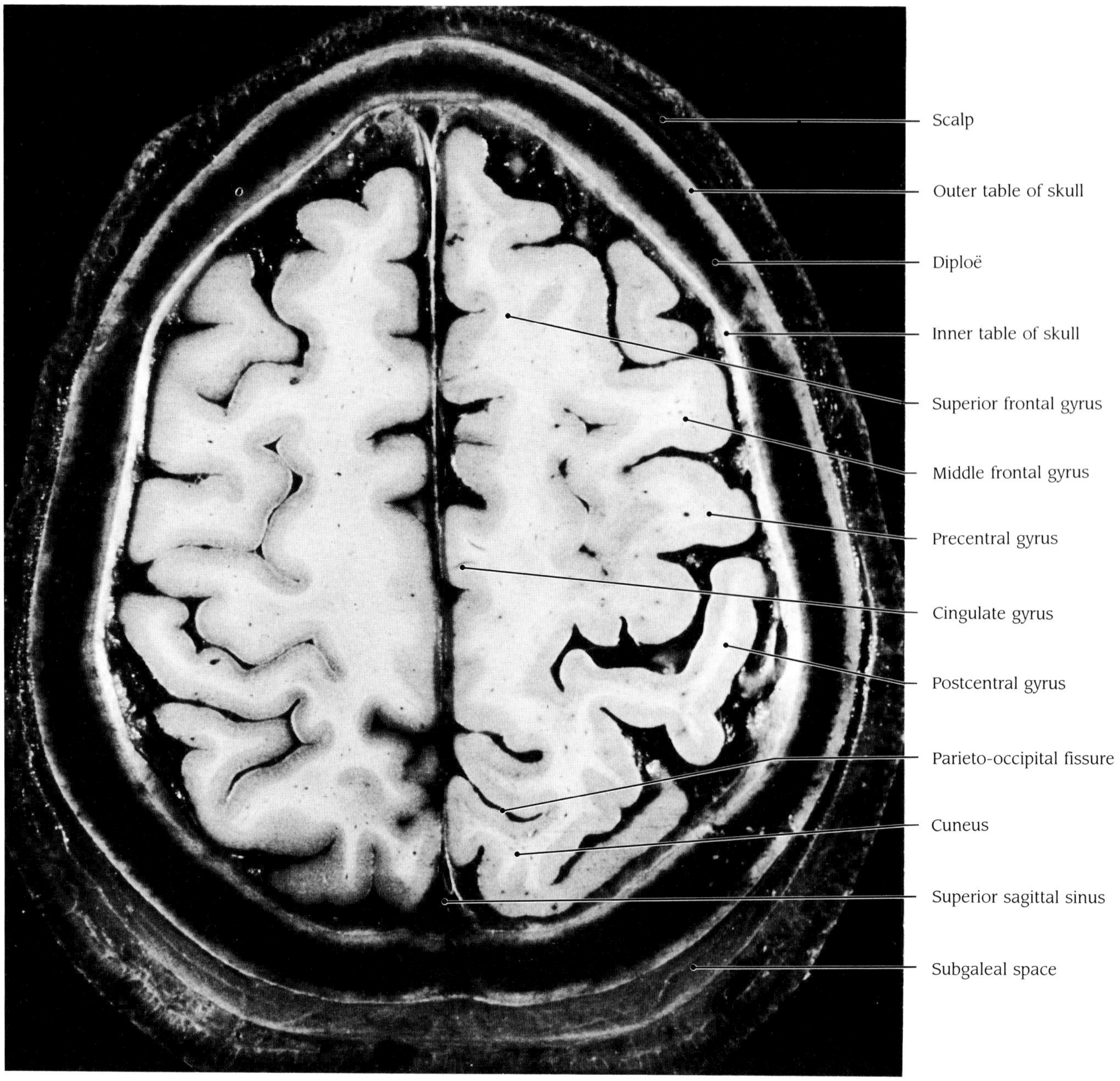

FIG. 2.13.

- Scalp
- Outer table of skull
- Diploë
- Inner table of skull
- Superior frontal gyrus
- Middle frontal gyrus
- Precentral gyrus
- Cingulate gyrus
- Postcentral gyrus
- Parieto-occipital fissure
- Cuneus
- Superior sagittal sinus
- Subgaleal space

- The three layers of the calvaria consist of a marrow-containing diploic cavity between two compact layers of bone, the inner and outer tables. Magnetic resonance images show these layers as a high intensity diploic space delimited by the linear low intensities of the inner and outer tables.

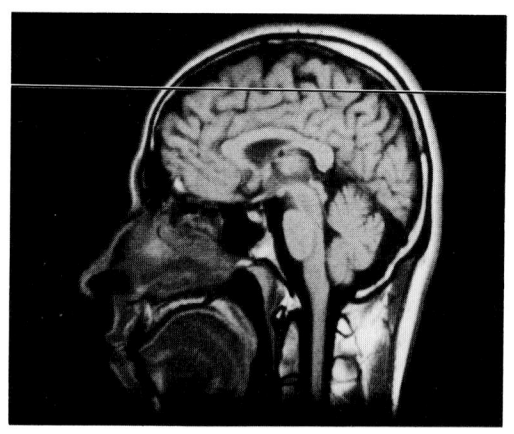

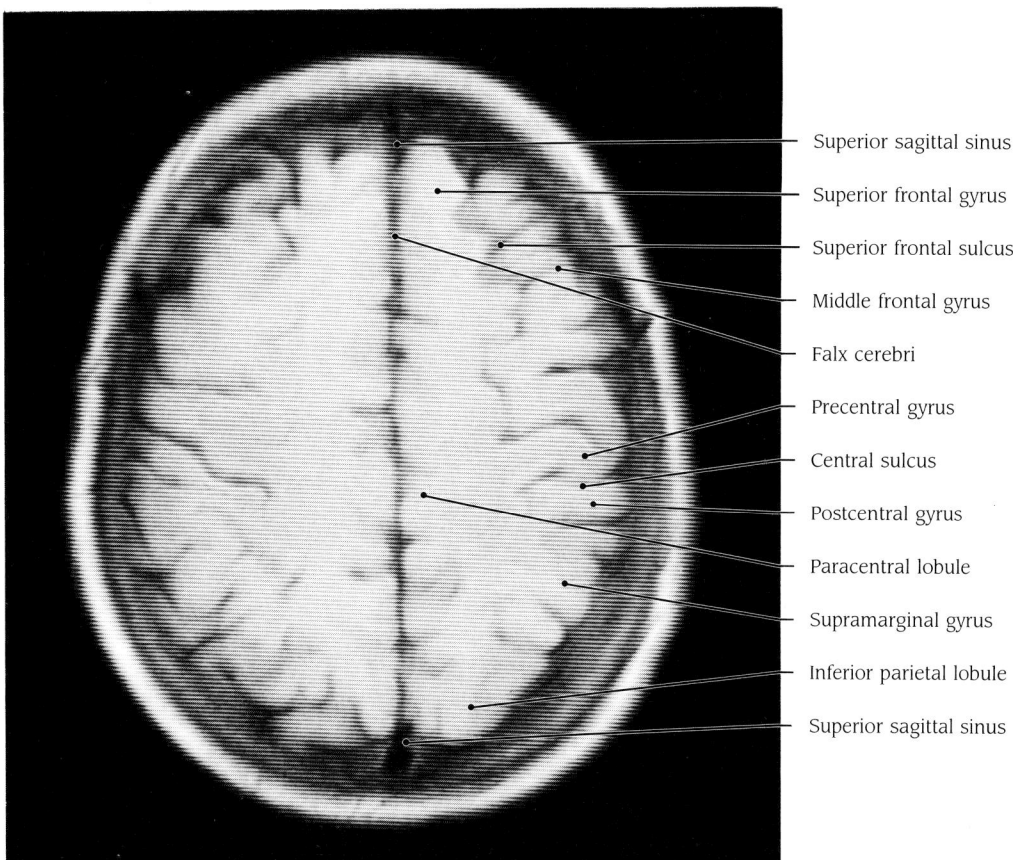

FIG. 2.14. TR = 500 msec, TE = 28 msec.

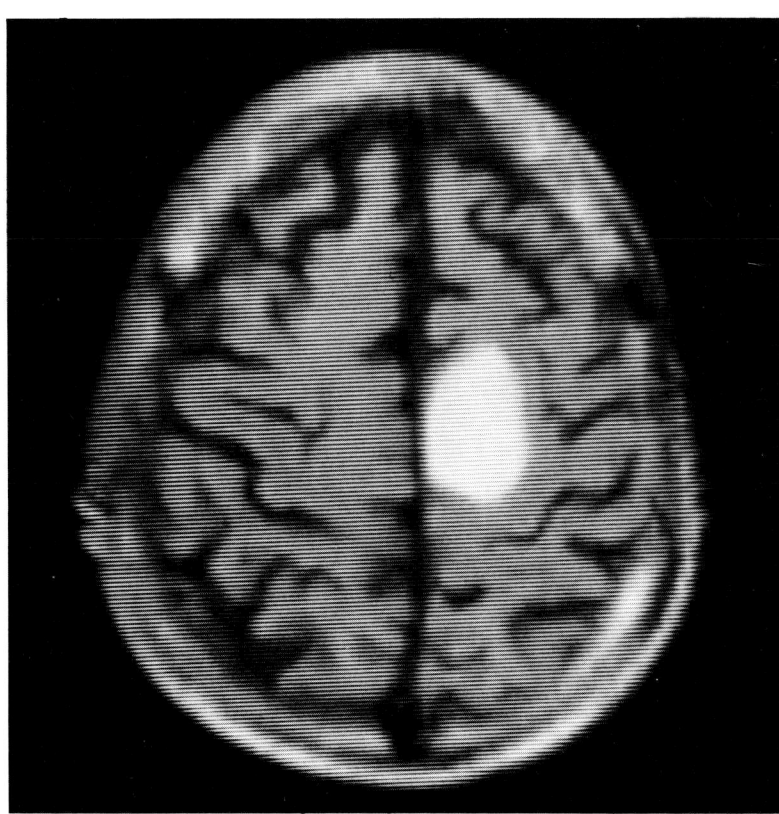

FIG. 2.15. TR = 500 msec, TE = 28 msec. This hemorrhagic metastasis from carcinoma of the lung causes sulcal effacement and exhibits the high signal intensity characteristic of subacute hemorrhage.

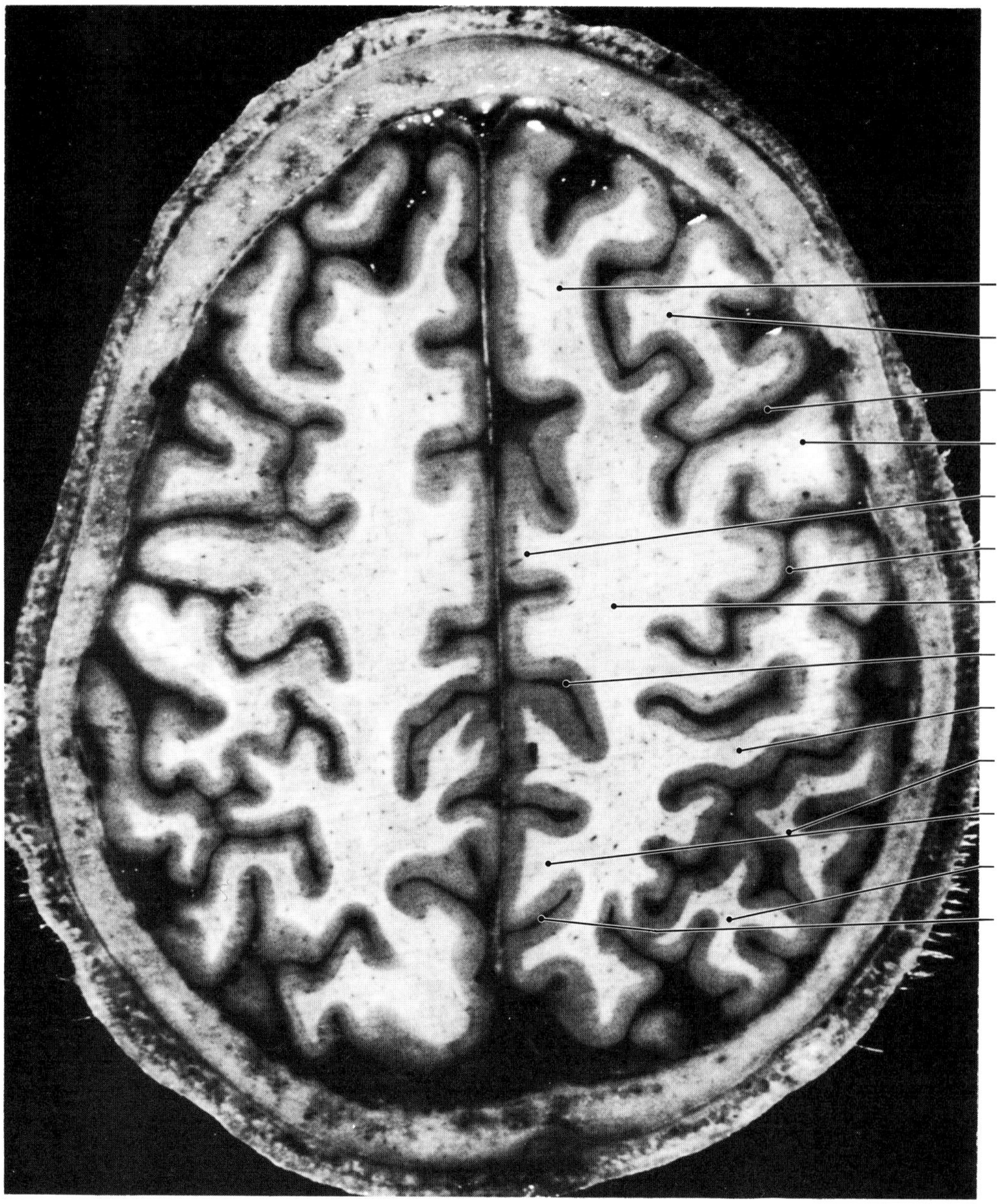

FIG. 2.16.

- Superior frontal gyrus
- Middle frontal gyrus
- Precentral sulcus
- Precentral gyrus
- Cingulate gyrus
- Central sulcus
- Centrum semiovale
- Cingulate sulcus
- Superior parietal lobule
- Supramarginal gyrus
- Precuneus
- Inferior parietal lobule
- Parieto-occipital fissure

- The supramarginal gyrus of the inferior parietal lobule defines the most cephalad extent of the temporal lobe.
- The centrum semiovale is composed of three categories of fiber systems: (1) the projection fibers to or from specific cortical areas, such as the corticospinal tract; (2) long and short association fibers, such as the fronto-occipital fasciculus; and (3) the callosal fibers, which interconnect the cortices of the two hemispheres.

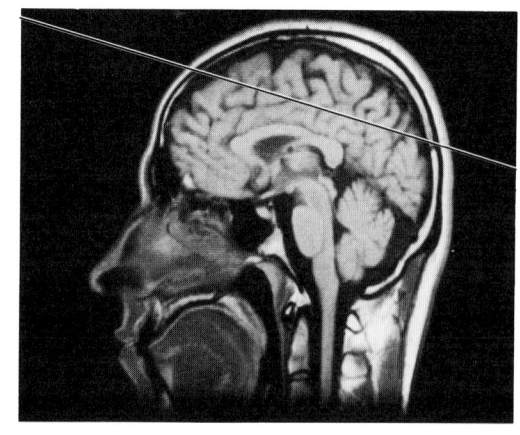

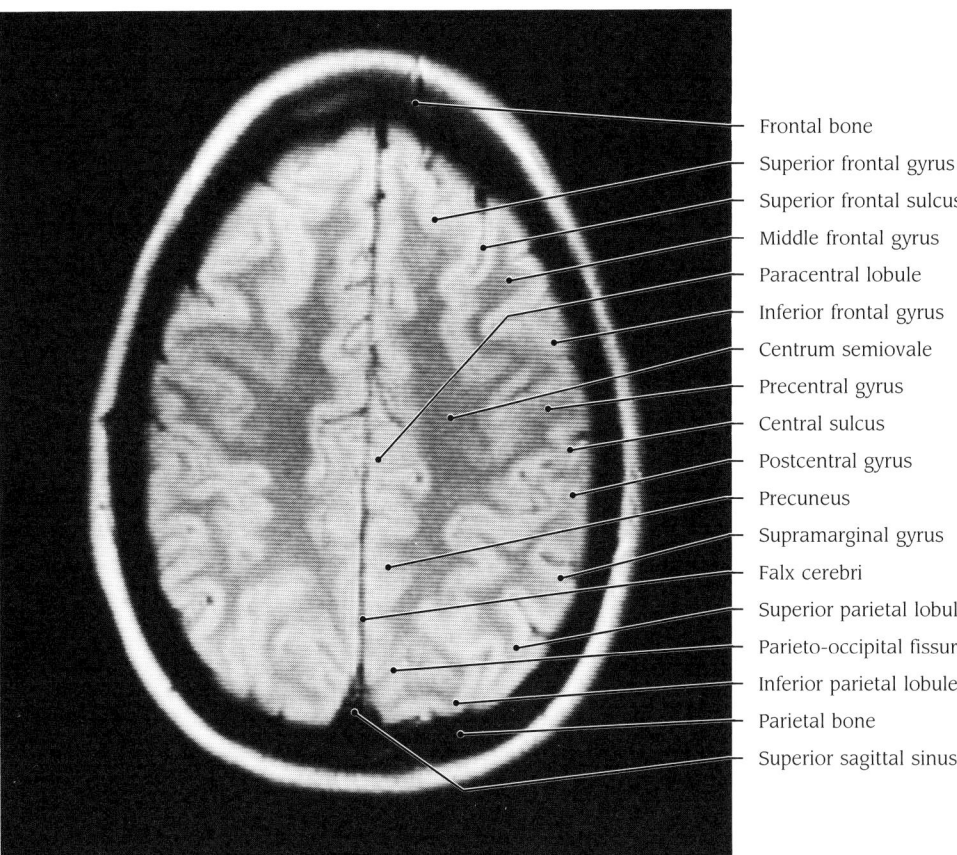

FIG. 2.17. TR = 2000 msec, TE = 28 msec.

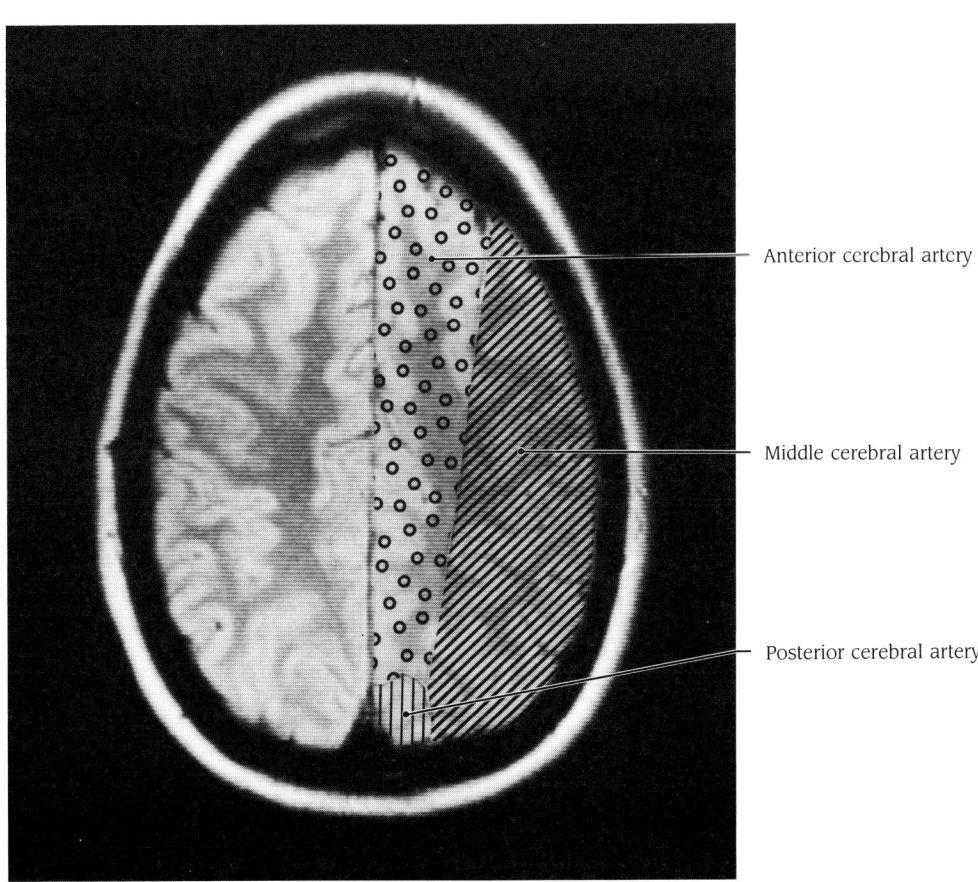

FIG. 2.18. TR = 2000 msec, TE = 28 msec.

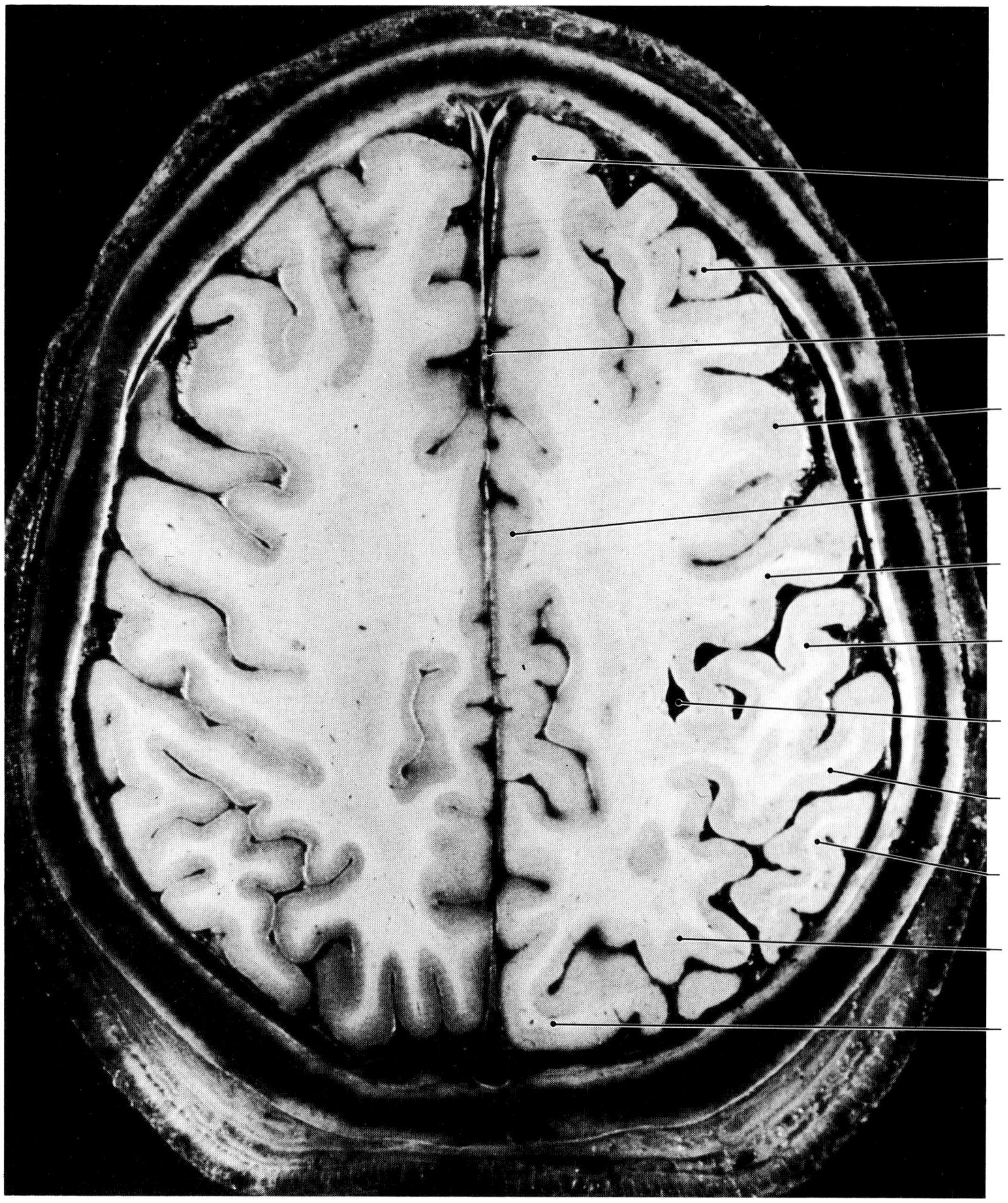

- Superior frontal gyrus
- Middle frontal gyrus
- Falx in interhemispheric fissure
- Inferior frontal gyrus
- Anterior cingulate gyrus
- Precentral gyrus
- Postcentral gyrus
- Artifact
- Superior parietal lobule
- Angular gyrus
- Precuneus
- Occipital gyrus

FIG. 2.19.

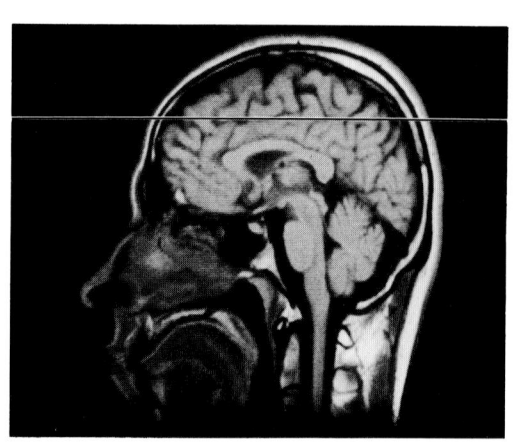

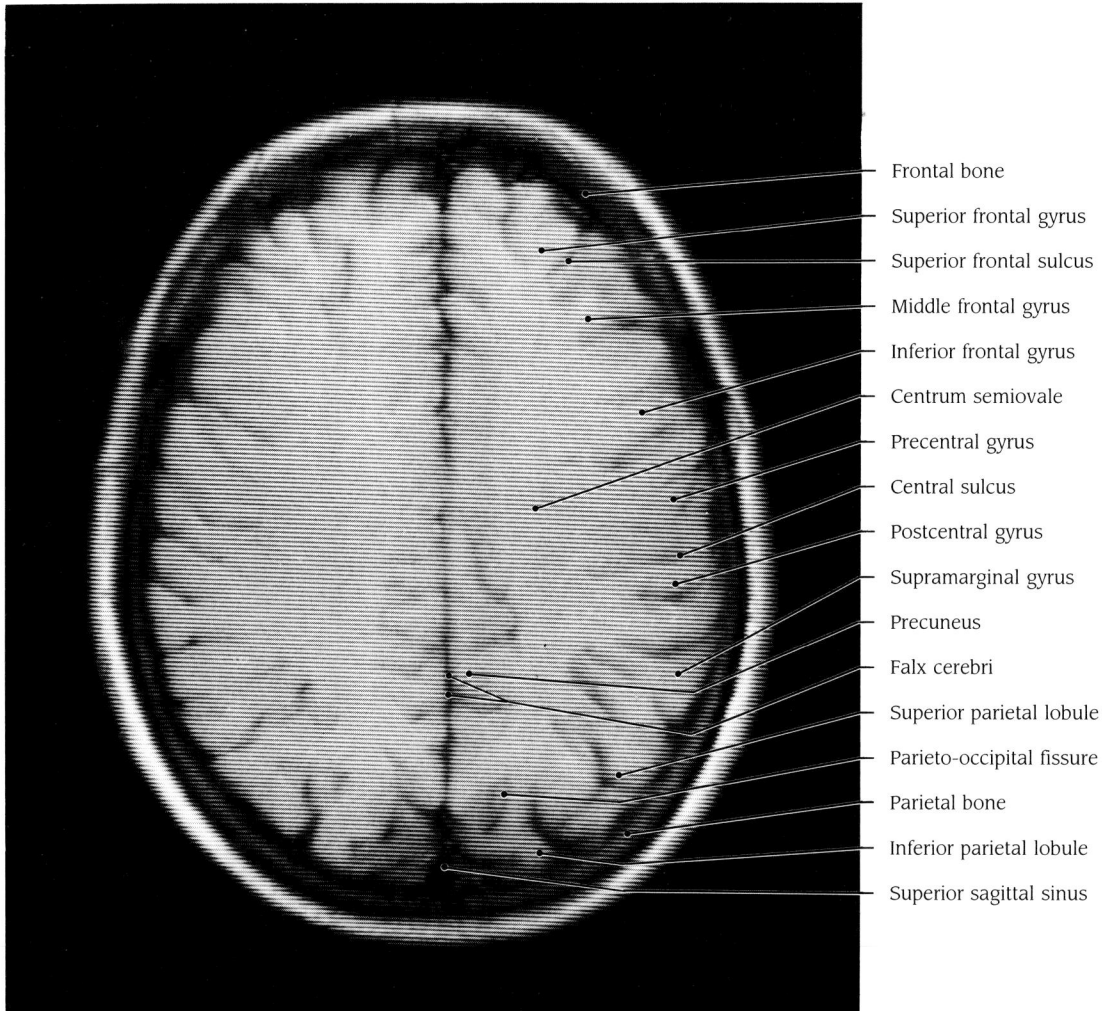

FIG. 2.20. TR = 500 msec, TE = 28 msec.

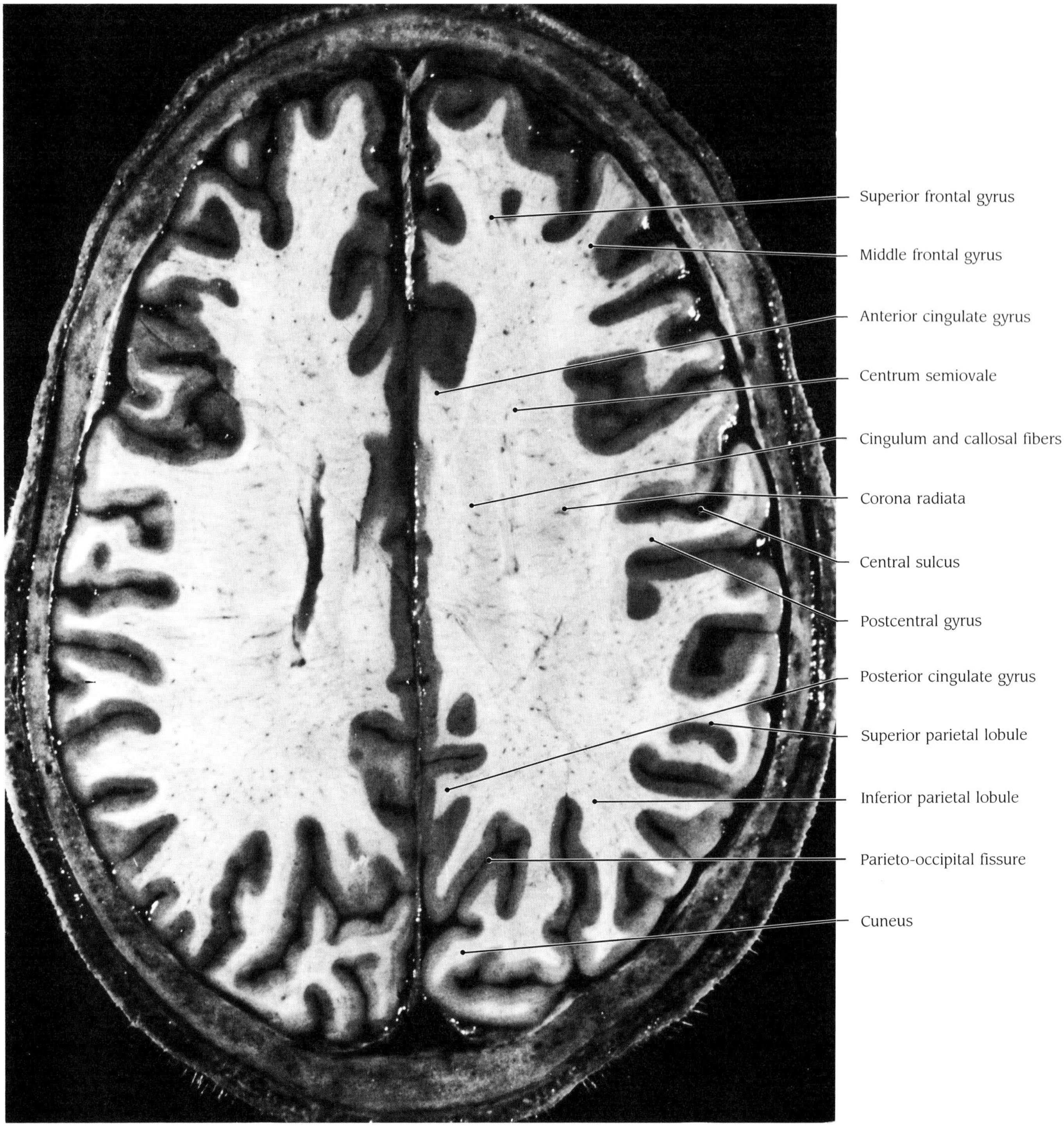

FIG. 2.21.

- The callosomarginal artery, a branch of the anterior cerebral artery, is visualized within the cingulate sulcus.
- The corona radiata is identified within the centrum semiovale. In addition, the cingulum, a long association bundle between the frontal and temporal lobes, may be distinguished in the white matter of the cingulate gyrus.

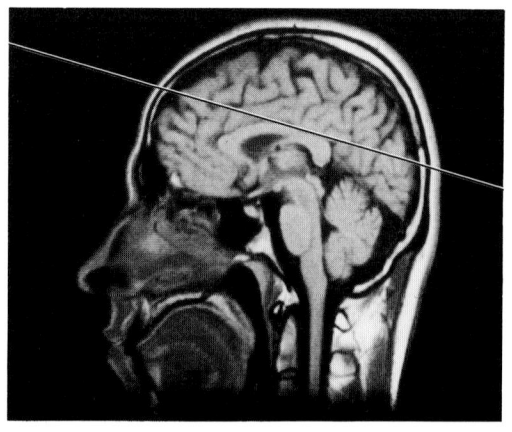

16

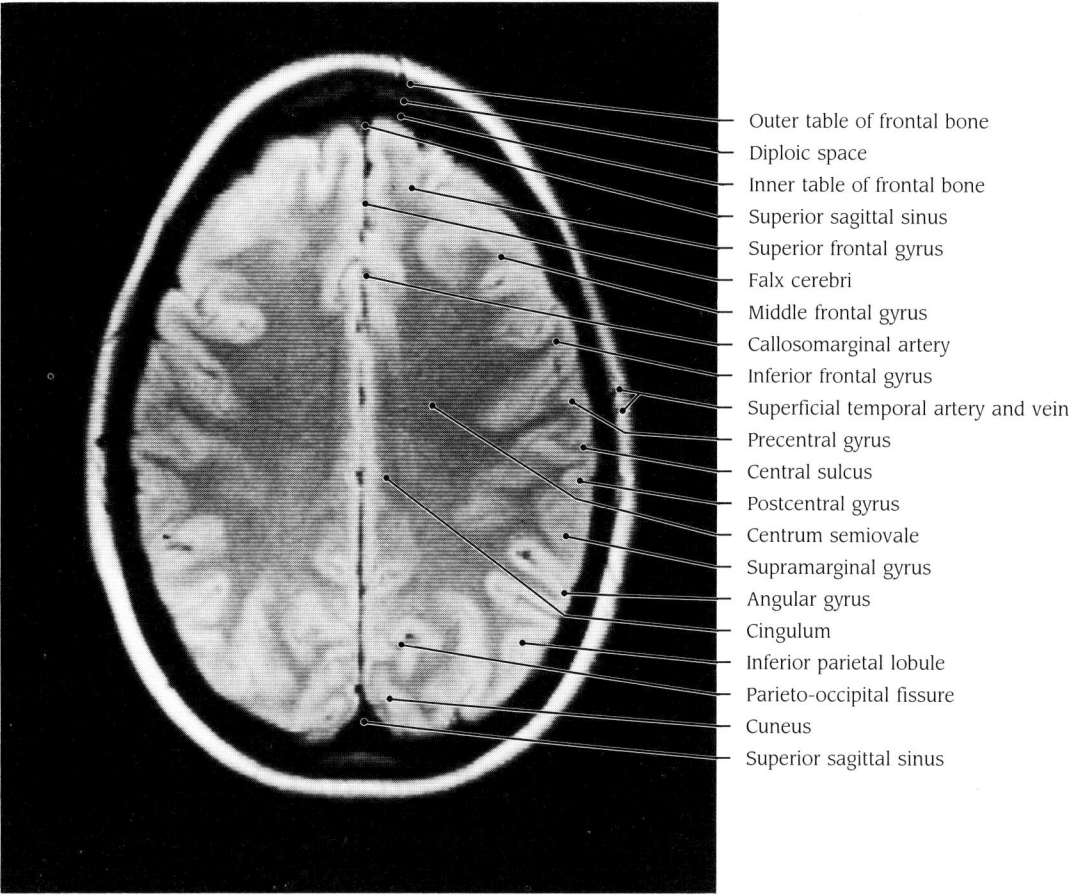

FIG. 2.22. TR = 2000 msec, TE = 28 msec.

- Outer table of frontal bone
- Diploic space
- Inner table of frontal bone
- Superior sagittal sinus
- Superior frontal gyrus
- Falx cerebri
- Middle frontal gyrus
- Callosomarginal artery
- Inferior frontal gyrus
- Superficial temporal artery and vein
- Precentral gyrus
- Central sulcus
- Postcentral gyrus
- Centrum semiovale
- Supramarginal gyrus
- Angular gyrus
- Cingulum
- Inferior parietal lobule
- Parieto-occipital fissure
- Cuneus
- Superior sagittal sinus

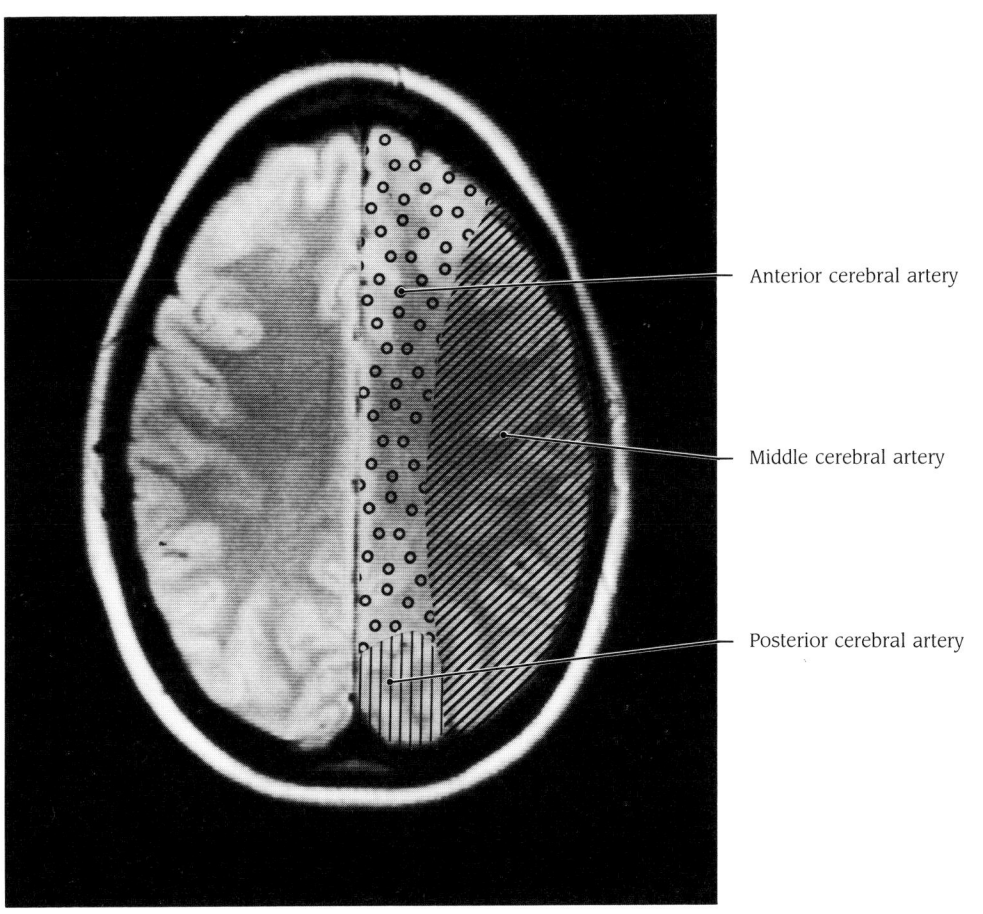

FIG. 2.23. TR = 2000 msec, TE = 28 msec.

- Anterior cerebral artery
- Middle cerebral artery
- Posterior cerebral artery

17

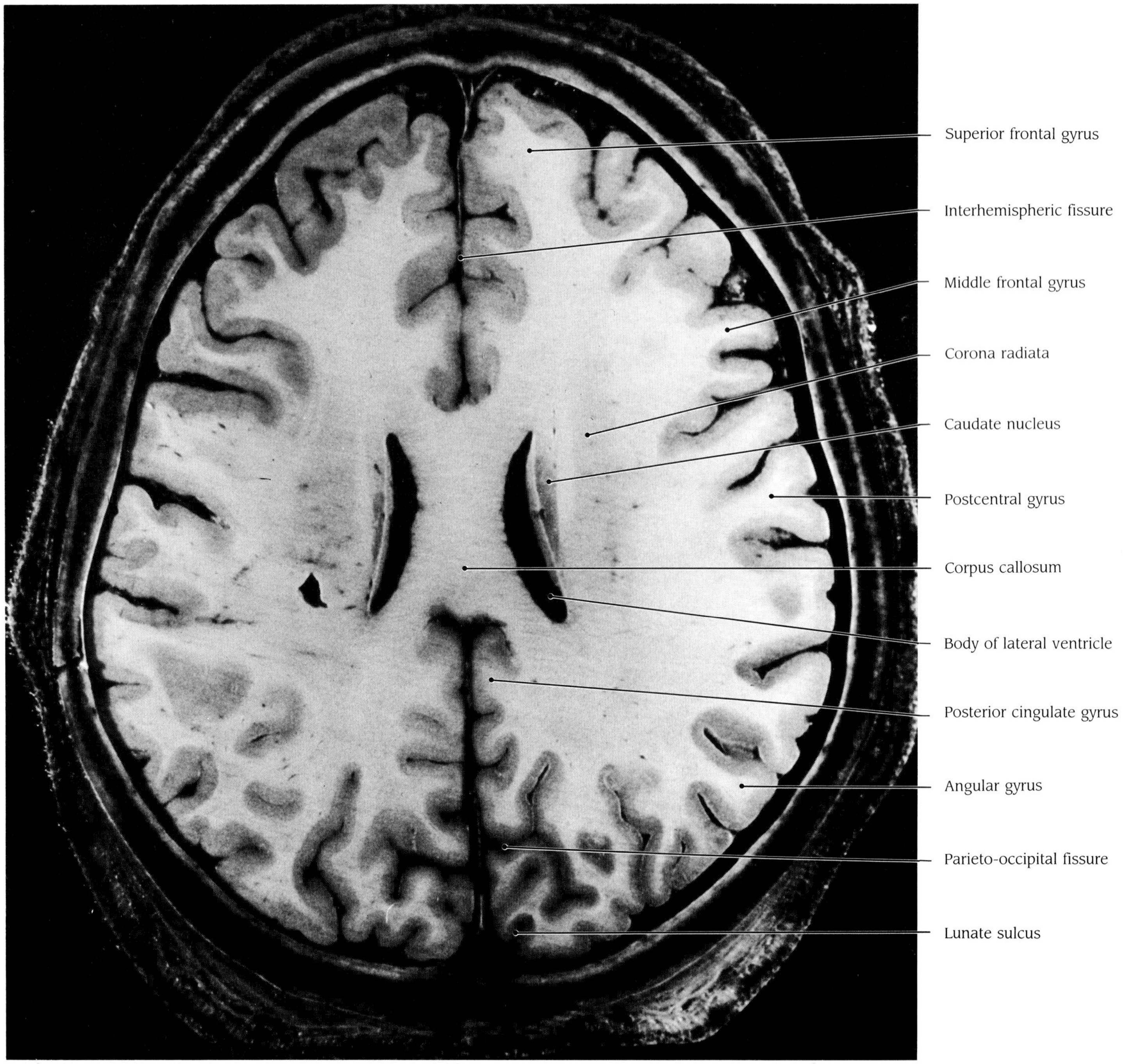

- Superior frontal gyrus
- Interhemispheric fissure
- Middle frontal gyrus
- Corona radiata
- Caudate nucleus
- Postcentral gyrus
- Corpus callosum
- Body of lateral ventricle
- Posterior cingulate gyrus
- Angular gyrus
- Parieto-occipital fissure
- Lunate sulcus

FIG. 2.24.

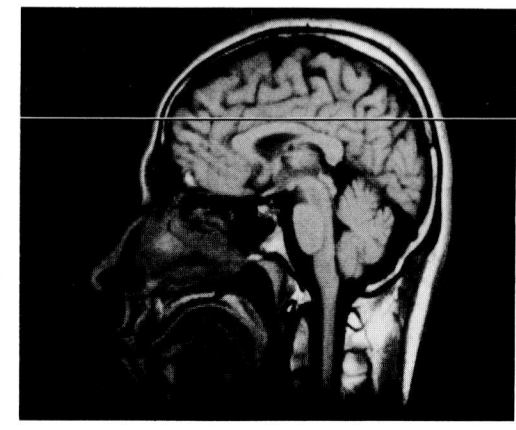

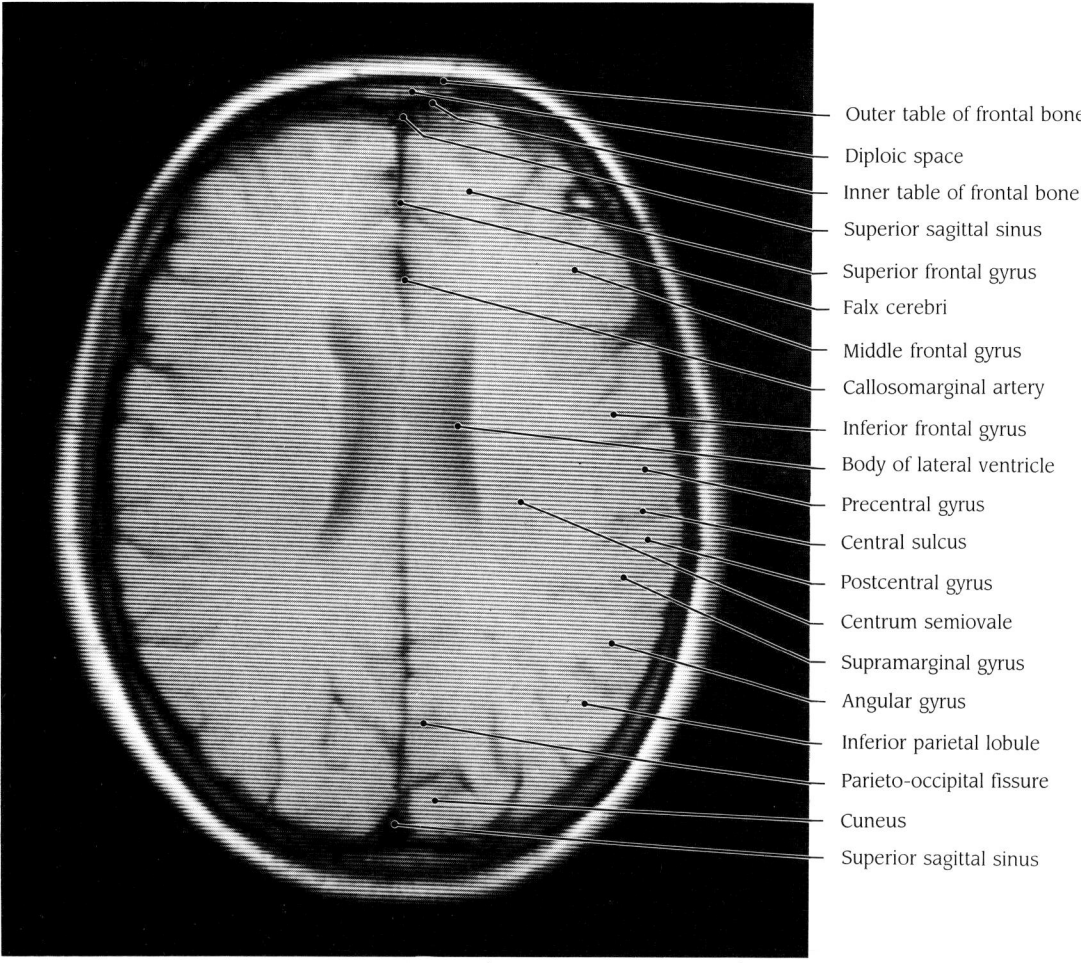

FIG. 2.25. TR = 500 msec, TE = 28 msec.

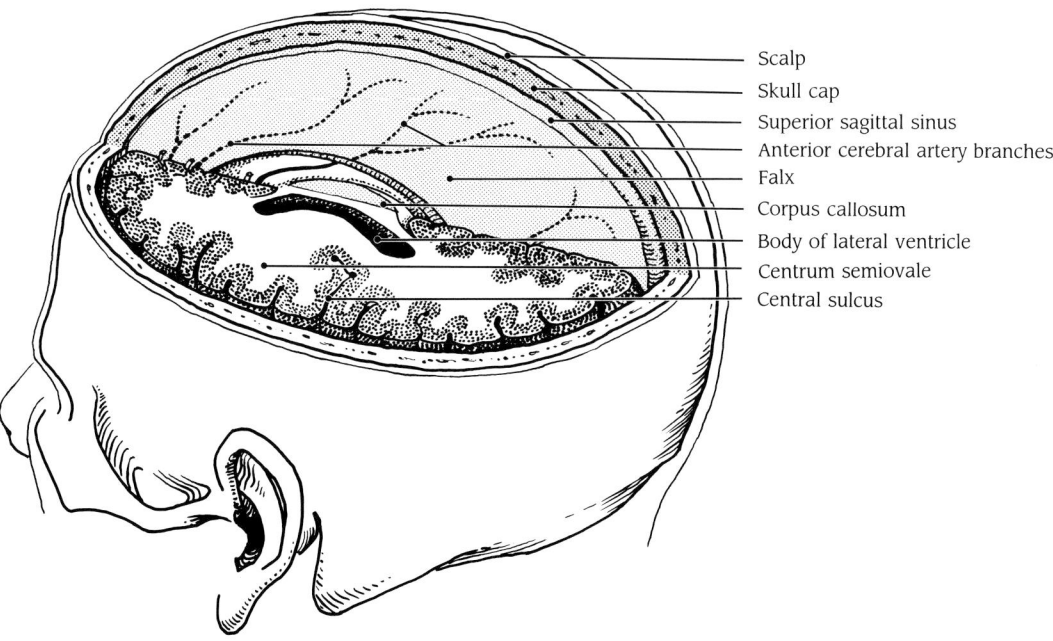

FIG. 2.26. Drawing of an axial slice at the level of the body of the lateral ventricle. (From de Groot, J.: Correlative Neuroanatomy of Computed Tomography and Magnetic Resonance Imaging. Philadelphia, Lea & Febiger, 1984.)

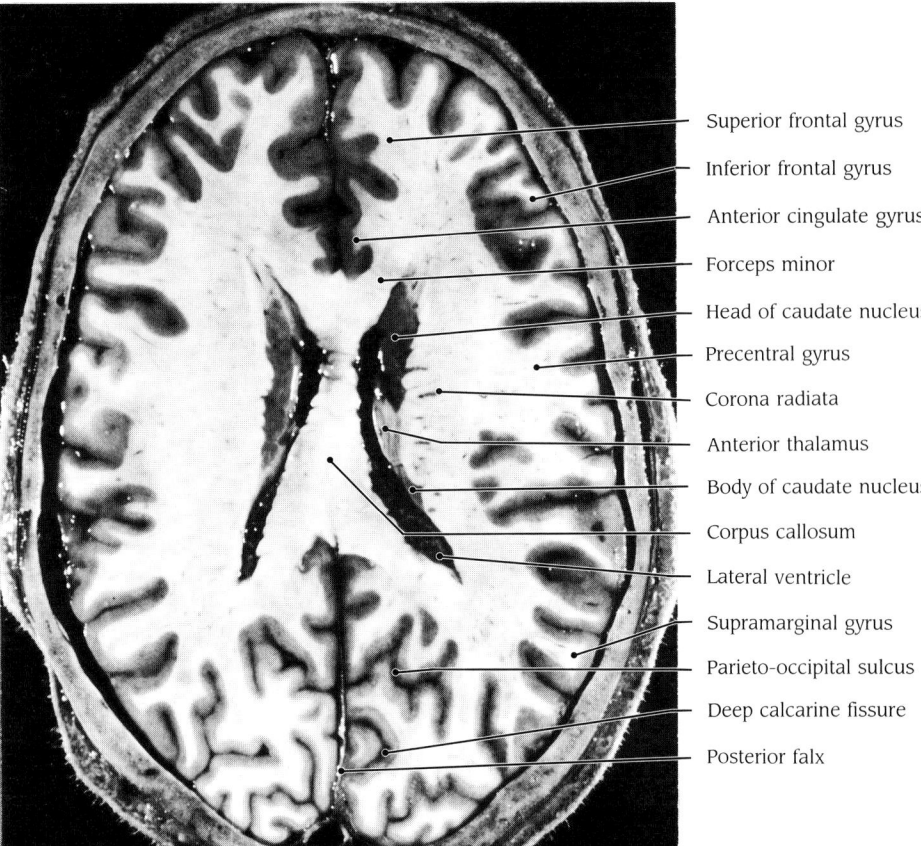

FIG. 2.27.

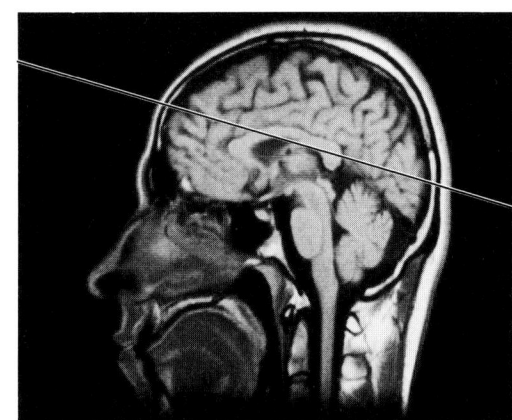

- The body of the comma-shaped caudate nucleus, a part of the basal ganglia, is adjacent to the body of the lateral ventricle.
- Variations among individuals may show the body of the lateral ventricle to be either superior to or at the level of the body of the corpus callosum.

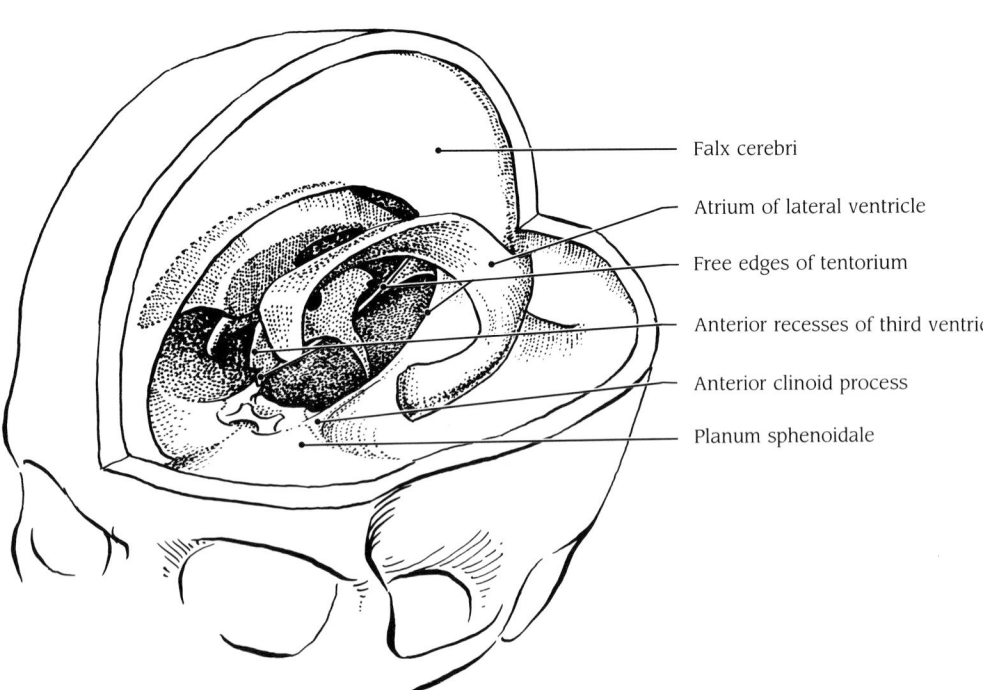

FIG. 2.28. Schematic illustration of the relationships between the ventricular system, the falx cerebri, and tentorium cerebelli within the skull.

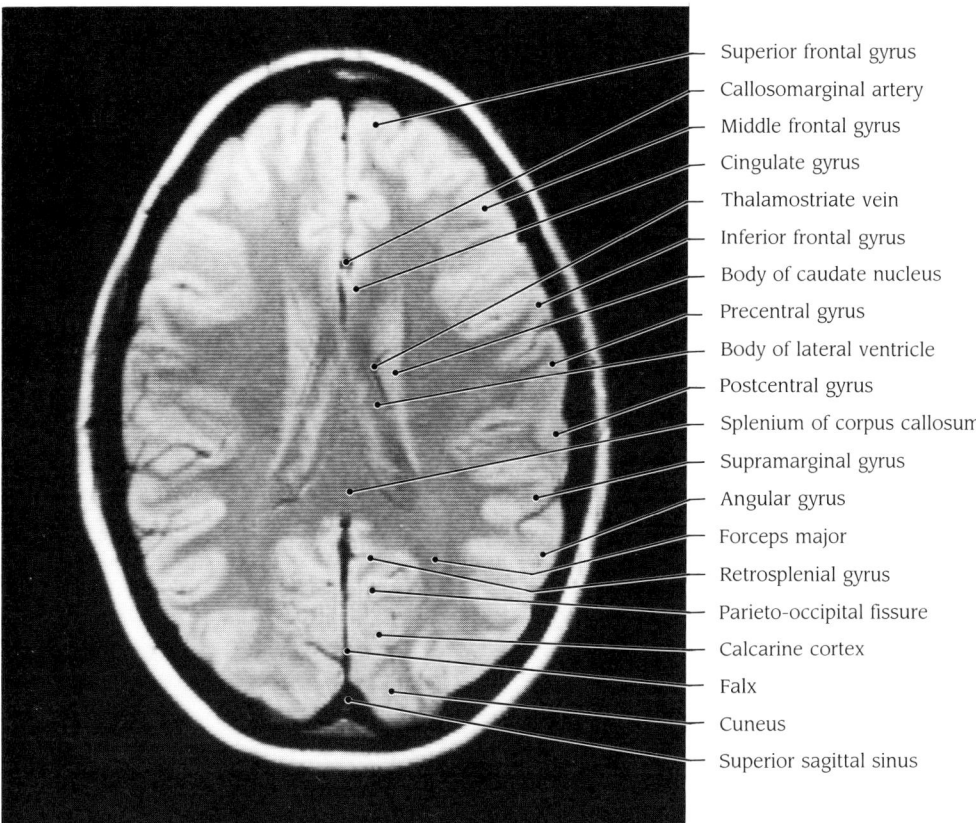

FIG. 2.29. TR = 2000 msec, TE = 28 msec.

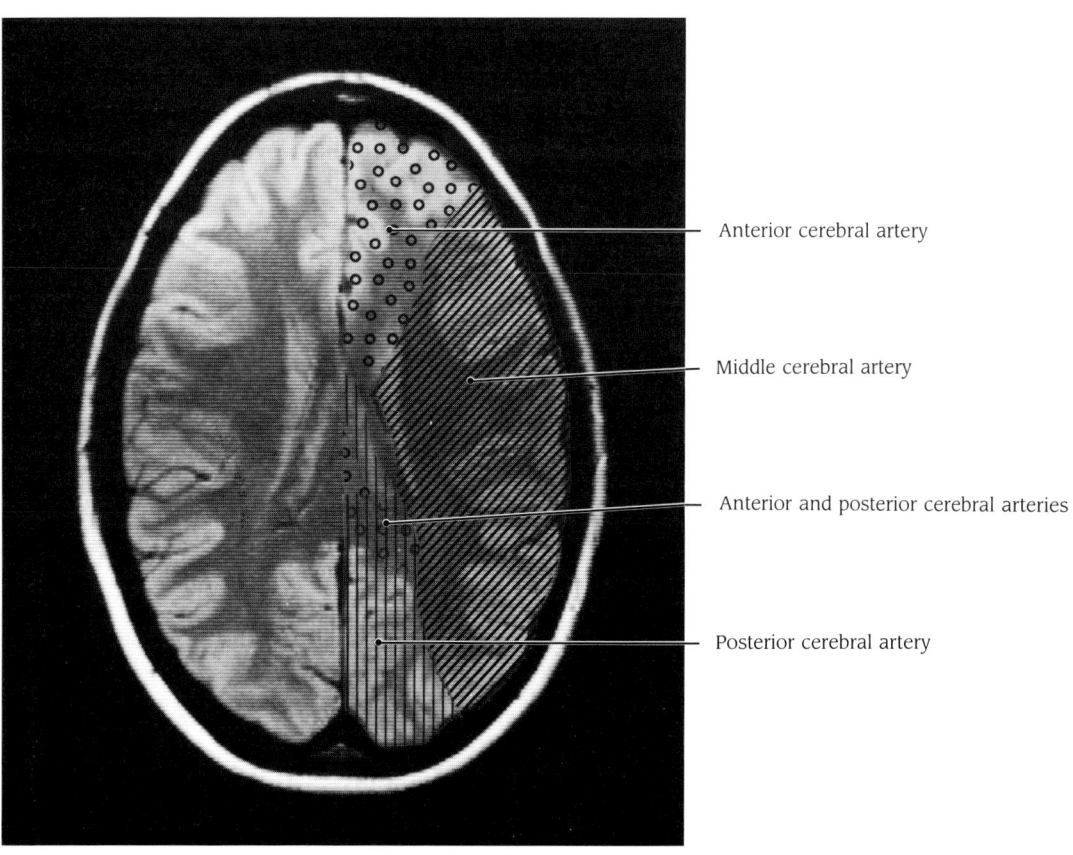

FIG. 2.30. TR = 2000 msec, TE = 28 msec. The splenium of the corpus callosum is supplied by branches of both the anterior and the posterior cerebral arteries.

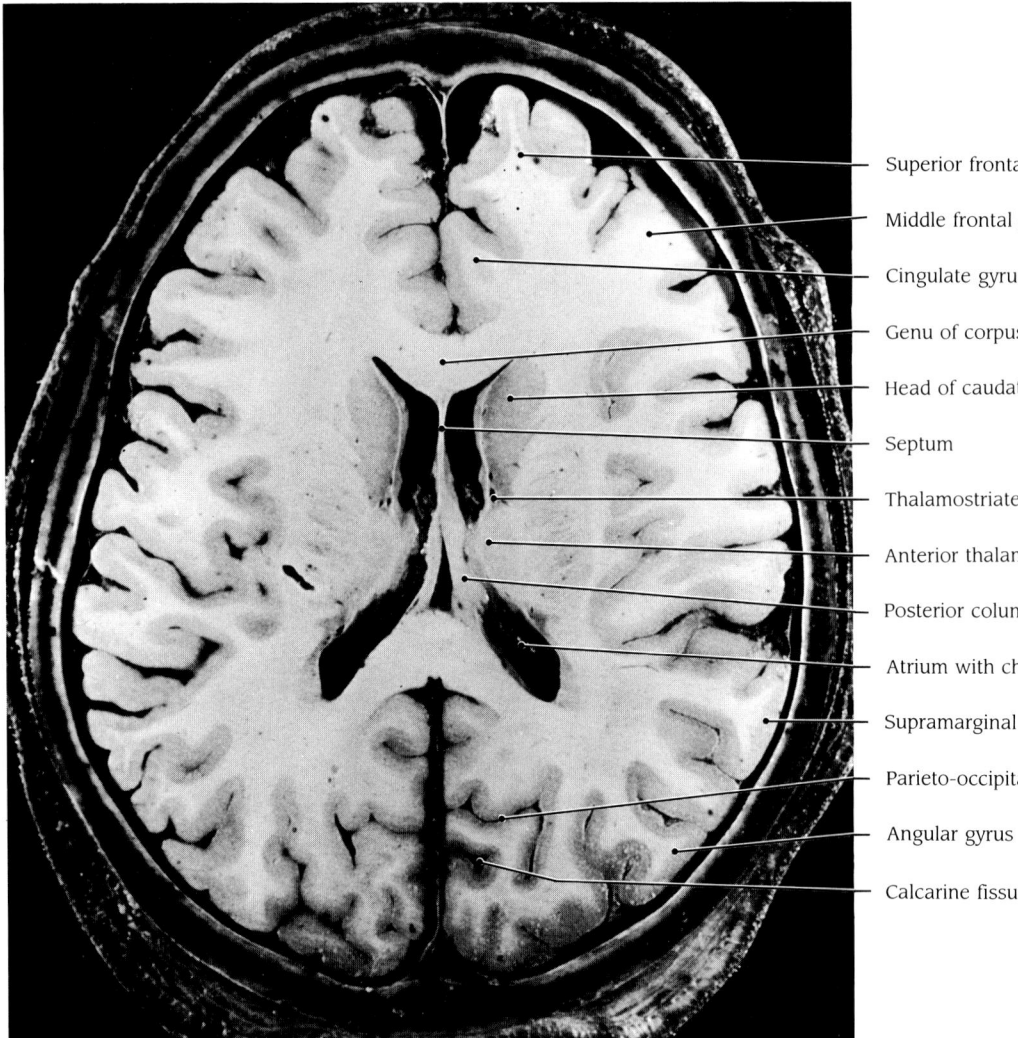

- Superior frontal gyrus
- Middle frontal gyrus
- Cingulate gyrus
- Genu of corpus callosum
- Head of caudate nucleus
- Septum
- Thalamostriate vein
- Anterior thalamus
- Posterior column of fornix
- Atrium with choroid plexus
- Supramarginal gyrus
- Parieto-occipital fissure
- Angular gyrus
- Calcarine fissure (upper part)

FIG. 2.31.

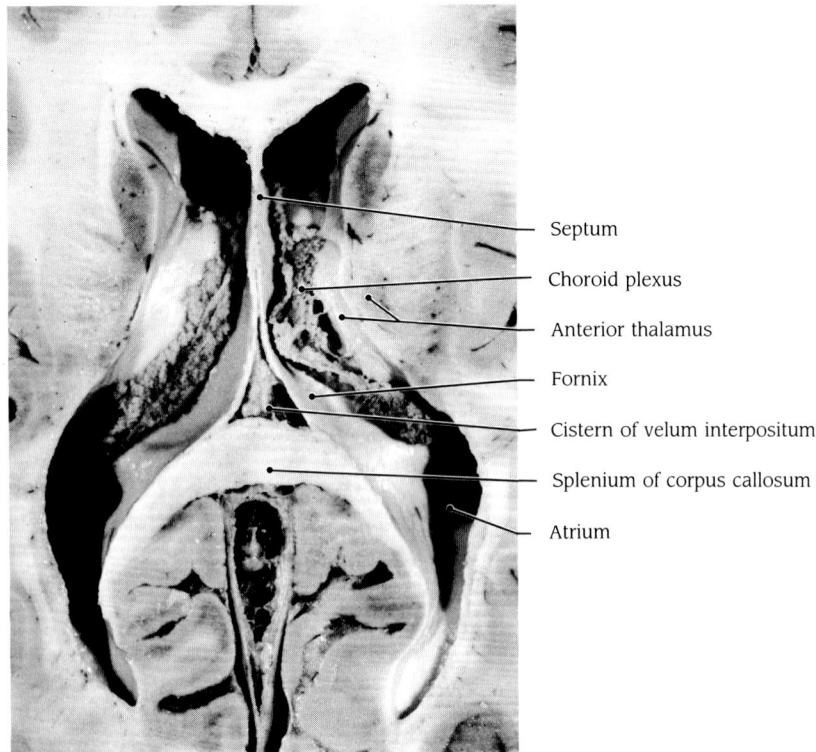

- Septum
- Choroid plexus
- Anterior thalamus
- Fornix
- Cistern of velum interpositum
- Splenium of corpus callosum
- Atrium

FIG. 2.32.

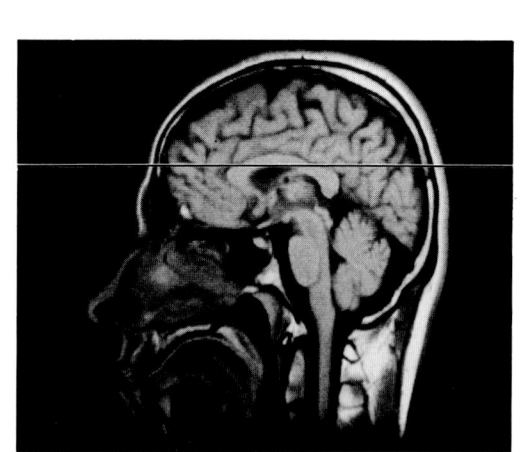

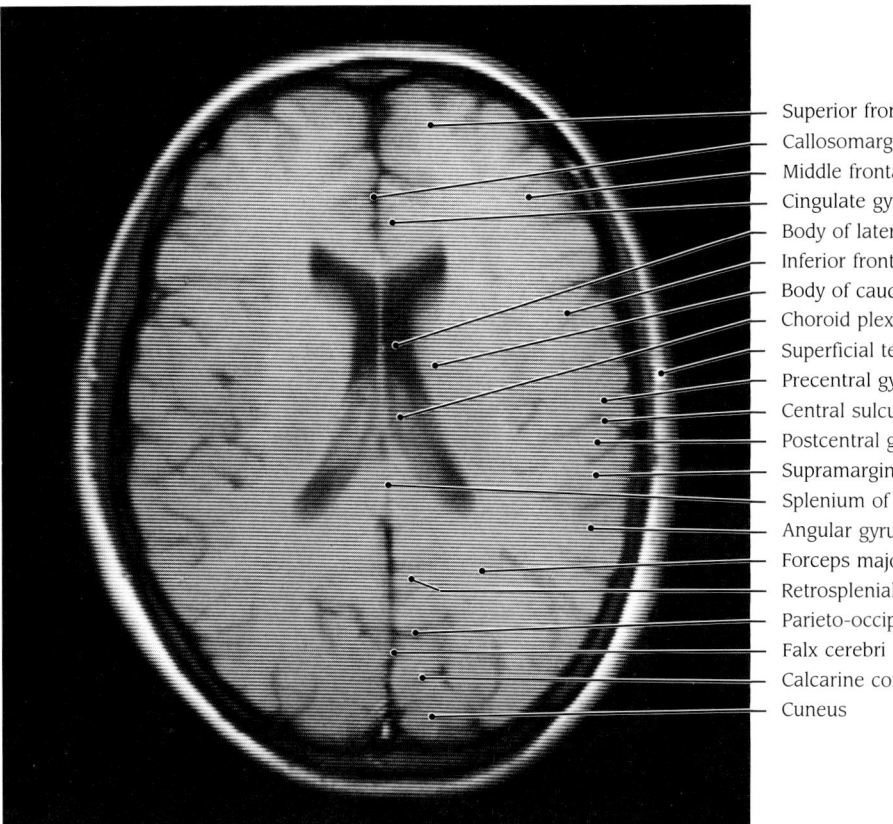

FIG. 2.33. TR = 500 msec, TE = 28 msec.

- Superior frontal gyrus
- Callosomarginal artery
- Middle frontal gyrus
- Cingulate gyrus
- Body of lateral ventricle
- Inferior frontal gyrus
- Body of caudate nucleus
- Choroid plexus
- Superficial temporal vein
- Precentral gyrus
- Central sulcus
- Postcentral gyrus
- Supramarginal gyrus
- Splenium of corpus callosum
- Angular gyrus
- Forceps major
- Retrosplenial gyrus
- Parieto-occipital fissure
- Falx cerebri
- Calcarine cortex
- Cuneus

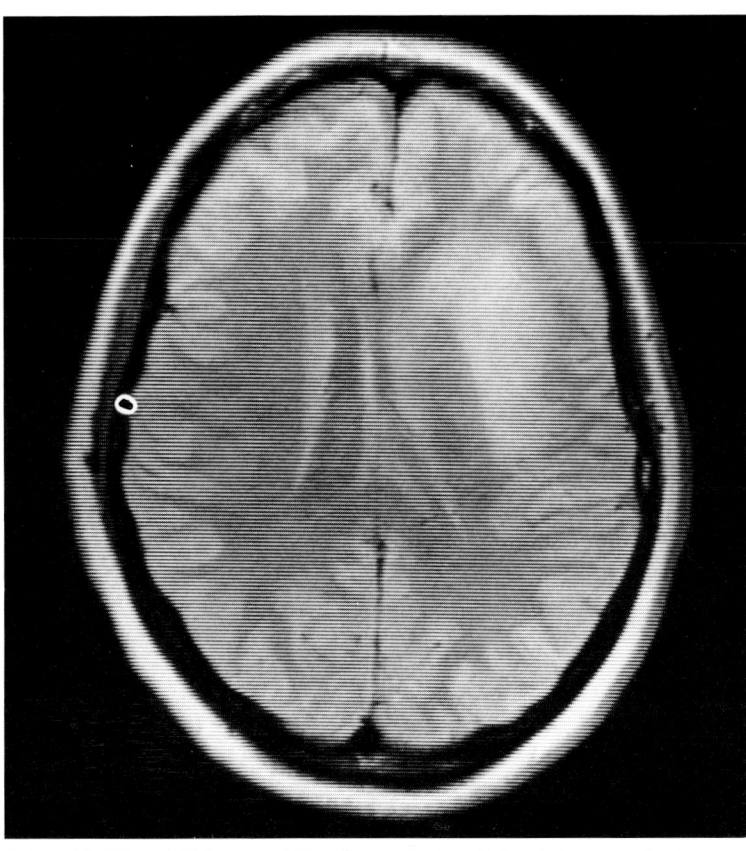

FIG. 2.34. TR = 2000 msec, TE = 28 msec. A left frontotemporal astrocytoma effaces the left lateral ventricle and causes a left-to-right shift.

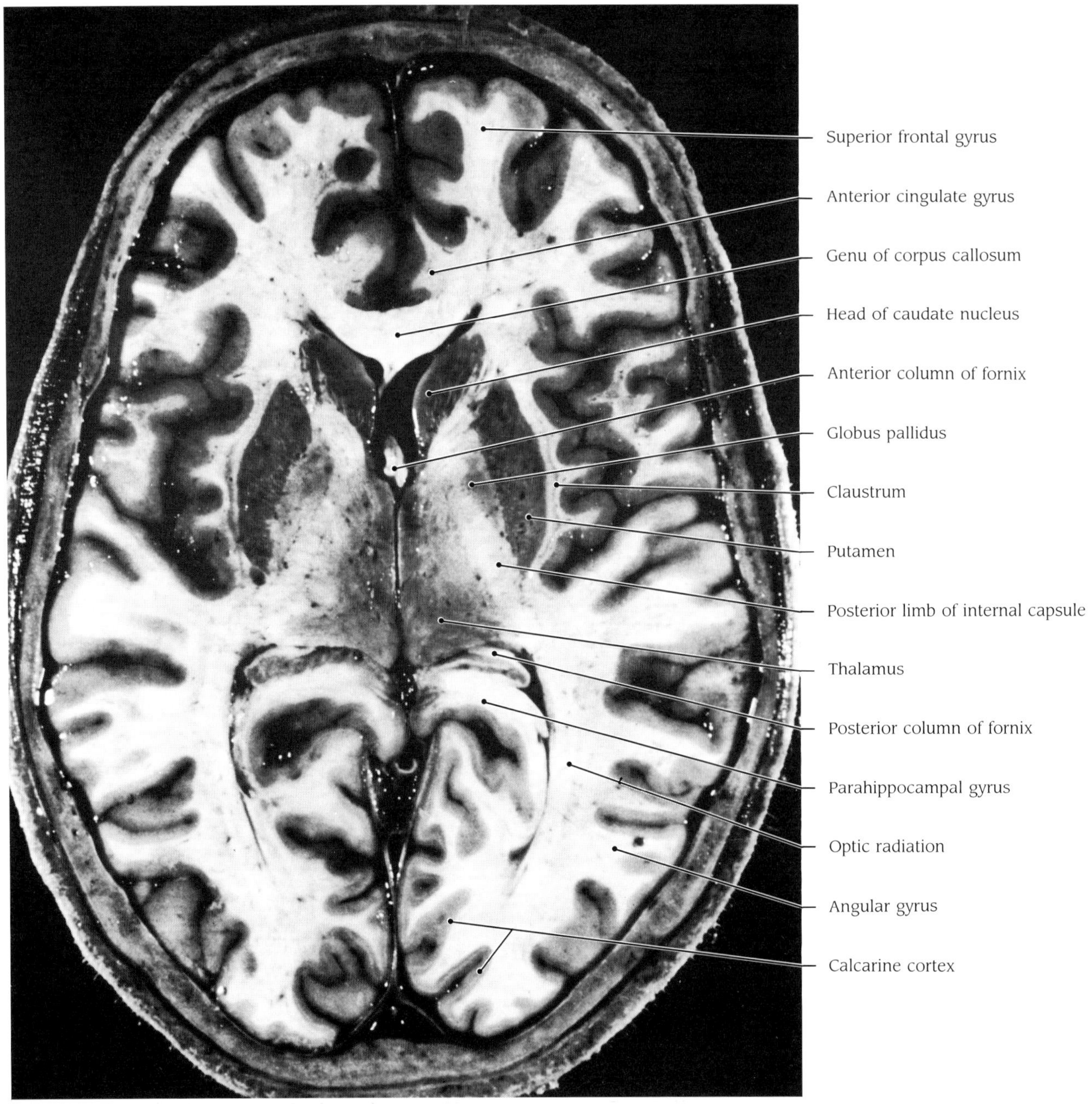

FIG. 2.35.

- Superior frontal gyrus
- Anterior cingulate gyrus
- Genu of corpus callosum
- Head of caudate nucleus
- Anterior column of fornix
- Globus pallidus
- Claustrum
- Putamen
- Posterior limb of internal capsule
- Thalamus
- Posterior column of fornix
- Parahippocampal gyrus
- Optic radiation
- Angular gyrus
- Calcarine cortex

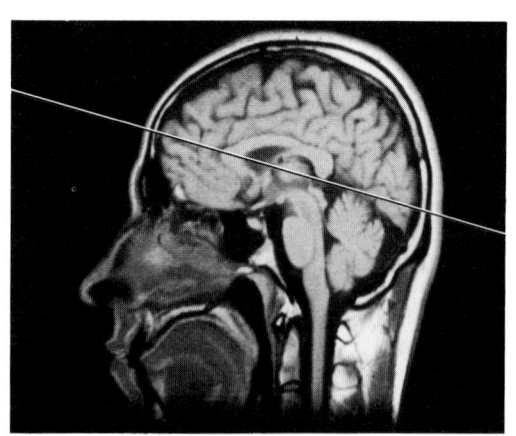

- The internal capsule is composed of ascending and descending fiber systems that form two distinct limbs. The anterior limb, which includes the genu, lies between the caudate nucleus and the lentiform nucleus, whereas the posterior limb lies between the thalamus and the lentiform nucleus.
- Recent research findings show that the anterior limb and genu contain descending fibers from the cortex to the caudate nucleus and to the pons, as well as ascending fibers from the thalamus to the cortex. The posterior limb contains descending corticobulbar and corticospinal fibers and additional corticopontine fibers, as well as ascending thalamocortical fibers.
- The septum pellucidum is composed of two parallel laminae that extend from the genu of the corpus callosum to the columns of the fornix. The cavum of the septum pellucidum, a normal variation commonly seen in younger individuals, is formed by the separation of the two laminae.

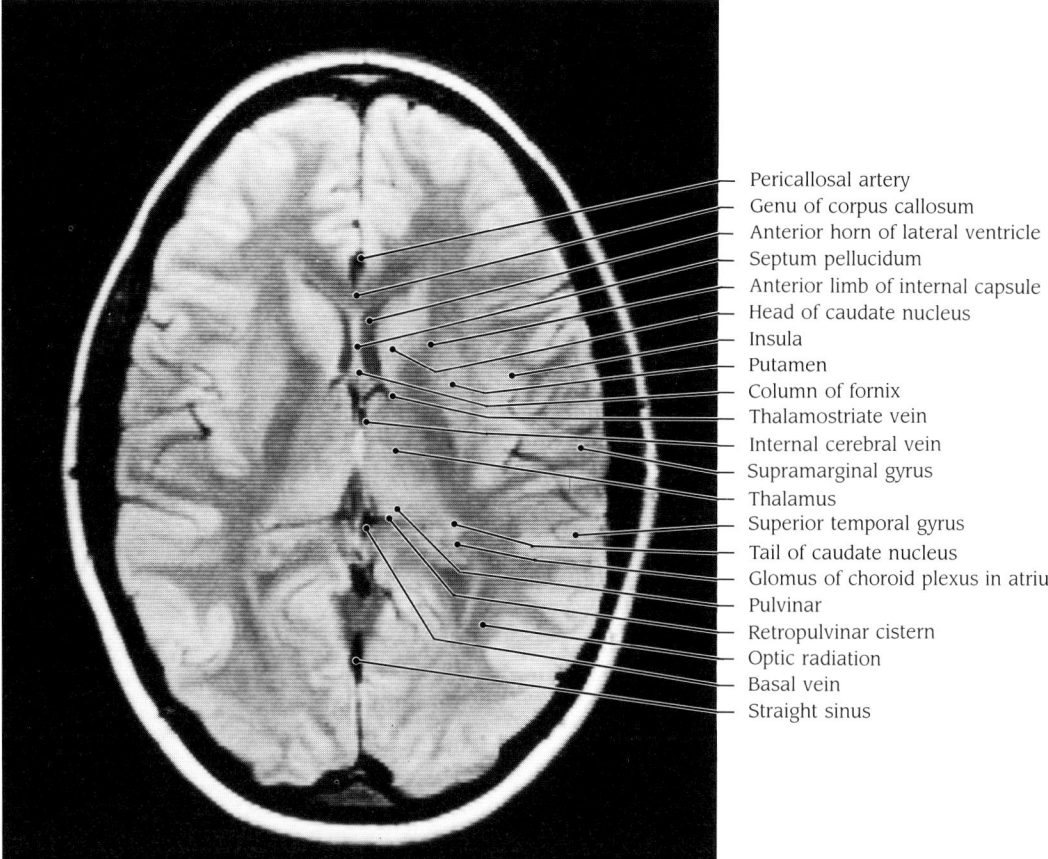

FIG. 2.36. TR = 2000 msec, TE = 28 msec.

- Pericallosal artery
- Genu of corpus callosum
- Anterior horn of lateral ventricle
- Septum pellucidum
- Anterior limb of internal capsule
- Head of caudate nucleus
- Insula
- Putamen
- Column of fornix
- Thalamostriate vein
- Internal cerebral vein
- Supramarginal gyrus
- Thalamus
- Superior temporal gyrus
- Tail of caudate nucleus
- Glomus of choroid plexus in atrium
- Pulvinar
- Retropulvinar cistern
- Optic radiation
- Basal vein
- Straight sinus

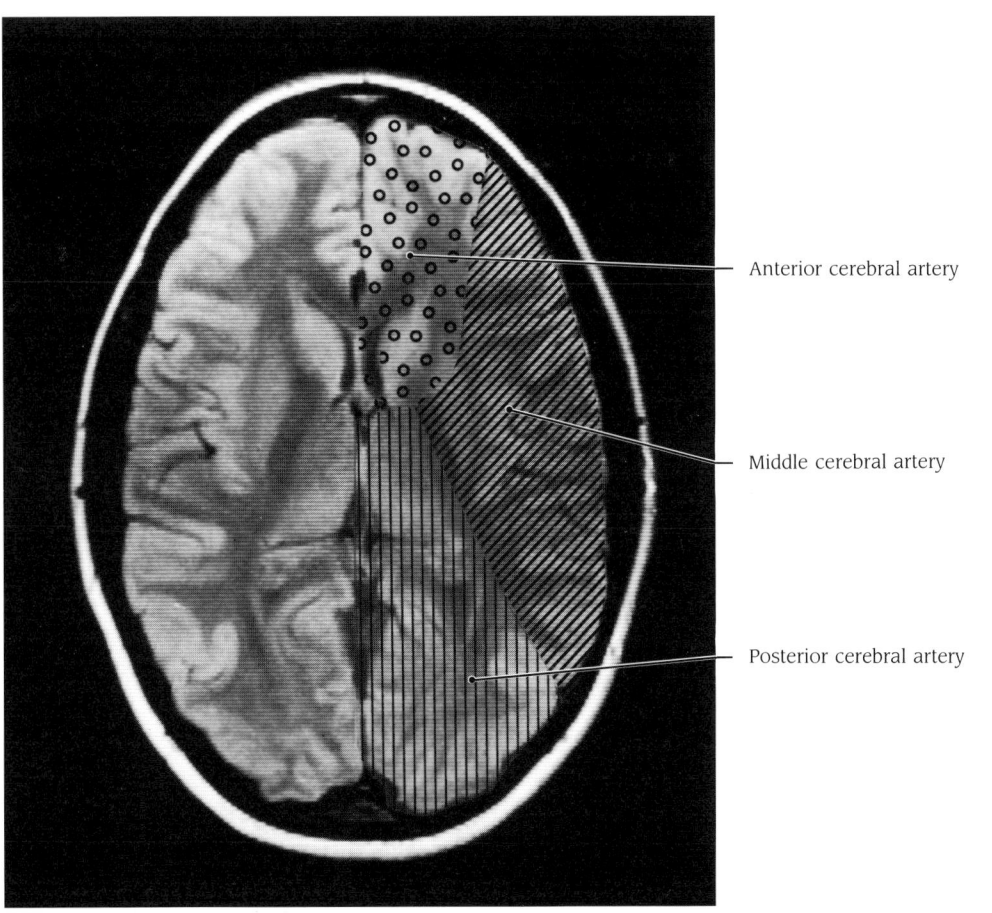

FIG. 2.37. TR = 2000 msec, TE = 28 msec.

- Anterior cerebral artery
- Middle cerebral artery
- Posterior cerebral artery

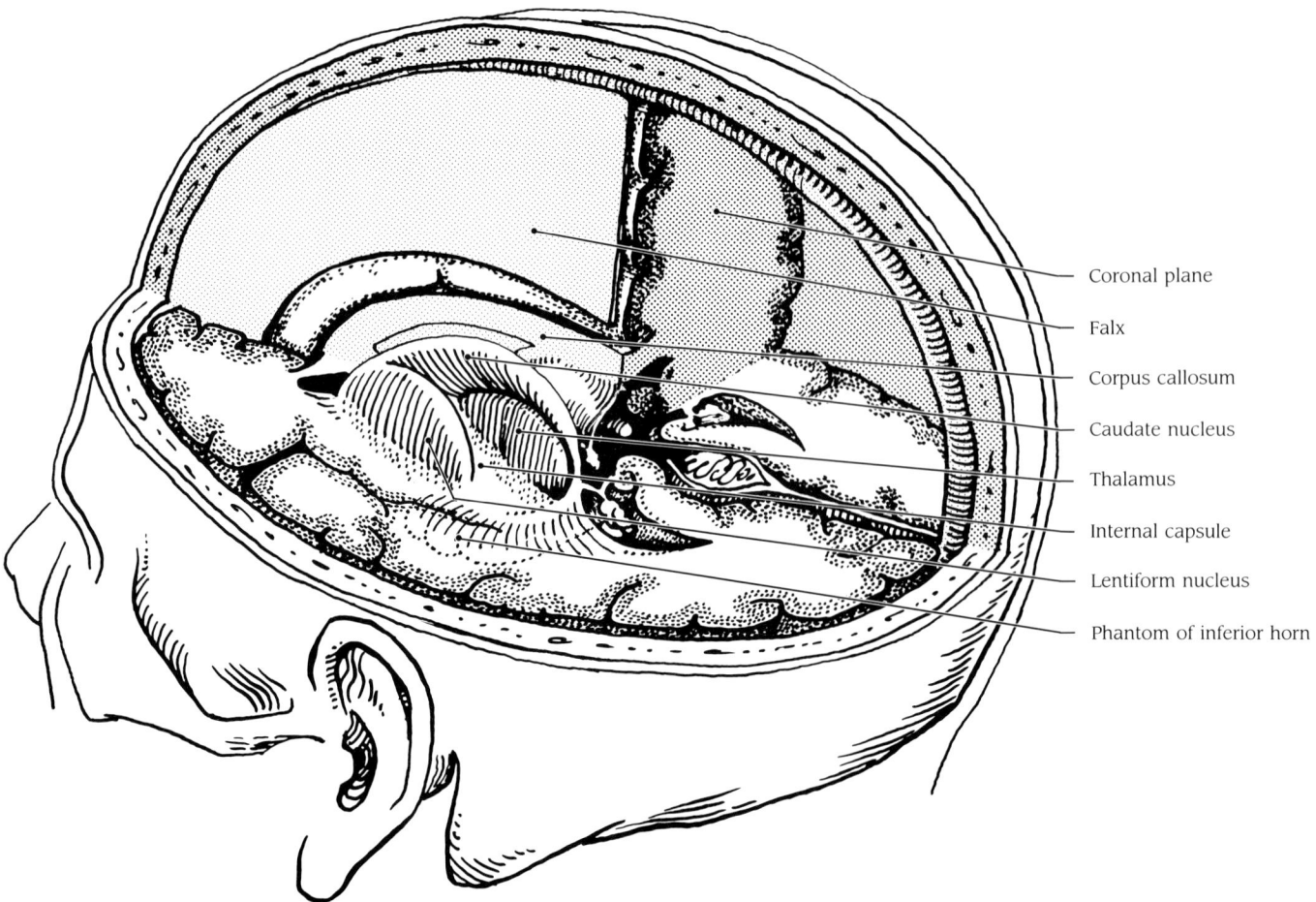

FIG. 2.38. Illustration of the relationships of the central gray masses to a midthalamic axial plane. (From de Groot, J.: Correlative Neuroanatomy of Computed Tomography and Magnetic Resonance Imaging. Philadelphia, Lea & Febiger, 1984.)

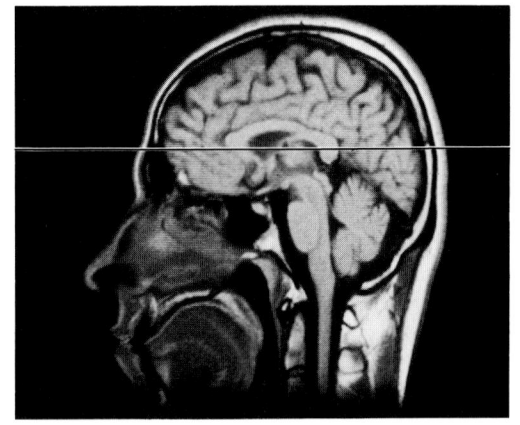

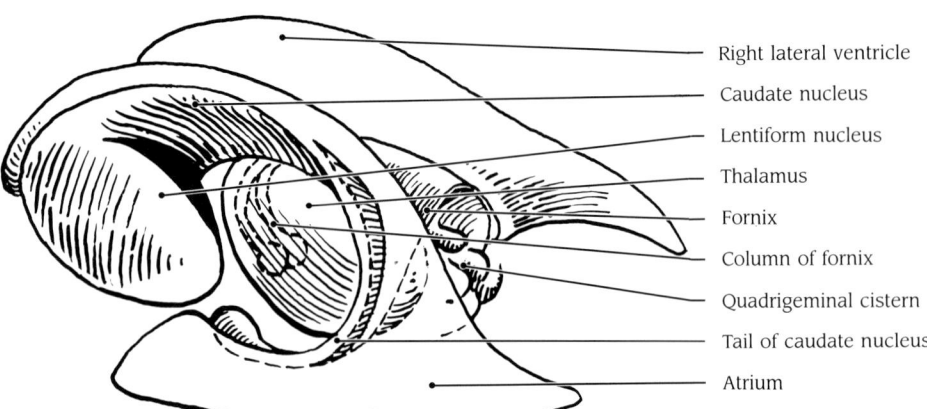

FIG. 2.39. Schematic illustration of the relationship between the basal ganglia and the lateral ventricles. (From de Groot, J.: Correlative Neuroanatomy of Computed Tomography and Magnetic Resonance Imaging. Philadelphia, Lea & Febiger, 1984.)

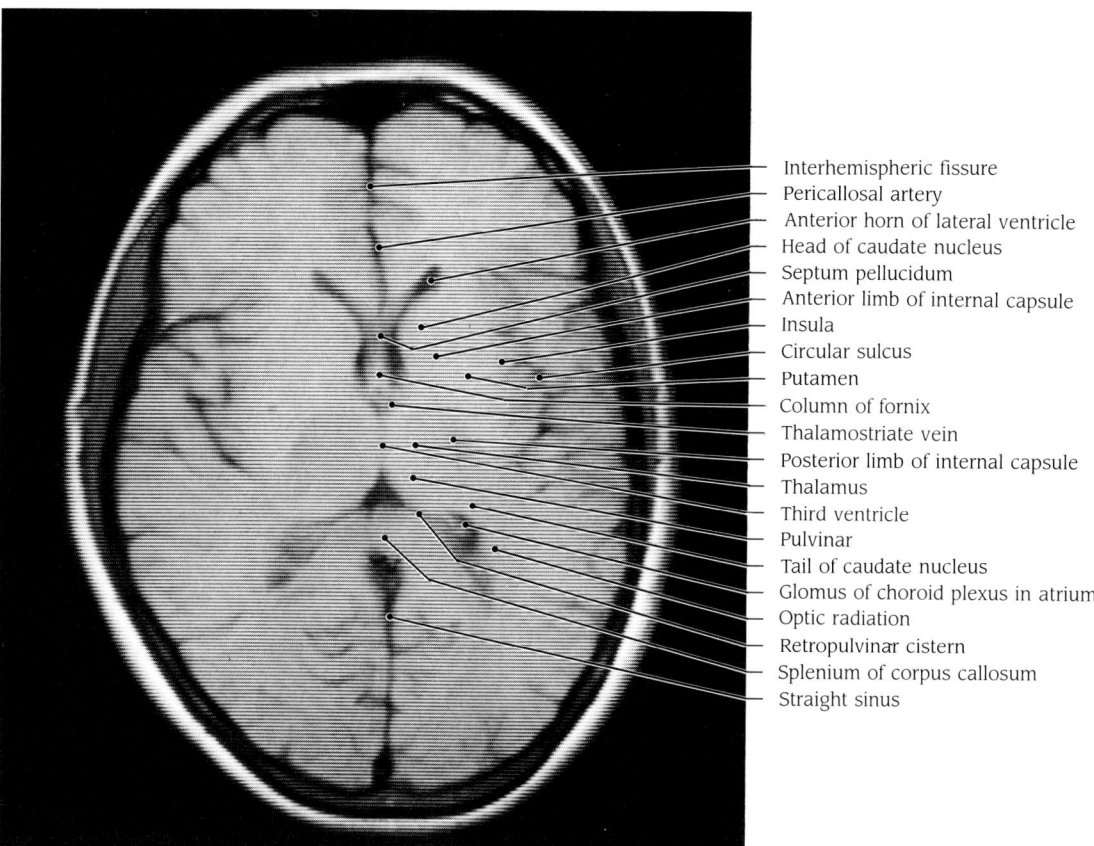

FIG. 2.40. TR = 500 msec, TE = 28 msec.

- Interhemispheric fissure
- Pericallosal artery
- Anterior horn of lateral ventricle
- Head of caudate nucleus
- Septum pellucidum
- Anterior limb of internal capsule
- Insula
- Circular sulcus
- Putamen
- Column of fornix
- Thalamostriate vein
- Posterior limb of internal capsule
- Thalamus
- Third ventricle
- Pulvinar
- Tail of caudate nucleus
- Glomus of choroid plexus in atrium
- Optic radiation
- Retropulvinar cistern
- Splenium of corpus callosum
- Straight sinus

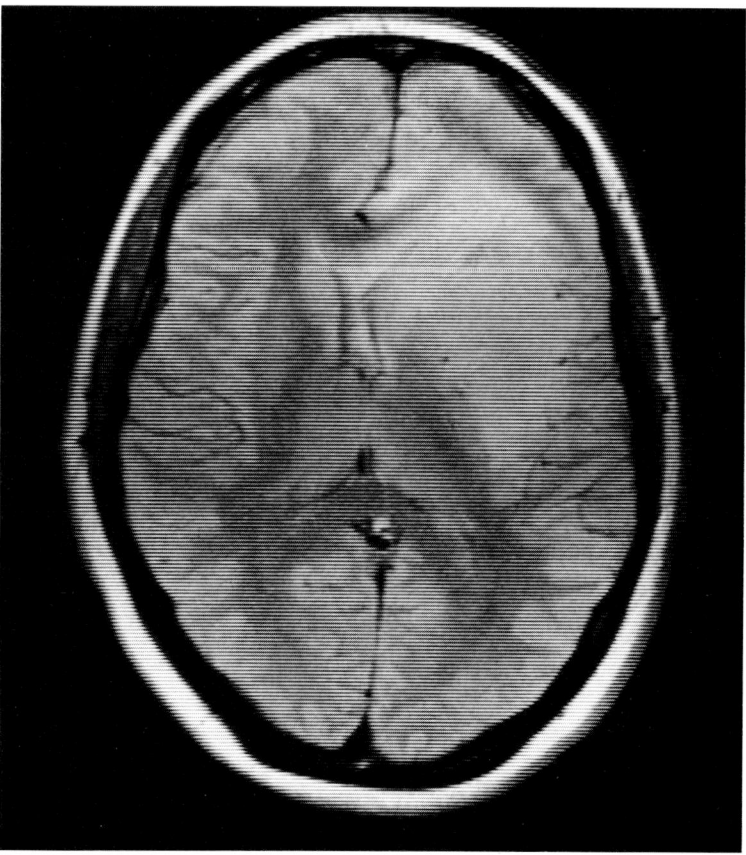

FIG. 2.41. TR = 2000 msec, TE = 28 msec. A left frontotemporal astrocytoma extends into the genu of the corpus callosum and the septum pellucidum.

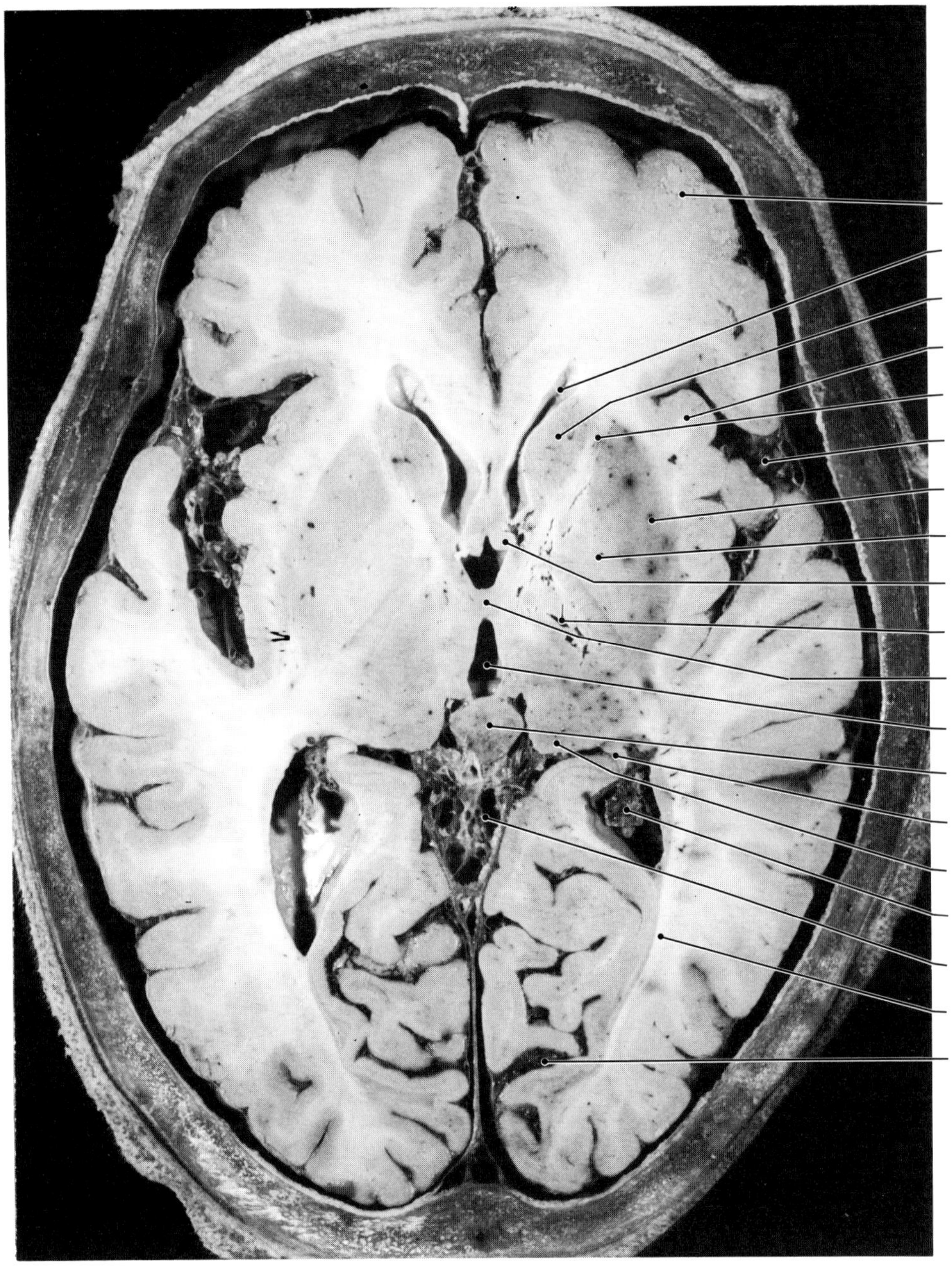

FIG. 2.42.

- Middle frontal gyrus
- Anterior horn
- Head of caudate nucleus
- Insula
- Anterior limb of internal capsule
- Lateral fissure
- Putamen
- Globus pallidus
- Anterior column of fornix
- Posterior limb of internal capsule
- Interthalamic adhesion
- Third ventricle
- Pineal gland
- Posterior column of fornix
- Pulvinar
- Atrium with choroid plexus
- Quadrigeminal cistern
- Optic radiation
- Calcarine fissure

- The lentiform nucleus, a part of the basal ganglia, has two components: the medially located globus pallidus, and the putamen, which is lateral.
- The culmen of the vermis, the most superior structure within the posterior fossa, is seen at this level between the tentorial margins.

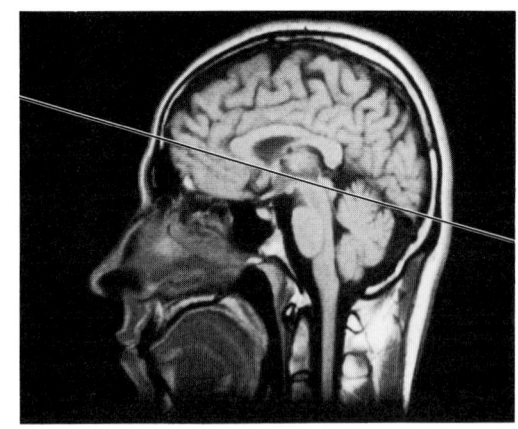

28

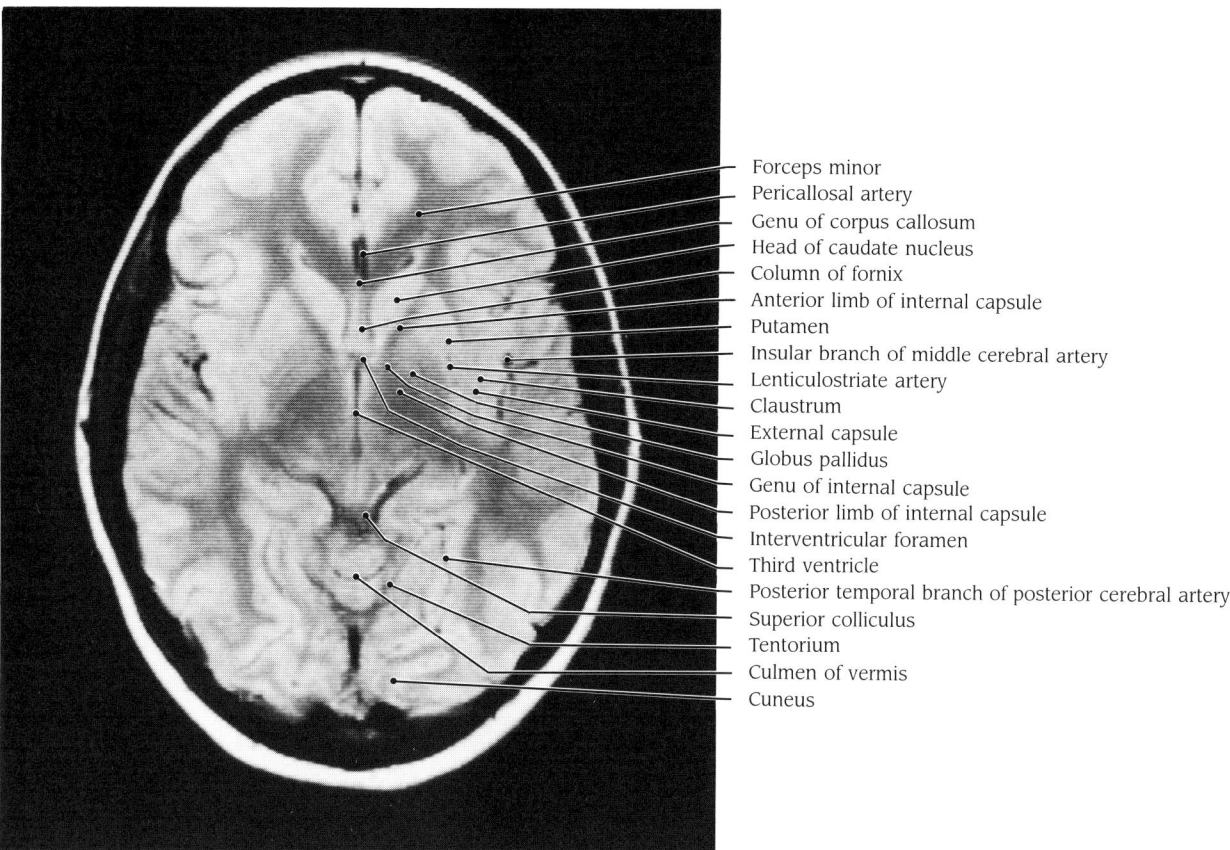

FIG. 2.43. TR = 2000 msec, TE = 28 msec.

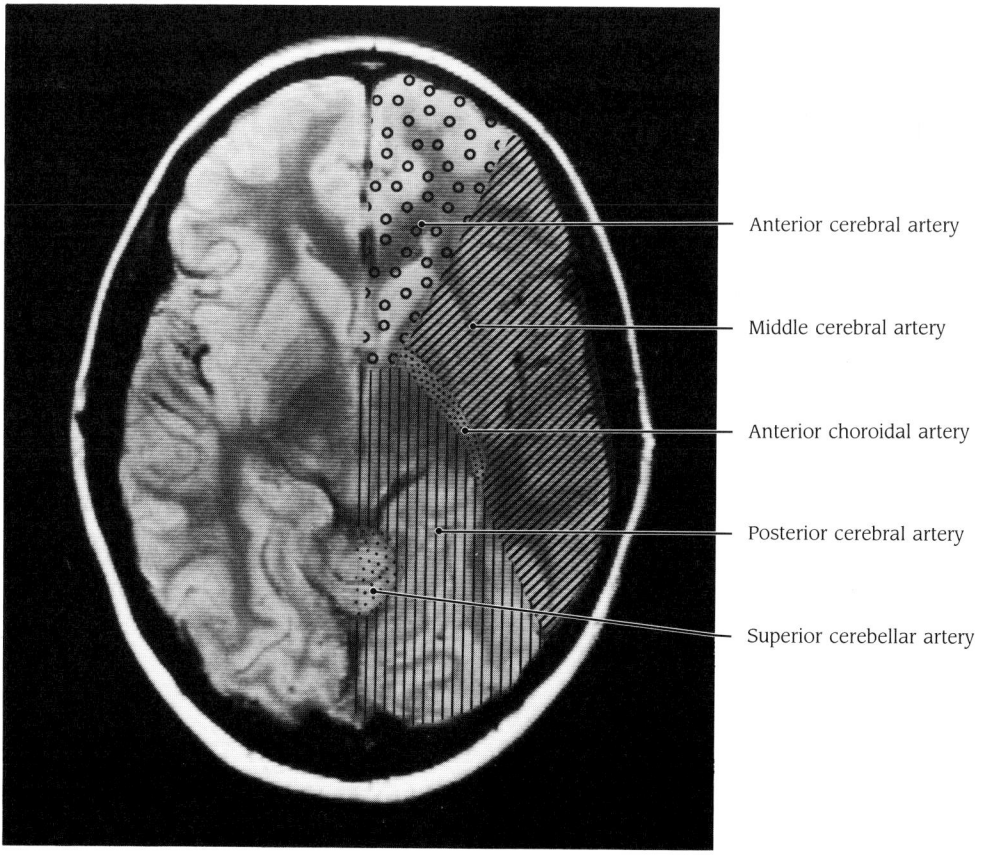

FIG. 2.44. TR = 2000 msec, TE = 28 msec.

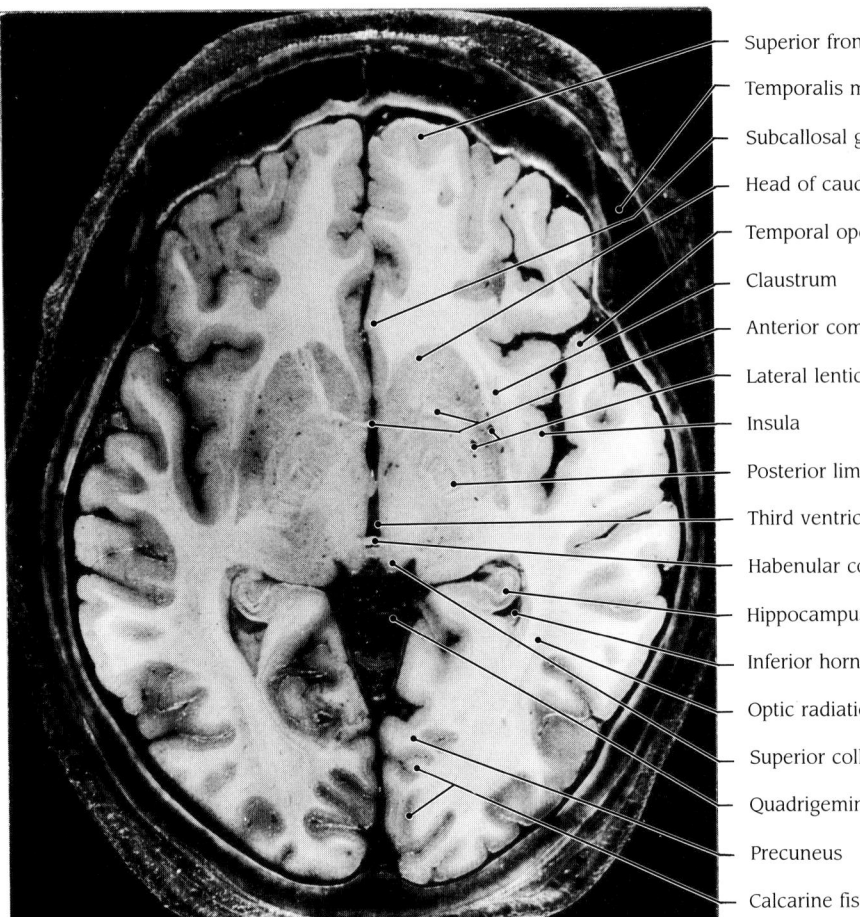

FIG. 2.45.

- Superior frontal gyrus
- Temporalis muscle
- Subcallosal gyrus
- Head of caudate nucleus
- Temporal operculum
- Claustrum
- Anterior commissure (twice)
- Lateral lenticulostriate arteries
- Insula
- Posterior limb of internal capsule
- Third ventricle
- Habenular commissure
- Hippocampus
- Inferior horn
- Optic radiation
- Superior colliculus
- Quadrigeminal cistern
- Precuneus
- Calcarine fissure

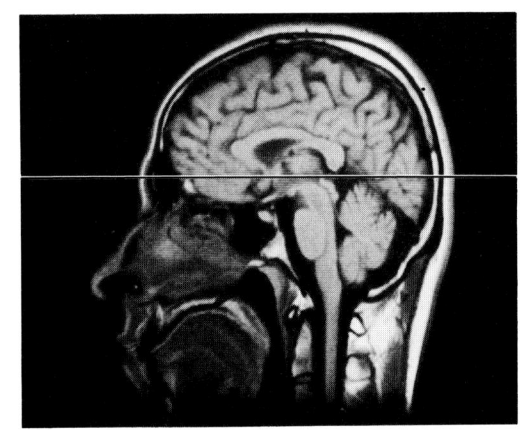

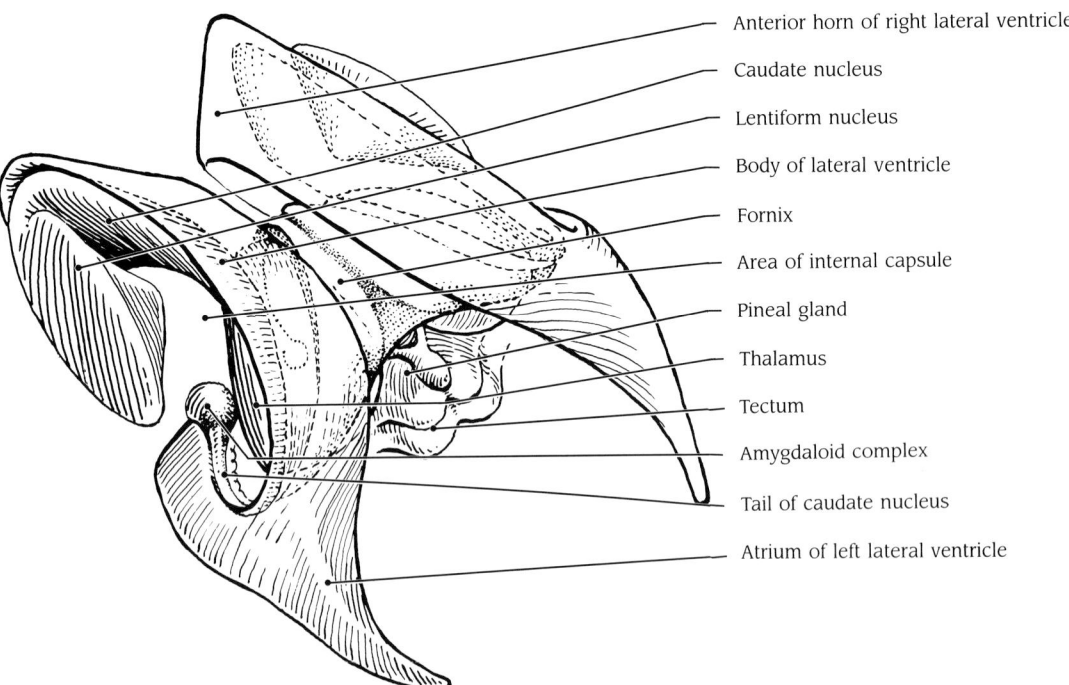

- Anterior horn of right lateral ventricle
- Caudate nucleus
- Lentiform nucleus
- Body of lateral ventricle
- Fornix
- Area of internal capsule
- Pineal gland
- Thalamus
- Tectum
- Amygdaloid complex
- Tail of caudate nucleus
- Atrium of left lateral ventricle

FIG. 2.46. Illustration of the relationships of the central gray masses to the lateral ventricle (oblique view). (From de Groot, J.: Correlative Neuroanatomy of Computed Tomography and Magnetic Resonance Imaging. Philadelphia, Lea & Febiger, 1984.)

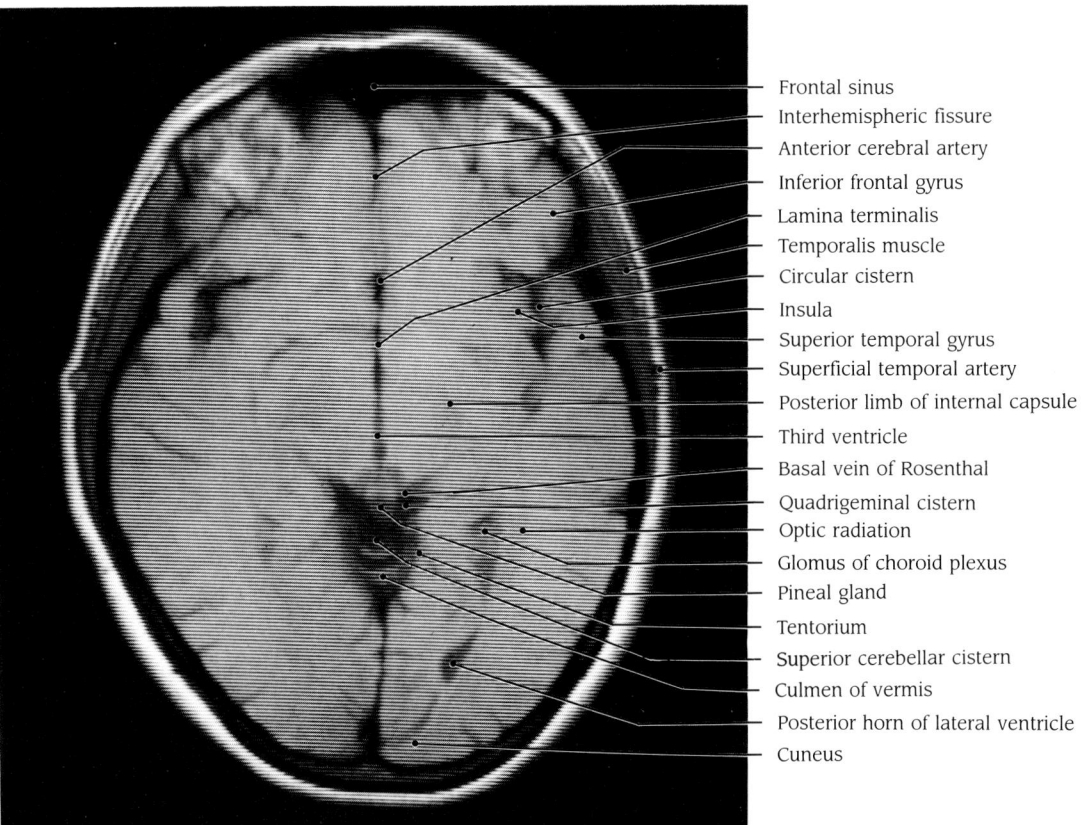

FIG. 2.47. TR = 500 msec, TE = 28 msec.

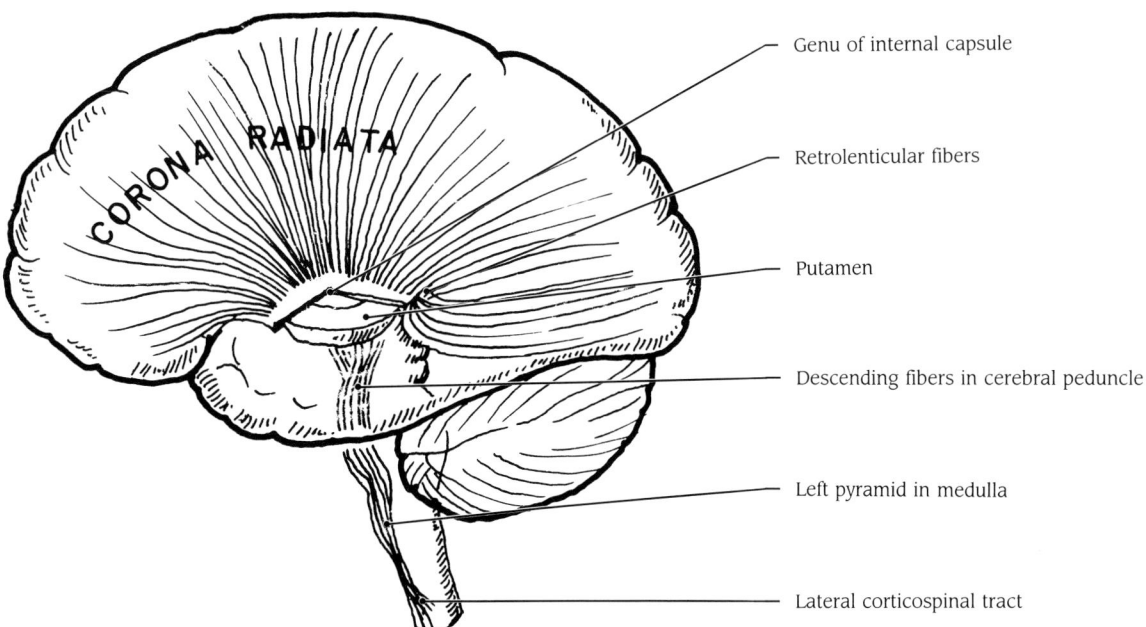

FIG. 2.48. Illustration of descending fiber systems in the left hemisphere and brain stem. (From de Groot, J.: Correlative Neuroanatomy of Computed Tomography and Magnetic Resonance Imaging. Philadelphia, Lea & Febiger, 1984.)

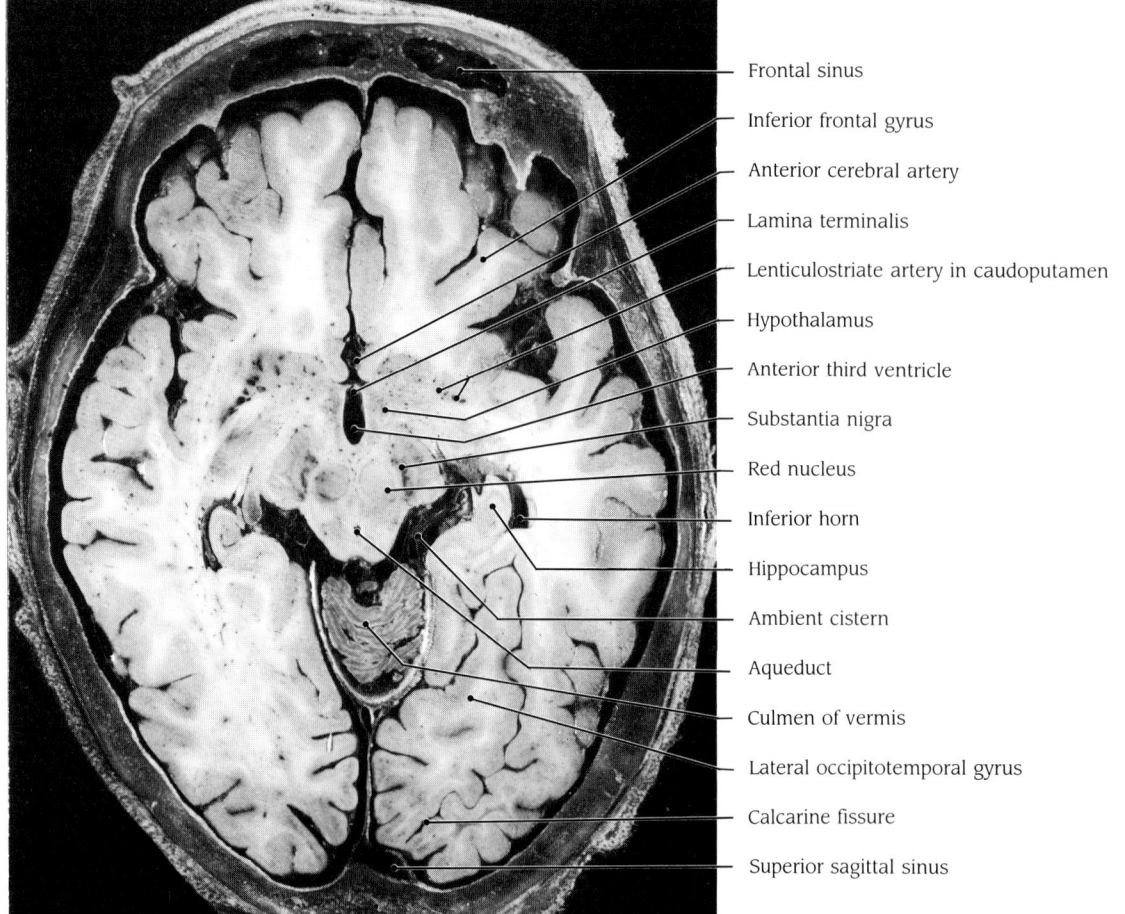

FIG. 2.49.

- The optic tracts extend posterolaterally from the optic chiasm to the lateral geniculate bodies.
- The anterior recesses of the third ventricle extend more inferiorly than the posterior recesses and, therefore, are visualized in the same axial plane as is the cerebral aqueduct.

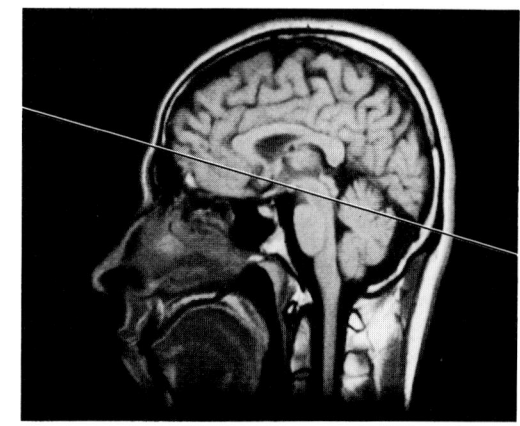

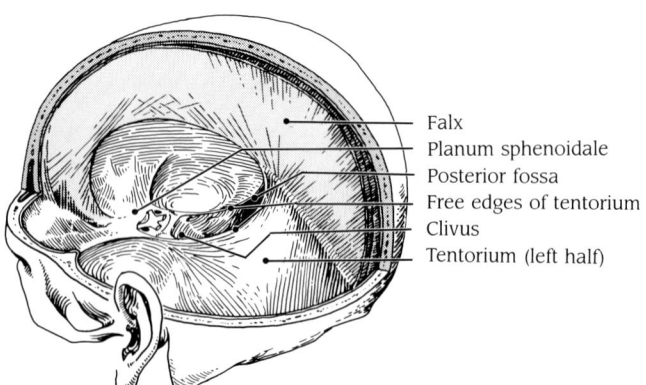

FIG. 2.50. Schematic illustration of the relationships between the falx, the tentorium, the skull, and the brain. Brain entirely removed to show the dural compartments. (From de Groot, J.: Correlative Neuroanatomy of Computed Tomography and Magnetic Resonance Imaging. Philadelphia, Lea & Febiger, 1984.)

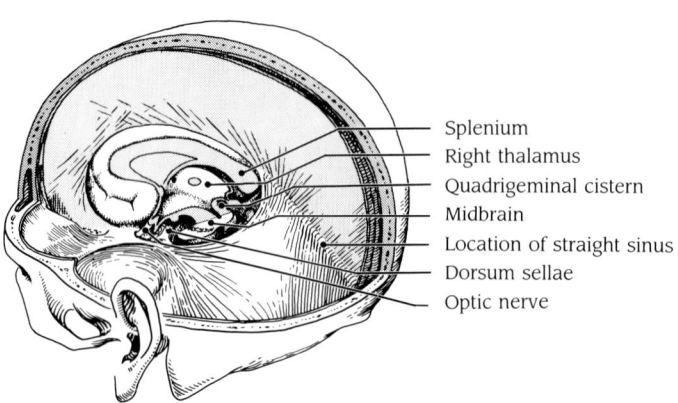

FIG. 2.51. Right hemisphere and brain stem in situ. (From de Groot, J.: Correlative Neuroanatomy of Computed Tomography and Magnetic Resonance Imaging. Philadelphia, Lea & Febiger, 1984.)

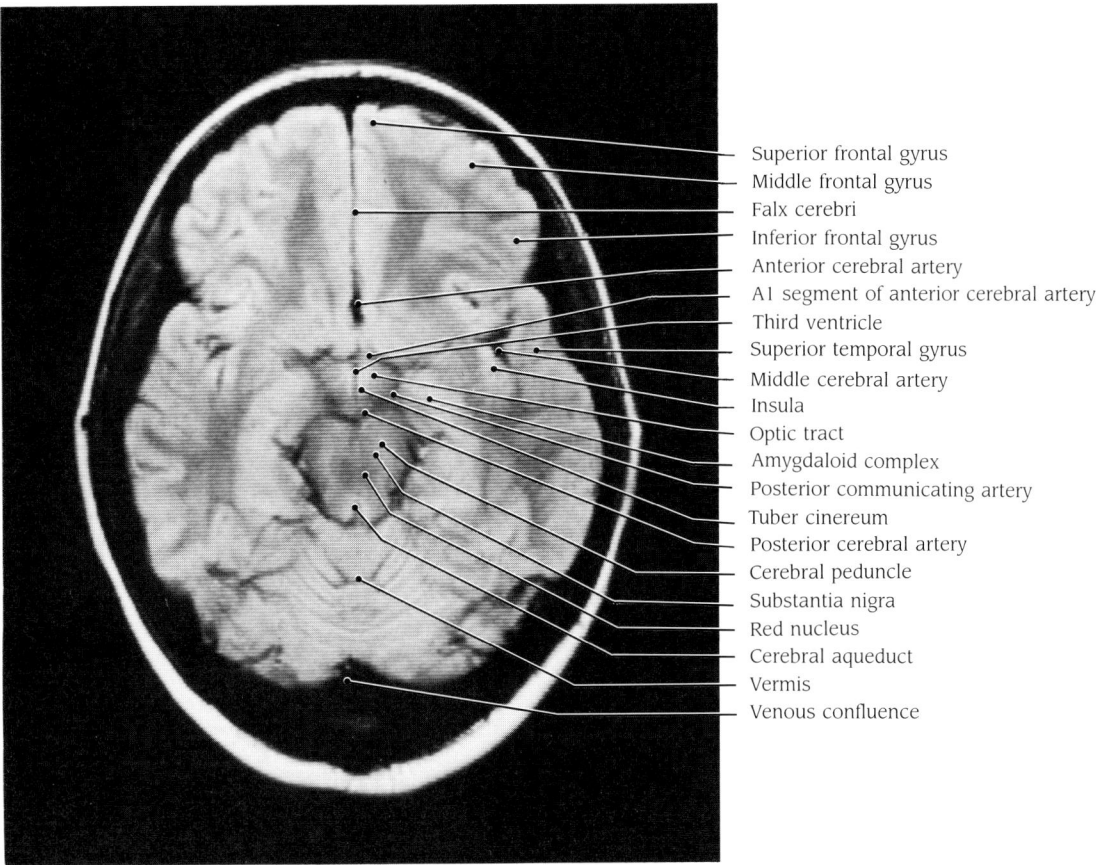

FIG. 2.52. TR = 2000 msec, TE = 28 msec.

- Superior frontal gyrus
- Middle frontal gyrus
- Falx cerebri
- Inferior frontal gyrus
- Anterior cerebral artery
- A1 segment of anterior cerebral artery
- Third ventricle
- Superior temporal gyrus
- Middle cerebral artery
- Insula
- Optic tract
- Amygdaloid complex
- Posterior communicating artery
- Tuber cinereum
- Posterior cerebral artery
- Cerebral peduncle
- Substantia nigra
- Red nucleus
- Cerebral aqueduct
- Vermis
- Venous confluence

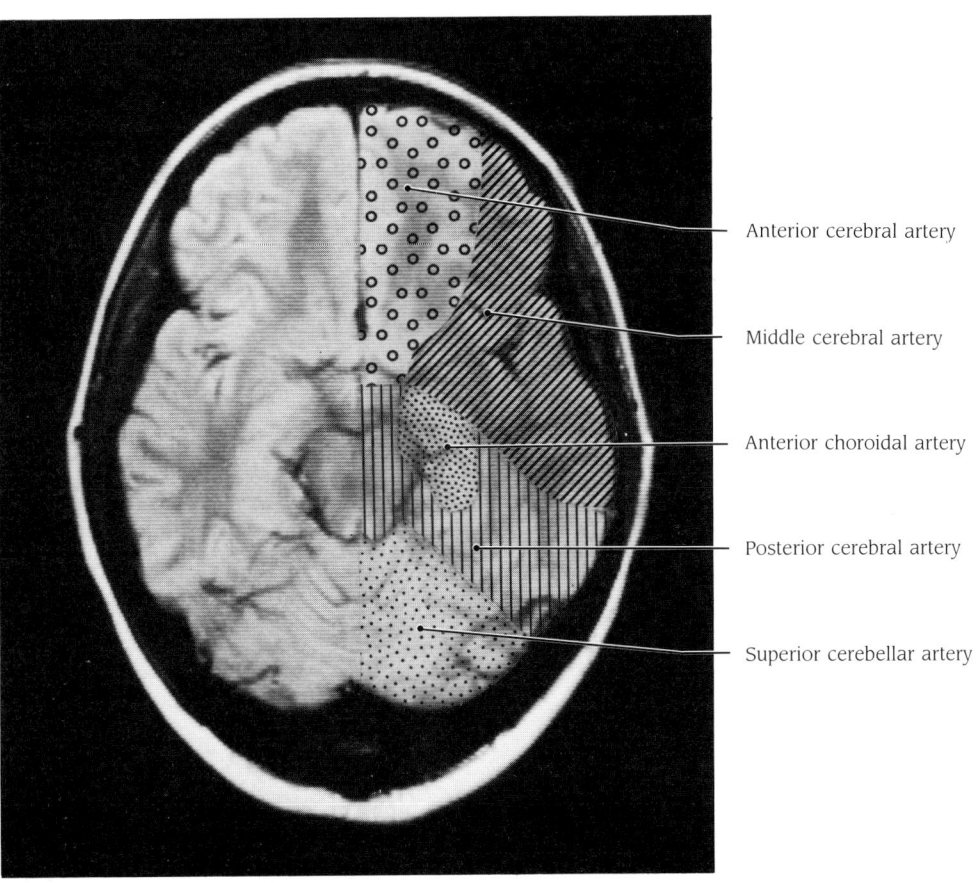

FIG. 2.53. TR = 2000 msec, TE = 28 msec.

- Anterior cerebral artery
- Middle cerebral artery
- Anterior choroidal artery
- Posterior cerebral artery
- Superior cerebellar artery

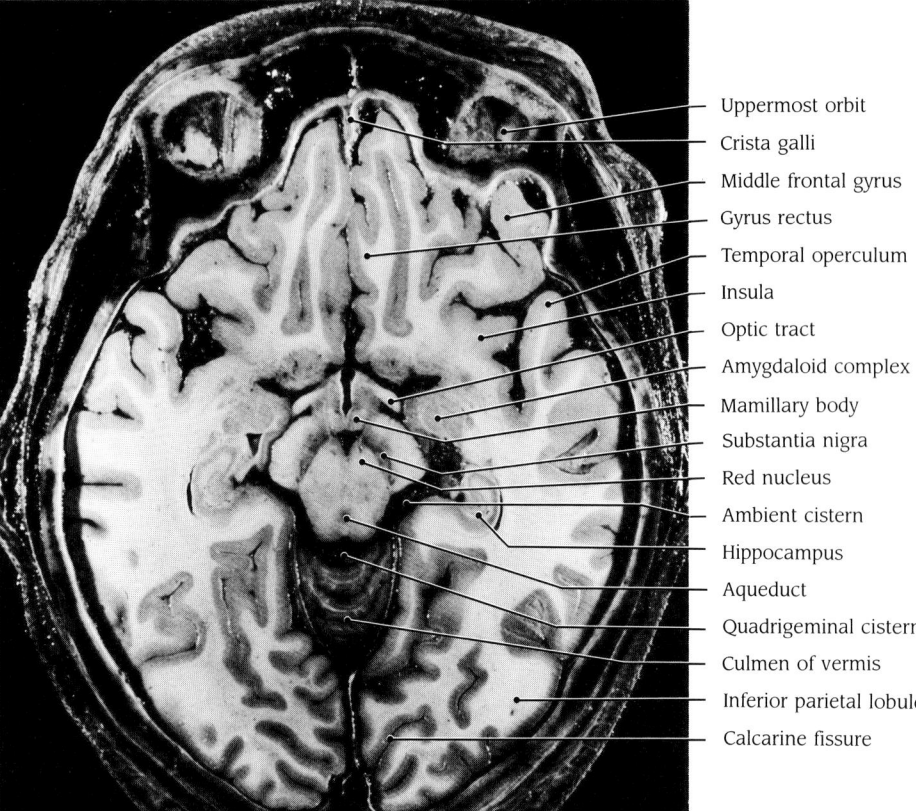
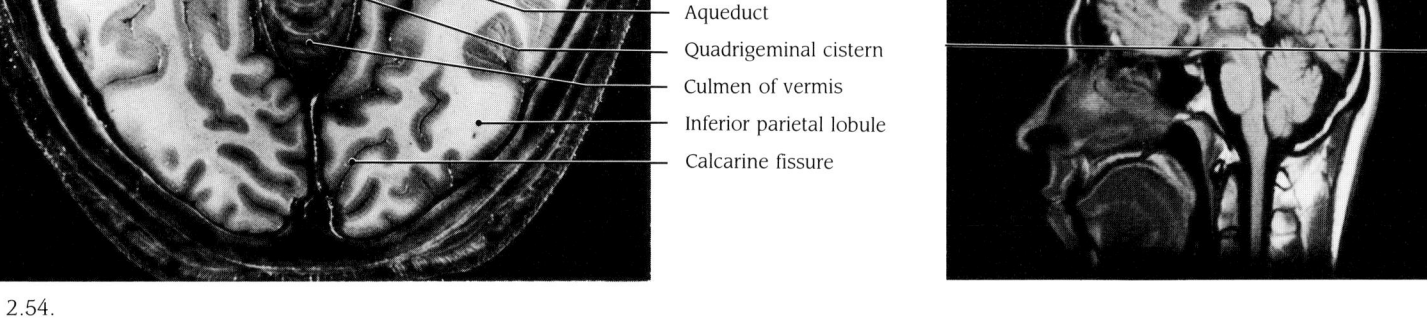

FIG. 2.54.

- Uppermost orbit
- Crista galli
- Middle frontal gyrus
- Gyrus rectus
- Temporal operculum
- Insula
- Optic tract
- Amygdaloid complex
- Mamillary body
- Substantia nigra
- Red nucleus
- Ambient cistern
- Hippocampus
- Aqueduct
- Quadrigeminal cistern
- Culmen of vermis
- Inferior parietal lobule
- Calcarine fissure

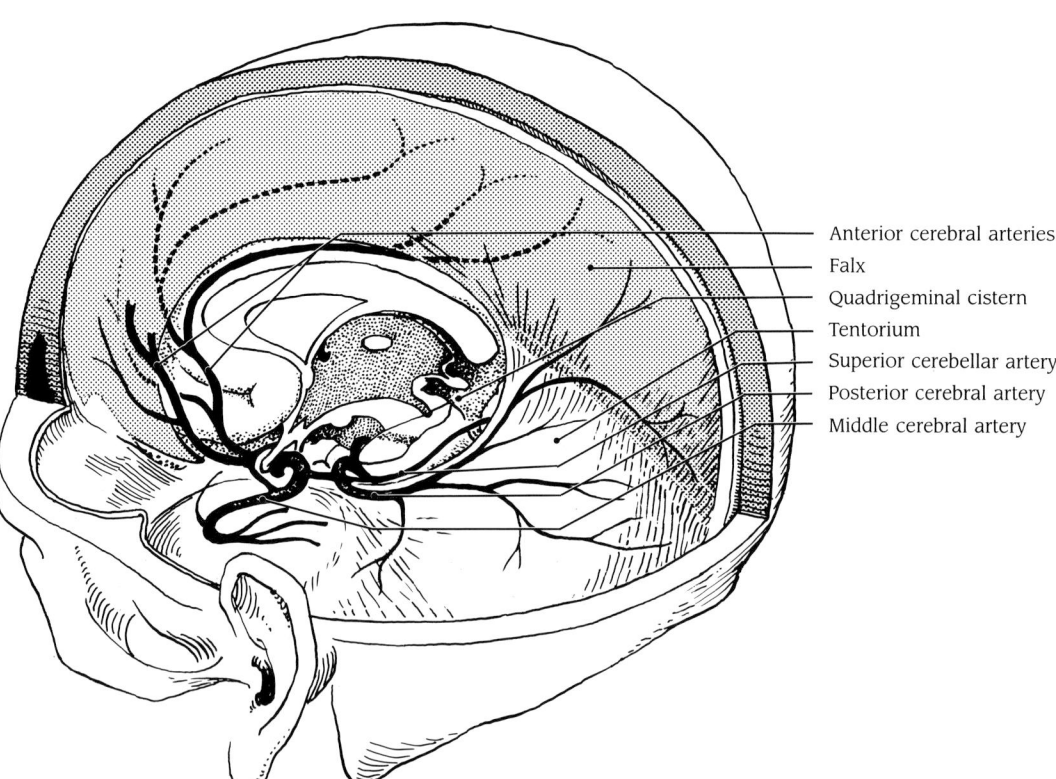

FIG. 2.55. Schematic illustration of the relationships between the major cerebral vessels, the falx, and the tentorium. (From de Groot, J.: Correlative Neuroanatomy of Computed Tomography and Magnetic Resonance Imaging. Philadelphia, Lea & Febiger, 1984.)

- Anterior cerebral arteries
- Falx
- Quadrigeminal cistern
- Tentorium
- Superior cerebellar artery
- Posterior cerebral artery
- Middle cerebral artery

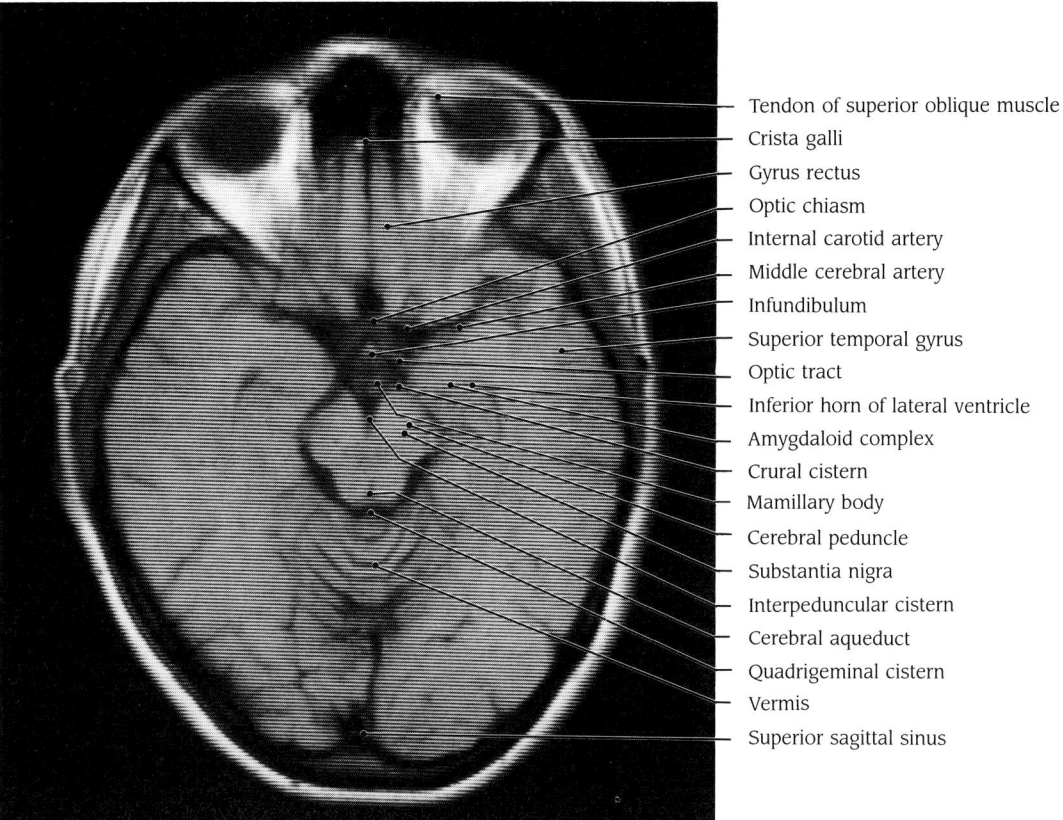

FIG. 2.56. TR = 500 msec, TE = 28 msec.

- Tendon of superior oblique muscle
- Crista galli
- Gyrus rectus
- Optic chiasm
- Internal carotid artery
- Middle cerebral artery
- Infundibulum
- Superior temporal gyrus
- Optic tract
- Inferior horn of lateral ventricle
- Amygdaloid complex
- Crural cistern
- Mamillary body
- Cerebral peduncle
- Substantia nigra
- Interpeduncular cistern
- Cerebral aqueduct
- Quadrigeminal cistern
- Vermis
- Superior sagittal sinus

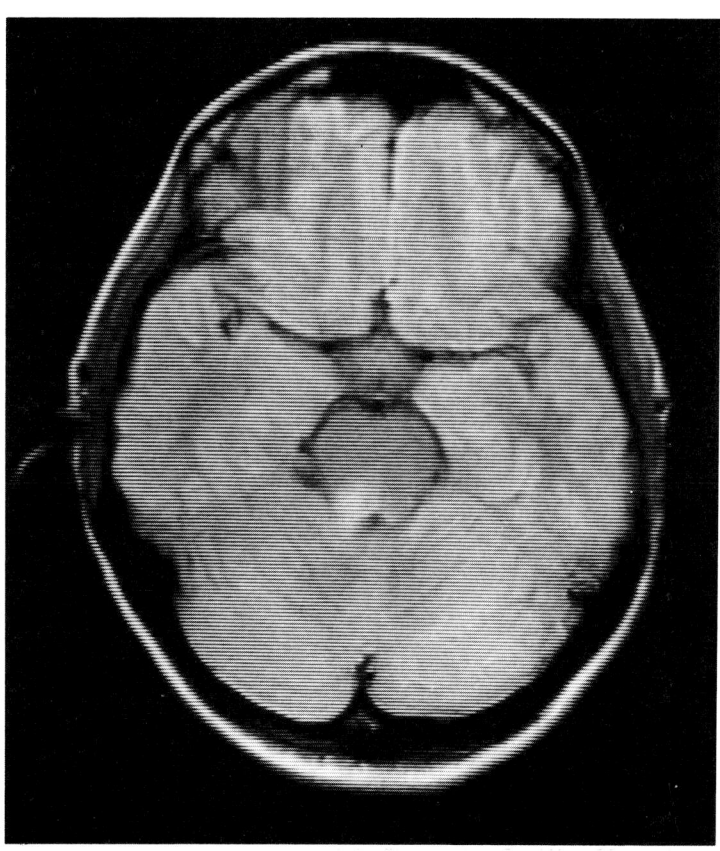

FIG. 2.57. TR = 2000 msec, TE = 28 msec. A lesion of multiple sclerosis in the tectum is identified as abnormal increased signal intensity.

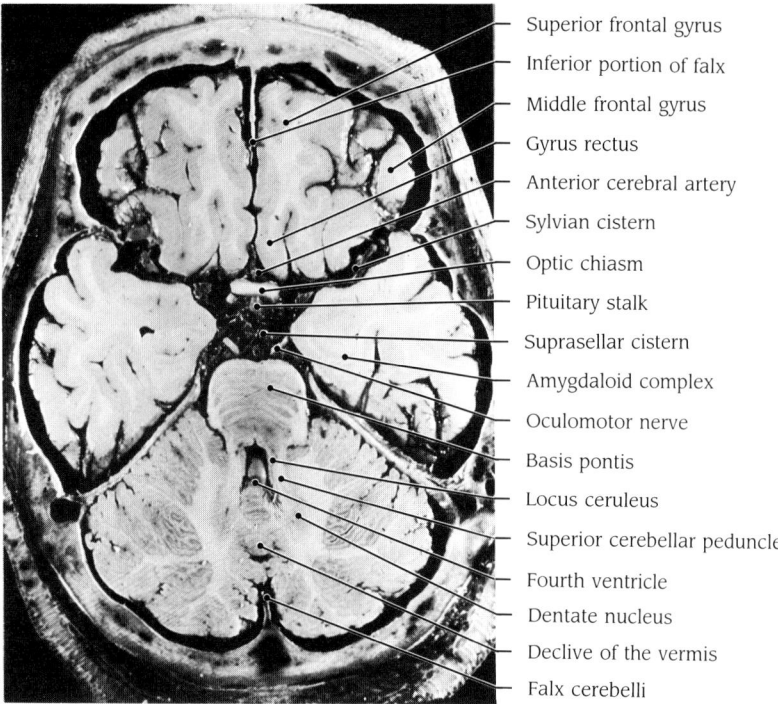

FIG. 2.58.
- Superior frontal gyrus
- Inferior portion of falx
- Middle frontal gyrus
- Gyrus rectus
- Anterior cerebral artery
- Sylvian cistern
- Optic chiasm
- Pituitary stalk
- Suprasellar cistern
- Amygdaloid complex
- Oculomotor nerve
- Basis pontis
- Locus ceruleus
- Superior cerebellar peduncle
- Fourth ventricle
- Dentate nucleus
- Declive of the vermis
- Falx cerebelli

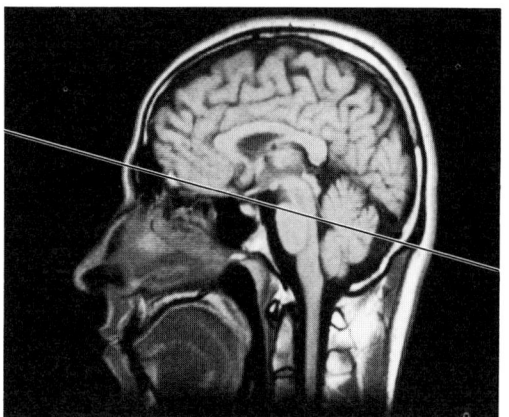

- Partial volume effects show the orbital structures and the orbital gyri in the same section plane.

- The dorsum sellae separates the prepontine cistern with the basilar artery from the cavernous sinus and pituitary gland.

- The tentorium cerebelli, composed of two layers of dura mater, separates the cerebral hemispheres from the cerebellum and brain stem. The free edges of the tentorium extend to the anterior clinoid processes (see Fig. 2.50).

- The medial portion of the temporal lobe consists of the uncus, the hippocampus, and the amygdaloid complex. The uncus normally extends slightly beyond the free edge of the tentorium.

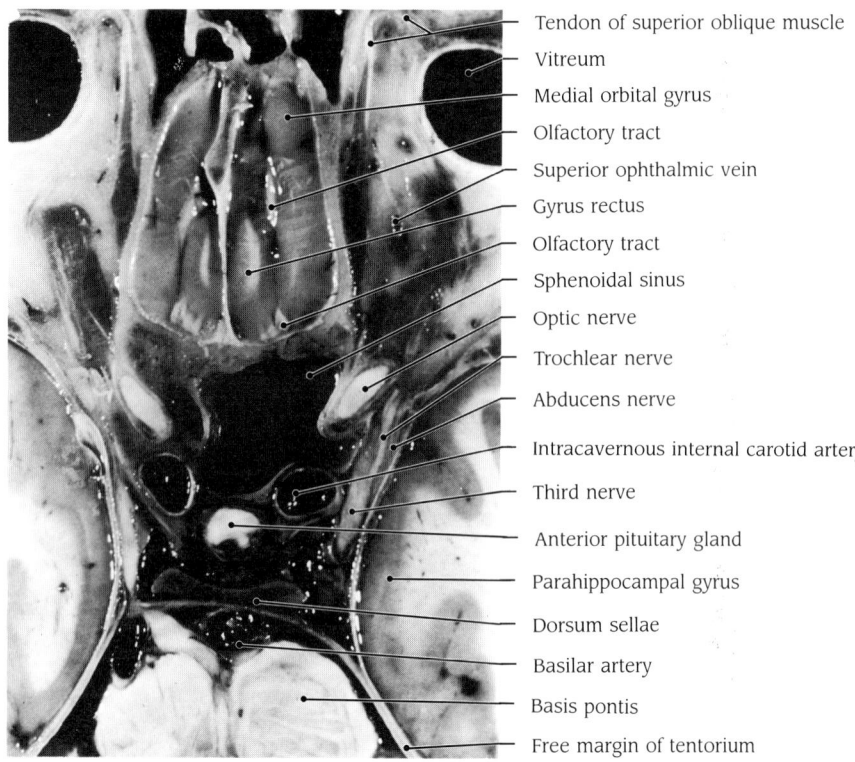

FIG. 2.59.
- Tendon of superior oblique muscle
- Vitreum
- Medial orbital gyrus
- Olfactory tract
- Superior ophthalmic vein
- Gyrus rectus
- Olfactory tract
- Sphenoidal sinus
- Optic nerve
- Trochlear nerve
- Abducens nerve
- Intracavernous internal carotid artery
- Third nerve
- Anterior pituitary gland
- Parahippocampal gyrus
- Dorsum sellae
- Basilar artery
- Basis pontis
- Free margin of tentorium

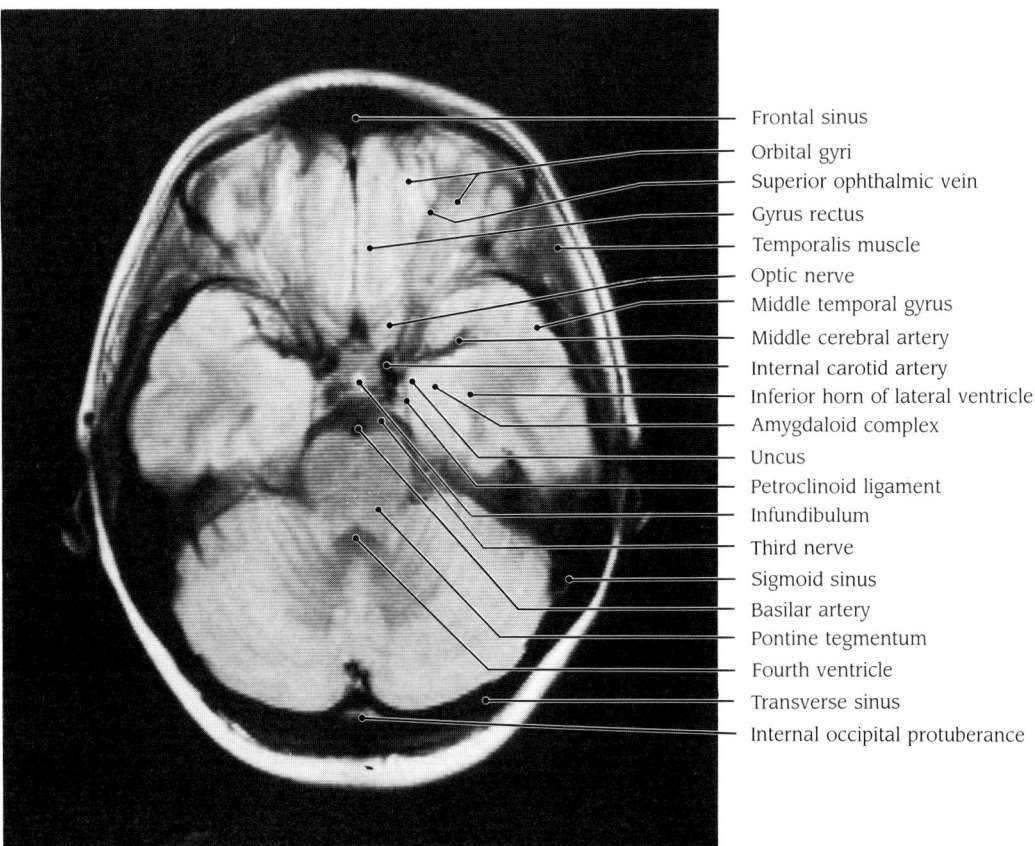

FIG. 2.60. TR = 2000 msec, TE = 28 msec.

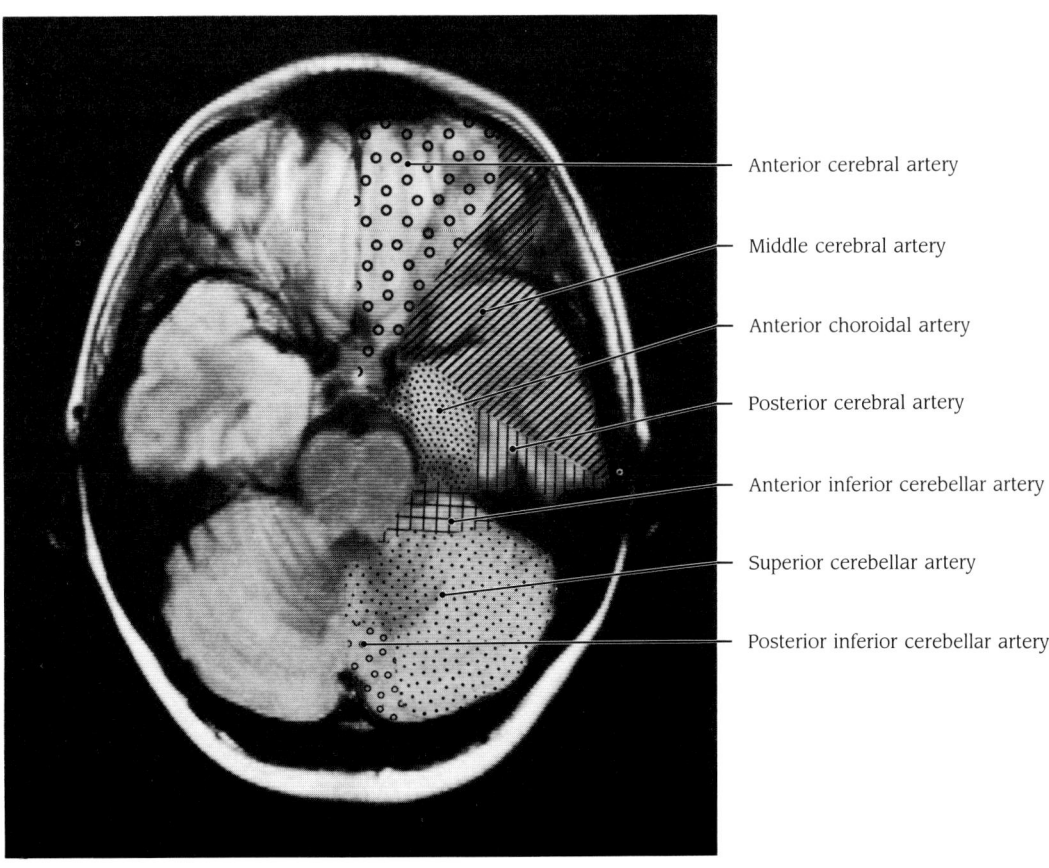

FIG. 2.61. TR = 2000 msec, TE = 28 msec.

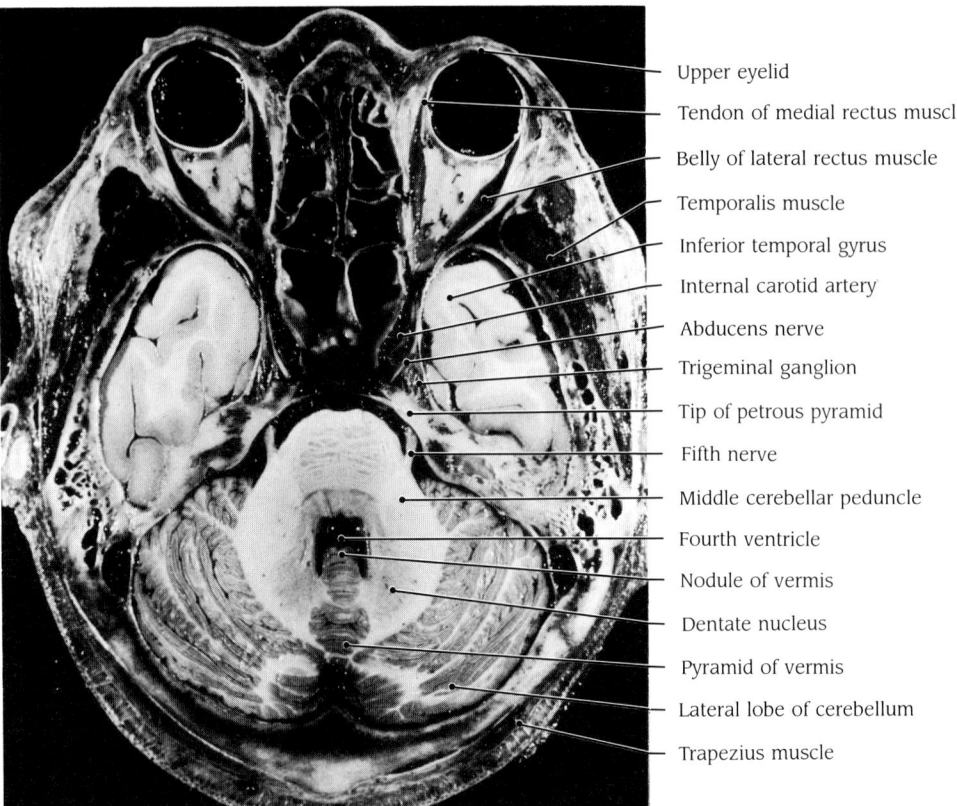

FIG. 2.62.

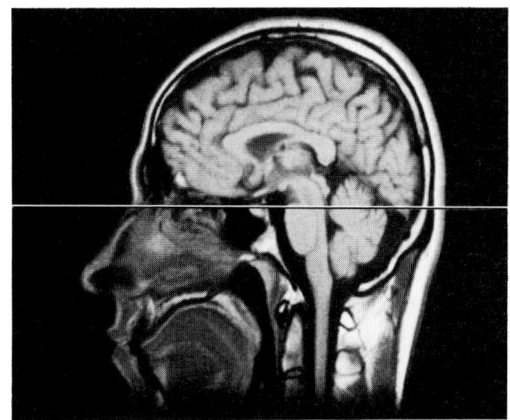

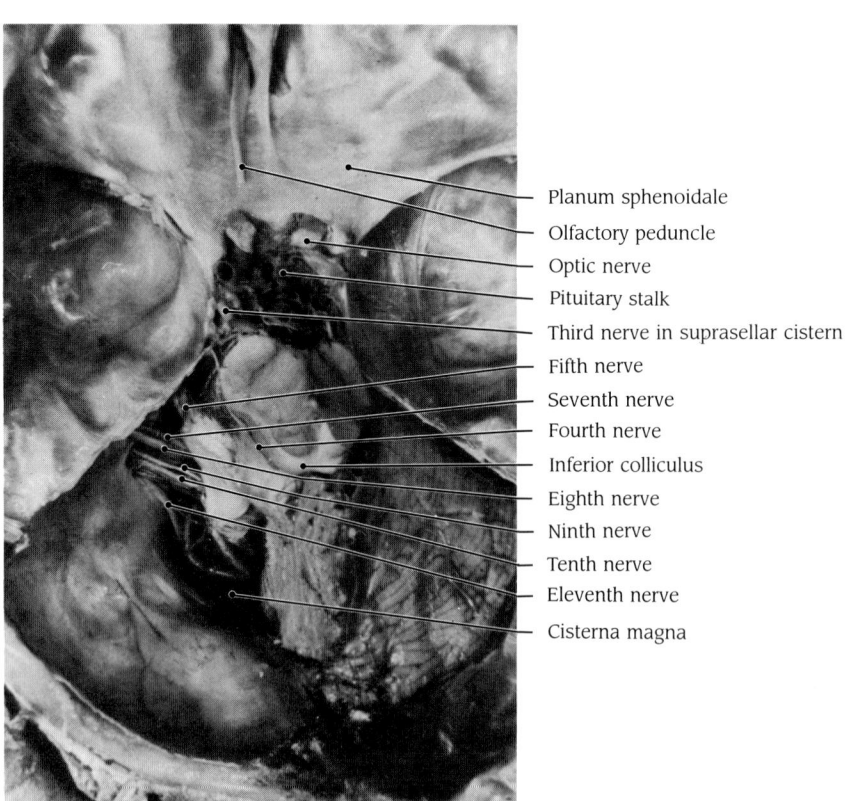

FIG. 2.63. Anatomic image of exposed cranial nerves in the posterior fossa and suprasellar cistern. (From de Groot, J.: Correlative Neuroanatomy of Computed Tomography and Magnetic Resonance Imaging. Philadelphia, Lea & Febiger, 1984.)

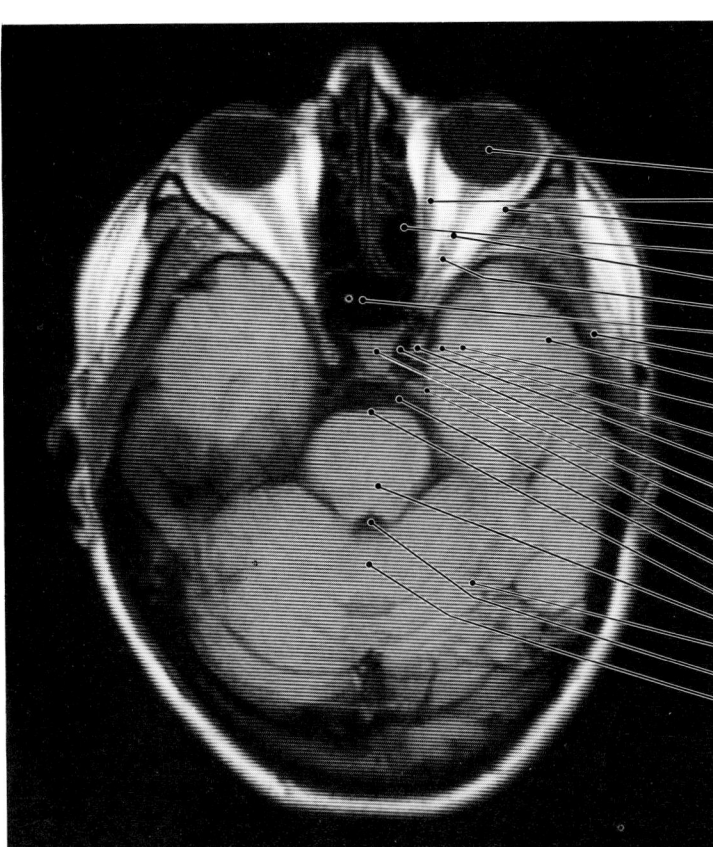

FIG. 2.64. TR = 500 msec, TE = 28 msec.

- Vitreous body
- Medial rectus muscle
- Lateral rectus muscle
- Ethmoidal sinus
- Optic nerve
- Ophthalmic artery
- Sphenoidal sinus
- Temporalis muscle
- Middle temporal gyrus
- Amygdaloid complex
- Uncus
- Cavernous sinus
- Internal carotid artery
- Pituitary gland
- Petroclinoid ligament
- Prepontine cistern
- Basilar artery
- Pontine tegmentum
- Cerebellar hemisphere
- Fourth ventricle
- Vermis

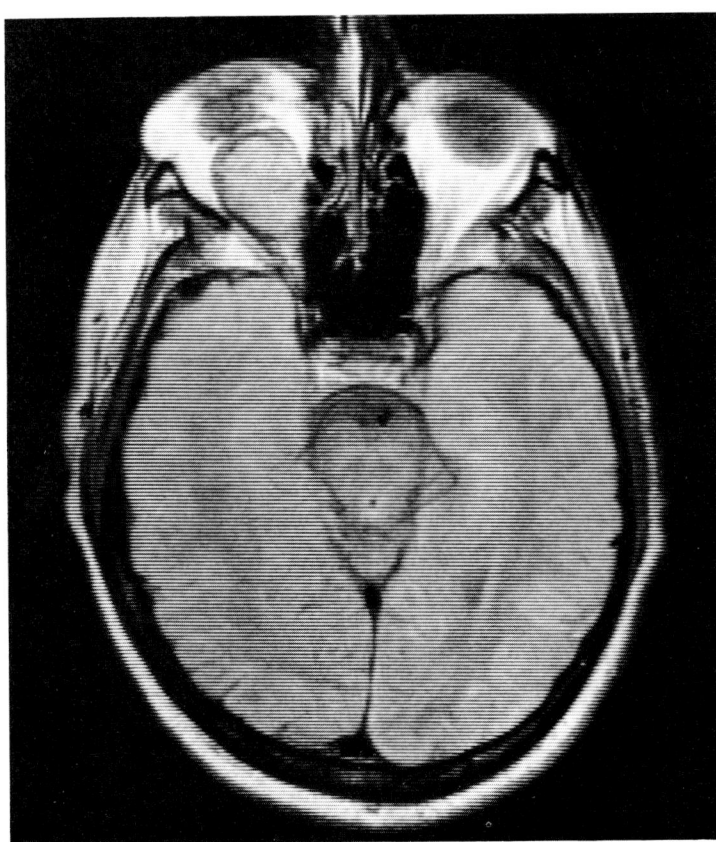

FIG. 2.65. TR = 2000 msec, TE = 28 msec. A right orbital metastasis from renal cell carcinoma has a rim of low signal intensity indicating either calcification or a fibrous capsule.

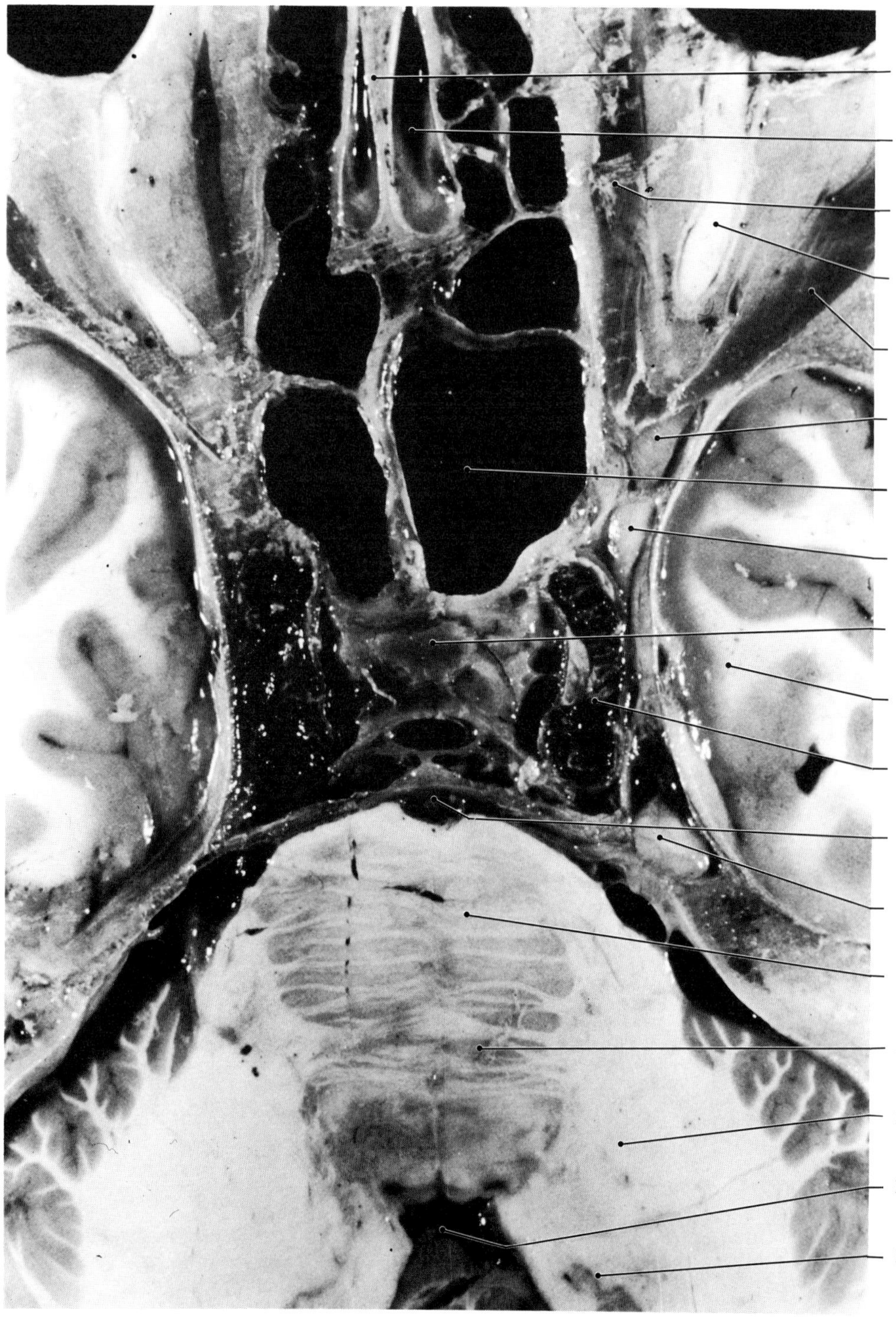

FIG. 2.66.

- Crista galli
- Cribriform plate
- Superior oblique muscle
- Optic nerve
- Lateral rectus muscle
- Oculomotor nerve
- Sphenoidal sinus
- Fat in superior orbital fissure
- Pituitary gland
- Inferior temporal gyrus
- Intracavernous internal carotid artery
- Basilar artery
- Meckel's cave and fifth nerve ganglion
- Basis pontis
- Medial lemniscus
- Middle cerebellar peduncle
- Fourth ventricle
- Dentate nucleus

- The internal carotid artery and the abducens nerve are within the cavernous sinus, whereas the oculomotor, the trochlear, the ophthalmic, and, often, the maxillary nerves lie between the dura of the medial temporal fossa and the sinus itself. All nerves are covered by a layer of connective tissue (perineurium) and a layer of endothelium and, therefore, are not in direct contact with blood.
- The trigeminal ganglion is located within an evagination of the dura of the posterior fossa, called the trigeminal recess, or Meckel's cave. The cerebrospinal fluid in this cavity communicates with the prepontine cistern.

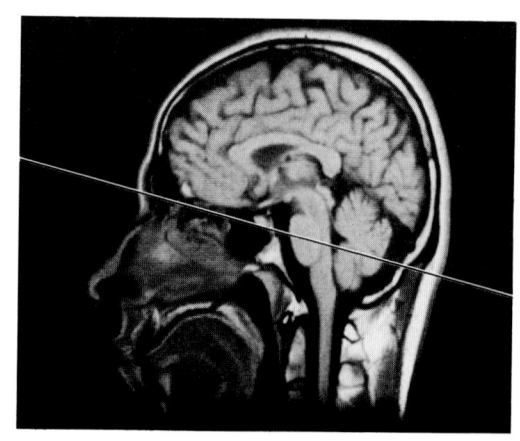

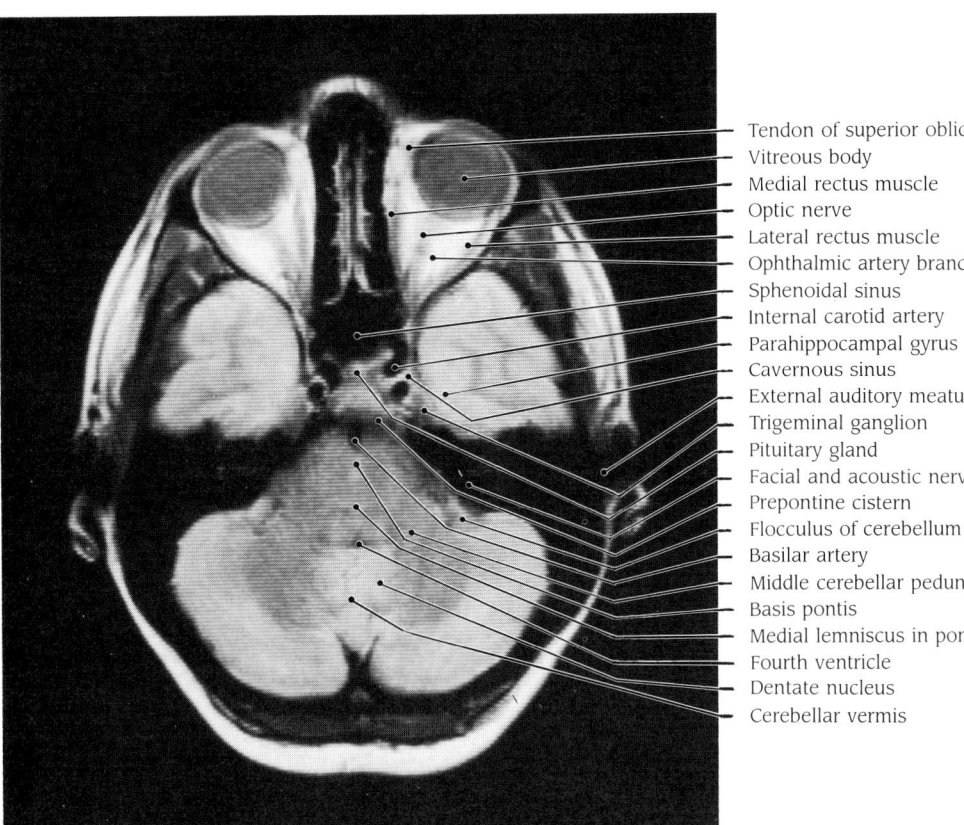

FIG. 2.67. TR = 2000 msec, TE = 28 msec.

- Tendon of superior oblique muscle
- Vitreous body
- Medial rectus muscle
- Optic nerve
- Lateral rectus muscle
- Ophthalmic artery branch
- Sphenoidal sinus
- Internal carotid artery
- Parahippocampal gyrus
- Cavernous sinus
- External auditory meatus
- Trigeminal ganglion
- Pituitary gland
- Facial and acoustic nerves
- Prepontine cistern
- Flocculus of cerebellum
- Basilar artery
- Middle cerebellar peduncle
- Basis pontis
- Medial lemniscus in pontine tegmentum
- Fourth ventricle
- Dentate nucleus
- Cerebellar vermis

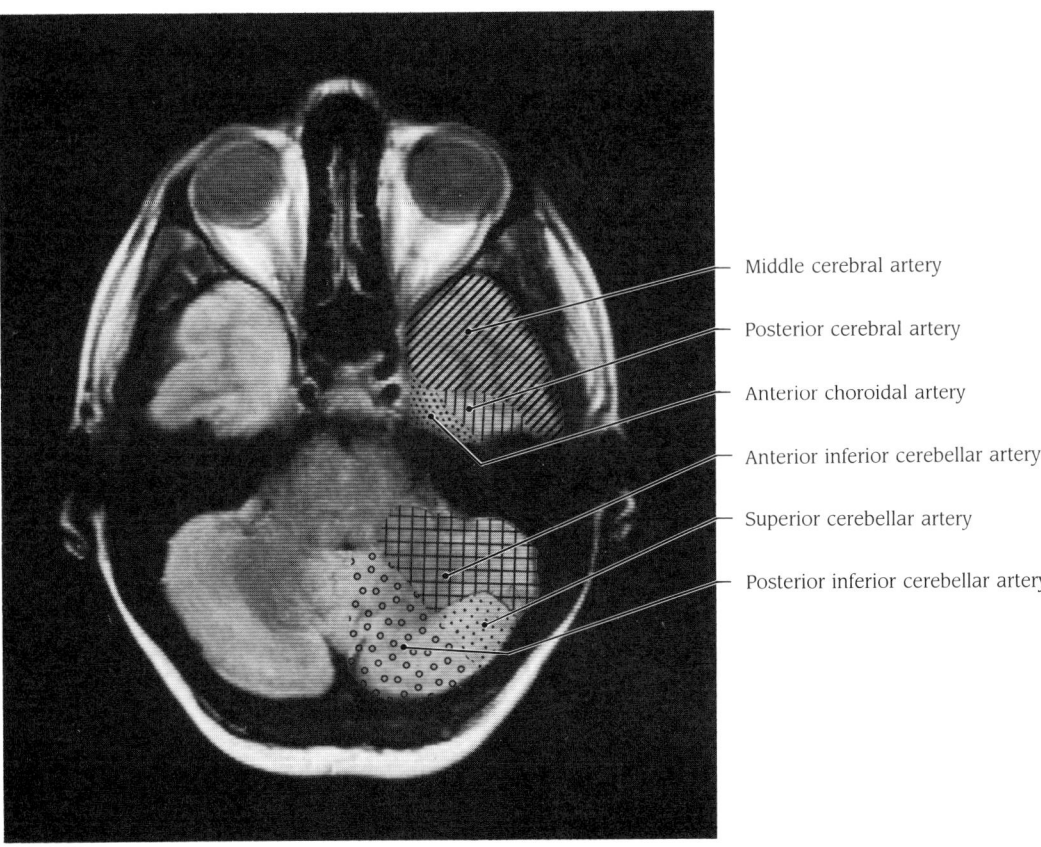

FIG. 2.68. TR = 2000 msec, TE = 28 msec.

- Middle cerebral artery
- Posterior cerebral artery
- Anterior choroidal artery
- Anterior inferior cerebellar artery
- Superior cerebellar artery
- Posterior inferior cerebellar artery

41

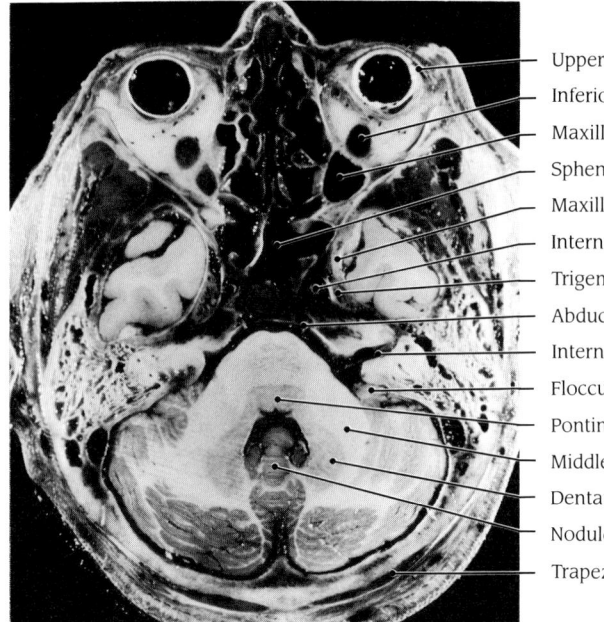

- Upper eyelid
- Inferior rectus muscle
- Maxillary sinus
- Sphenoidal sinus
- Maxillary nerve
- Internal carotid artery
- Trigeminal ganglion
- Abducens nerve
- Internal auditory meatus
- Flocculus
- Pontine tegmentum
- Middle cerebellar peduncle
- Dentate nucleus
- Nodule of vermis
- Trapezius muscle

FIG. 2.69.

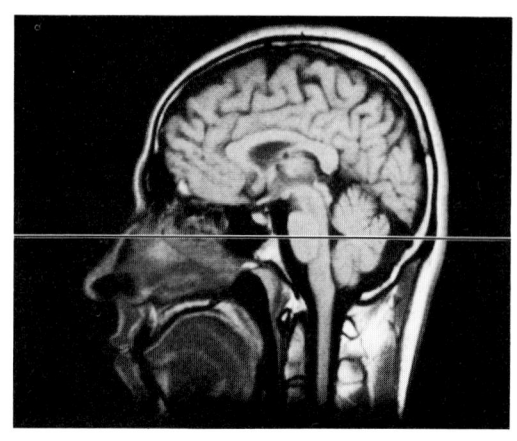

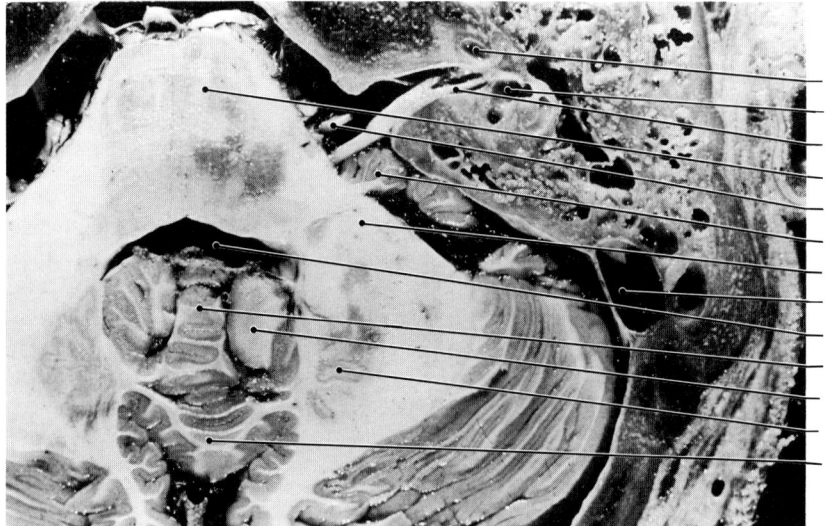

- Cochlea
- Vestibule
- Vestibular division of eighth nerve
- Pons
- Seventh nerve
- Flocculus
- Middle cerebellar peduncle
- Sigmoid sinus
- Fourth ventricle
- Nodule of vermis
- Cerebellar tonsil
- Dentate nucleus
- Tuber of vermis

FIG. 2.70.

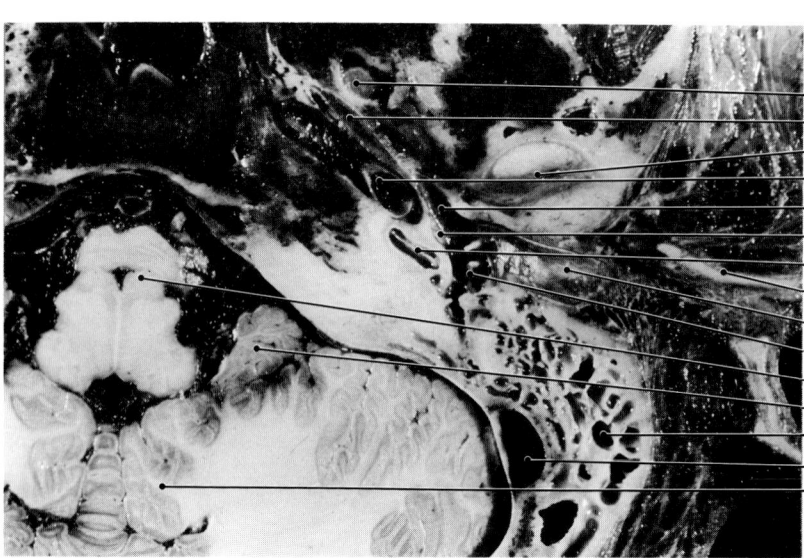

- Foramen ovale
- Tensor tympani muscle
- Temporomandibular joint
- Internal carotid artery
- Tuba auditiva
- Facial nerve
- Cochlea
- Ear cartilage
- External auditory canal
- Middle ear cavity
- Pontomedullary junction
- Flocculus
- Mastoid air cells
- Sigmoid sinus
- Cerebellar tonsil

FIG. 2.71.

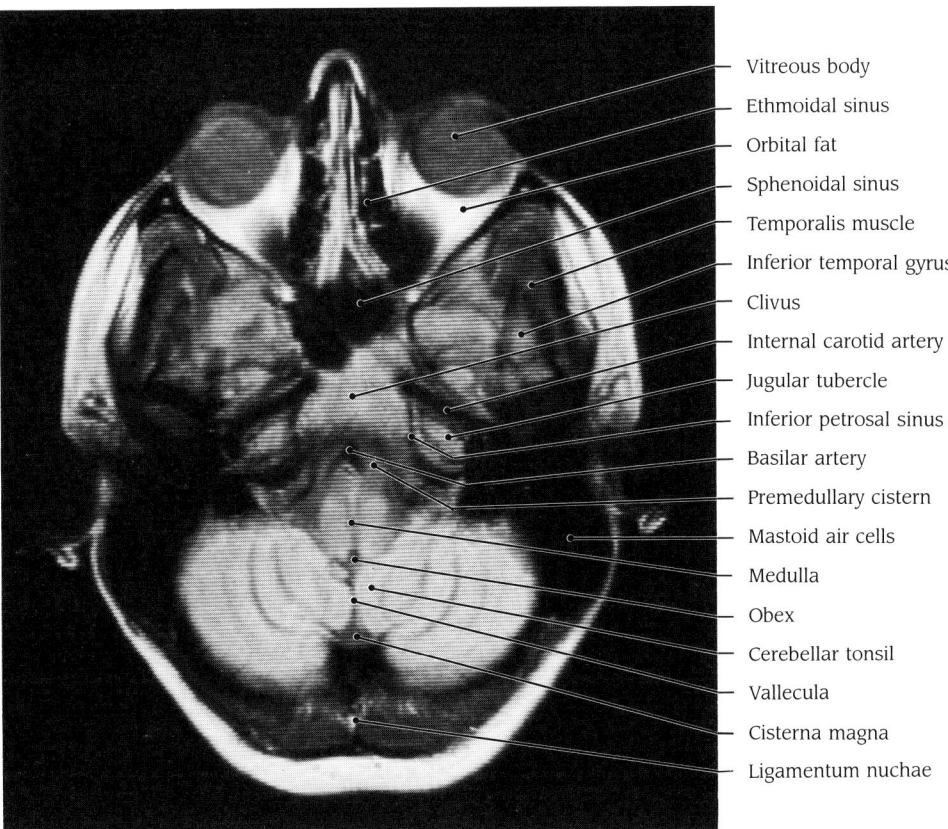

FIG. 2.76. TR = 2000 msec, TE = 28 msec.

- Vitreous body
- Ethmoidal sinus
- Orbital fat
- Sphenoidal sinus
- Temporalis muscle
- Inferior temporal gyrus
- Clivus
- Internal carotid artery
- Jugular tubercle
- Inferior petrosal sinus
- Basilar artery
- Premedullary cistern
- Mastoid air cells
- Medulla
- Obex
- Cerebellar tonsil
- Vallecula
- Cisterna magna
- Ligamentum nuchae

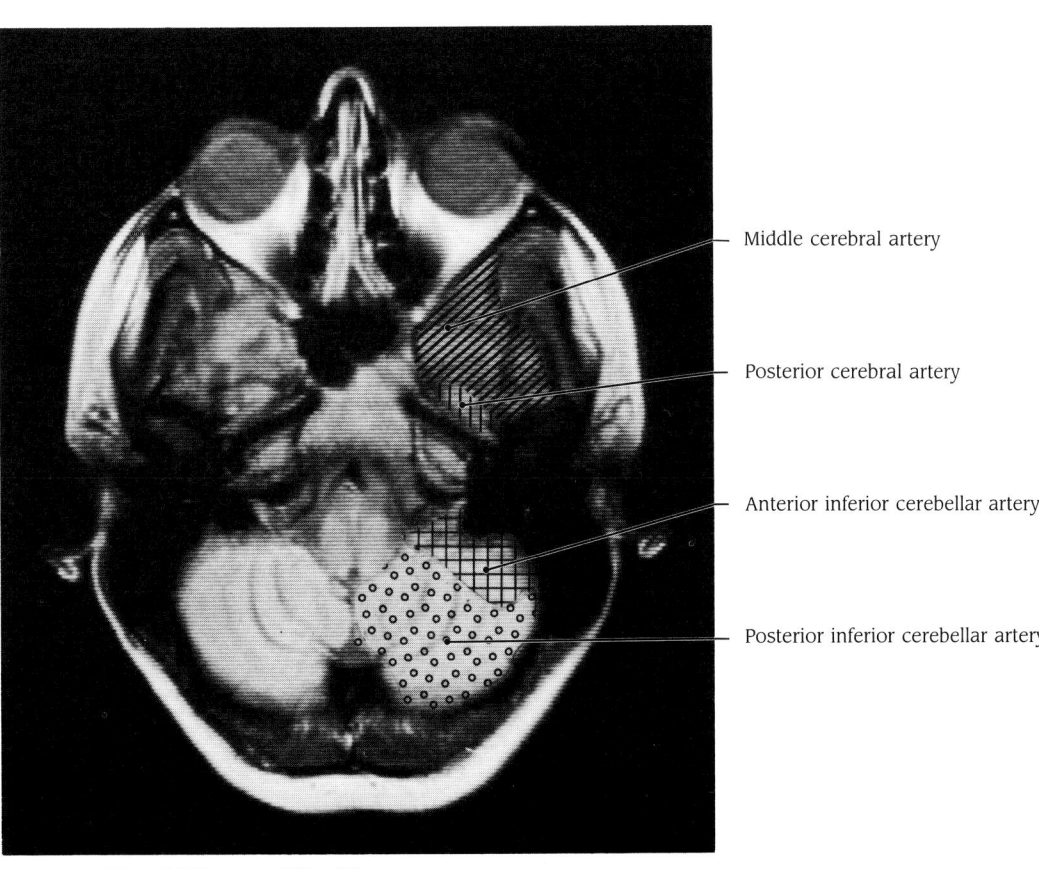

FIG. 2.77. TR = 2000 msec, TE = 28 msec.

- Middle cerebral artery
- Posterior cerebral artery
- Anterior inferior cerebellar artery
- Posterior inferior cerebellar artery

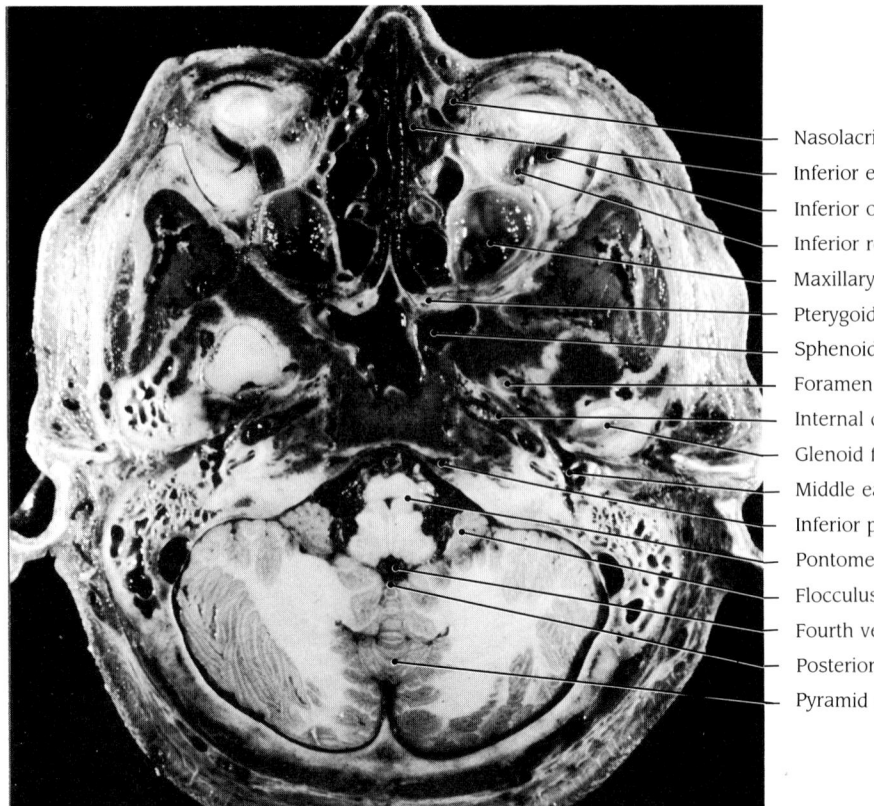

FIG. 2.78.

- Nasolacrimal duct
- Inferior ethmoid cells
- Inferior oblique muscle
- Inferior rectus muscle
- Maxillary sinus
- Pterygoid process
- Sphenoidal sinus
- Foramen ovale
- Internal carotid artery
- Glenoid fossa
- Middle ear cavity with ossicles
- Inferior petrosal sinus
- Pontomedullary junction
- Flocculus
- Fourth ventricle
- Posterior inferior cerebellar artery
- Pyramid of vermis

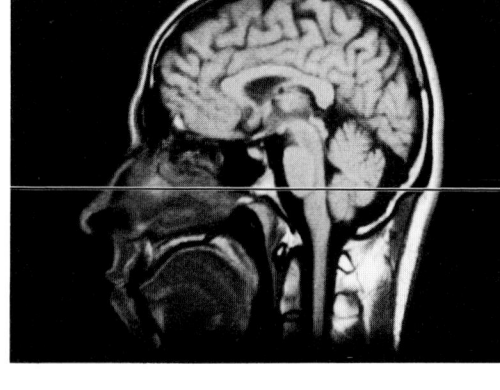

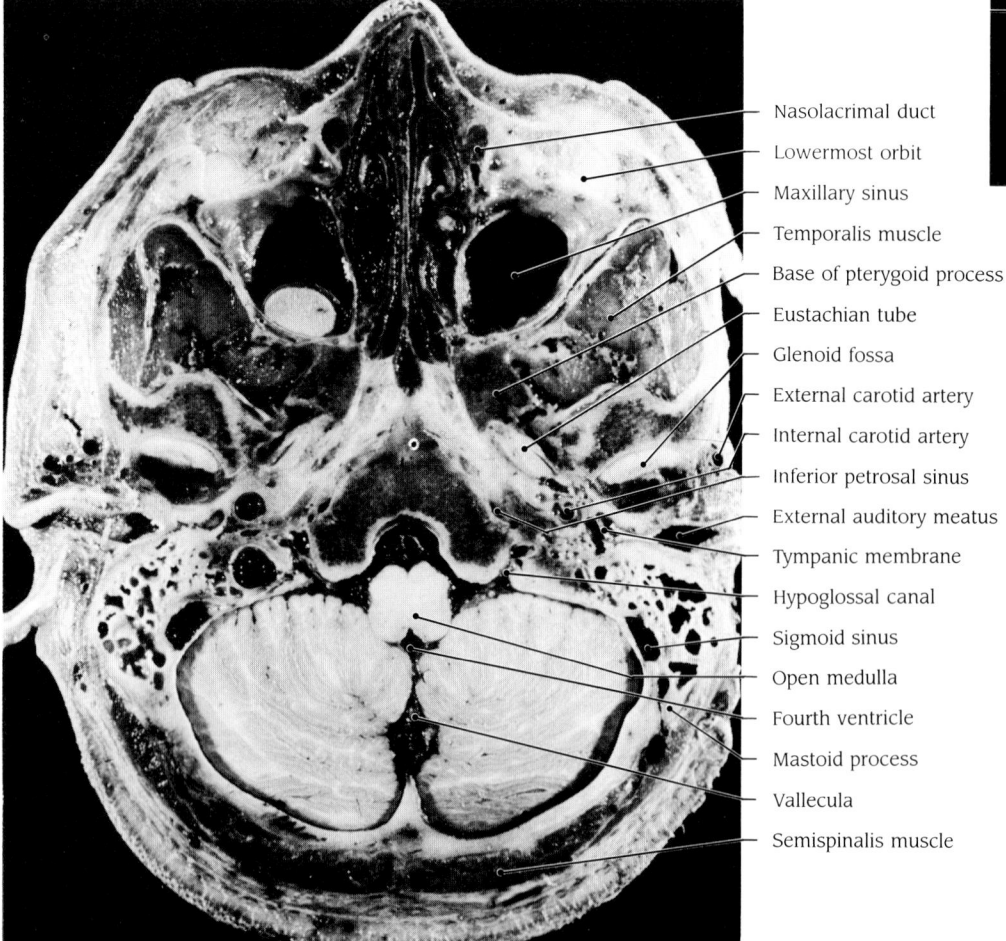

FIG. 2.79.

- Nasolacrimal duct
- Lowermost orbit
- Maxillary sinus
- Temporalis muscle
- Base of pterygoid process
- Eustachian tube
- Glenoid fossa
- External carotid artery
- Internal carotid artery
- Inferior petrosal sinus
- External auditory meatus
- Tympanic membrane
- Hypoglossal canal
- Sigmoid sinus
- Open medulla
- Fourth ventricle
- Mastoid process
- Vallecula
- Semispinalis muscle

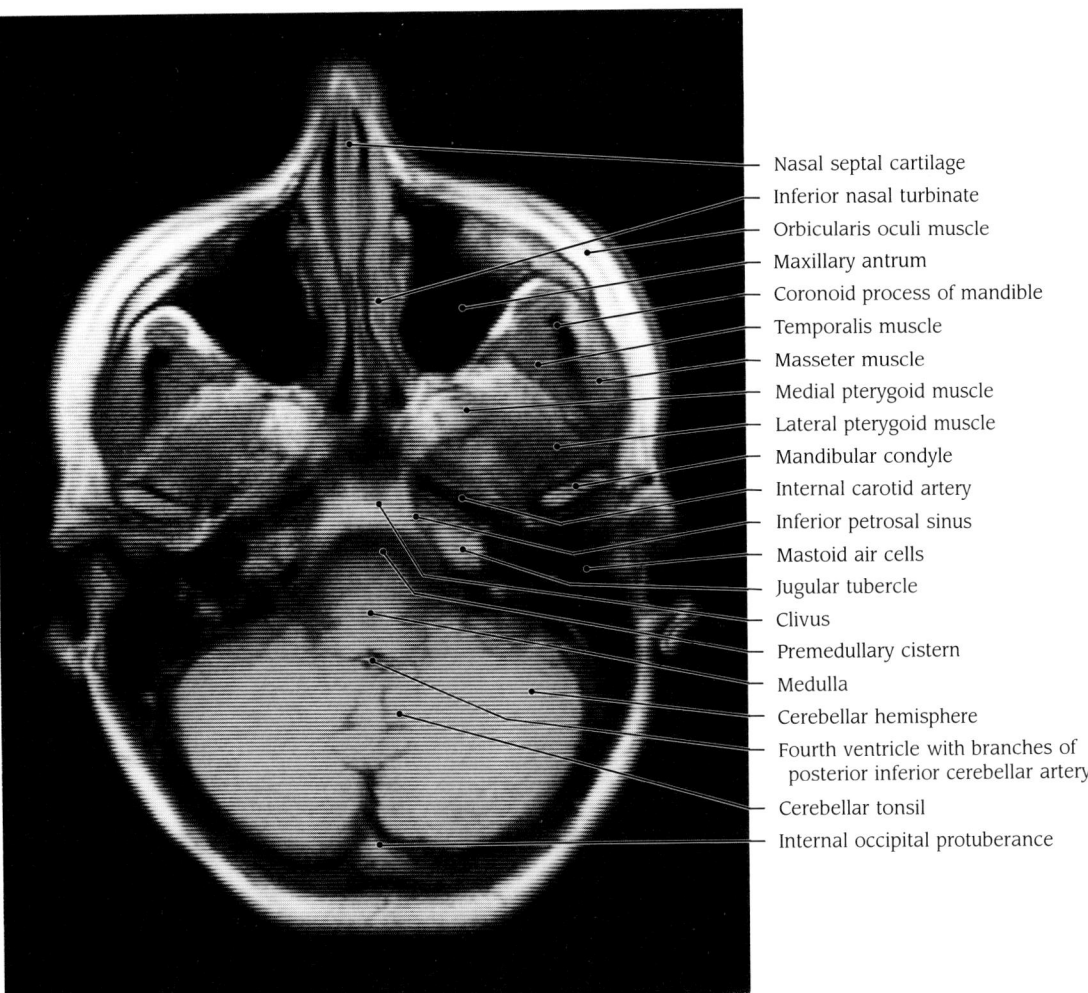

FIG. 2.80. TR = 500 msec, TE = 28 msec.

- Nasal septal cartilage
- Inferior nasal turbinate
- Orbicularis oculi muscle
- Maxillary antrum
- Coronoid process of mandible
- Temporalis muscle
- Masseter muscle
- Medial pterygoid muscle
- Lateral pterygoid muscle
- Mandibular condyle
- Internal carotid artery
- Inferior petrosal sinus
- Mastoid air cells
- Jugular tubercle
- Clivus
- Premedullary cistern
- Medulla
- Cerebellar hemisphere
- Fourth ventricle with branches of posterior inferior cerebellar artery
- Cerebellar tonsil
- Internal occipital protuberance

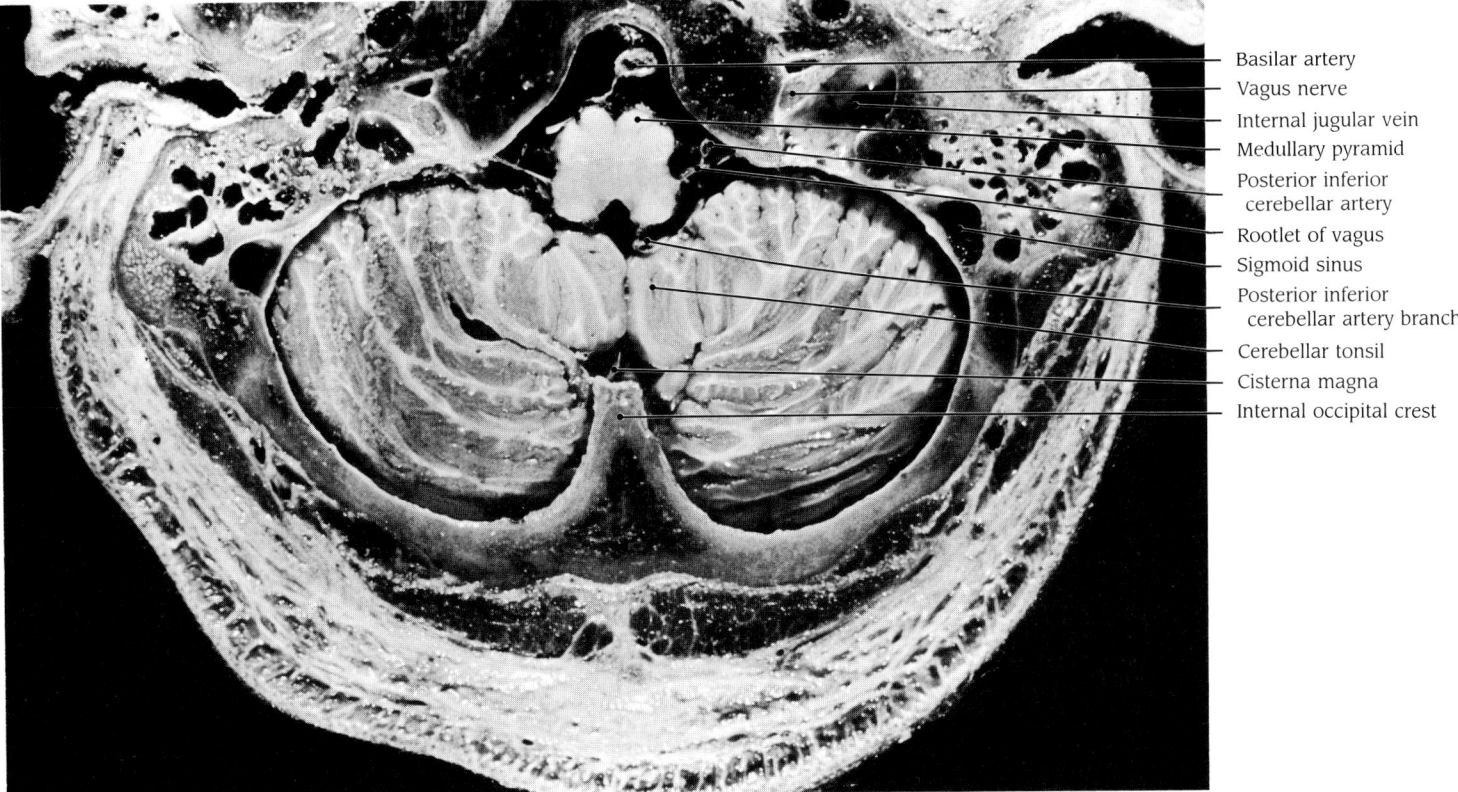

FIG. 2.81.

- Basilar artery
- Vagus nerve
- Internal jugular vein
- Medullary pyramid
- Posterior inferior cerebellar artery
- Rootlet of vagus
- Sigmoid sinus
- Posterior inferior cerebellar artery branch
- Cerebellar tonsil
- Cisterna magna
- Internal occipital crest

47

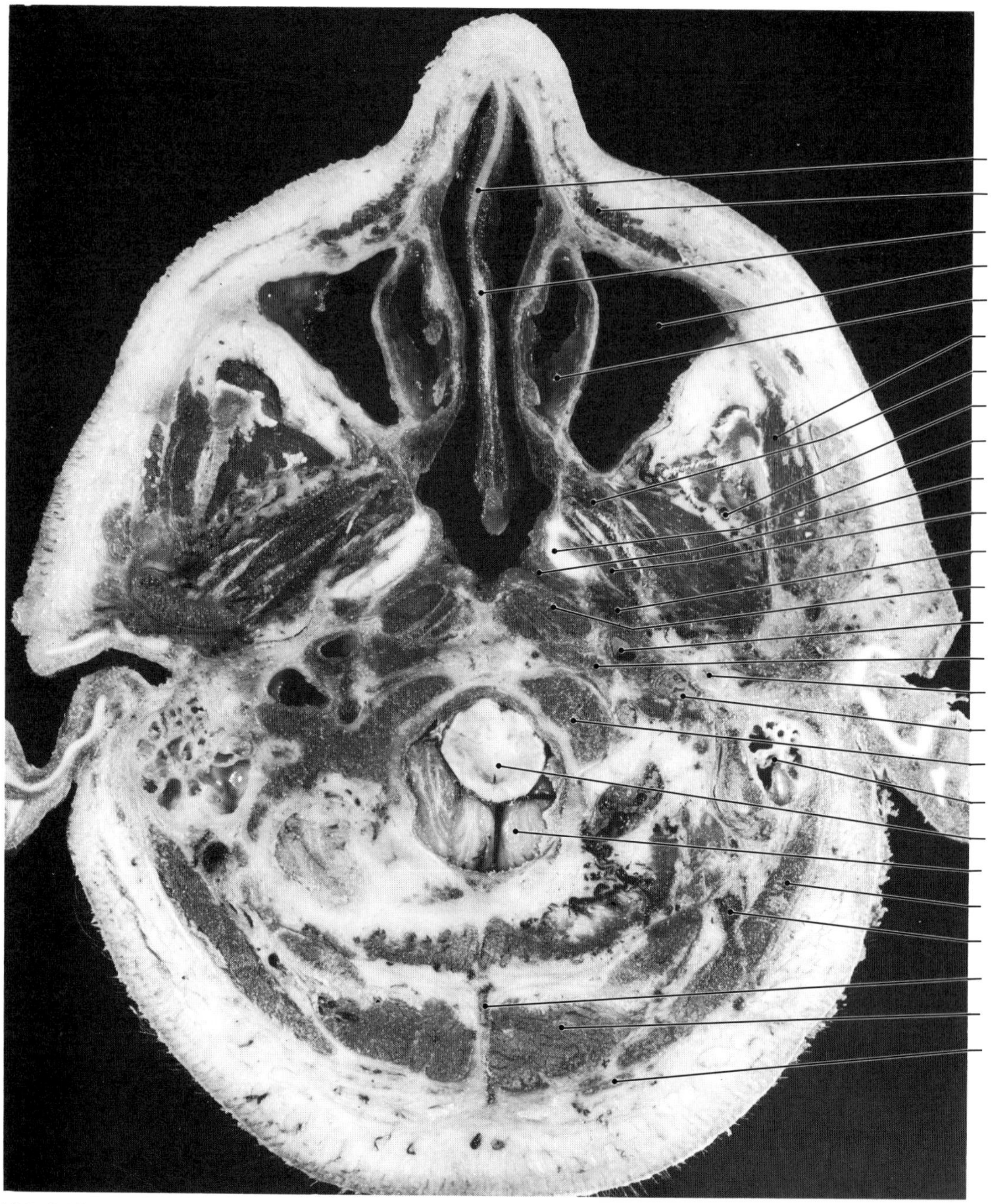

FIG. 2.82.

- Nasal septum
- Quadratus labii superioris muscle
- Vomer
- Maxillary sinus
- Middle turbinate
- Masseter muscle
- Medial pterygoid muscle
- Maxillary artery
- Eustachian tube
- Pharyngeal recess
- Tensor veli palatini muscle
- Levator veli palatini muscle
- Longus capitis muscle
- Internal carotid artery
- Rectus capitis anterior muscle
- Styloid process
- Internal jugular vein
- Occipital condyle
- Mastoid process
- Closed medulla
- Cerebellar tonsil
- Sternocleidomastoid muscle
- Deep cervical vein
- Ligamentum nuchae
- Semispinalis capitis muscle
- Trapezius muscle

- One internal jugular vein may be larger in diameter than the other because of the size difference between the sigmoid sinuses. The bulb of the larger internal jugular vein extends farther upward into the petrous bone than does the smaller vein. The jugular bulb frequently is identified as a high signal intensity structure in or above the lateral part of the jugular fossa.
- Normally, the cerebellar tonsils do not extend below the lower aperture of the foramen magnum.
- The medulla is divided at the level of the obex into two portions: the open medulla extends upward to the pontomedullary junction, and the closed medulla extends inferiorly to the lower rim of the foramen magnum.

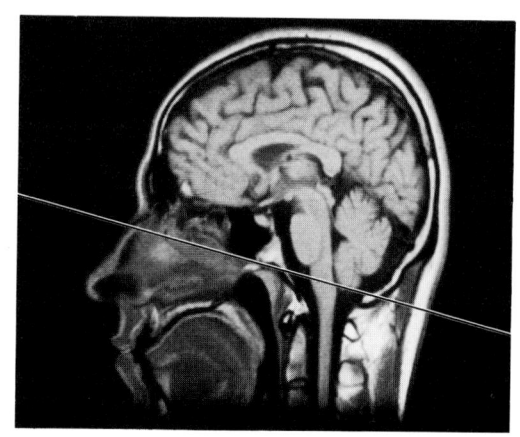

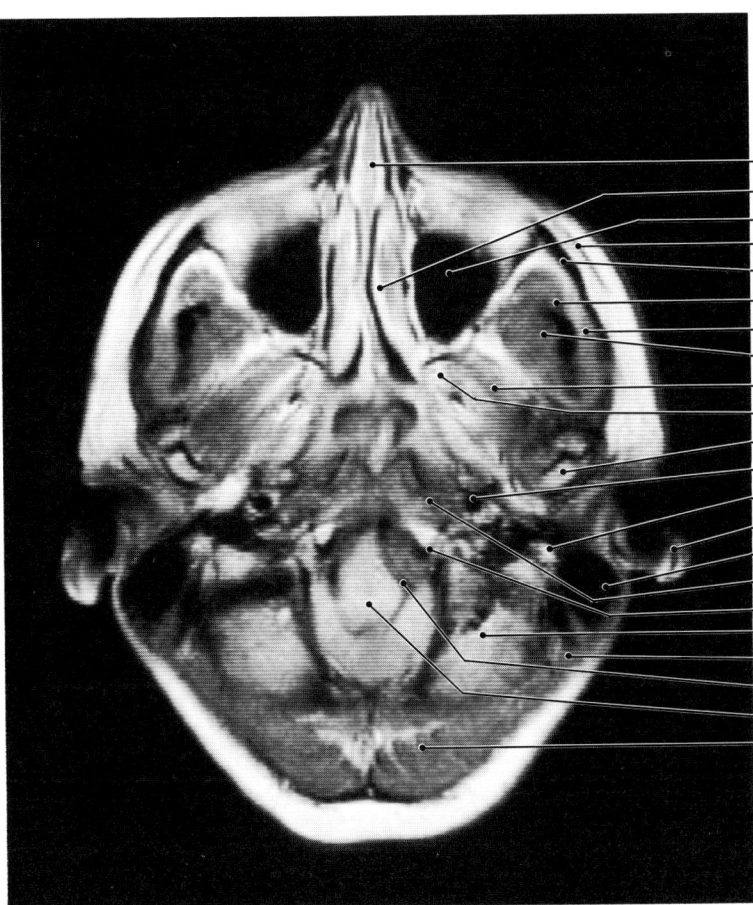

FIG. 2.83. TR = 2000 msec, TE = 28 msec.

- Nasal cartilage
- Superior nasal turbinate
- Maxillary antrum
- Orbicularis oculi muscle
- Zygomatic arch
- Coronoid process of mandible
- Masseter muscle
- Temporalis muscle
- Lateral pterygoid muscle
- Medial pterygoid muscle
- Mandibular condyle
- Internal carotid artery
- Internal jugular vein
- Auricular cartilage
- Mastoid air cells
- Rectus capitis anterior muscle
- Hypoglossal canal
- Cerebellar hemisphere
- Splenius capitis muscle
- Vertebral artery
- Medulla
- Semispinalis capitis muscle

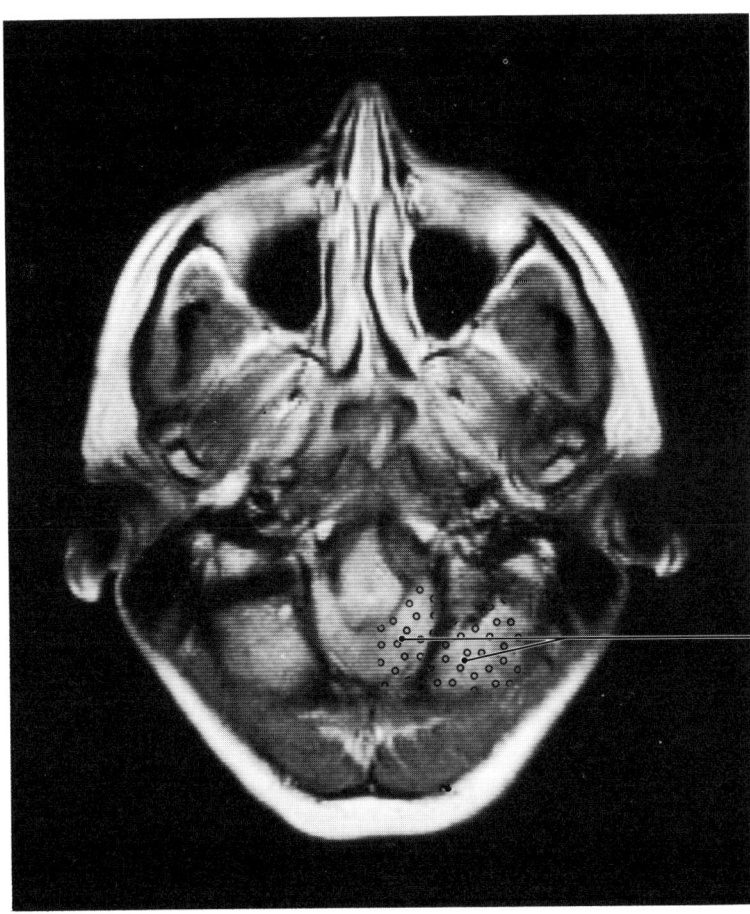

- Posterior inferior cerebellar artery

FIG. 2.84. TR = 2000 msec, TE = 28 msec.

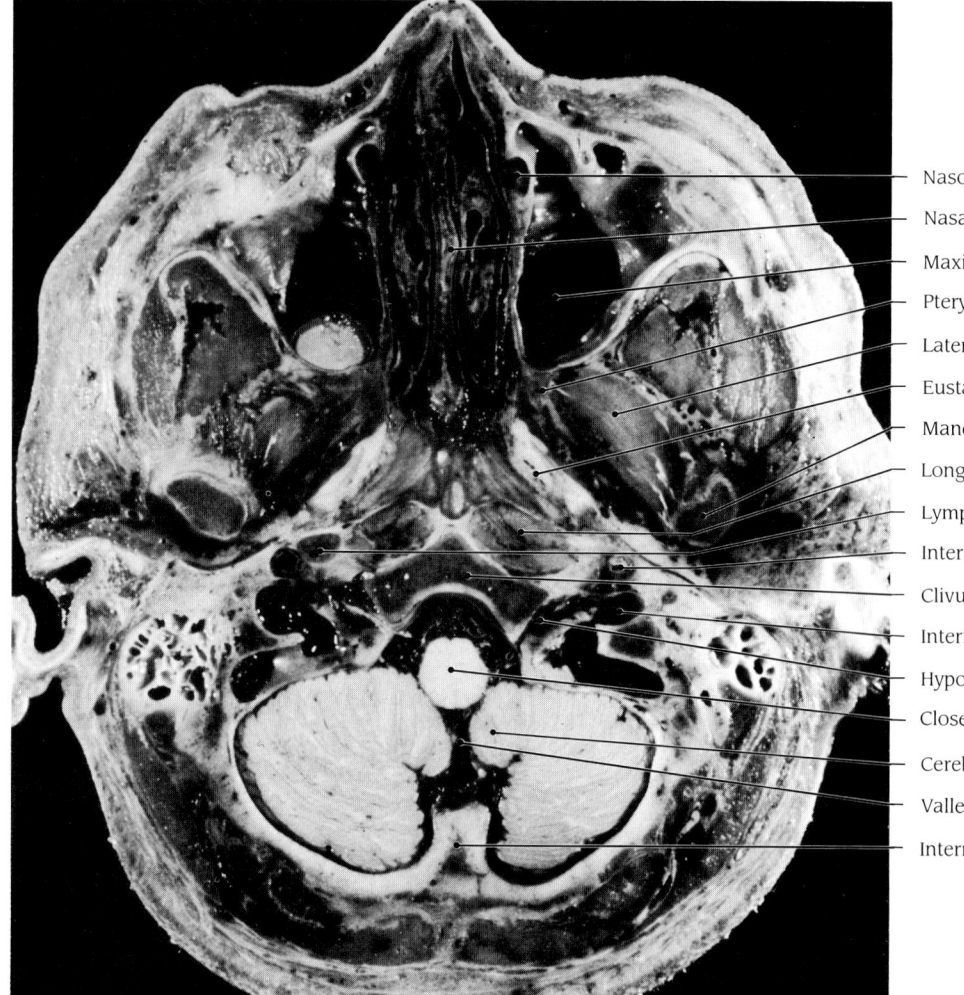

FIG. 2.85.

- Nasolacrimal duct
- Nasal septum
- Maxillary sinus
- Pterygoid plate
- Lateral pterygoid muscle
- Eustachian tube
- Mandible
- Longus capitis muscle
- Lymph node
- Internal carotid artery
- Clivus
- Internal jugular vein
- Hypoglossal canal
- Closed medulla
- Cerebellar tonsil
- Vallecula
- Internal occipital protuberance

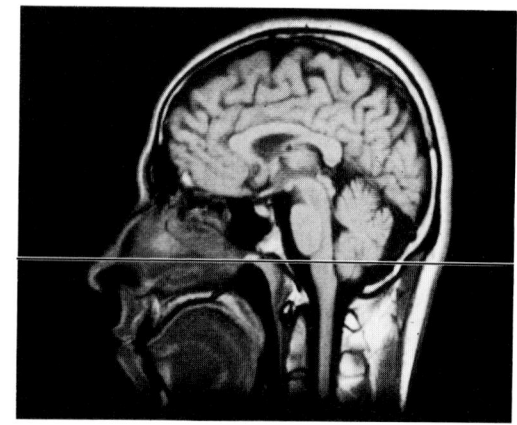

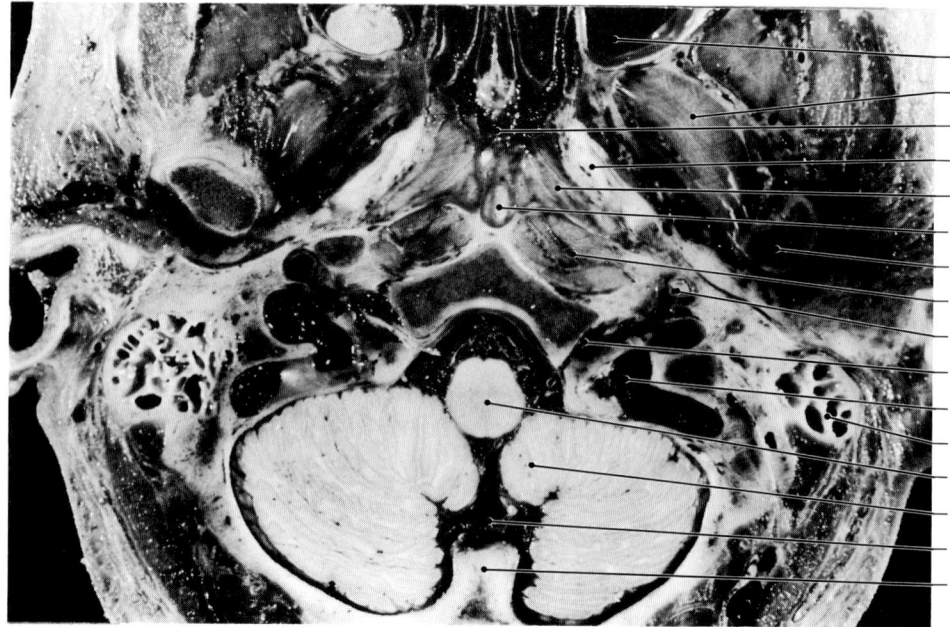

FIG. 2.86.

- Maxillary sinus
- Lateral pterygoid muscle
- Nasopharynx
- Tuba auditiva
- Swollen mucosa
- Lymph gland
- Mandible
- Longus capitis muscle
- Internal carotid artery
- Hypoglossal canal
- Jugular foramen
- Mastoid process
- Closed medulla
- Cerebellar tonsil
- Cisterna magna
- Internal occipital protuberance

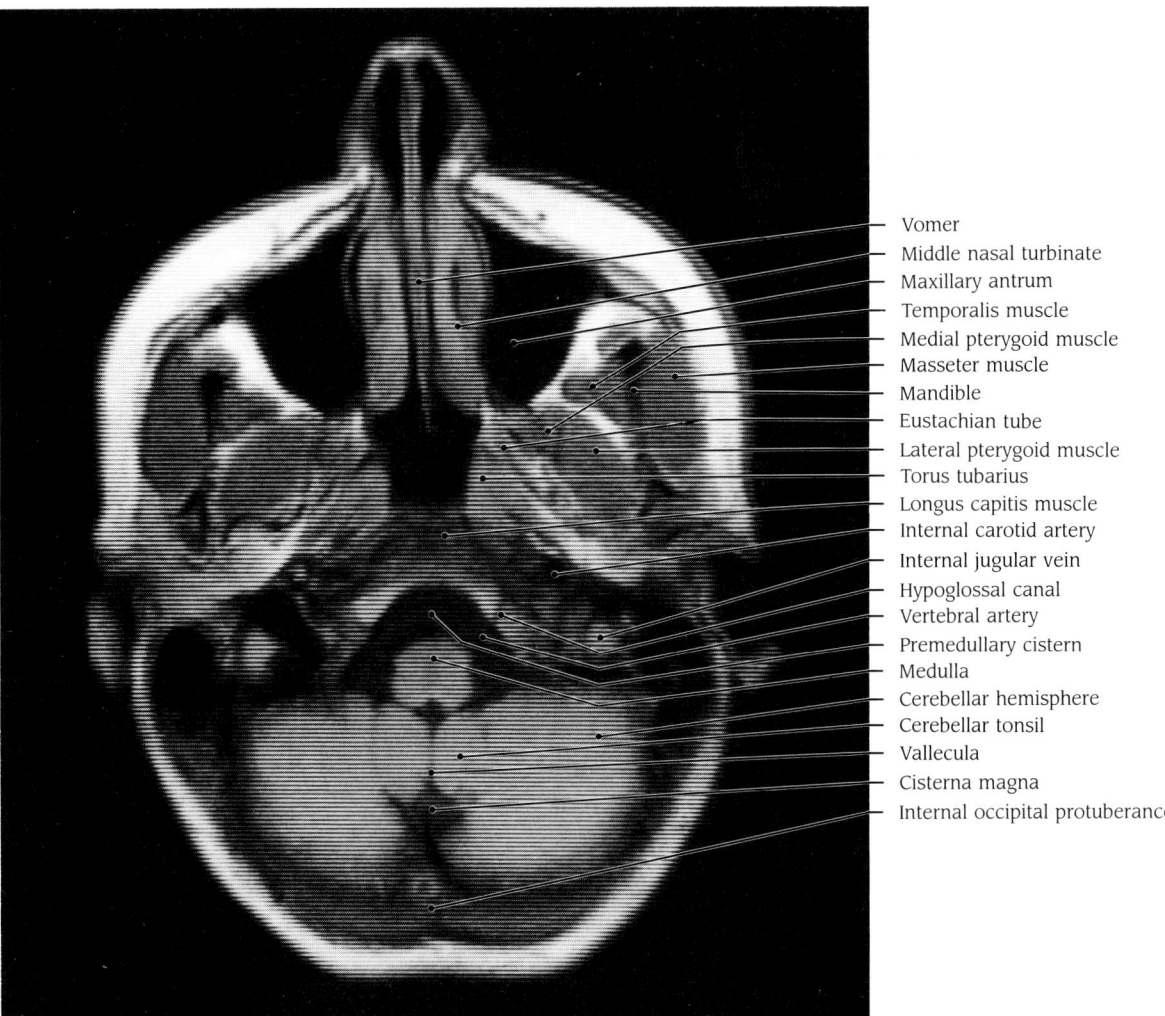

FIG. 2.87. TR = 500 msec, TE = 28 msec.

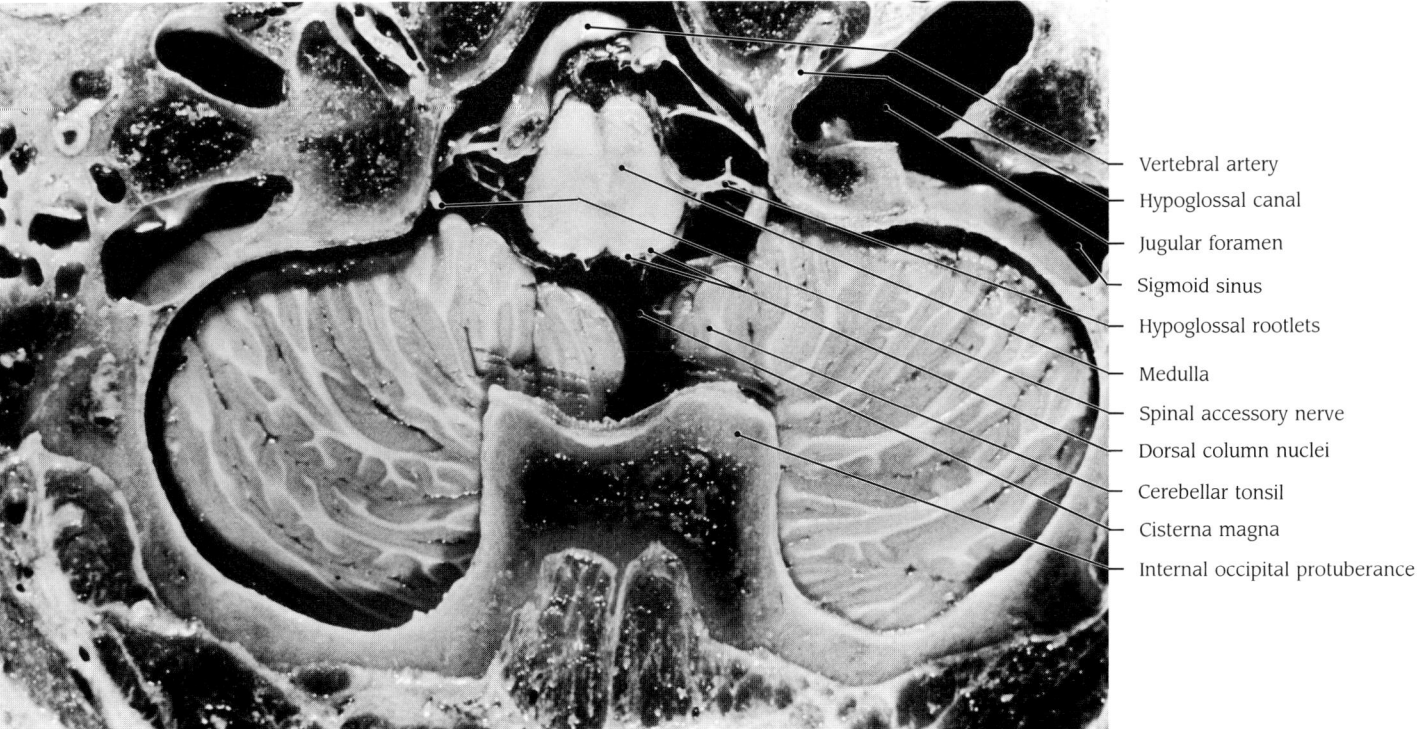

FIG. 2.88.

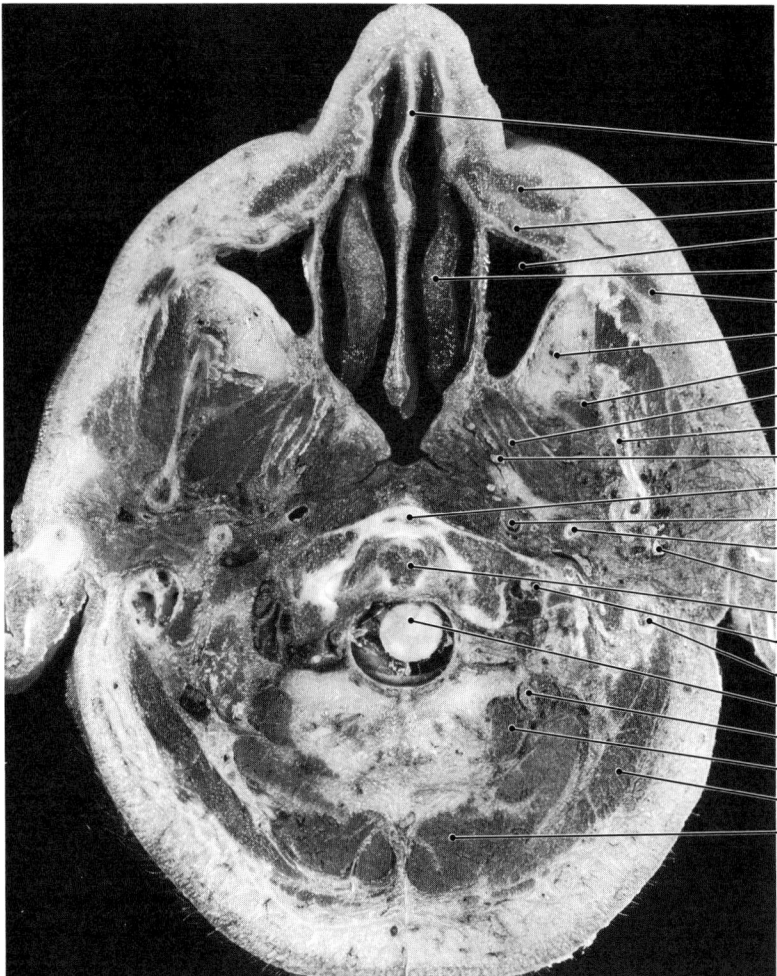

FIG. 2.89.

- Nasal septum
- Quadratus labii superioris muscle
- Canine muscle
- Maxillary sinus
- Middle turbinate
- Zygomatic muscle
- Retromandibular fat
- Temporalis muscle
- Medial pterygoid muscle
- Ramus of mandible
- Pharyngeal vein
- Anterior arch of C1
- Internal carotid artery
- Styloid process
- Posterior facial vein in parotid gland
- Odontoid process
- Vertebral artery
- Tip of mastoid process
- Pyramidal decussation
- Deep cervical vein
- Superior oblique capitis muscle
- Semispinalis capitis muscle
- Rectus capitis posterior major muscle

- The internal carotid artery is anteromedial to the internal jugular vein. The ninth, tenth, and eleventh cranial nerves lie between these two vessels.
- In the spinal cord, this level contains the decussation of the corticospinal tracts, as well as the uppermost part of the dorsal columns of the lemniscal system.

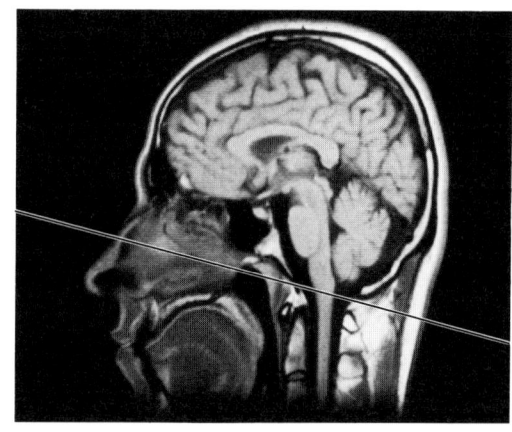

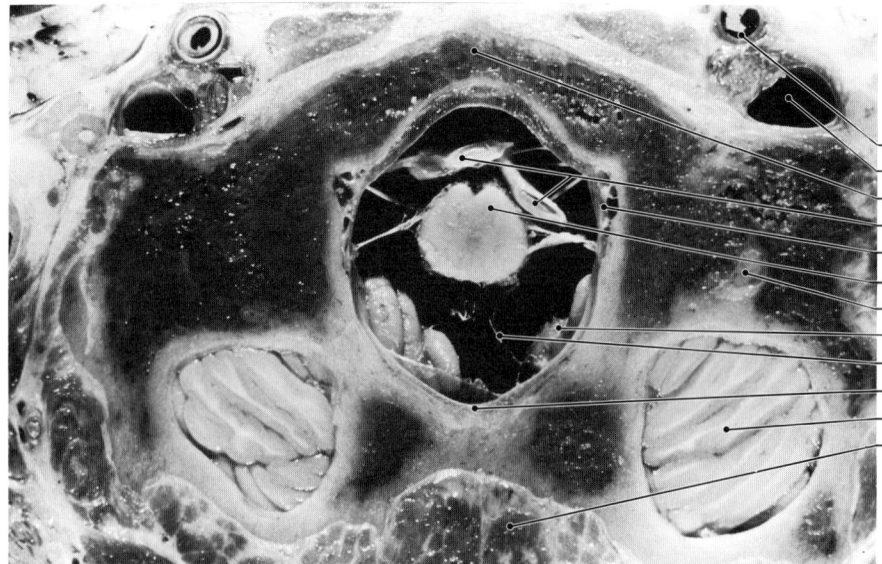

FIG. 2.90.

- Internal carotid artery
- Internal jugular vein
- Clivus
- Vertebral arteries
- Epidural veins
- Pyramid of medulla
- Posterior condylar emissary vein
- Cerebellar tonsil
- Cisterna magna
- Posterior rim of foramen magnum
- Lateral cerebellar lobe
- Suboccipital muscle

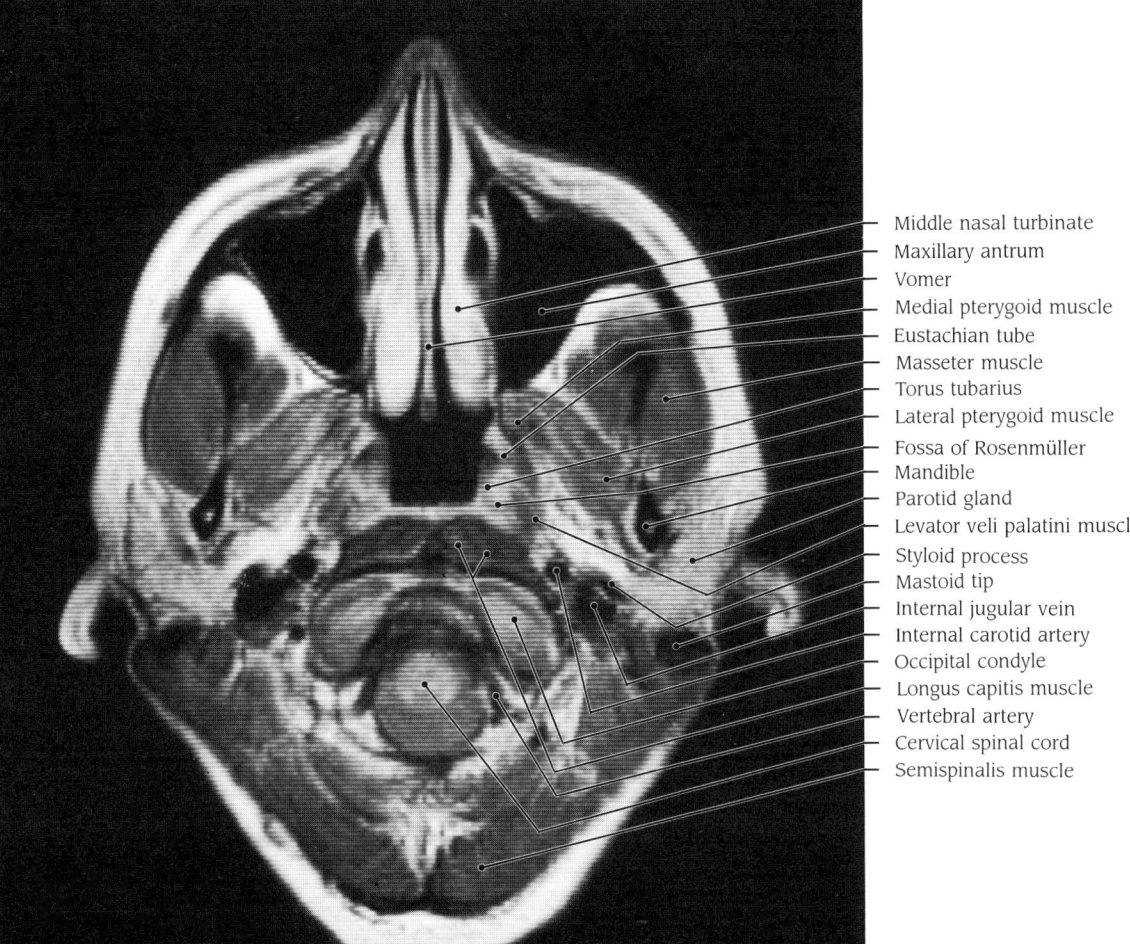

FIG. 2.91. TR = 2000 msec, TE = 28 msec.

- Middle nasal turbinate
- Maxillary antrum
- Vomer
- Medial pterygoid muscle
- Eustachian tube
- Masseter muscle
- Torus tubarius
- Lateral pterygoid muscle
- Fossa of Rosenmüller
- Mandible
- Parotid gland
- Levator veli palatini muscle
- Styloid process
- Mastoid tip
- Internal jugular vein
- Internal carotid artery
- Occipital condyle
- Longus capitis muscle
- Vertebral artery
- Cervical spinal cord
- Semispinalis muscle

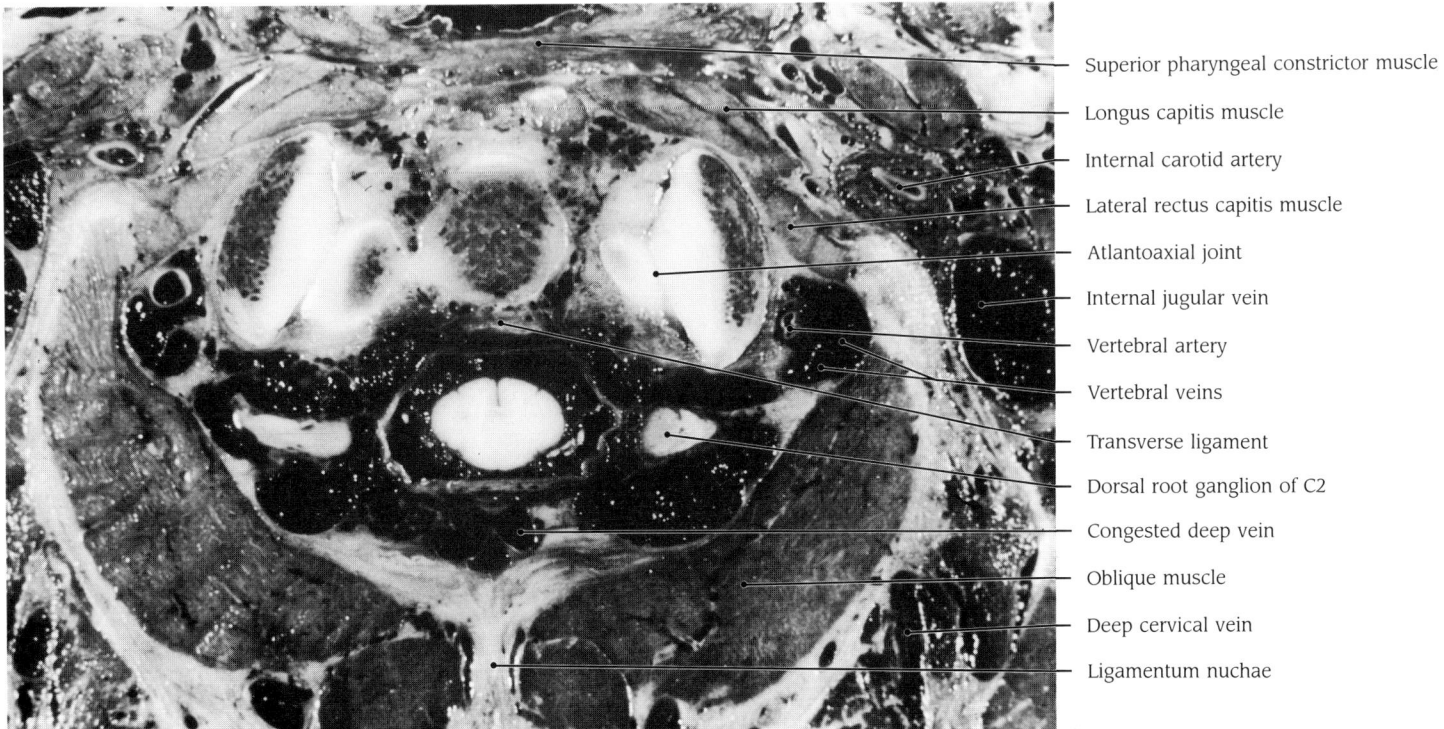

FIG. 2.92.

- Superior pharyngeal constrictor muscle
- Longus capitis muscle
- Internal carotid artery
- Lateral rectus capitis muscle
- Atlantoaxial joint
- Internal jugular vein
- Vertebral artery
- Vertebral veins
- Transverse ligament
- Dorsal root ganglion of C2
- Congested deep vein
- Oblique muscle
- Deep cervical vein
- Ligamentum nuchae

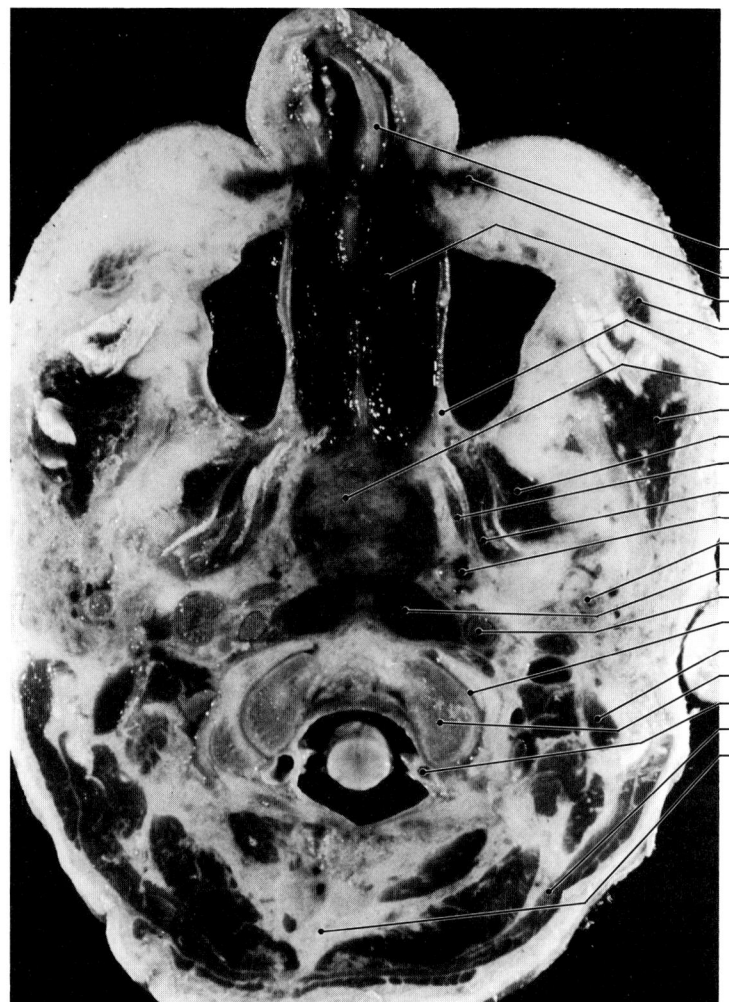

- Nasal septum
- Quadratus labii superioris muscle
- Nasal cavity
- Zygomatic muscle
- Base of pterygoid process
- Nasopharynx
- Masseter muscle
- External pterygoid muscle
- Tensor veli palatini muscle
- Internal pterygoid muscle
- Pharyngeal vein
- External carotid artery in parotid gland
- Longus capitis muscle
- Internal carotid artery
- Atlanto-occipital joint
- Digastric muscle
- Occipital condyle
- Vertebral artery
- Semispinalis capitis muscle
- Ligamentum nuchae

FIG. 2.93.

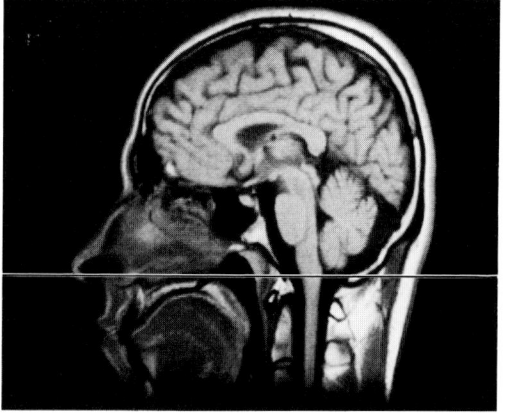

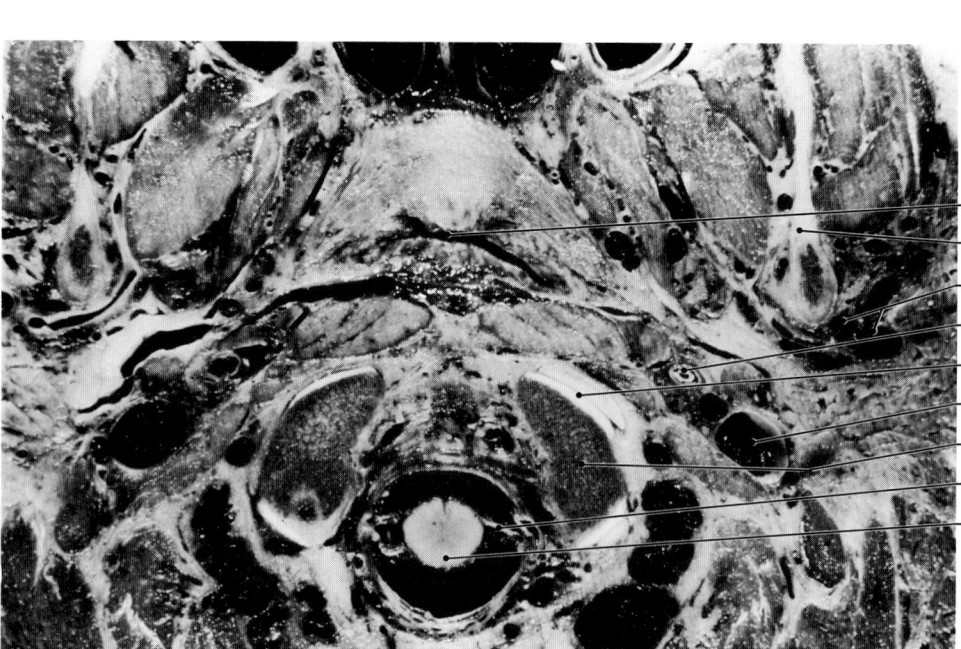

- Nasopharynx
- Ramus of mandible
- Retromandibular veins
- Internal carotid artery
- Atlanto-occipital joint
- Internal jugular vein
- Occipital condyle
- Rootlet of C1 nerve
- Dorsal columns of spinal cord

FIG. 2.94.

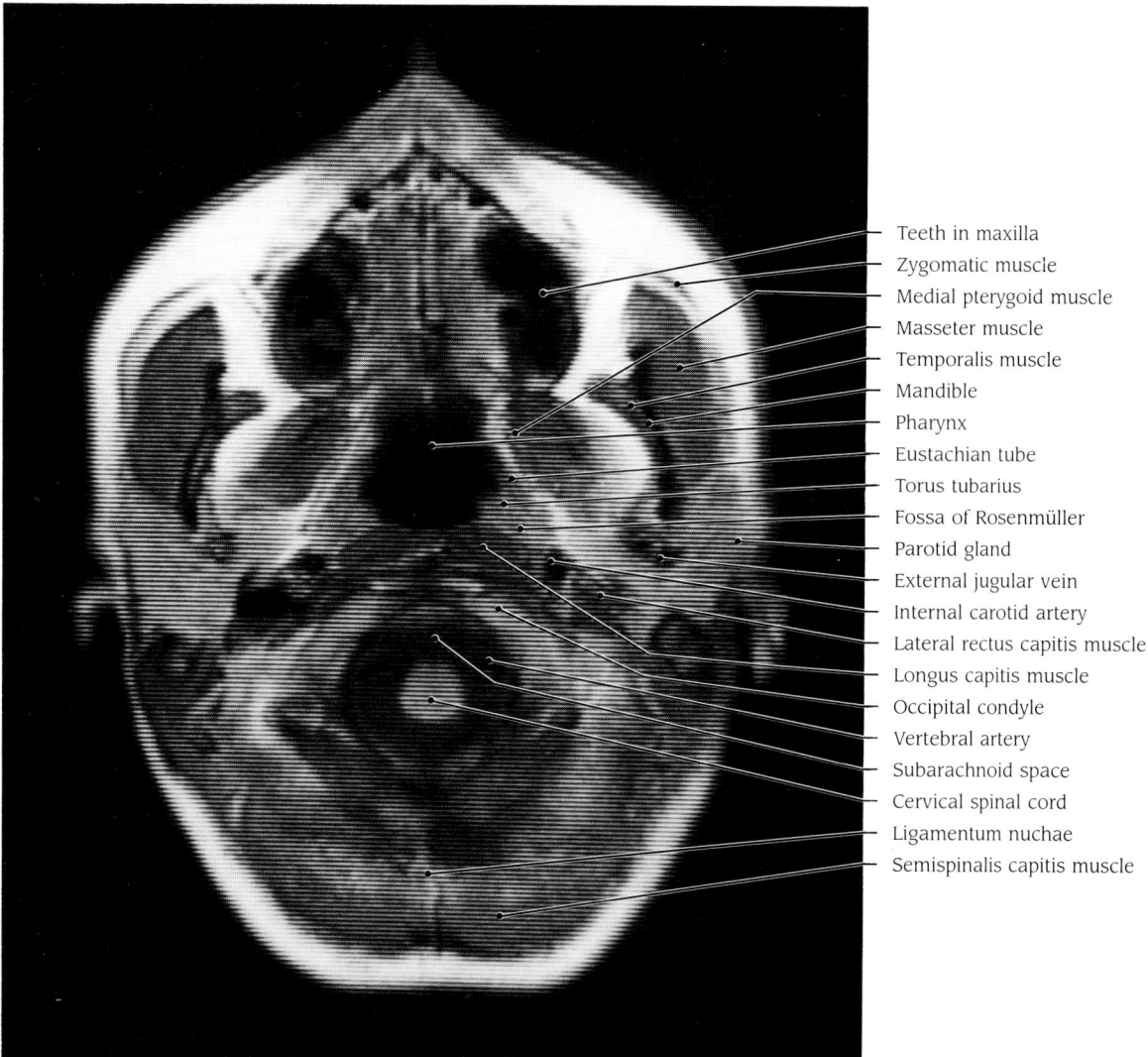

FIG. 2.95. TR = 500 msec, TE = 28 msec.

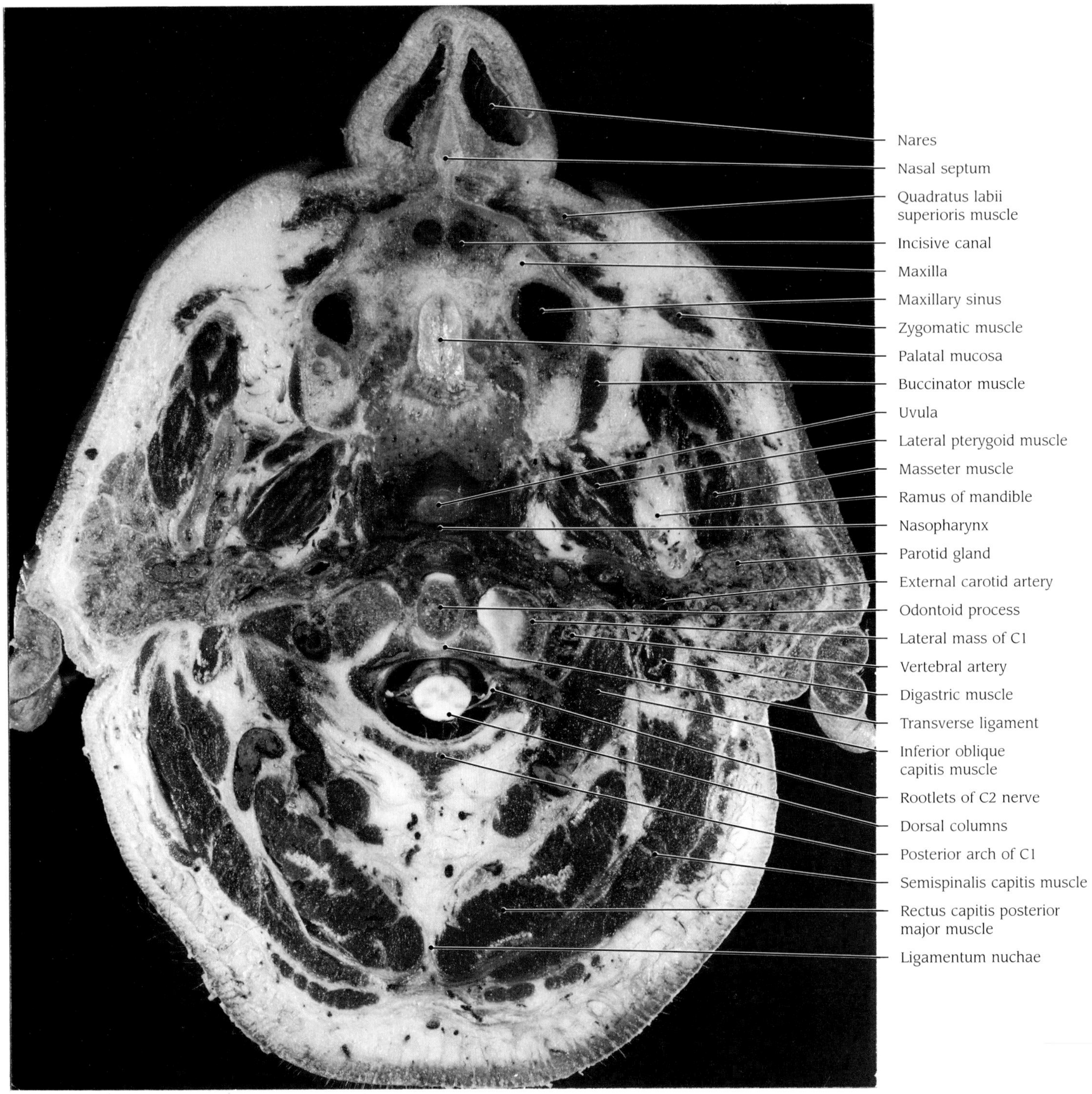

FIG. 2.96.

- The dens (odontoid process of C2) lies between the transverse atlantal ligament posteriorly and the anterior arch of C1 anteriorly. A small articulation between the dens and the anterior arch is called the anterior atlantoaxial joint.
- The pharyngeal tubercle on the rostral aspect of the anterior arch serves as one of the origins for the longus colli muscle.

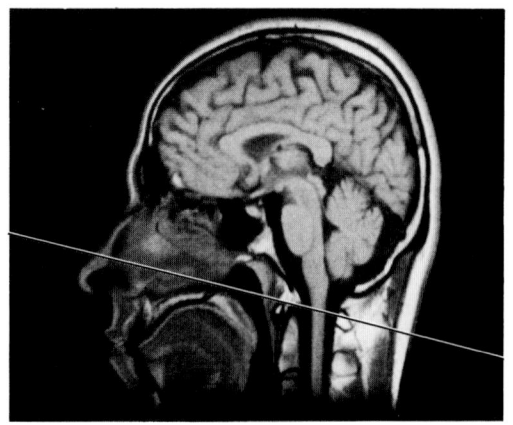

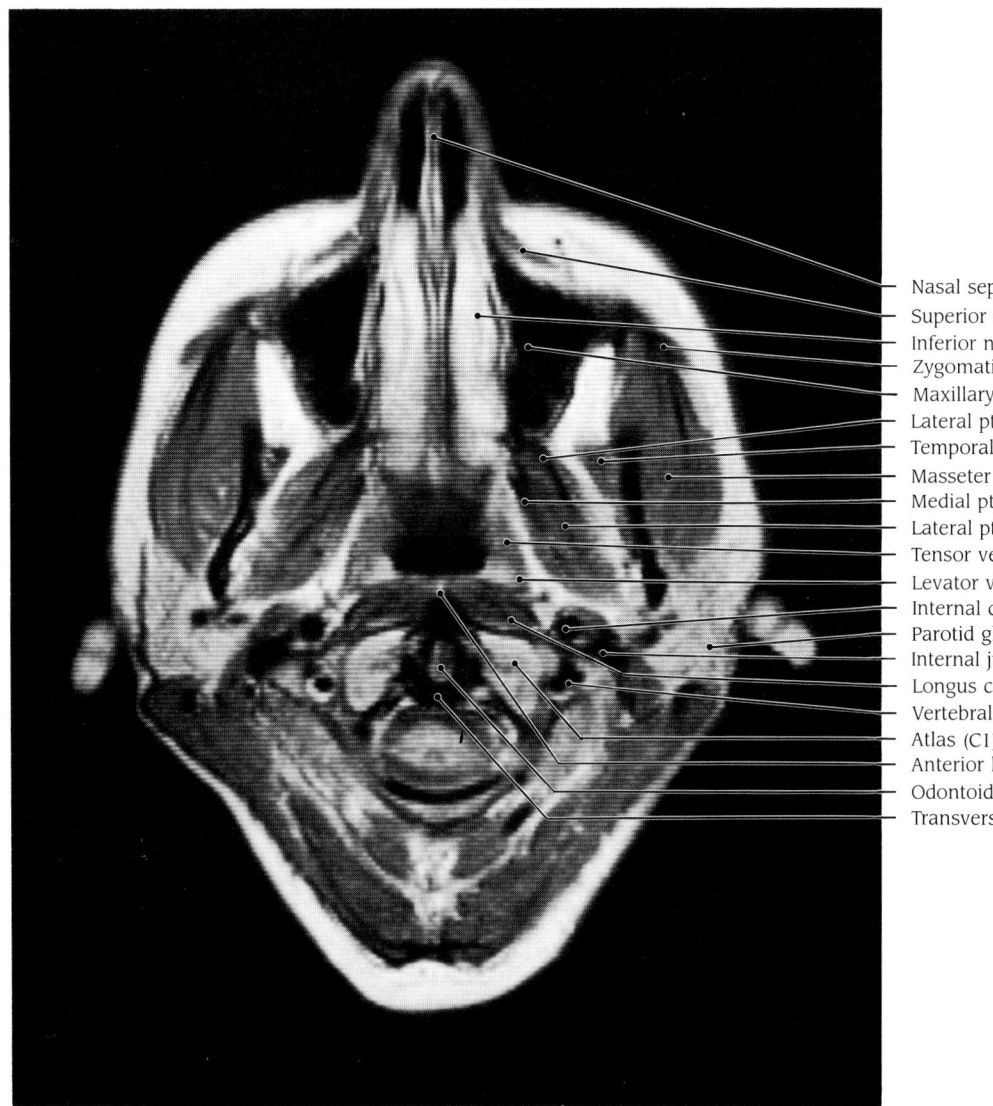

FIG. 2.97. TR = 2000 msec, TE = 28 msec.

- Nasal septum
- Superior quadratus labii muscle
- Inferior nasal turbinate
- Zygomatic muscle
- Maxillary antrum
- Lateral pterygoid plate
- Temporalis muscle
- Masseter muscle
- Medial pterygoid plate
- Lateral pterygoid muscle
- Tensor veli palatini muscle
- Levator veli palatini muscle
- Internal carotid artery
- Parotid gland
- Internal jugular vein
- Longus capitis muscle
- Vertebral artery
- Atlas (C1)
- Anterior longitudinal ligament
- Odontoid process
- Transverse atlantal ligament

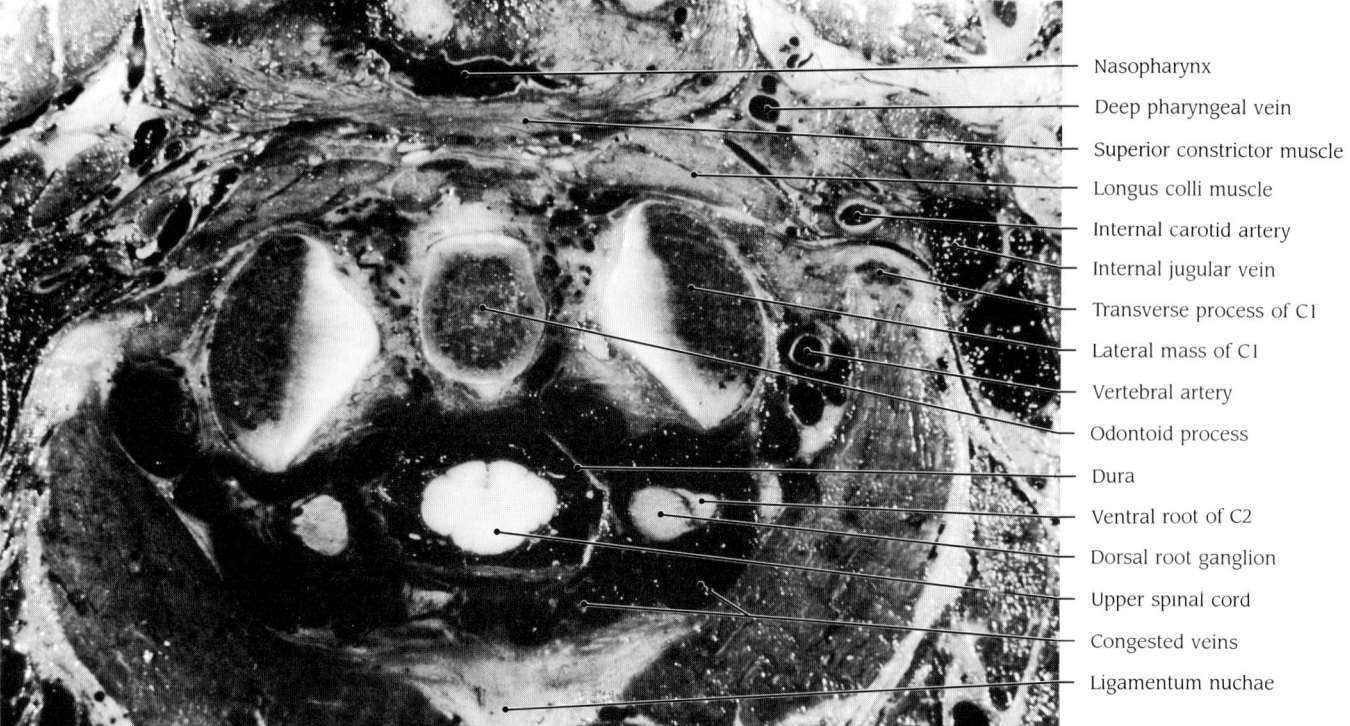

FIG. 2.98.

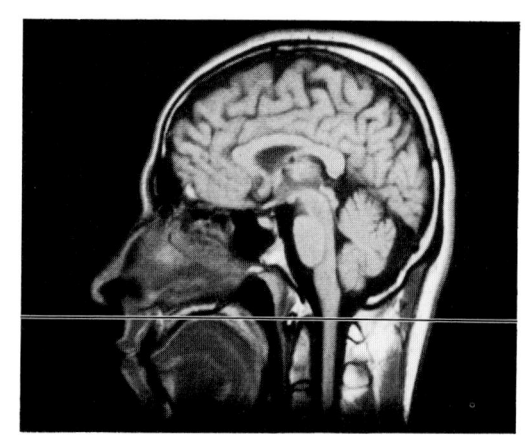

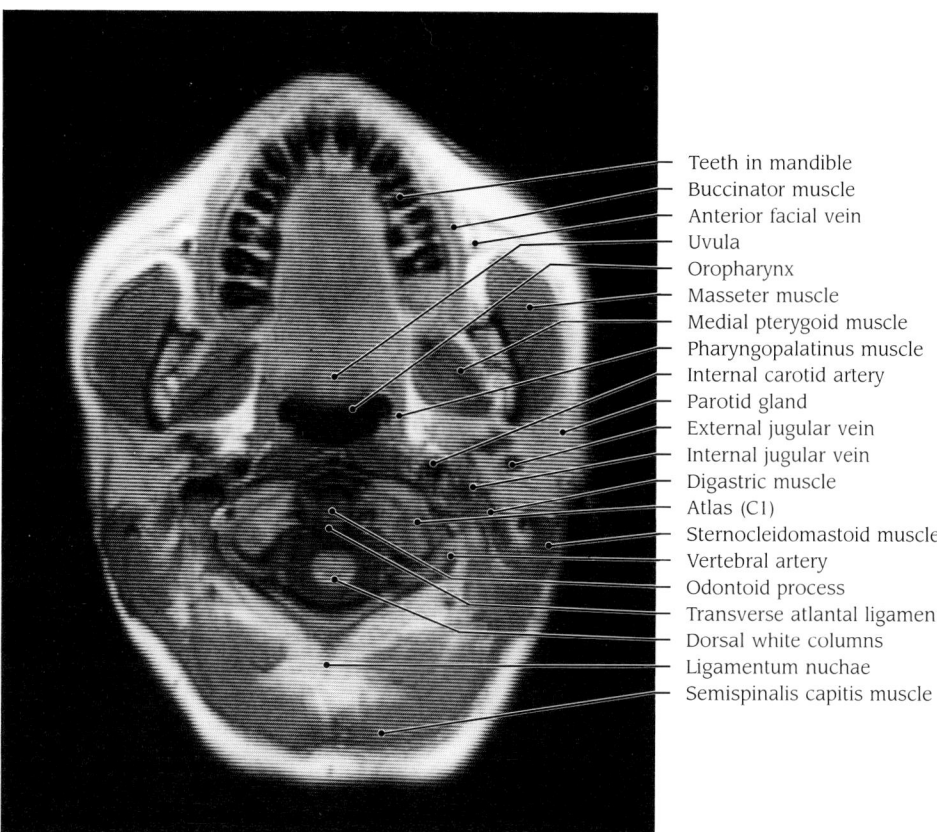

- Teeth in mandible
- Buccinator muscle
- Anterior facial vein
- Uvula
- Oropharynx
- Masseter muscle
- Medial pterygoid muscle
- Pharyngopalatinus muscle
- Internal carotid artery
- Parotid gland
- External jugular vein
- Internal jugular vein
- Digastric muscle
- Atlas (C1)
- Sternocleidomastoid muscle
- Vertebral artery
- Odontoid process
- Transverse atlantal ligament
- Dorsal white columns
- Ligamentum nuchae
- Semispinalis capitis muscle

FIG. 2.99. TR = 500 msec, TE = 28 msec.

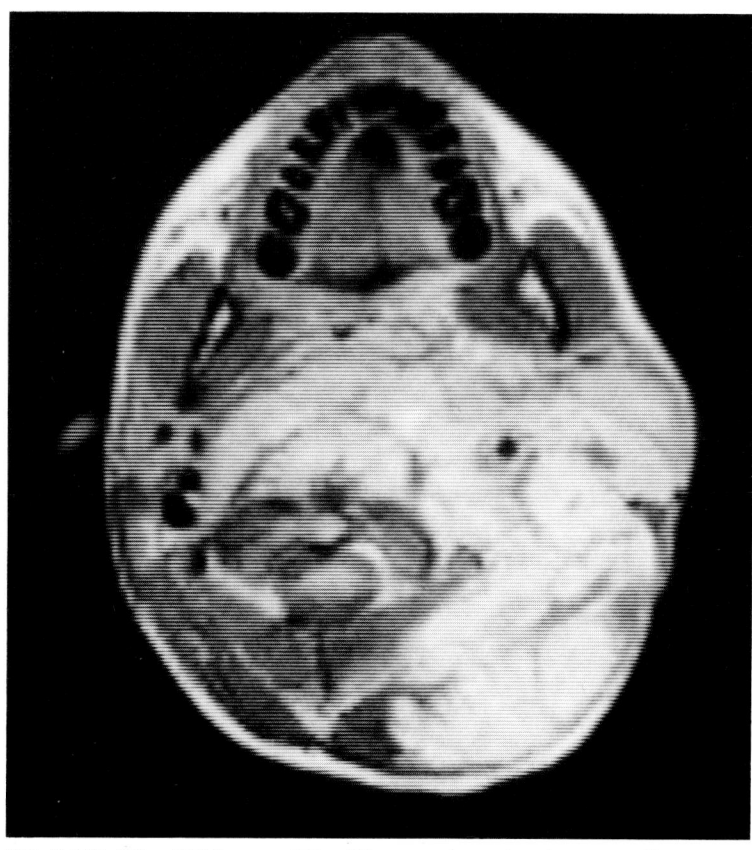

FIG. 2.100. TR = 2000 msec, TE = 28 msec. An extensive neurofibroma displaces the left internal carotid artery, occludes the left internal jugular vein, and effaces most of the oropharynx.

3

Head, Coronal Plane

Anatomic Level	Figures
Anterior to the corpus callosum	3.1–3.10
Genu of corpus callosum through foramen of Monro	3.11–3.23
Thalamus and posterior body of lateral ventricle	3.24–3.34
Splenium of corpus callosum and occipital lobe	3.35–3.57

A series of cadaveric coronal sections that extend from the frontal lobe through the occipital lobe are shown. These sections are matched with coronal magnetic resonance images of normal volunteers. The difference in the planes between the anatomic sections and the magnetic resonance images reflects the variability resulting from both angulation and positioning. The planes of the short and long repetition time images also are not identical because of slight differences both in the shape of the brain and in positioning. The locator image chosen is approximately through the center of both the long and the short repetition time images. Vascular territories are indicated by overlays on a companion image.

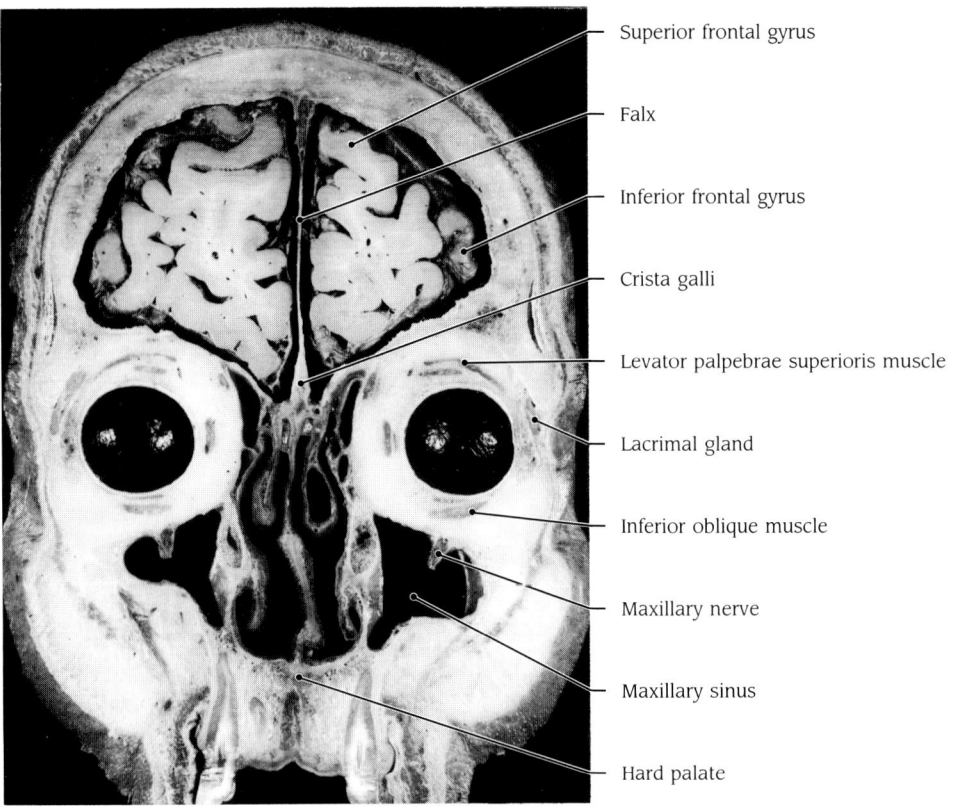
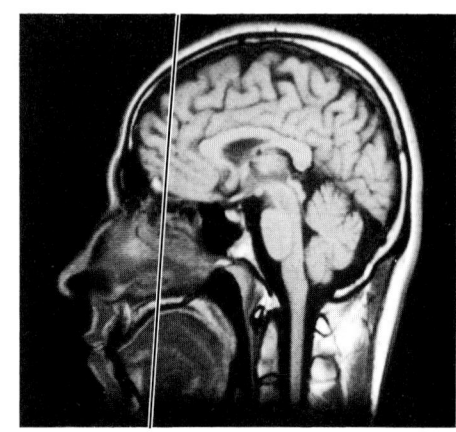

FIG. 3.1.

- The most anterior portion of the frontal lobe is positioned below the level of the upper border of the orbits. In axial sections, the gyrus rectus of the frontal lobe is seen between the orbits.
- The cribriform plate of the ethmoid bone forms a portion of the roof of the nasal cavity. Its thick, triangular, superior projection in the midline is called the crista galli, to which the falx cerebri attaches. The anterior border of the crista galli has two small projecting alae that articulate with the frontal bone to define the foramen caecum. This foramen may contain an emissary vein that connects the facial veins with the superior sagittal sinus. Lateral to the crista galli, the cribriform plate is depressed and contains numerous foramina for the passage of the olfactory nerves.
- The ethmoidal labyrinths located between the medial wall of the orbit and the lateral wall of the nasal cavity are composed of three groups of ethmoidal air cells, the anterior, middle, and posterior. The extremely thin medial wall of the orbit, the lamina papyracea, may permit infection to spread from the sinuses into the orbit.

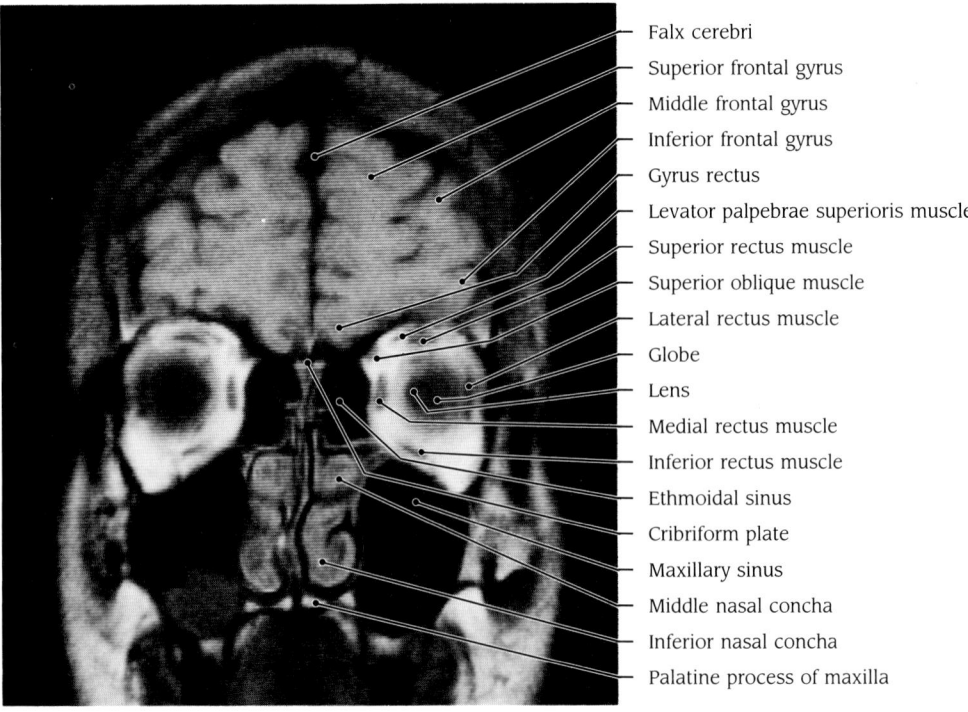

FIG. 3.2. TR = 500 msec, TE = 28 msec.

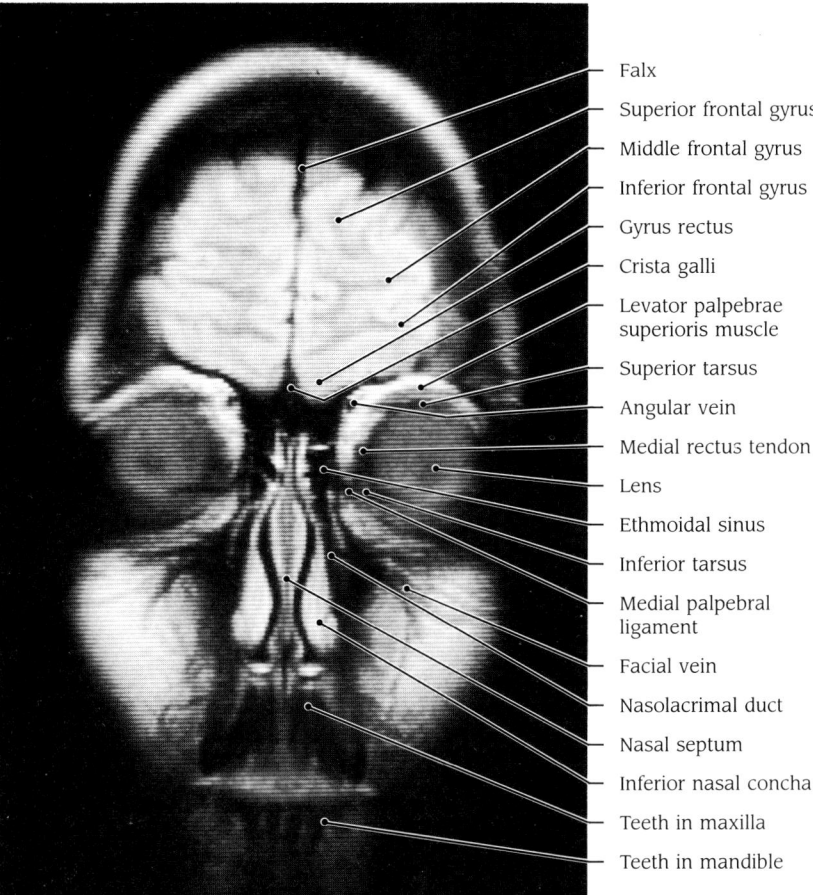

FIG. 3.3. TR = 2000 msec, TE = 28 msec.

- Falx
- Superior frontal gyrus
- Middle frontal gyrus
- Inferior frontal gyrus
- Gyrus rectus
- Crista galli
- Levator palpebrae superioris muscle
- Superior tarsus
- Angular vein
- Medial rectus tendon
- Lens
- Ethmoidal sinus
- Inferior tarsus
- Medial palpebral ligament
- Facial vein
- Nasolacrimal duct
- Nasal septum
- Inferior nasal concha
- Teeth in maxilla
- Teeth in mandible

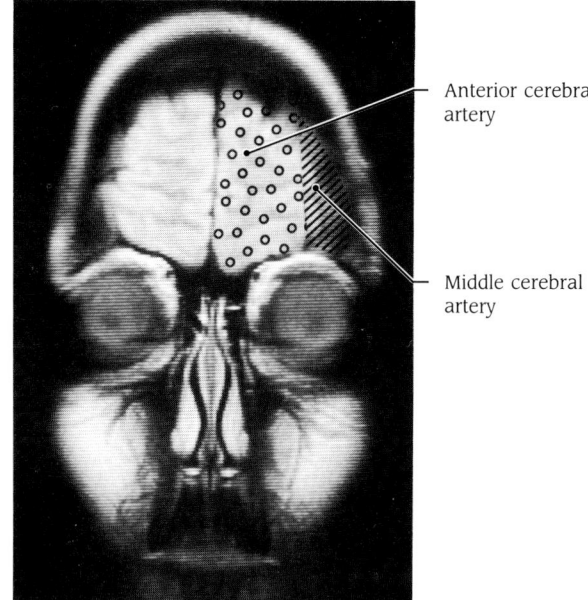

FIG. 3.4. TR = 2000 msec, TE = 28 msec.

- Anterior cerebral artery
- Middle cerebral artery

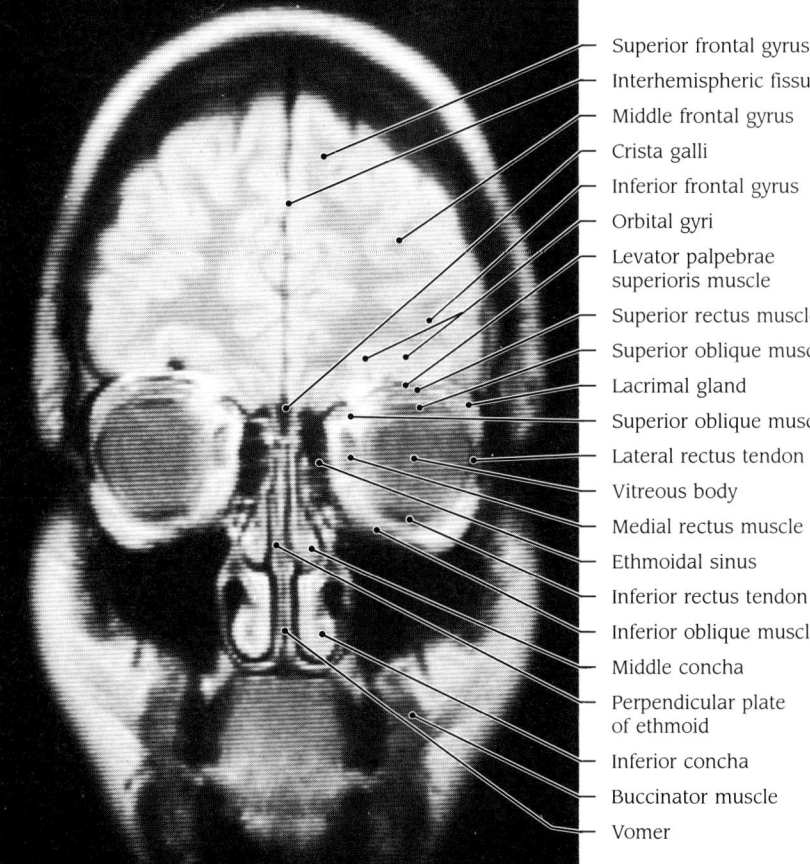

FIG. 3.5. TR = 2000 msec, TE = 28 msec.

- Superior frontal gyrus
- Interhemispheric fissure
- Middle frontal gyrus
- Crista galli
- Inferior frontal gyrus
- Orbital gyri
- Levator palpebrae superioris muscle
- Superior rectus muscle
- Superior oblique muscle
- Lacrimal gland
- Superior oblique muscle
- Lateral rectus tendon
- Vitreous body
- Medial rectus muscle
- Ethmoidal sinus
- Inferior rectus tendon
- Inferior oblique muscle
- Middle concha
- Perpendicular plate of ethmoid
- Inferior concha
- Buccinator muscle
- Vomer

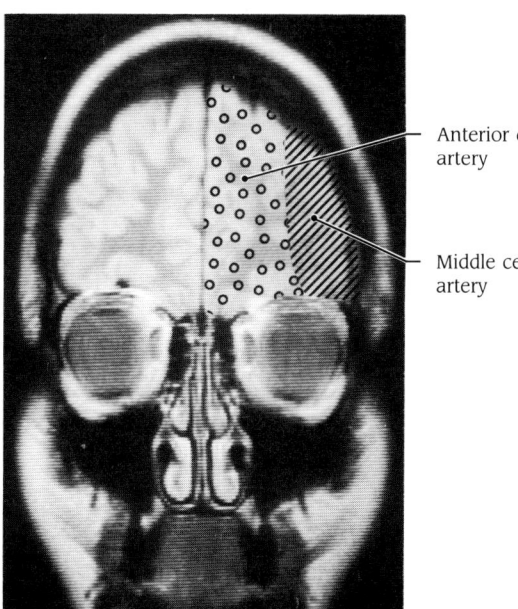

FIG. 3.6. TR = 2000 msec, TE = 28 msec.

- Anterior cerebral artery
- Middle cerebral artery

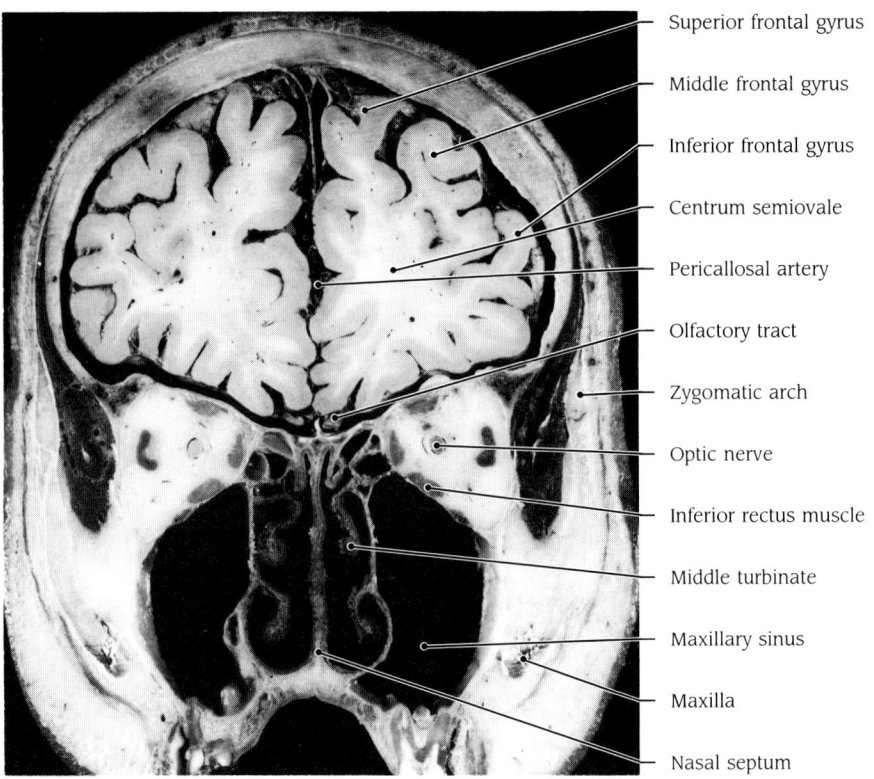
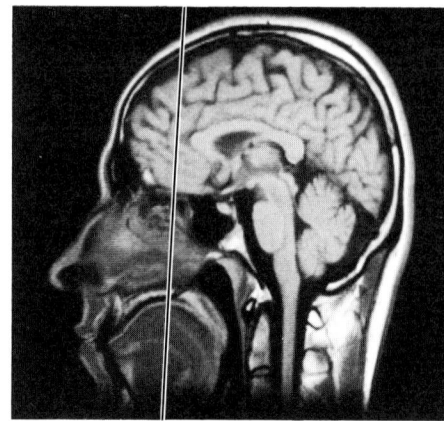

FIG. 3.7.

- The maxillary sinus, a thin-walled pyramidal cavity in the body of the maxilla, varies in size in different skulls and even in the two sides of the same skull. A tumor or infection within the sinus may expand the sinus and impinge upon the orbital floor, the nasal cavity, the infratemporal fossa, or the mouth because of the extreme thinness of the bony wall.
- Three bony projections, the inferior, middle, and superior nasal conchae (turbinates), project from the lateral wall of the nasal cavity. These conchae project inferiorly and medially, each forming the roof of a passage or meatus that freely communicates with the nasal cavity. The superior nasal concha often is small or absent.
- The anterior aspect of the falx attaches to the crista galli and separates the frontal lobes to a varying degree. The falx may simply be a narrow band of connective tissue within the interhemispheric fissure.

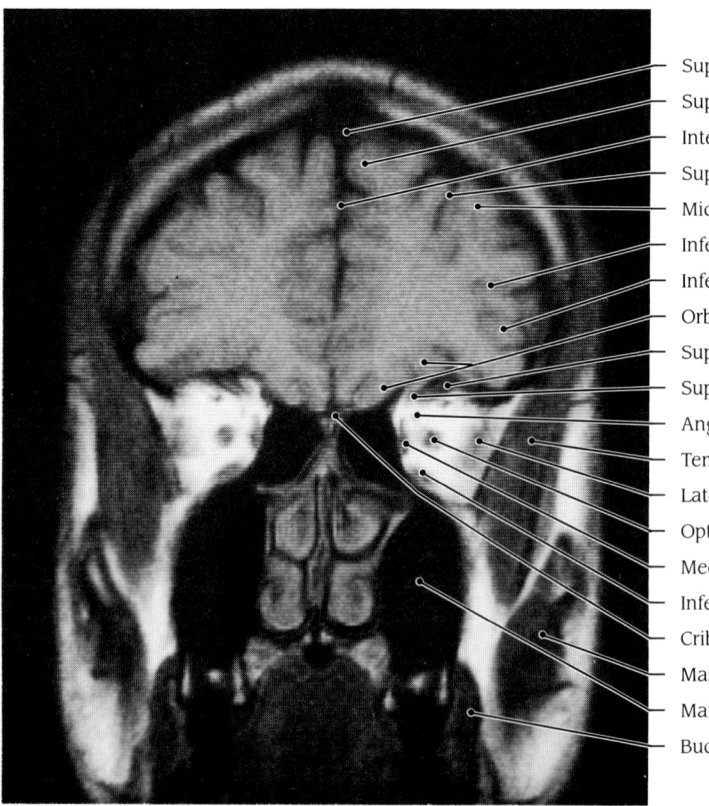

FIG. 3.8. TR = 500 msec, TE = 28 msec.

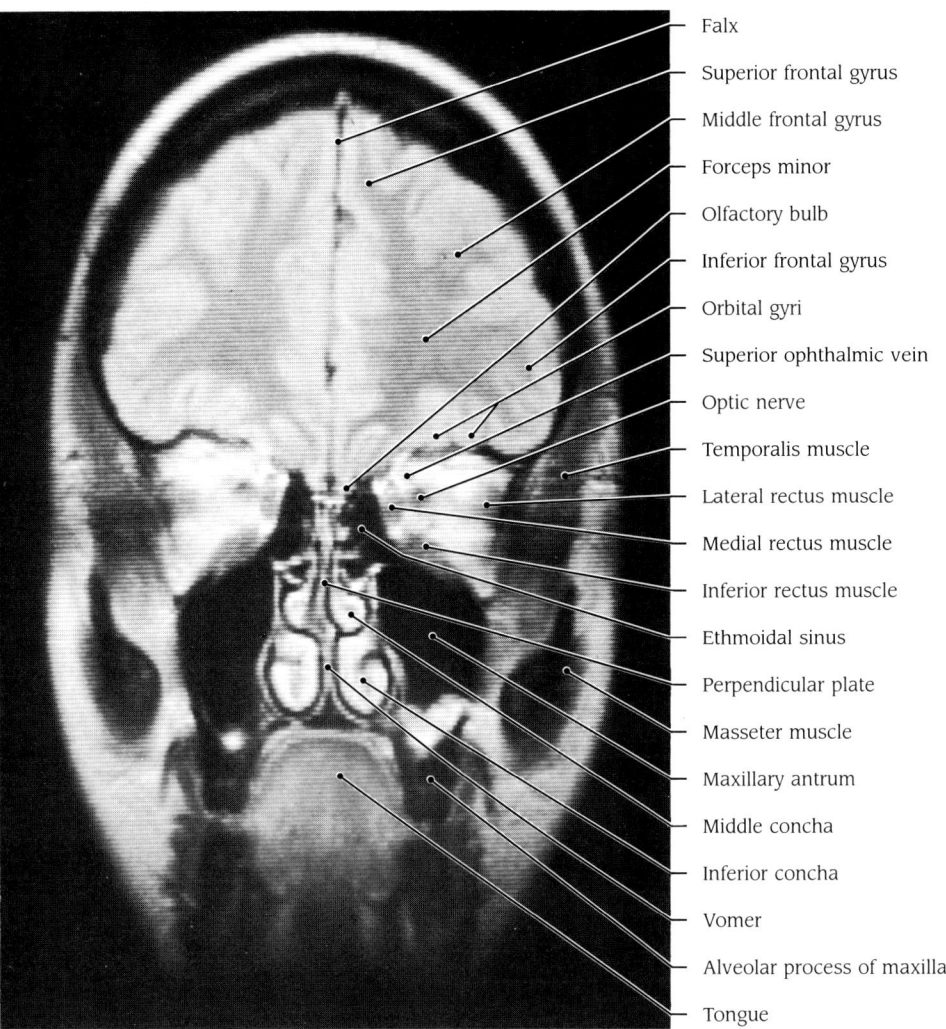

FIG. 3.9. TR = 2000 msec, TE = 28 msec.

- Falx
- Superior frontal gyrus
- Middle frontal gyrus
- Forceps minor
- Olfactory bulb
- Inferior frontal gyrus
- Orbital gyri
- Superior ophthalmic vein
- Optic nerve
- Temporalis muscle
- Lateral rectus muscle
- Medial rectus muscle
- Inferior rectus muscle
- Ethmoidal sinus
- Perpendicular plate
- Masseter muscle
- Maxillary antrum
- Middle concha
- Inferior concha
- Vomer
- Alveolar process of maxilla
- Tongue

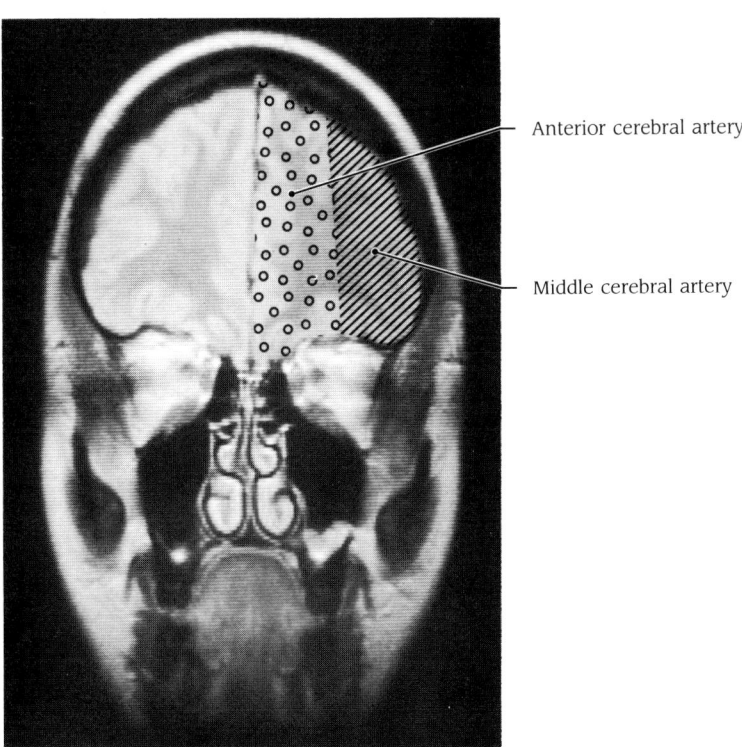

FIG. 3.10. TR = 2000 msec, TE = 28 msec.

- Anterior cerebral artery
- Middle cerebral artery

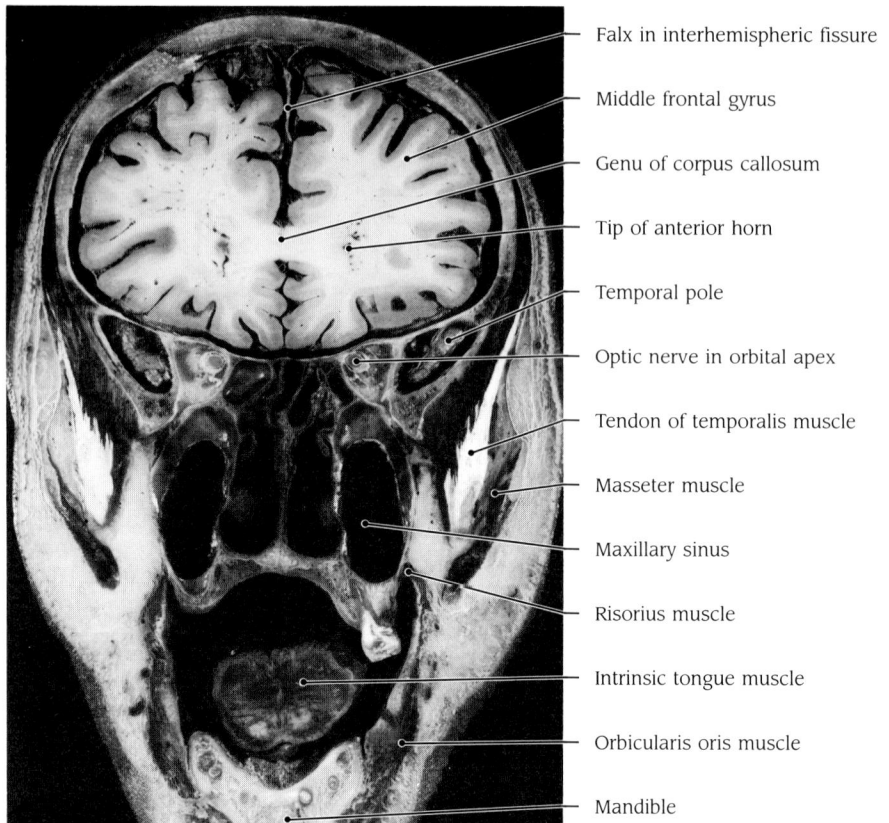
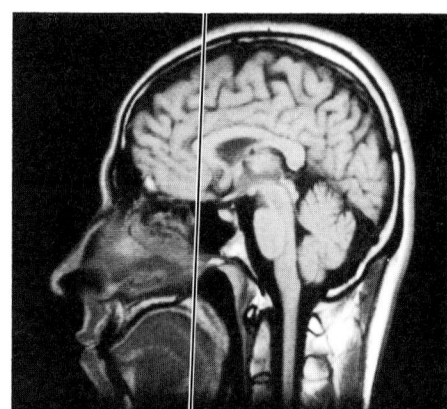

FIG. 3.11.

- The vomer extends from the inferior surface of the body of the sphenoid to the bony palate and forms the inferior and posterior portions of the nasal septum.
- The perpendicular plate of the ethmoid forms the superior and anterior parts of the nasal septum and is continuous with the cribriform plate superiorly.

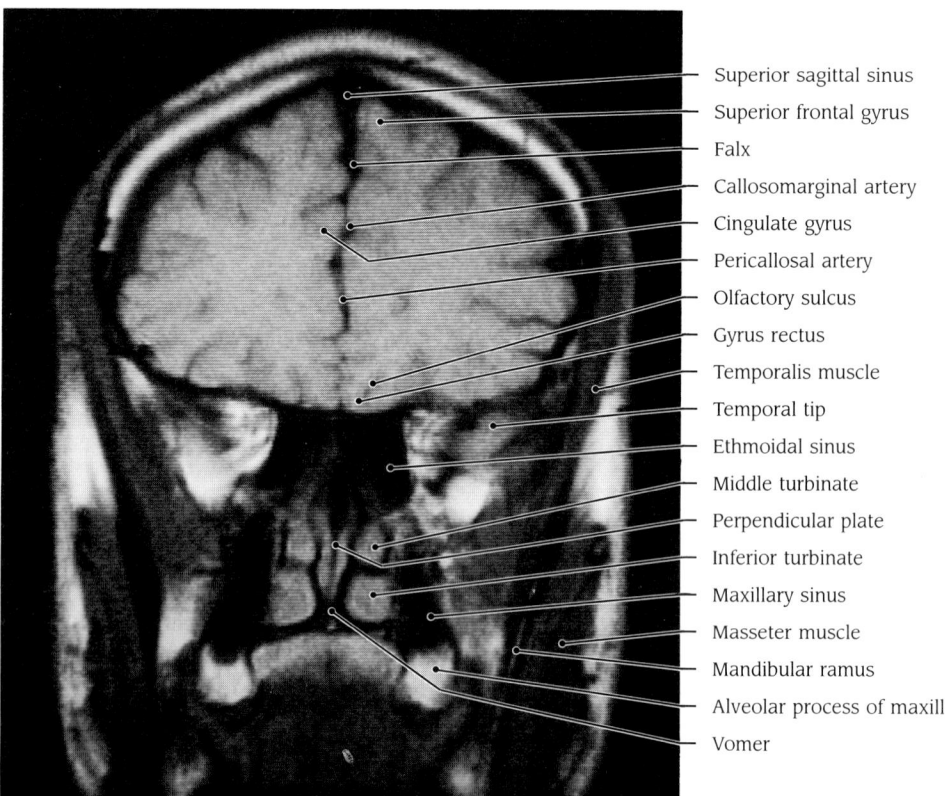

FIG. 3.12. TR = 500 msec, TE = 28 msec.

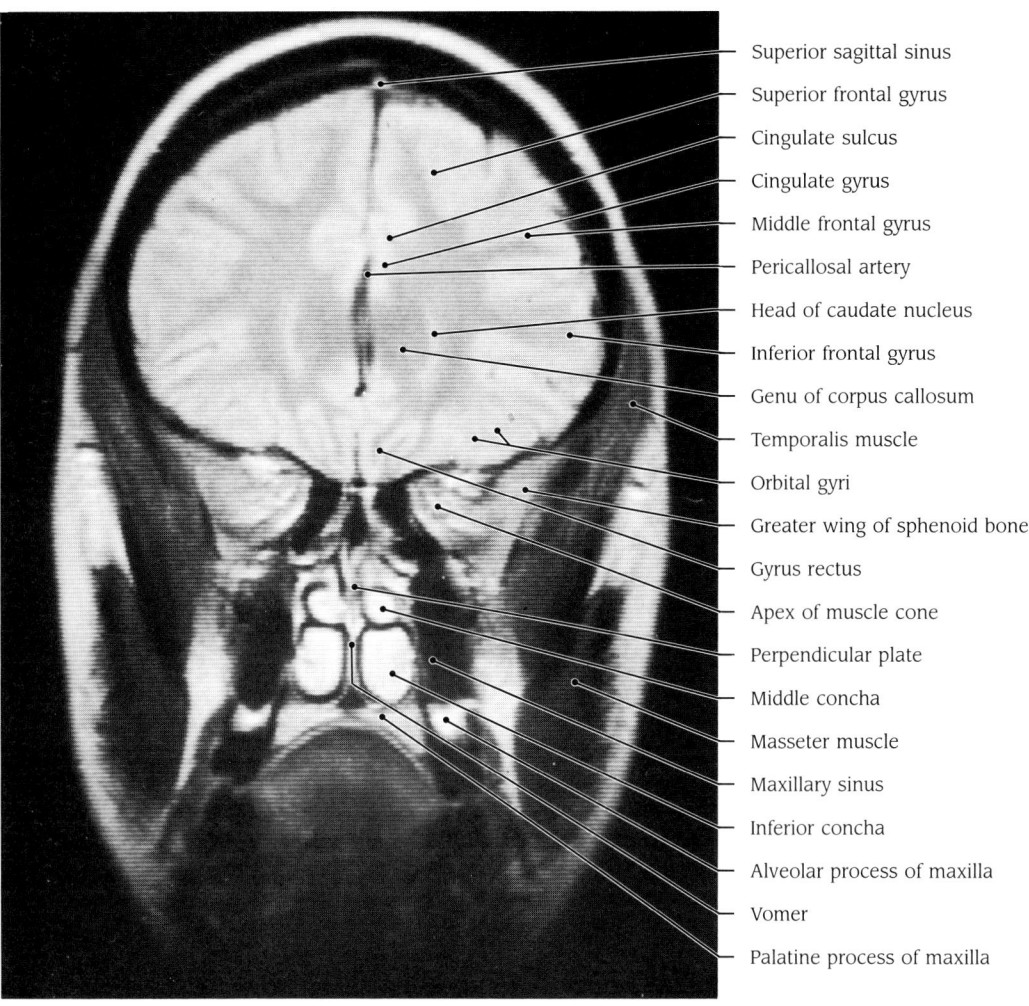

FIG. 3.13. TR = 2000 msec, TE = 28 msec.

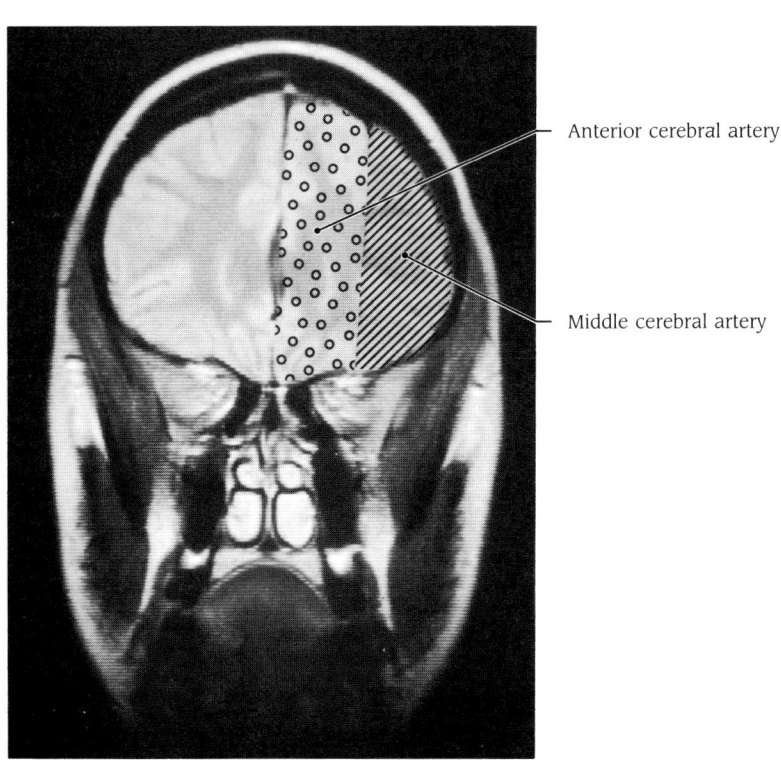

FIG. 3.14. TR = 2000 msec, TE = 28 msec.

67

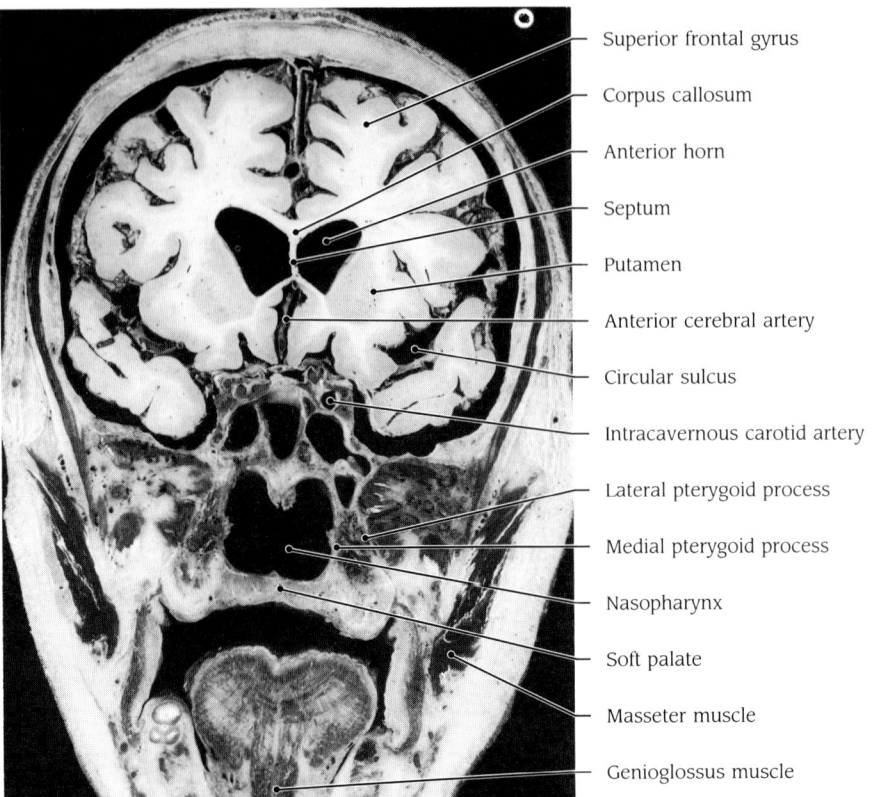
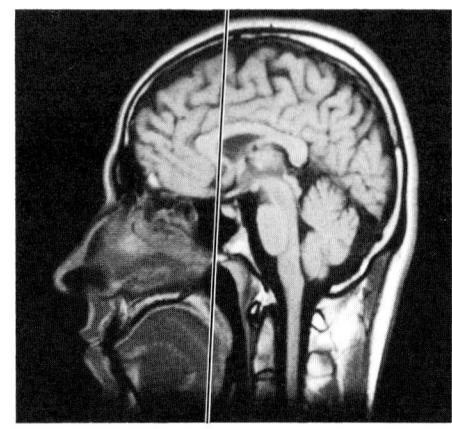

FIG. 3.15.

- The tip of the anterior horn normally extends slightly anteriorly to the rostral aspect of the genu of the corpus callosum.
- The sphenoid sinuses are two large, irregular cavities separated by a bony septum. They are seldom symmetric and may be divided partially by bony laminae. Each sinus may have a lateral recess that extends into the greater wing and lingula. Occasionally, the sphenoid sinus may partially surround the ipsilateral optic canal.
- In a coronal plane, the genu and rostrum of the corpus callosum show the configuration of the letter "X."

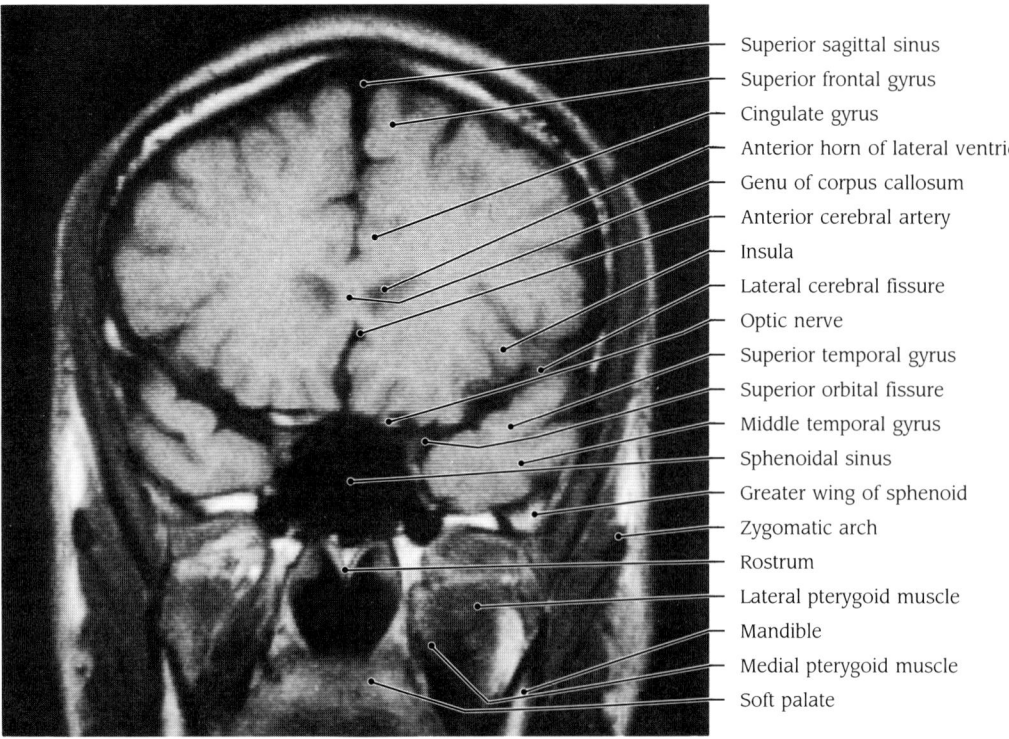

FIG. 3.16. TR = 500 msec, TE = 28 msec.

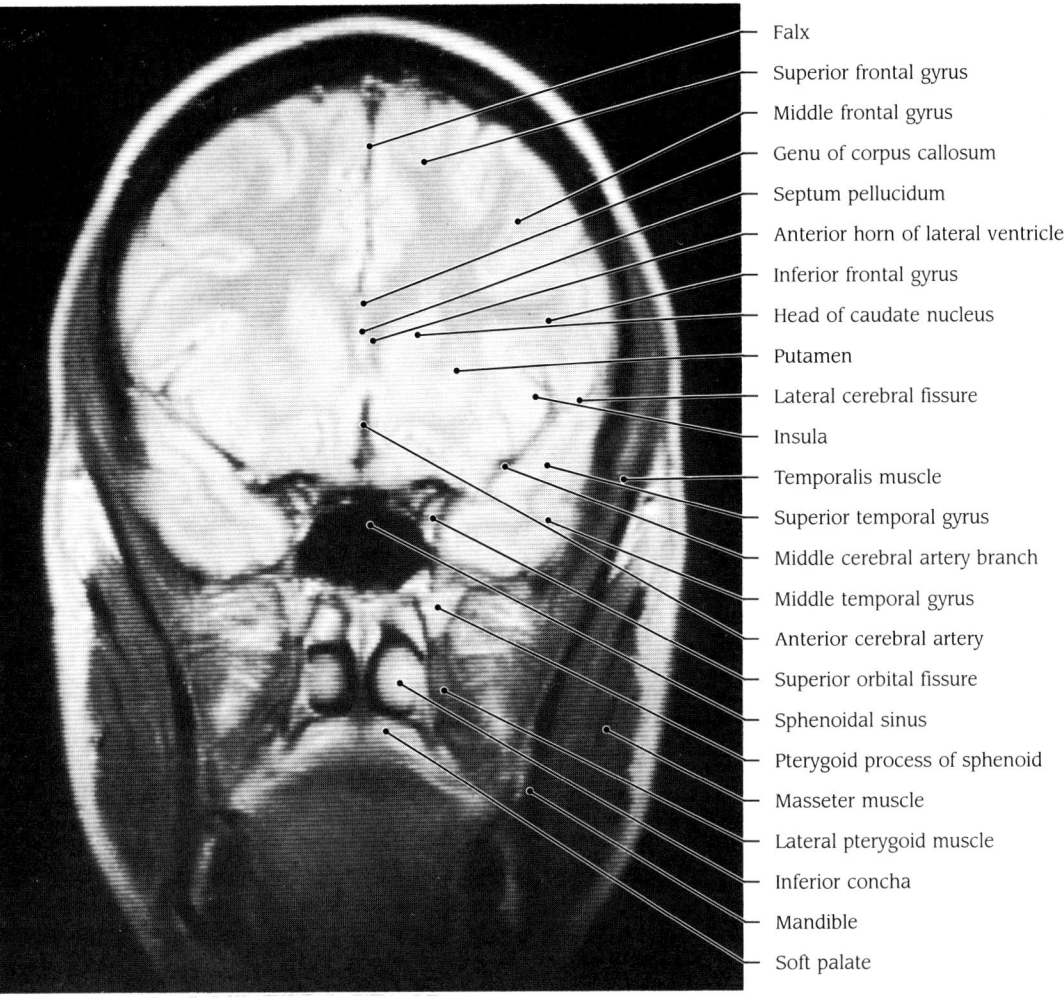

FIG. 3.17. TR = 2000 msec, TE = 28 msec.

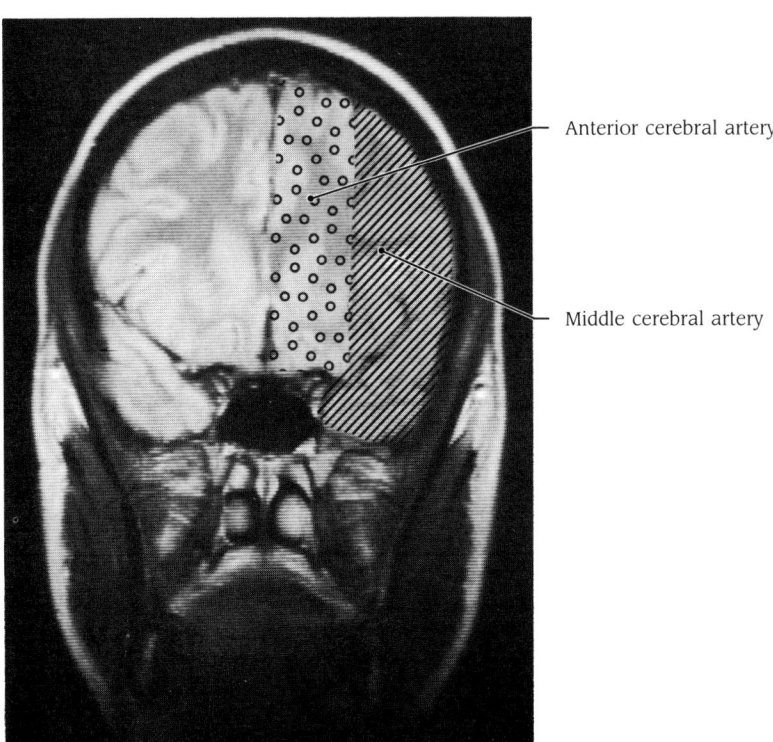

FIG. 3.18. TR = 2000 msec, TE = 28 msec.

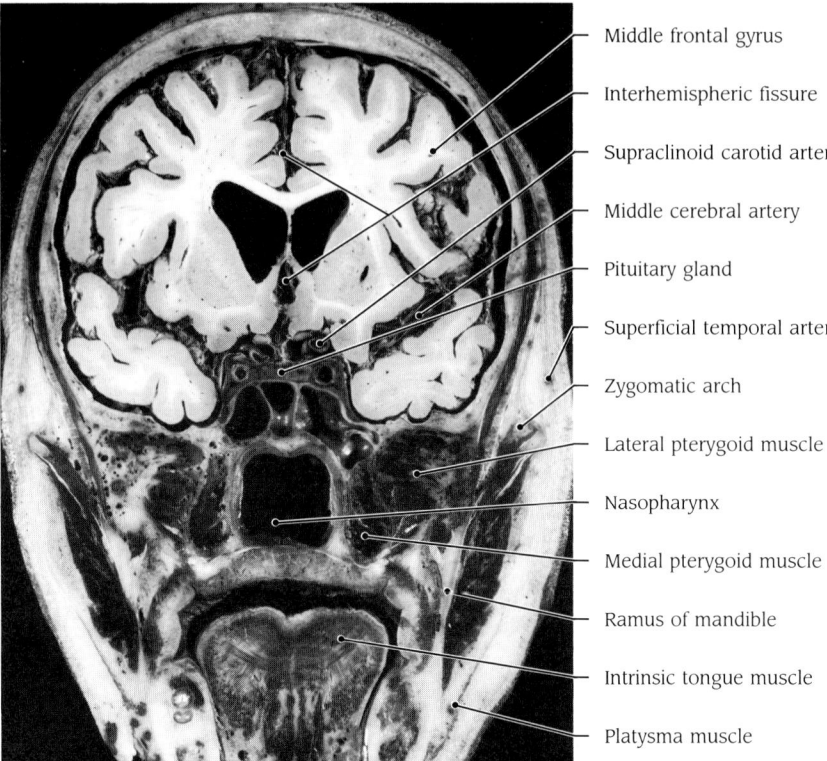
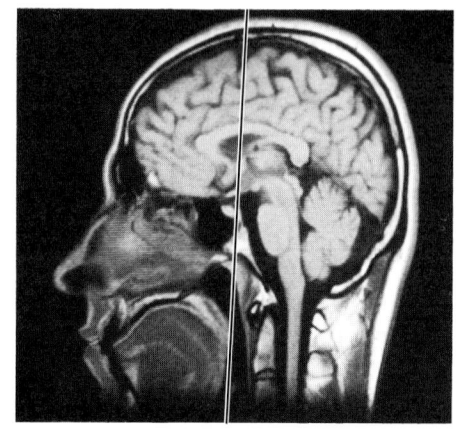

FIG. 3.19.

- In this anterior section, the caudate nucleus and the putamen are separated by the anterior limb of the internal capsule; these two gray masses sometimes are referred to as the corpus striatum.
- The optic chiasm, a quadrilateral bundle of nerve fibers, is situated at the junction of the anterior wall of the third ventricle with its floor. Its rich vascular supply is from a pial plexus composed of branches off the superior hypophyseal, internal carotid, anterior cerebral, anterior communicating, and, sometimes, the posterior communicating arteries.
- Pituitary tumors may extend through the diaphragm superiorly or into the sphenoid sinuses inferiorly. Lateral growth of the tumor may compress an adjacent cavernous sinus and, rarely, invade it.

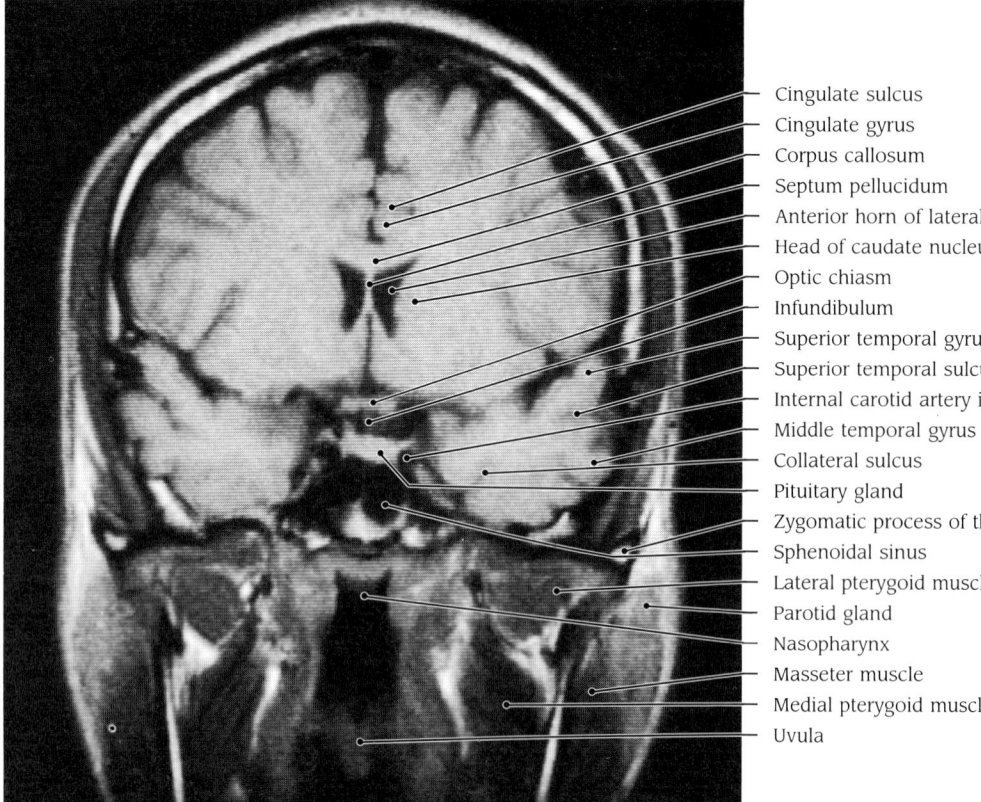

FIG. 3.20. TR = 500 msec, TE = 28 msec.

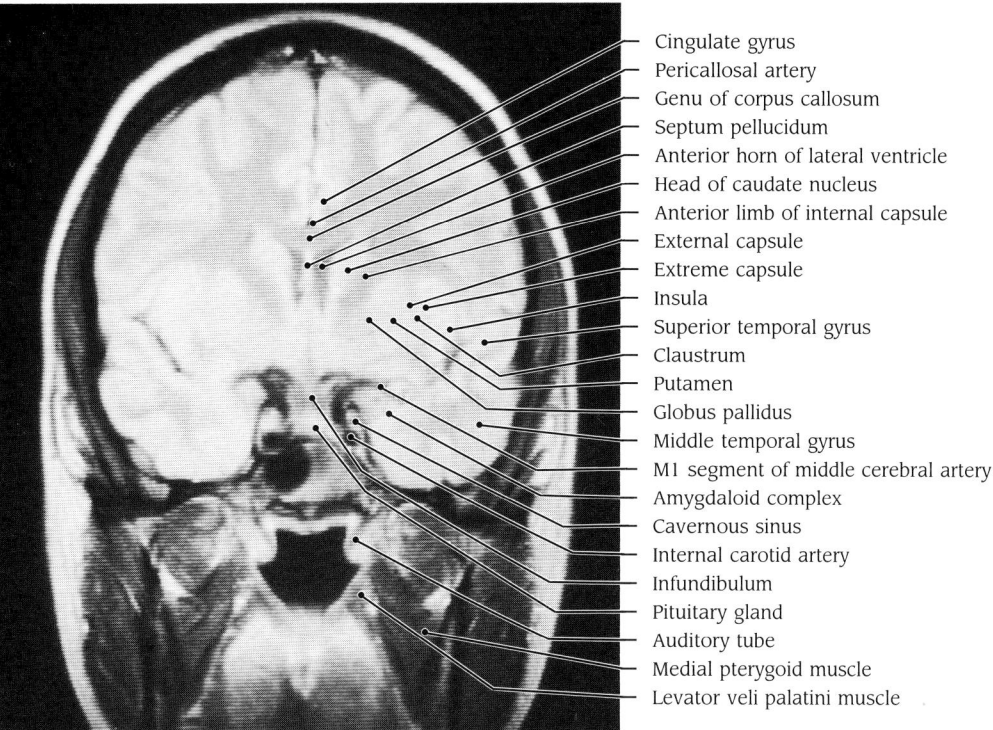

FIG. 3.21. TR = 2000 msec, TE = 28 msec.

- Cingulate gyrus
- Pericallosal artery
- Genu of corpus callosum
- Septum pellucidum
- Anterior horn of lateral ventricle
- Head of caudate nucleus
- Anterior limb of internal capsule
- External capsule
- Extreme capsule
- Insula
- Superior temporal gyrus
- Claustrum
- Putamen
- Globus pallidus
- Middle temporal gyrus
- M1 segment of middle cerebral artery
- Amygdaloid complex
- Cavernous sinus
- Internal carotid artery
- Infundibulum
- Pituitary gland
- Auditory tube
- Medial pterygoid muscle
- Levator veli palatini muscle

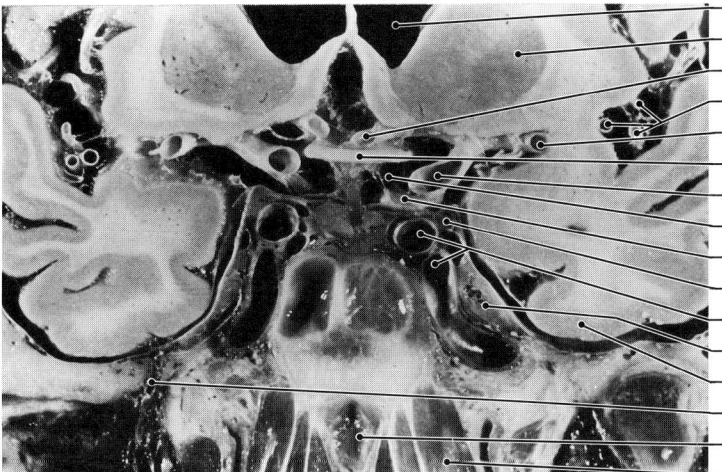

FIG. 3.22.

- Anterior horn of lateral ventricle
- Putamen
- Anterior cerebral artery
- Middle cerebral artery branches
- Middle cerebral artery
- Optic chiasm
- Internal carotid artery
- Suprasellar cistern
- Posterior communicating artery
- Oculomotor nerve
- Intracavernous carotid artery
- Fifth nerve ganglion
- Fusiform gyrus
- Middle meningeal artery
- Nasopharynx
- Longus capitis muscle

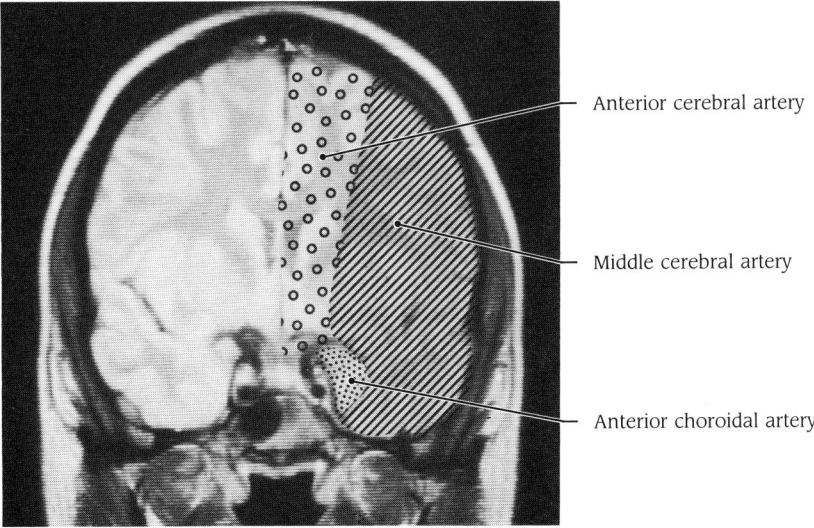

FIG. 3.23. TR = 2000 msec, TE = 28 msec.

- Anterior cerebral artery
- Middle cerebral artery
- Anterior choroidal artery

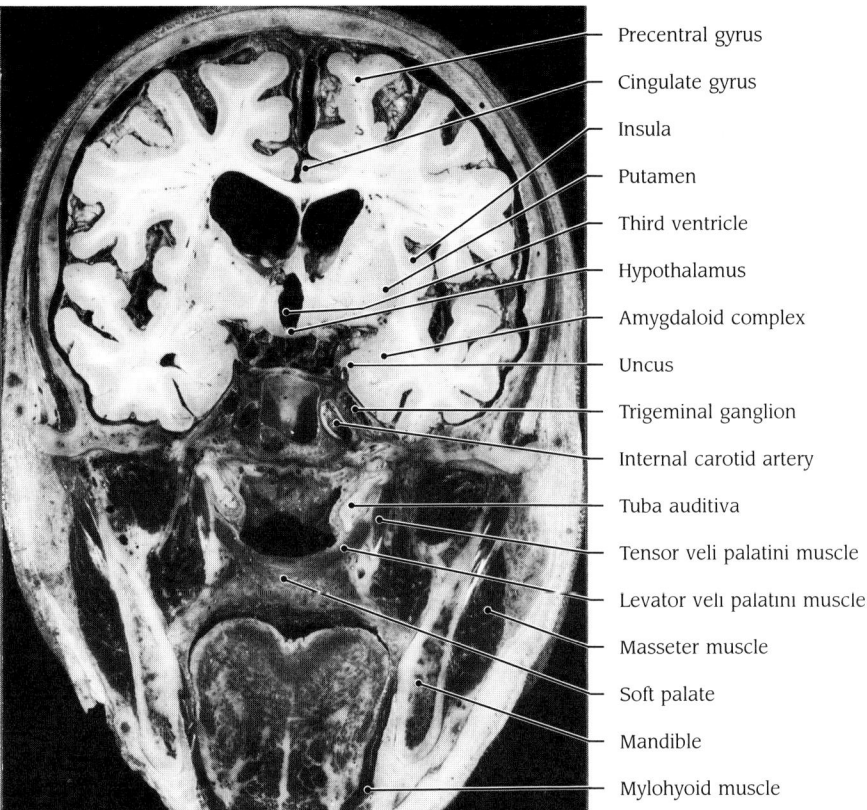
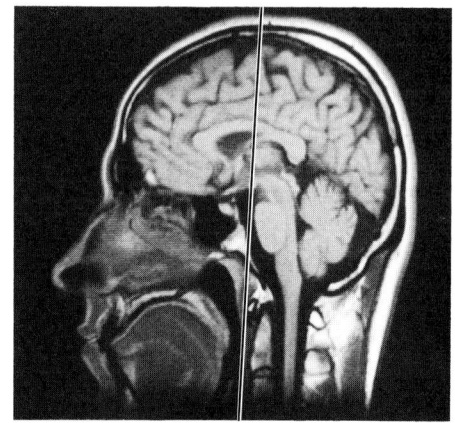

FIG. 3.24.

- The two crura of the fornix join anteriorly to form the body of the fornix, which is actually symmetric and bilateral. The body of the fornix lies above the tela choroidea and the ependyma of the third ventricle and is attached to the inferior aspect of the corpus callosum and the inferior border of the laminae of the septum pellucidum.

- The anterior aspect of the inferior horn of the lateral ventricle is bounded superiorly and anteriorly by the amygdaloid nuclear complex (amygdala) and inferiorly by the anterior portion of the hippocampus.

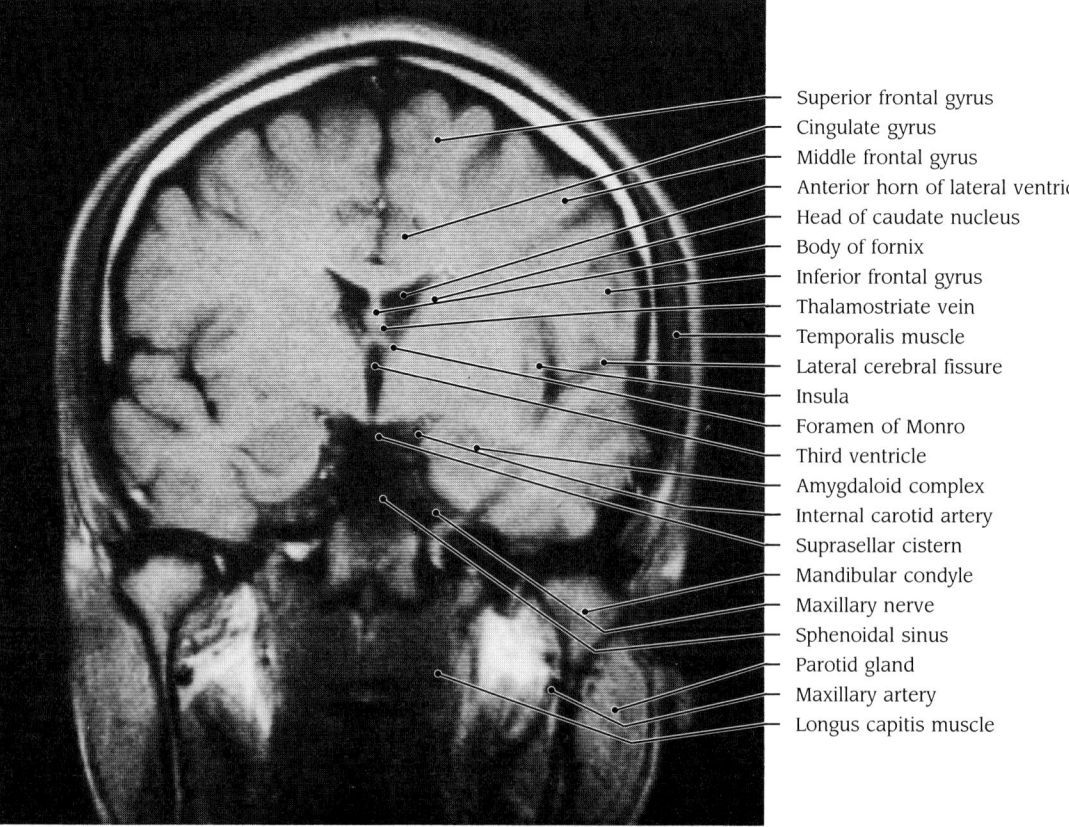

FIG. 3.25. TR = 500 msec, TE = 28 msec.

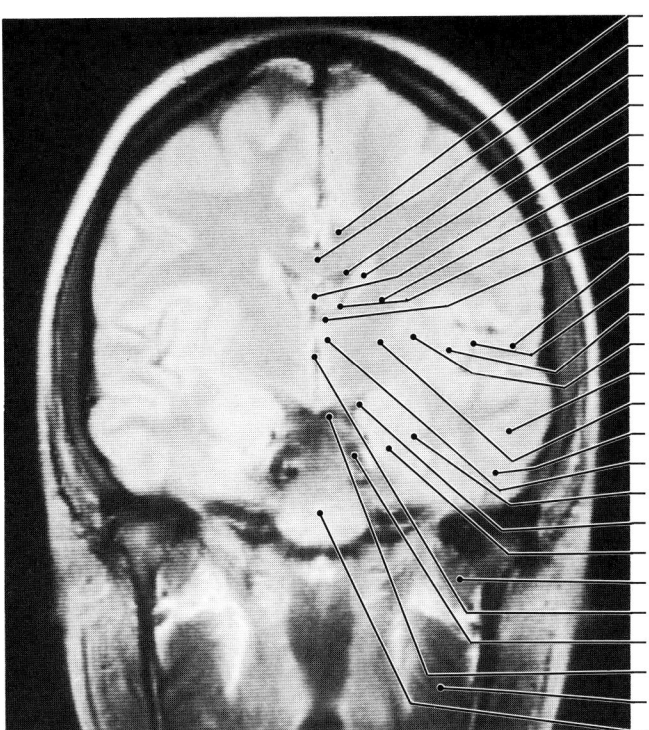

FIG. 3.26. TR = 2000 msec, TE = 28 msec.

- Cingulum
- Body of corpus callosum
- Body of lateral ventricle
- Body of caudate nucleus
- Body of fornix
- Posterior limb of internal capsule
- Thalamostriate vein
- Internal cerebral vein
- Superior temporal gyrus
- Circular sulcus
- Insula
- Putamen
- Middle temporal gyrus
- Globus pallidus
- Inferior temporal gyrus
- Thalamus
- Amygdaloid complex
- Anterior choroidal artery
- Parahippocampal gyrus
- Lateral pterygoid muscle
- Third ventricle
- Internal carotid artery
- Posterior cerebral artery
- Medial pterygoid muscle
- Clivus

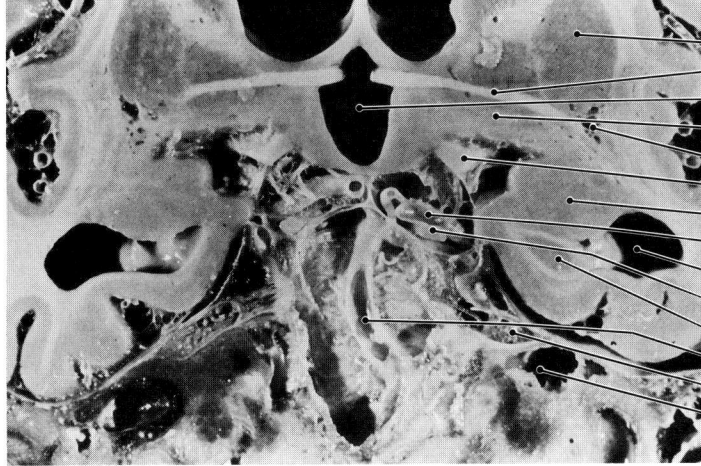

FIG. 3.27.

- Putamen
- Anterior commissure
- Third ventricle
- Nucleus basalis
- Lateral lenticulostriate artery
- Optic tract
- Amygdaloid complex
- Posterior cerebral artery
- Inferior horn
- Oculomotor nerve
- Hippocampus
- Basilar artery
- Mandibular nerve
- Internal carotid artery

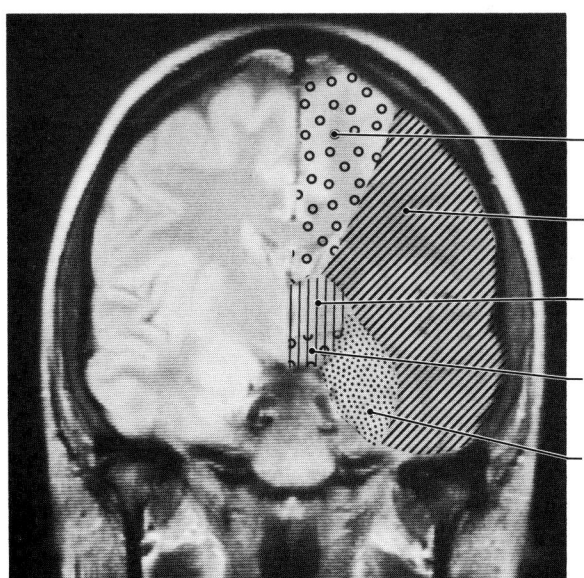

FIG. 3.28. TR = 2000 msec, TE = 28 msec.

- Anterior cerebral artery
- Middle cerebral artery
- Posterior cerebral artery
- Anterior and posterior cerebral arteries
- Anterior choroidal artery

73

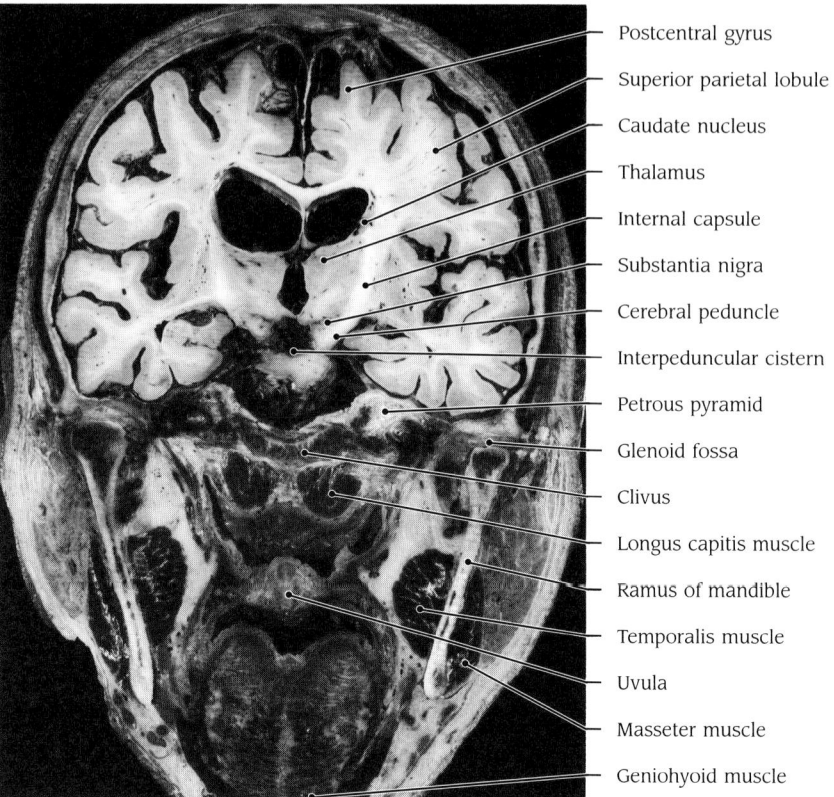
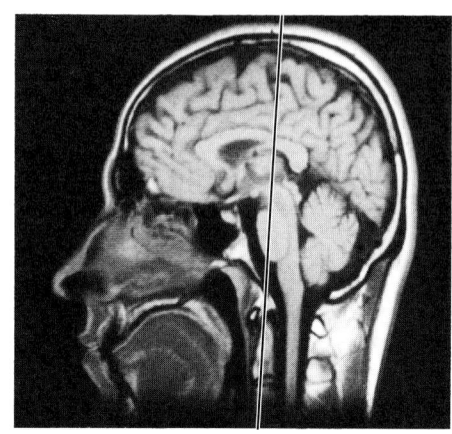

FIG. 3.29.

- The trigeminal ganglion lies lateral to the internal carotid artery, just posterior and inferior to the cavernous sinus; medial to the artery is the wall of the posterior portion of the sphenoid sinus, which may consist of thin bone or a thin layer of connective tissue under the mucosa.

- The massa intermedia is an adhesion between the two thalami and contains no crossing nerve fibers.

- The uncus is a recurved portion of the anterior aspect of the parahippocampal gyrus. The medial part of the uncus normally protrudes slightly over the anterior petroclinoid ligament (anterior continuation of the tentorium).

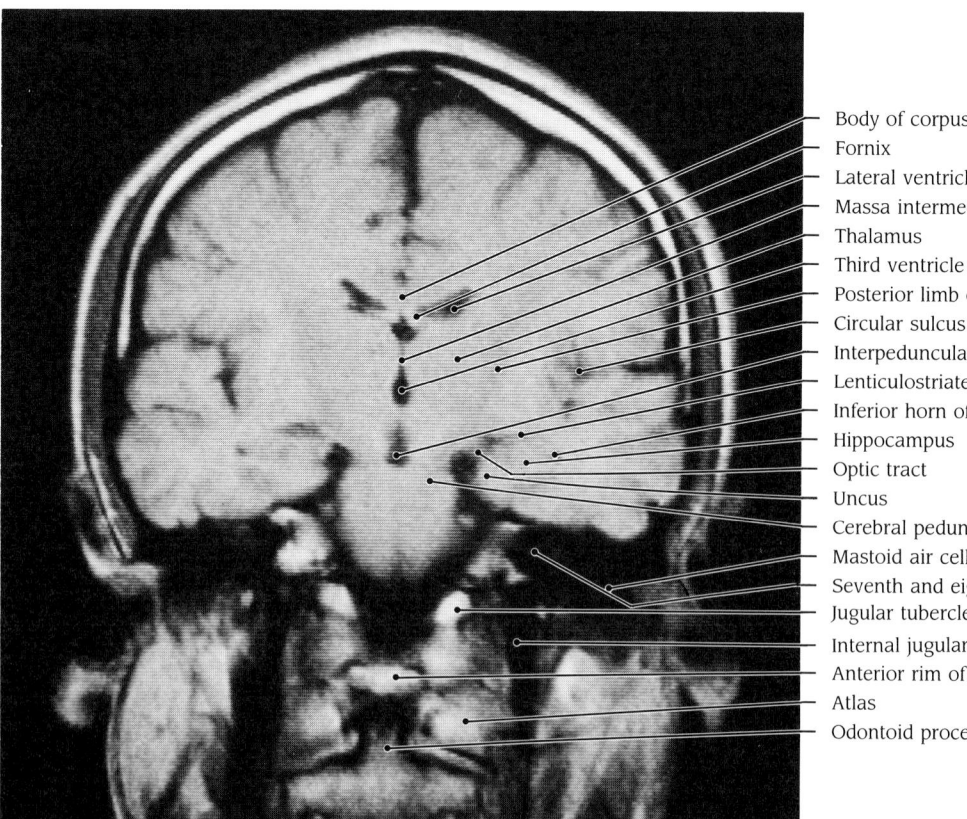

FIG. 3.30. TR = 500 msec, TE = 28 msec.

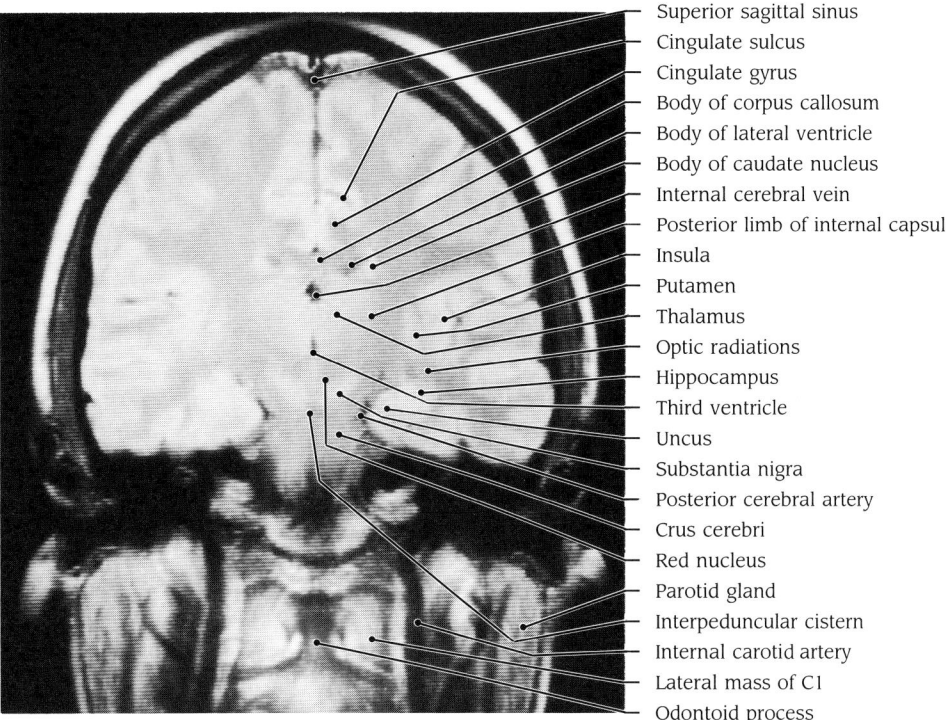

FIG. 3.31. TR = 2000 msec, TE = 28 msec.

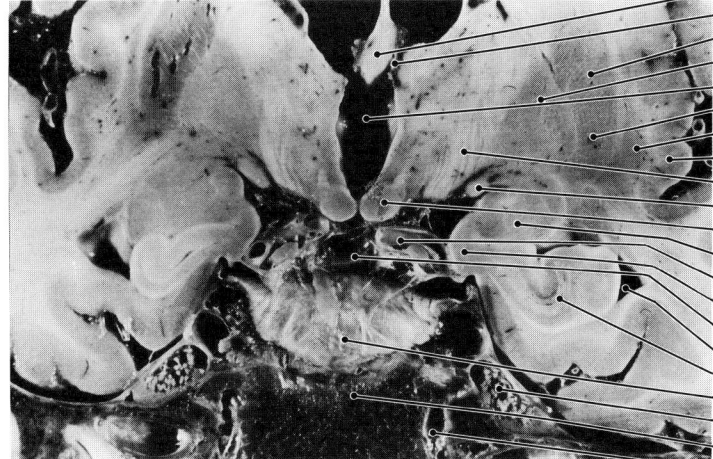

FIG. 3.32.

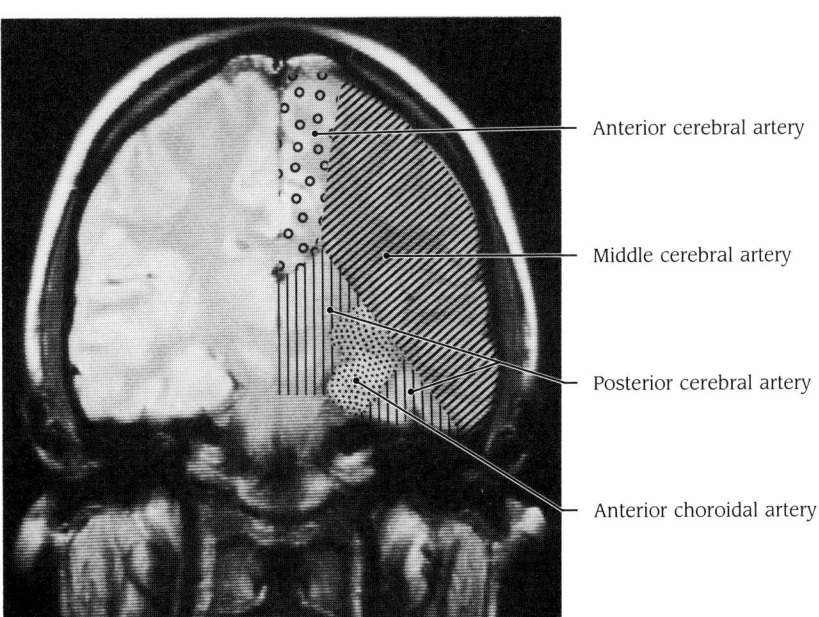

FIG. 3.33. TR = 2000 msec, TE = 28 msec.

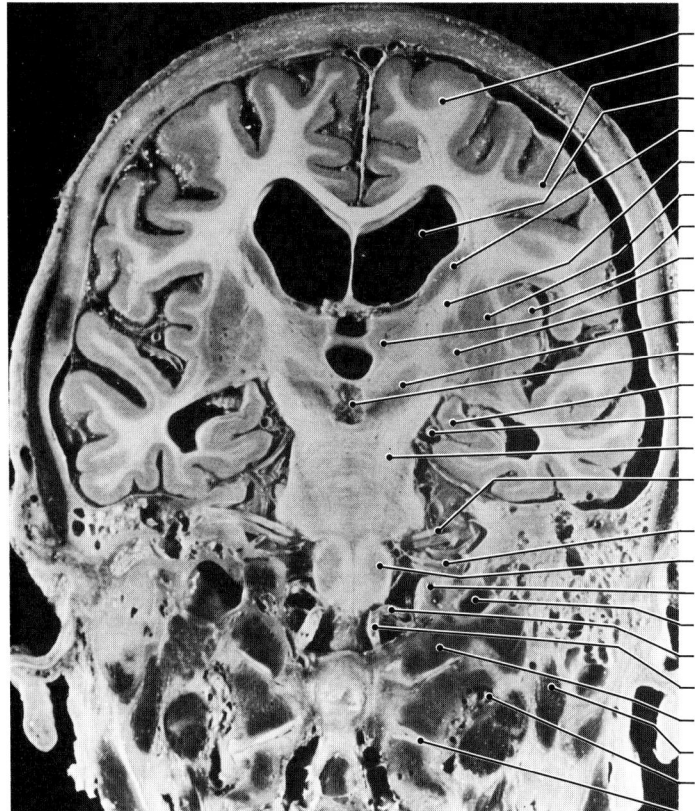
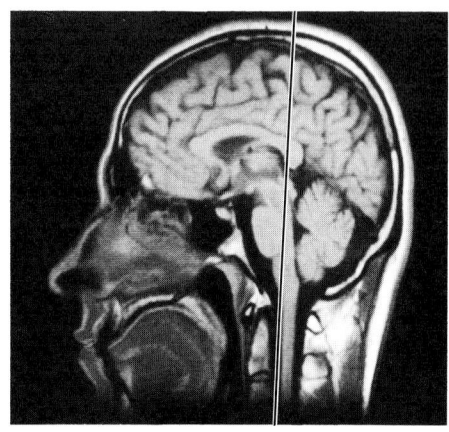

- Postcentral gyrus
- Supramarginal gyrus
- Lateral ventricle
- Caudate nucleus
- Internal capsule
- Putamen
- Insula
- Thalamus
- Globus pallidus
- Substantia nigra
- Interpeduncular cistern
- Hippocampus
- Posterior cerebral artery
- Corticospinal tract in pons
- Cerebellopontine angle with seventh and eighth nerves
- Ninth cranial nerve
- Inferior olivary nucleus
- Jugular tubercle
- Internal jugular vein
- Posterior inferior cerebellar artery
- Vertebral artery
- Occipital condyle
- Digastric muscle
- Vertebral artery
- Atlantoaxial joint

FIG. 3.34.

- The descending portion of the internal capsule continues below the lentiform nucleus as the cerebral peduncle. The fibers in the peduncle then extend into the pons, where the corticopontine fibers terminate, while the corticospinal and corticobulbar fibers continue their descending course (see Chap. 6).
- The red nucleus is an ovoid mass of nerve cells with a pink or red tinge, which is caused both by the presence of an iron-containing pigment in many of the cells and by its dense capillary network. The afferent connections of the red nucleus include the corticorubral projection, nerve fibers from the superior colliculi, and the deep nuclei of the cerebellum. The principal efferent pathways are the rubro-thalamocortical tract and the rubrospinal tract. The rubrospinal tract is considered one of the descending components of the upper motor neuron complex.

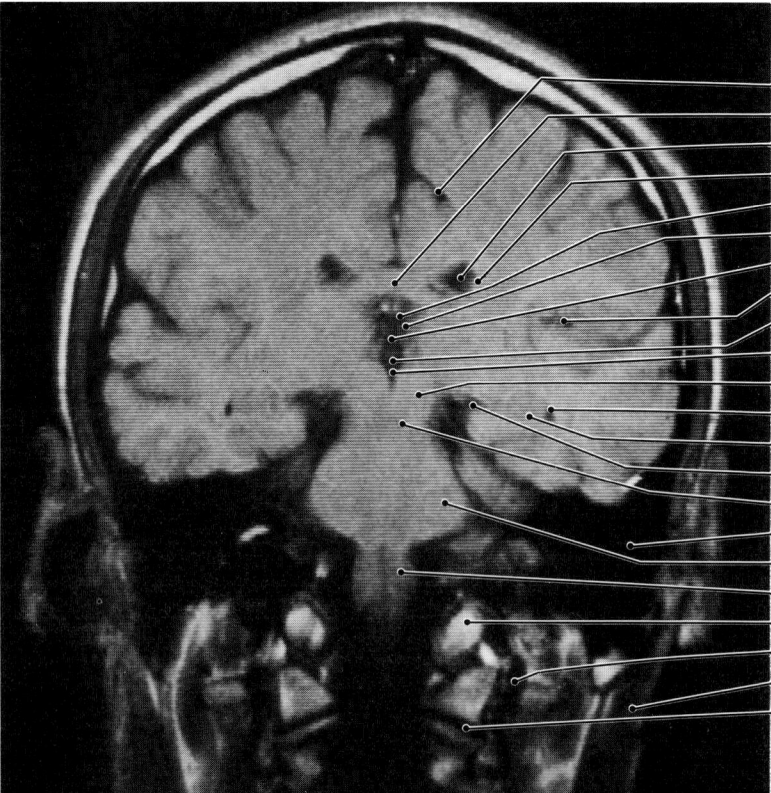

- Cingulate sulcus
- Corpus callosum
- Lateral ventricle
- Caudate nucleus
- Internal cerebral vein
- Basal vein of Rosenthal
- Suprapineal recess of third ventricle
- Angular artery
- Pineal gland
- Pineal recess of third ventricle
- Cerebral peduncle
- Inferior horn of lateral ventricle
- Hippocampus
- Choroidal fissure
- Red nucleus
- Mastoid air cells
- Middle cerebellar peduncle
- Inferior olivary nucleus
- Occipital condyle
- Vertebral artery
- Sternocleidomastoid muscle
- Atlantoaxial joint

FIG. 3.35. TR = 500 msec, TE = 28 msec.

76

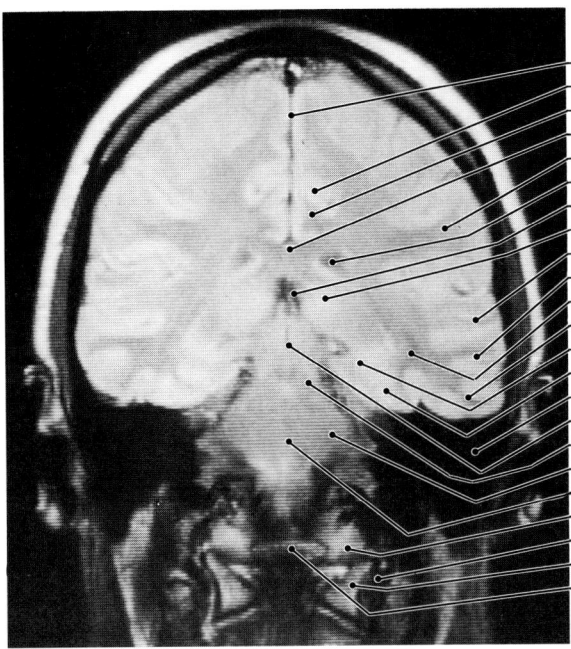

FIG. 3.36. TR = 2000 msec, TE = 28 msec.

- Falx cerebri
- Cingulate sulcus
- Cingulate gyrus
- Splenium of corpus callosum
- Supramarginal gyrus
- Atrium of lateral ventricle
- Internal cerebral vein
- Pulvinar of thalamus
- Superior temporal gyrus
- Middle temporal gyrus
- Optic radiations
- Inferior temporal gyrus
- Parahippocampal gyrus
- Lateral occipitotemporal gyrus
- Mastoid air cells
- Cerebral aqueduct
- Cerebral peduncle
- Middle cerebellar peduncle
- Pons
- Occipital condyle
- Vertebral artery
- Lateral mass of C1
- Anterior rim of foramen magnum

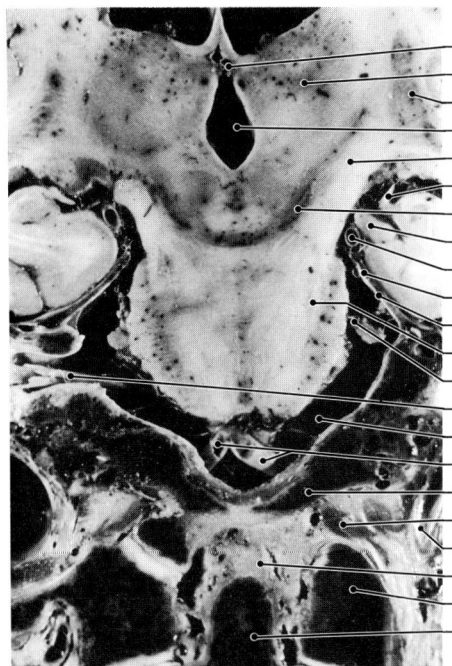

FIG. 3.37.

- Internal cerebral vein
- Thalamus
- Putamen
- Posterior third ventricle
- Cerebral peduncle
- Fimbria
- Substantia nigra
- Uncus
- Posterior cerebral artery
- Superior cerebellar artery
- Tentorium
- Corticospinal tract in pons
- Anterior inferior cerebellar artery
- Internal auditory meatus
- Pontine cistern
- Vertebral arteries
- Clivus
- Longus capitis muscle
- Internal carotid artery
- Apical ligament
- Lateral mass of C1
- Odontoid process

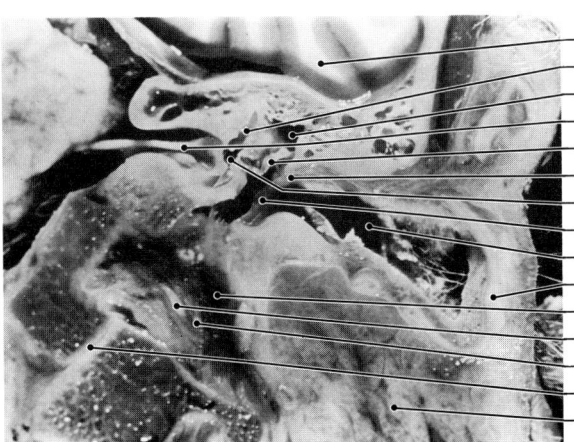

FIG. 3.38.

- Lateral occipitotemporal gyrus
- Semicircular canal
- Aditus ad antrum
- Facial nerve
- Incus
- Scutum
- Sacculus
- Tympanic membrane
- External auditory canal
- Cartilage of ear
- Internal jugular vein
- Ninth cranial nerve
- Tenth cranial nerve
- Atlanto-occipital joint
- Parotid gland

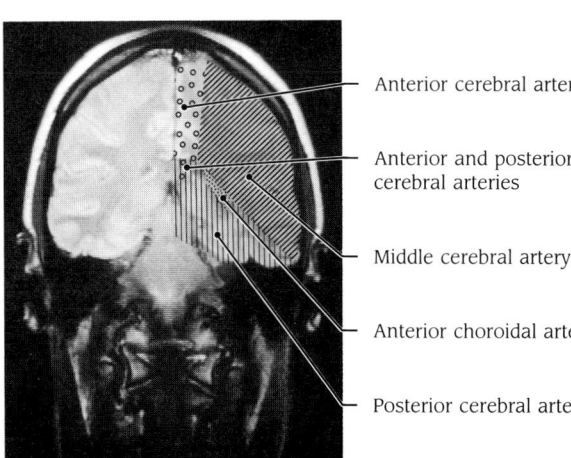

FIG. 3.39. TR = 2000 msec, TE = 28 msec.

- Anterior cerebral artery
- Anterior and posterior cerebral arteries
- Middle cerebral artery
- Anterior choroidal artery
- Posterior cerebral artery

77

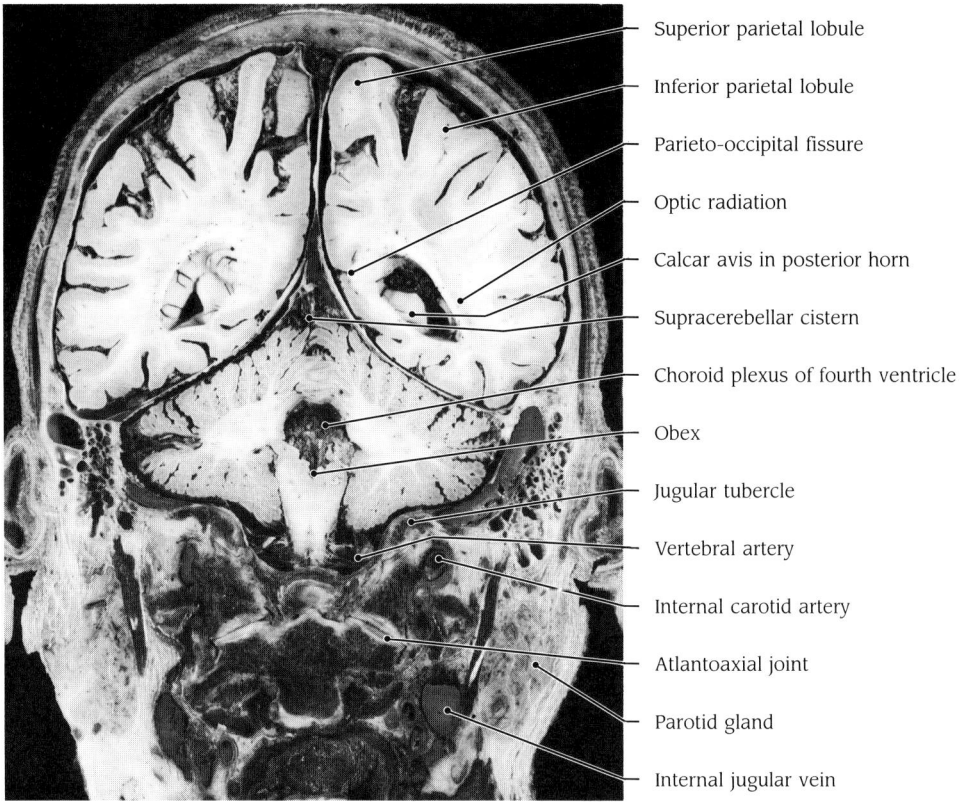
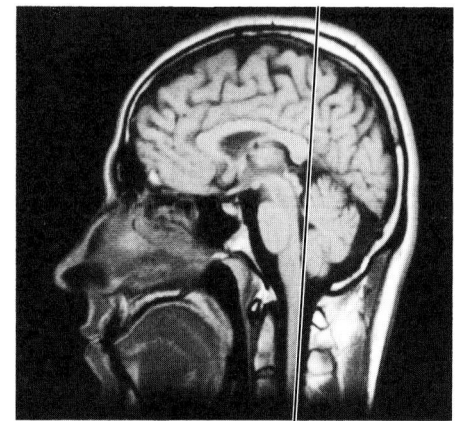

FIG. 3.40.

- The superior cerebellar peduncle (brachium conjunctivum) is the largest cerebellar efferent bundle and is formed by fibers arising from the deep nuclei of the cerebellum. The fiber bundle emerges from the hilus of the dentate nucleus and passes into the upper pons, where it forms a compact bundle along the dorsolateral wall of the fourth ventricle.
- The middle cerebellar peduncle (brachium pontis) is larger than the superior and inferior peduncles; it passes lateral to both of these peduncles as it continues from the dorsolateral region of the pons to become continuous with the white matter of the cerebellar hemisphere. The middle cerebellar peduncle represents the last portion of the extensive corticopontocerebellar pathway.
- The inferior cerebellar peduncle is ill-defined and lies far lateral in the medulla. It is composed of fibers from the spinal cord, the vestibular nuclei, and the inferior olivary nucleus (see Chap. 6).

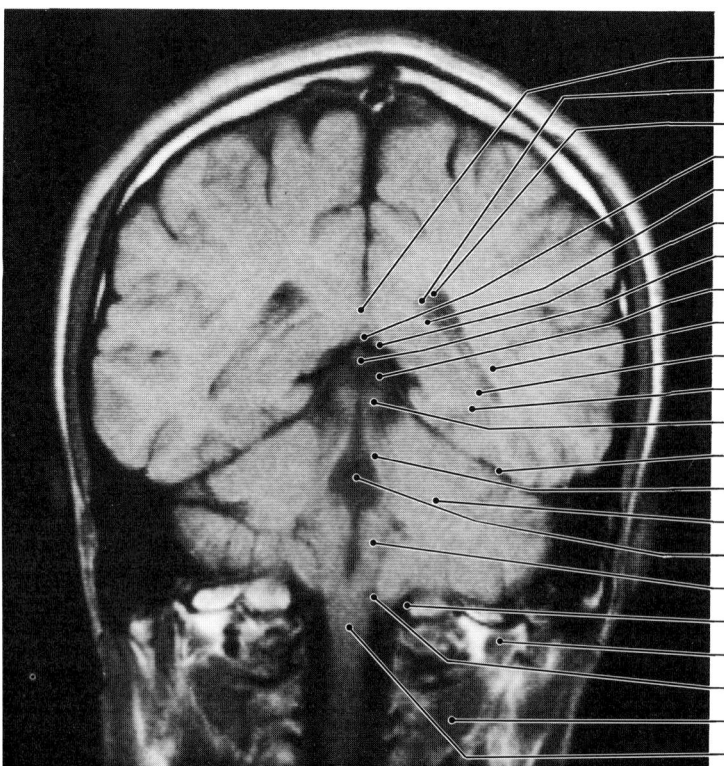

FIG. 3.41. TR = 500 msec, TE = 28 msec.

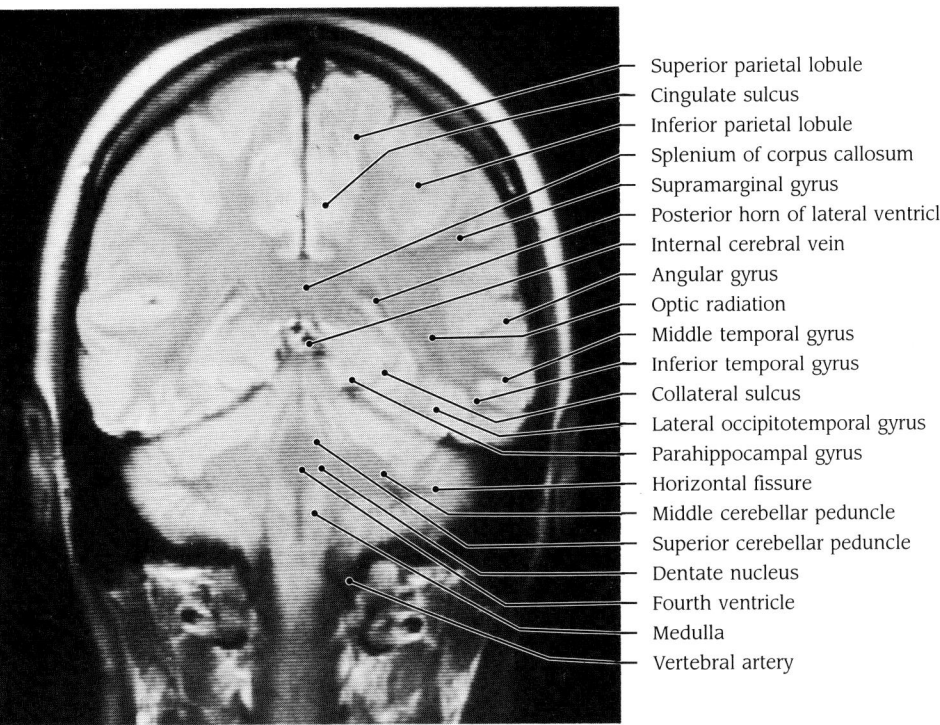

- Superior parietal lobule
- Cingulate sulcus
- Inferior parietal lobule
- Splenium of corpus callosum
- Supramarginal gyrus
- Posterior horn of lateral ventricle
- Internal cerebral vein
- Angular gyrus
- Optic radiation
- Middle temporal gyrus
- Inferior temporal gyrus
- Collateral sulcus
- Lateral occipitotemporal gyrus
- Parahippocampal gyrus
- Horizontal fissure
- Middle cerebellar peduncle
- Superior cerebellar peduncle
- Dentate nucleus
- Fourth ventricle
- Medulla
- Vertebral artery

FIG. 3.42. TR = 2000 msec, TE = 28 msec.

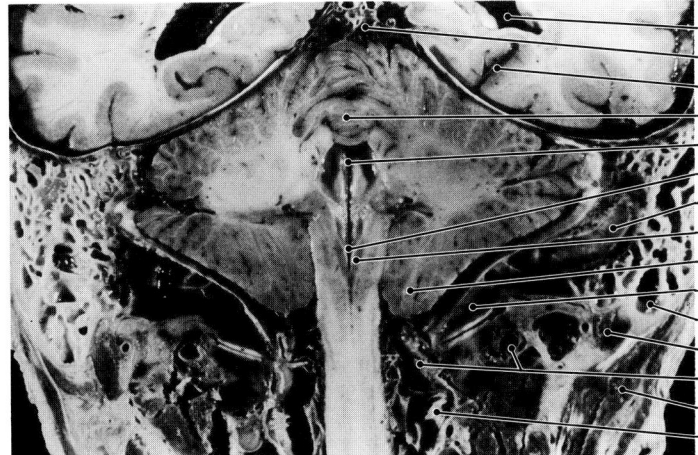

- Lateral ventricle
- Internal cerebral vein
- Collateral sulcus
- Central lobule of vermis
- Fourth ventricle
- Obex
- Sigmoid sinus
- Hypoglossal nucleus
- Tonsil
- Occipital condyle
- Mastoid air cell
- Digastric muscle
- Vertebral artery (twice)
- Sternocleidomastoid muscle
- Rootlets of C2 nerve

FIG. 3.43.

- Anterior cerebral artery
- Middle cerebral artery
- Posterior cerebral and anterior cerebral arteries
- Posterior cerebral artery
- Superior cerebellar artery
- Anterior inferior cerebellar artery
- Posterior inferior cerebellar artery

FIG. 3.44. TR = 2000 msec, TE = 28 msec.

79

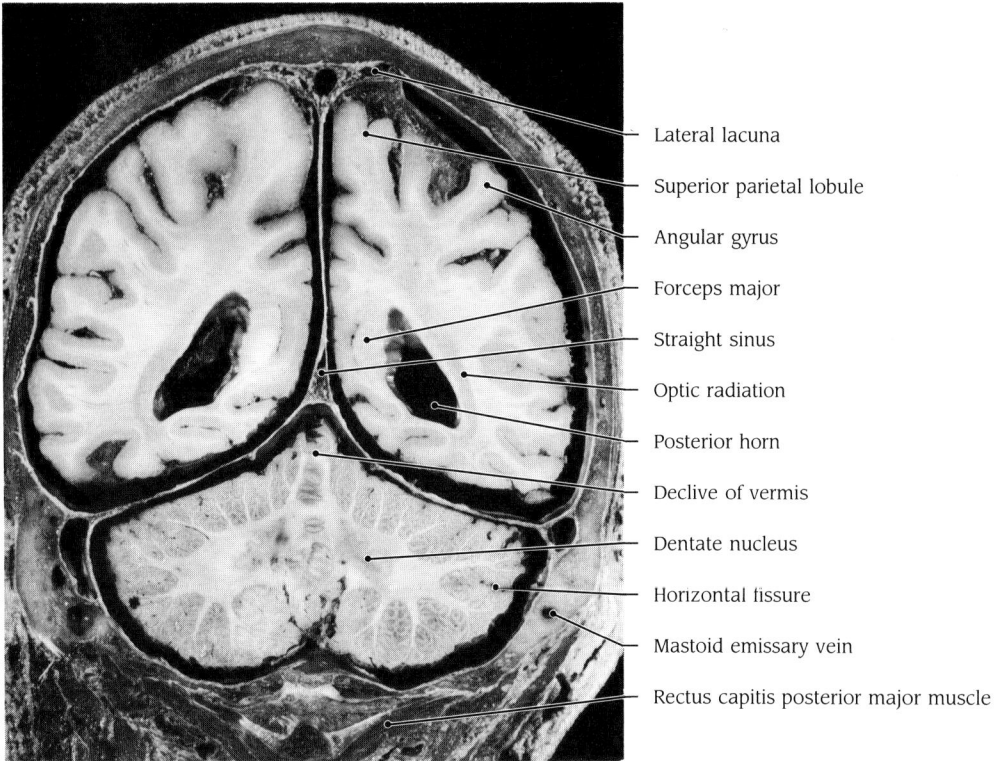

FIG. 3.45.

- The dentate nucleus is located slightly medial to the center of the white matter of the cerebellar hemisphere. Its fibers form a large portion of the superior cerebellar peduncle.

- The optic or geniculocortical radiation is composed of second-order fibers of the visual system. The radiation curves posteriorly and medially to reach the cortex of the occipital lobe. The optic radiation parallels the position of the posterior horn of the lateral ventricle, from which it is separated by the tapetum of the corpus callosum.

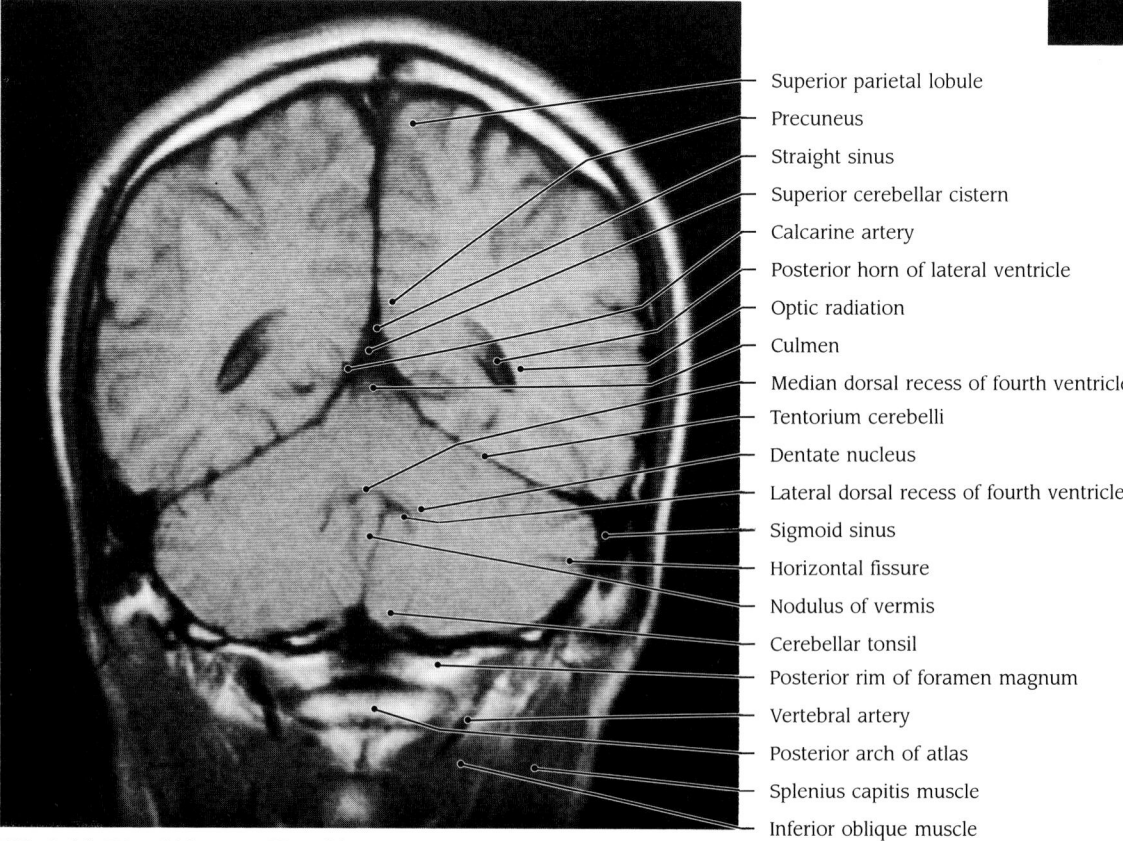

FIG. 3.46. TR = 500 msec, TE = 28 msec.

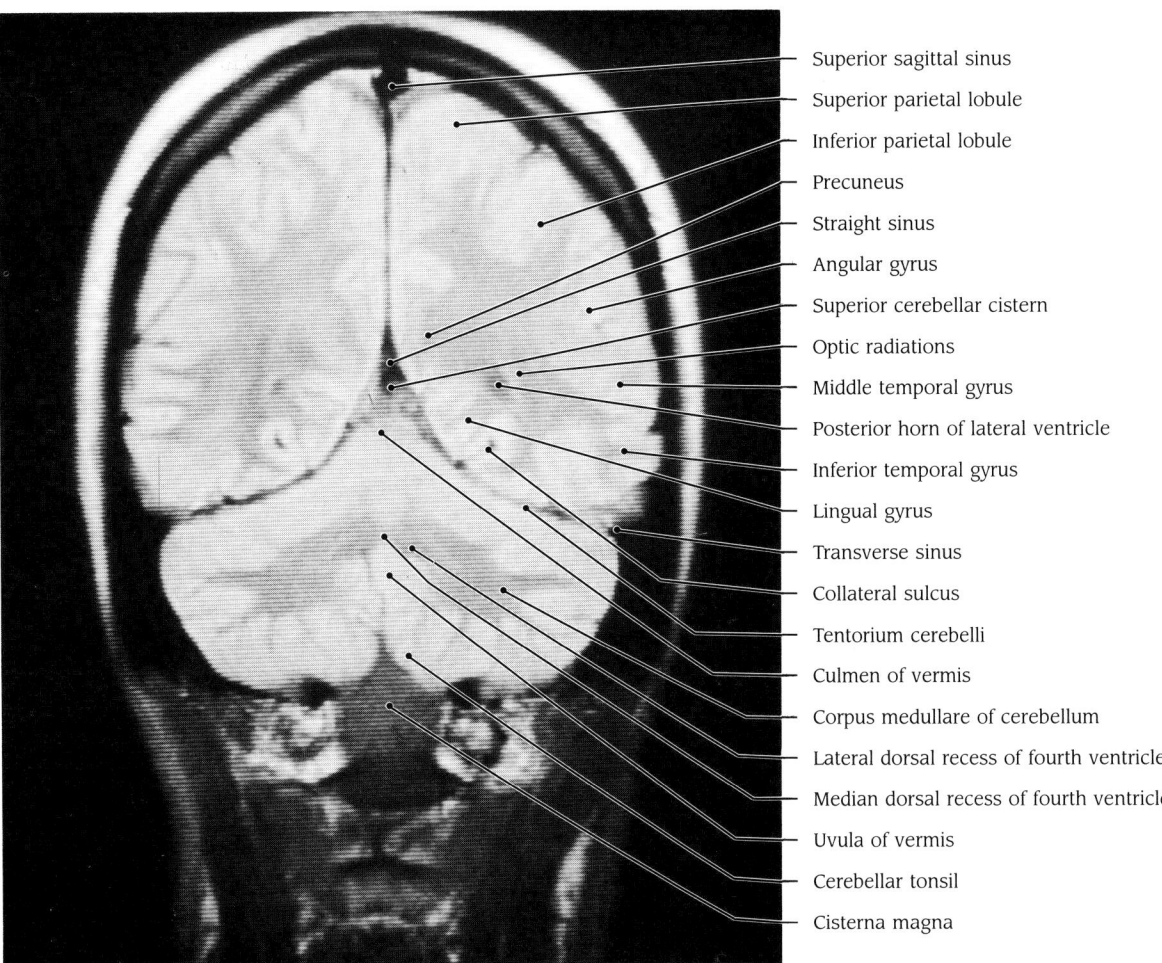

FIG. 3.47. TR = 2000 msec, TE = 28 msec.

- Superior sagittal sinus
- Superior parietal lobule
- Inferior parietal lobule
- Precuneus
- Straight sinus
- Angular gyrus
- Superior cerebellar cistern
- Optic radiations
- Middle temporal gyrus
- Posterior horn of lateral ventricle
- Inferior temporal gyrus
- Lingual gyrus
- Transverse sinus
- Collateral sulcus
- Tentorium cerebelli
- Culmen of vermis
- Corpus medullare of cerebellum
- Lateral dorsal recess of fourth ventricle
- Median dorsal recess of fourth ventricle
- Uvula of vermis
- Cerebellar tonsil
- Cisterna magna

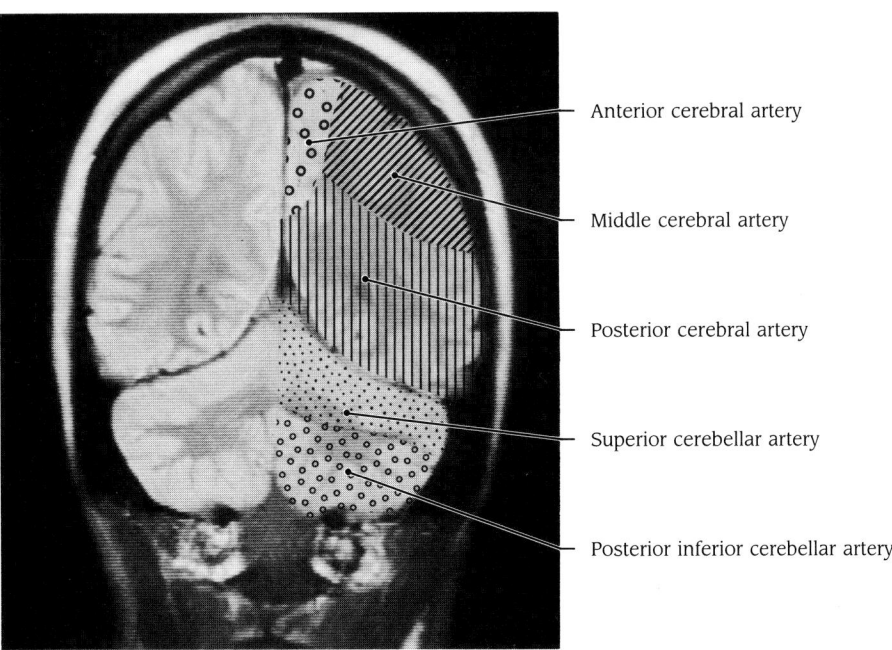

FIG. 3.48. TR = 2000 msec, TE = 28 msec.

- Anterior cerebral artery
- Middle cerebral artery
- Posterior cerebral artery
- Superior cerebellar artery
- Posterior inferior cerebellar artery

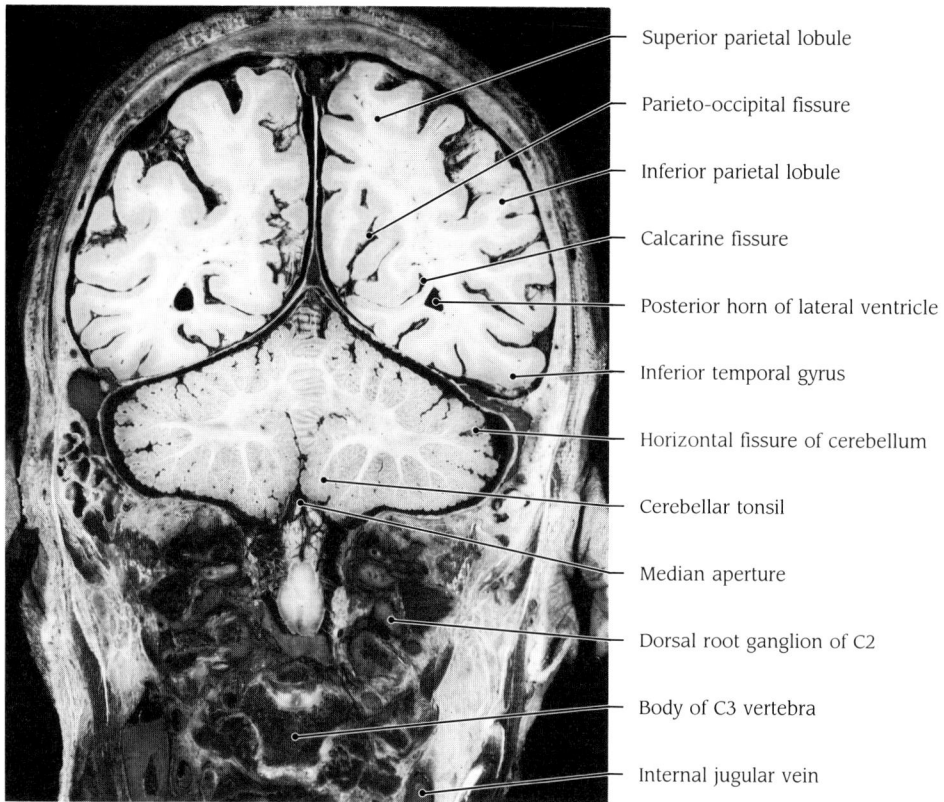

FIG. 3.49.

- The fourth ventricle communicates with the cisterna magna through three apertures: two small lateral (foramen of Luschka) and one variable median (foramen of Magendie). The median aperture lies between the cerebellar tonsils and is just posterior to the medulla.
- The parieto-occipital and calcarine fissures are extensions of a common groove, the anterior parieto-occipital fissure, which extends anteriorly to the coronal plane of the splenium.
- The posterior horns have a variable caudad extent; often, the horn in one hemisphere is longer and larger than that in the other hemisphere. There is no proven relationship between the side of the longer horn and hemispheric dominance.
- The straight sinus is in the junction of the falx cerebri and the tentorium cerebelli. It drains the inferior sagittal sinus, some of the superior cerebellar veins, and the great cerebral vein.

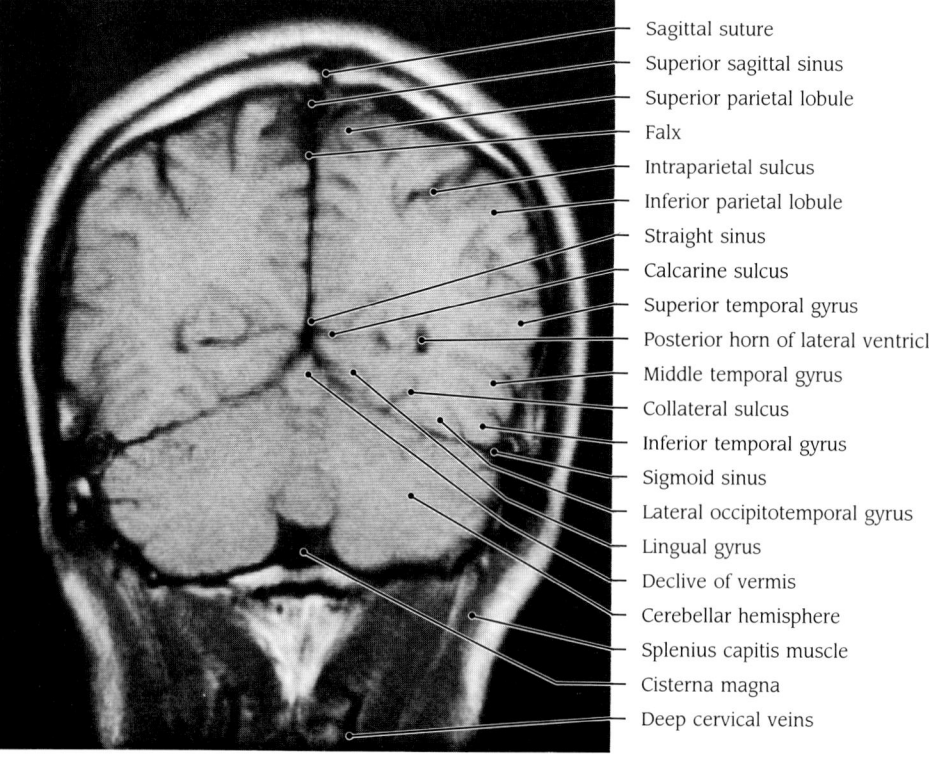

FIG. 3.50. TR = 500 msec, TE = 28 msec.

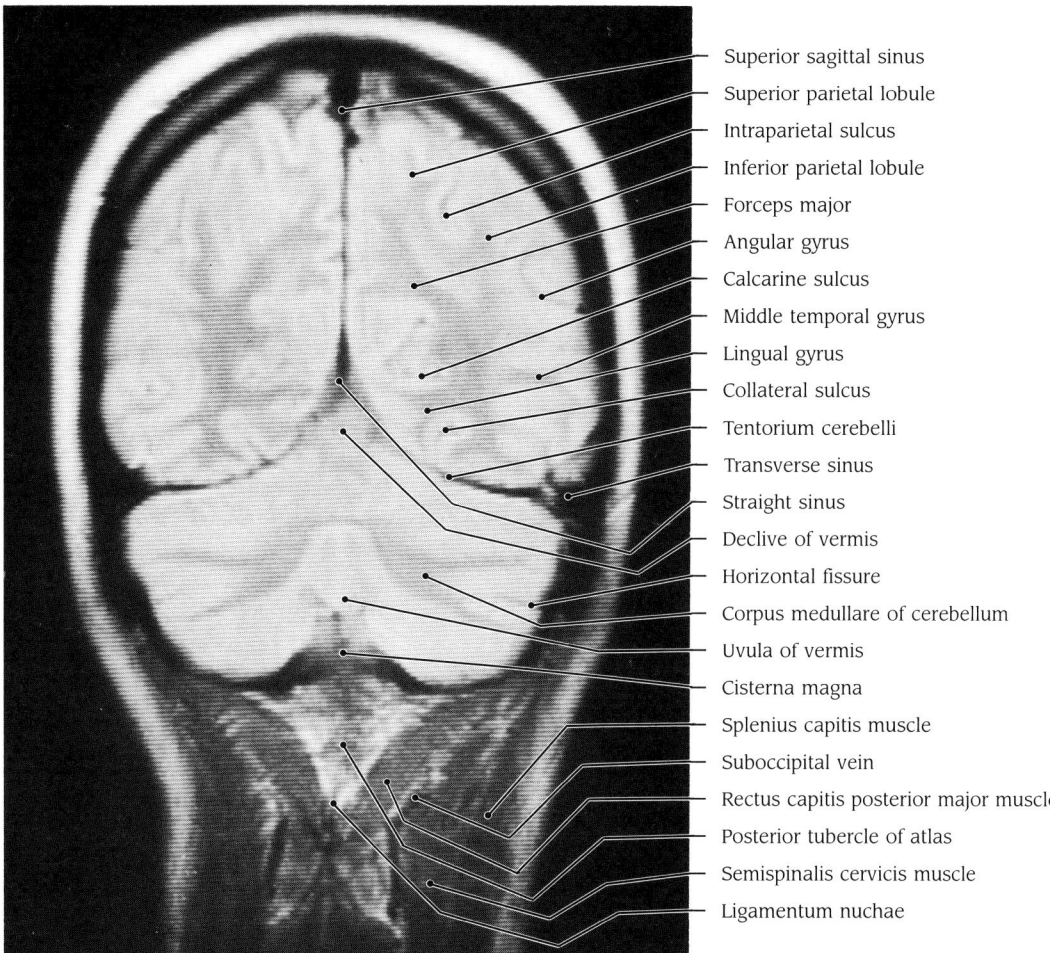

FIG. 3.51. TR = 2000 msec, TE = 28 msec.

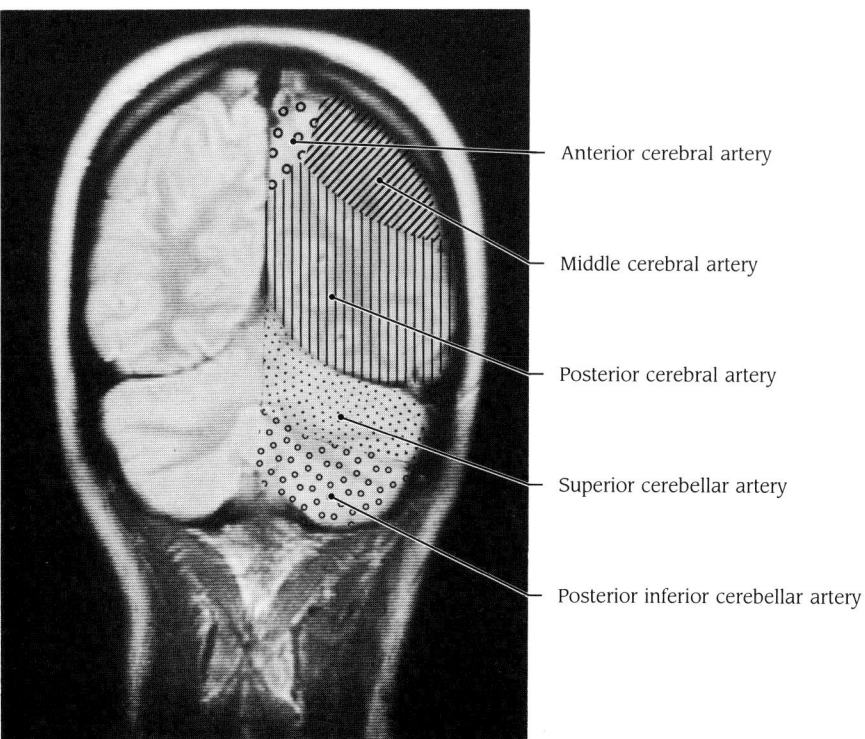

FIG. 3.52. TR = 2000 msec, TE = 28 msec.

83

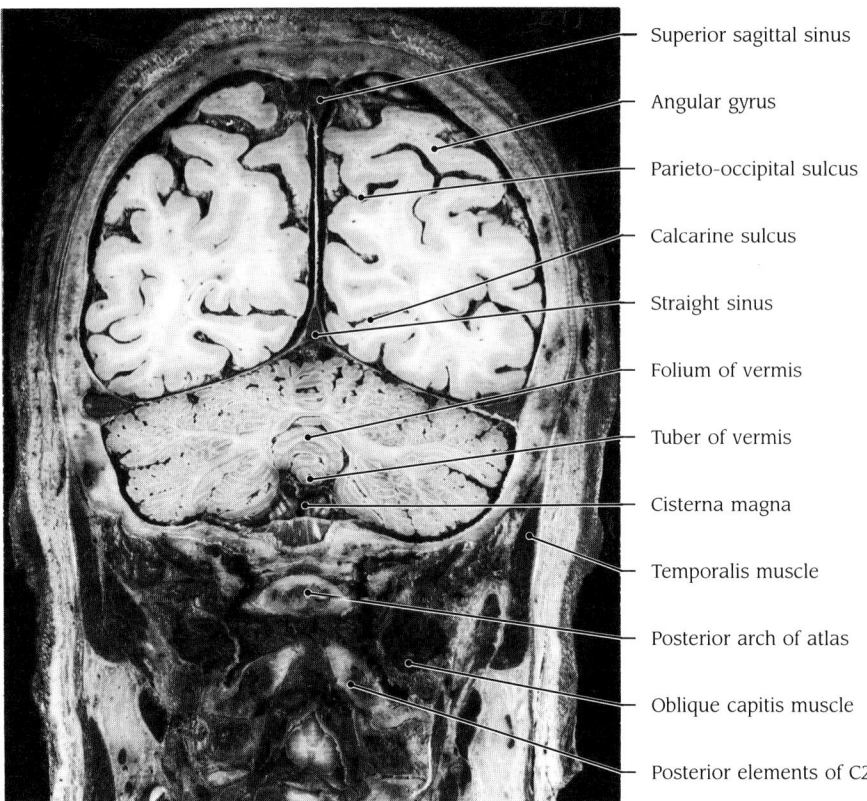
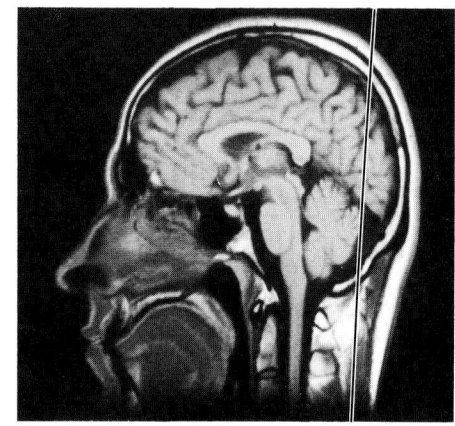

FIG. 3.53.

- The cisterna magna extends along the posterior aspect of the cerebellum to continue upward as the superior cerebellar cistern; the line separating these cisterns is variable and may be located quite far superiorly.
- The calcarine sulcus is an extensive, deep cleft with several side fissures; the total area of the cortical surface reflects the large extent of the primary visual cortex in man.

- The superior sagittal sinus communicates with irregularly shaped venous lacunae that are located in the dura mater. Three lacunae usually are on each side of the sinus: a small frontal, a large parietal, and an intermediate occipital. These lacunae tend to become continuous in elderly subjects as a long lacuna on either side.

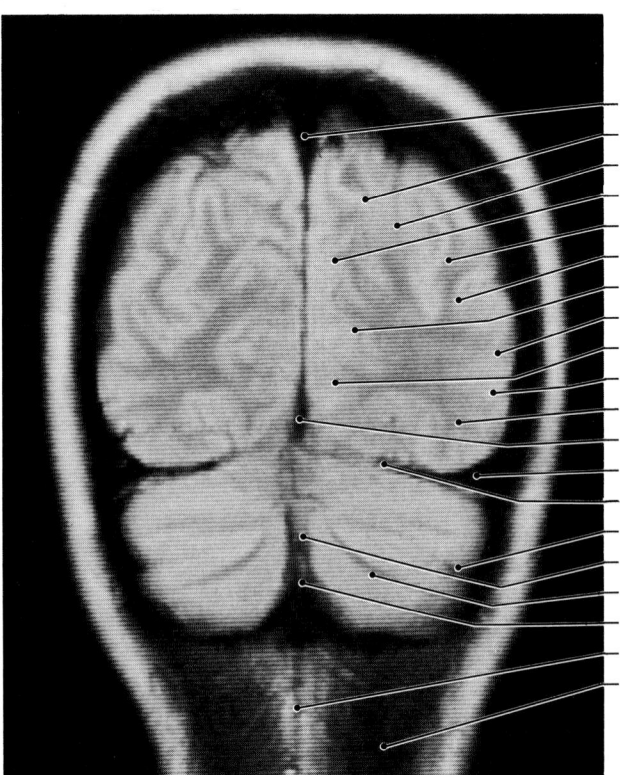

FIG. 3.54. TR = 2000 msec, TE = 28 msec.

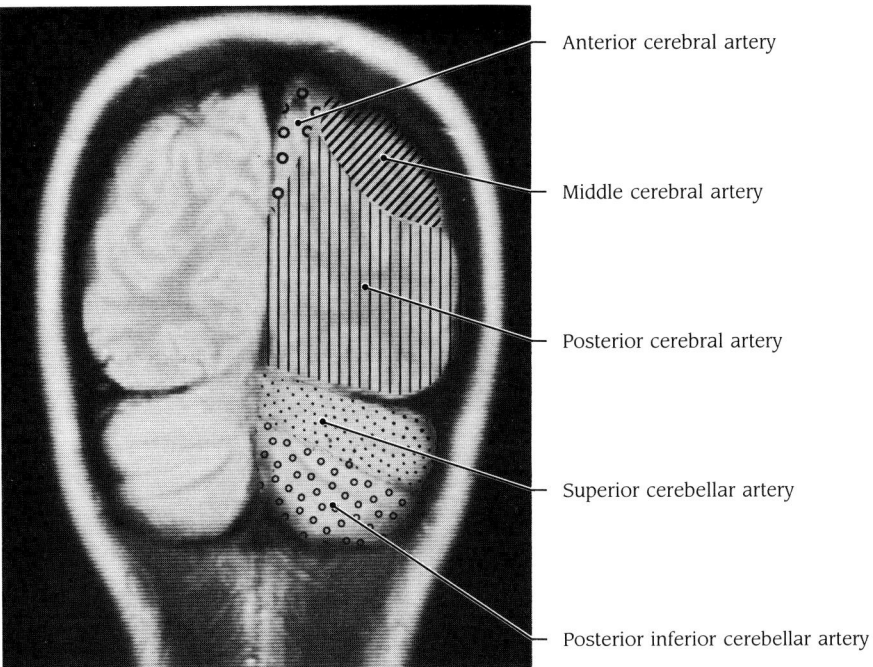

FIG. 3.55. TR = 2000 msec, TE = 28 msec.

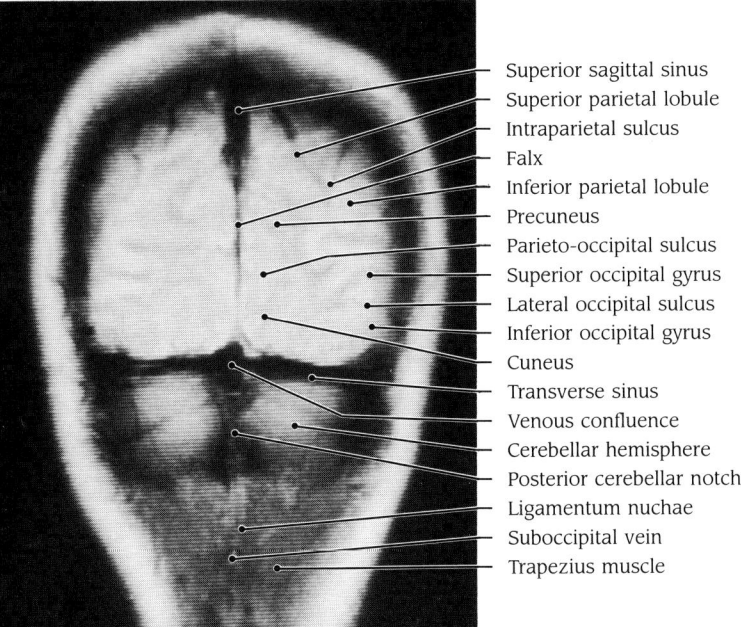

FIG. 3.56. TR = 2000 msec, TE = 28 msec.

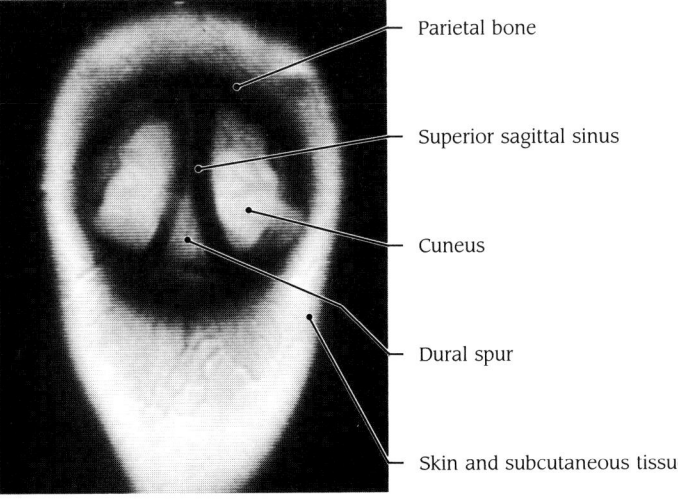

FIG. 3.57. TR = 2000 msec, TE = 28 msec.

4

Head, Sagittal Plane

Anatomic Level	Figures
Brainstem	4.1–4.13
Fifth cranial nerve; temporal pole	4.14–4.17
Internal auditory meatus; trigone	4.18–4.21
Lateral extent of basal ganglia	4.22–4.25
Insula	4.26–4.33
Superficial hemisphere	4.34–4.39

A series of cadaveric sagittal sections that extend from the midline through the temporal lobe are shown. These sections are matched with sagittal magnetic resonance images of normal volunteers. The planes of the short and long repetition time images are not identical because of slight differences both in the shape of the brain and in positioning. The locator image chosen is approximately through the center of both the long and short repetition time images. Vascular territories are indicated by overlays on a companion image.

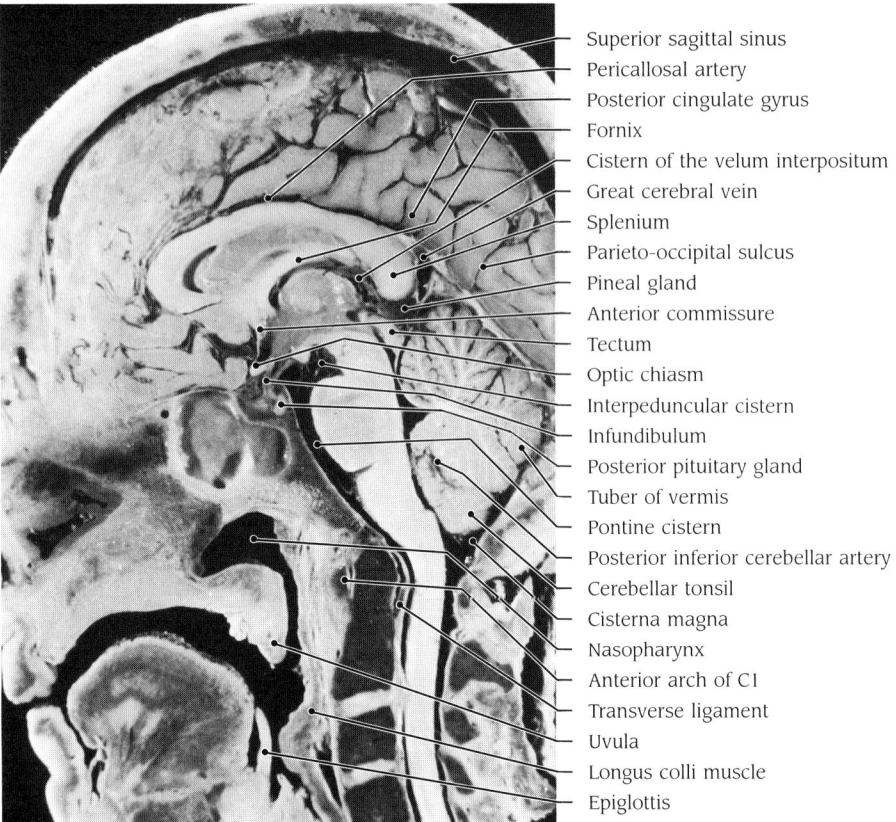
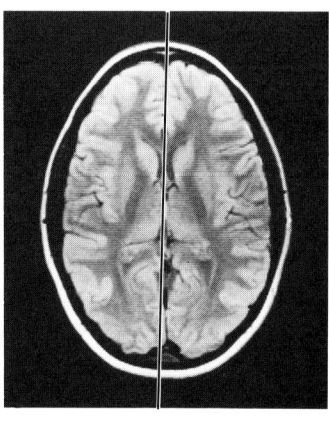

FIG. 4.1.

- The angle between the brainstem and the upper cervical cord is variable, depending on the position of the head during imaging or postmortem fixation.

- The midbrain, or mesencephalon, is the shortest segment of the brainstem, not more than 2 cm in length. It connects the pons and the cerebellum with the forebrain. The midbrain is divided into right and left halves, the cerebral peduncles, each of which is subdivided by the substantia nigra into the ventral crus cerebri and the dorsal tegmental portion. The portion of the tegmentum posterior to the cerebral aqueduct is called the tectum, which comprises the colliculi.

- The colliculi, or corpora quadrigemina, are four rounded eminences that are arranged in superior and inferior pairs and are separated from one another by a cruciform sulcus. The superior colliculi are larger and constitute centers for visual reflexes. The inferior colliculi are somewhat more prominent than the superior colliculi, although they are smaller. The inferior colliculi are associated with the auditory pathway and reflexes.

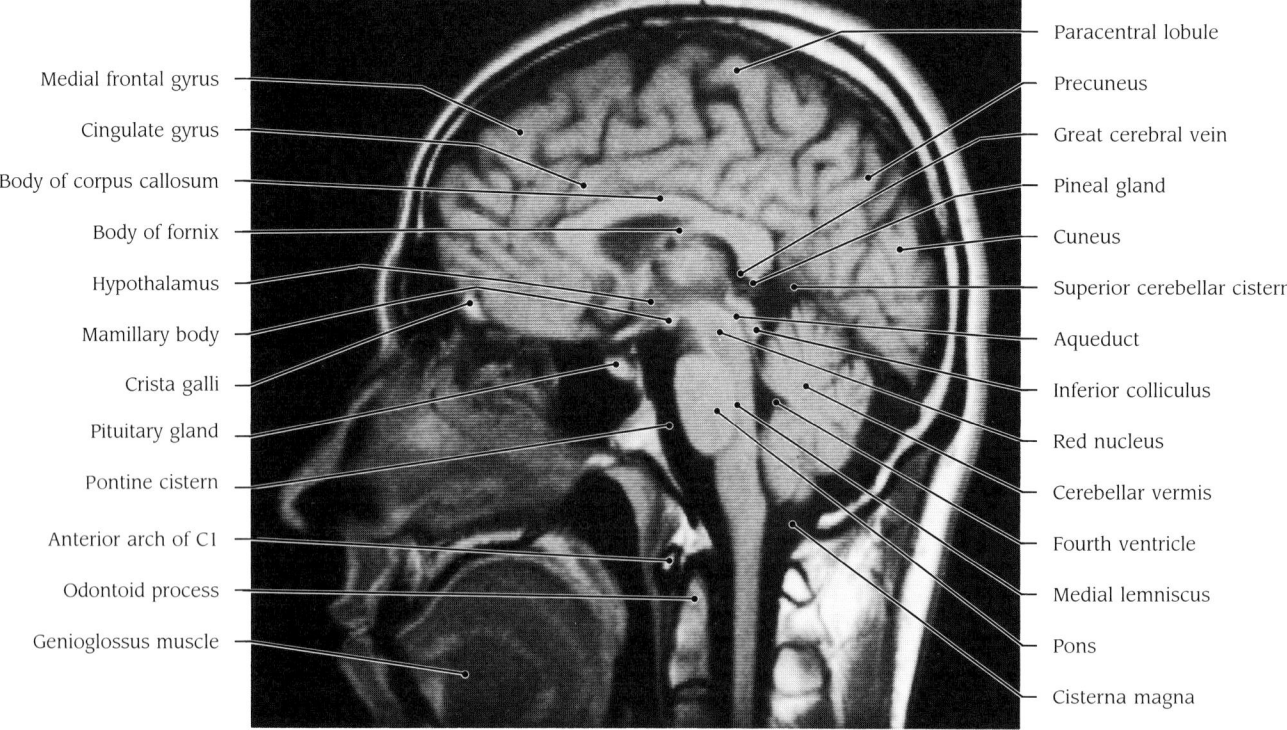

FIG. 4.2. TR = 500 msec, TE = 28 msec.

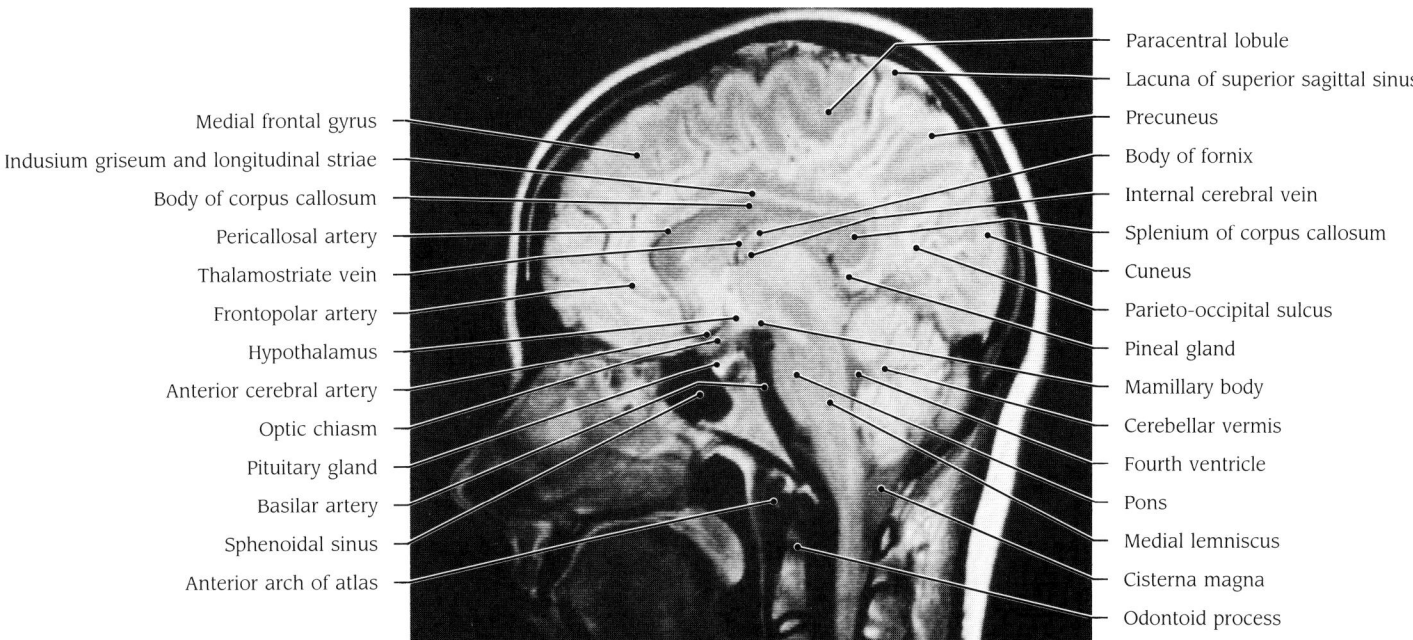

FIG. 4.3. TR = 2000 msec, TE = 28 msec.

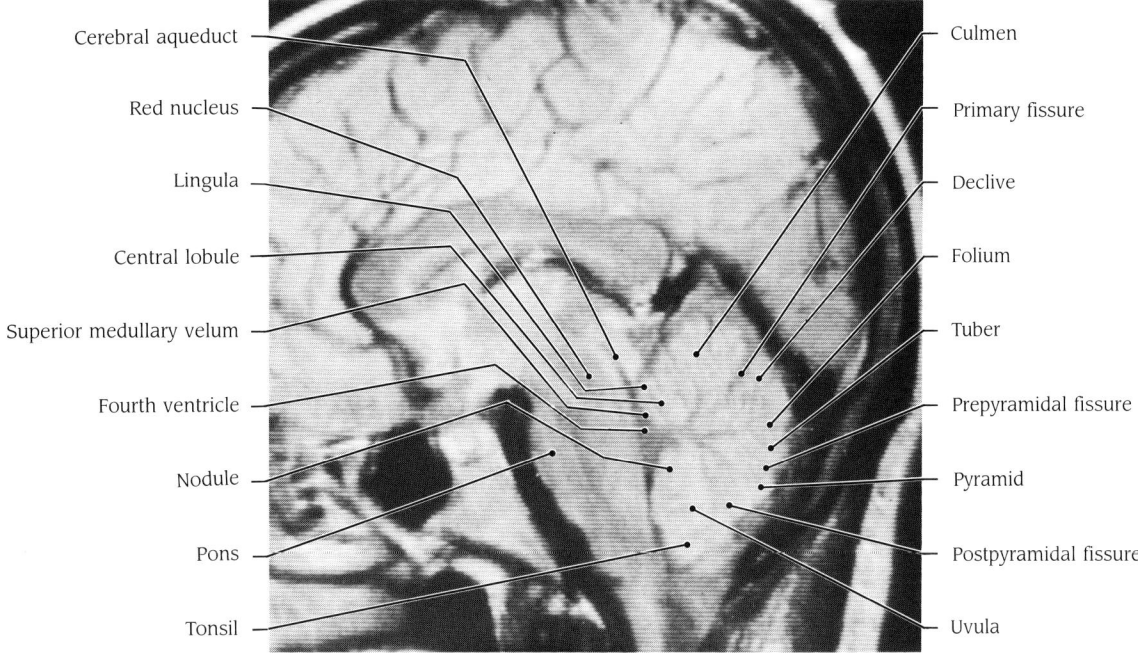

FIG. 4.4. TR = 2000 msec, TE = 28 msec.

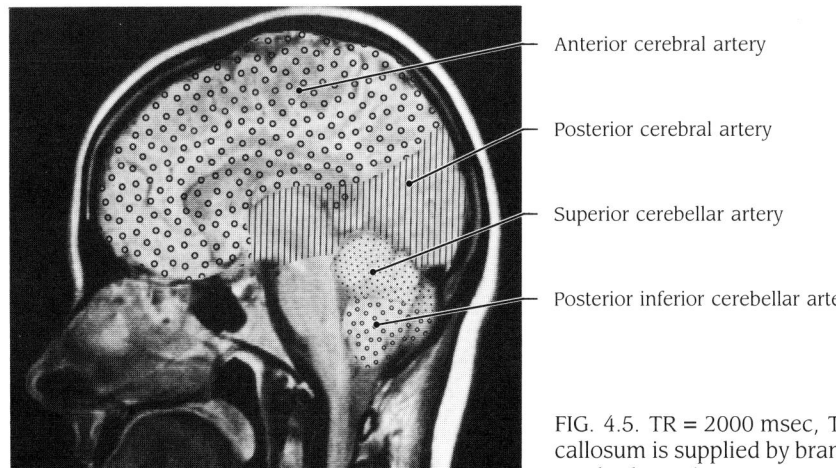

FIG. 4.5. TR = 2000 msec, TE = 28 msec. The splenium of the corpus callosum is supplied by branches of both the anterior and the posterior cerebral arteries.

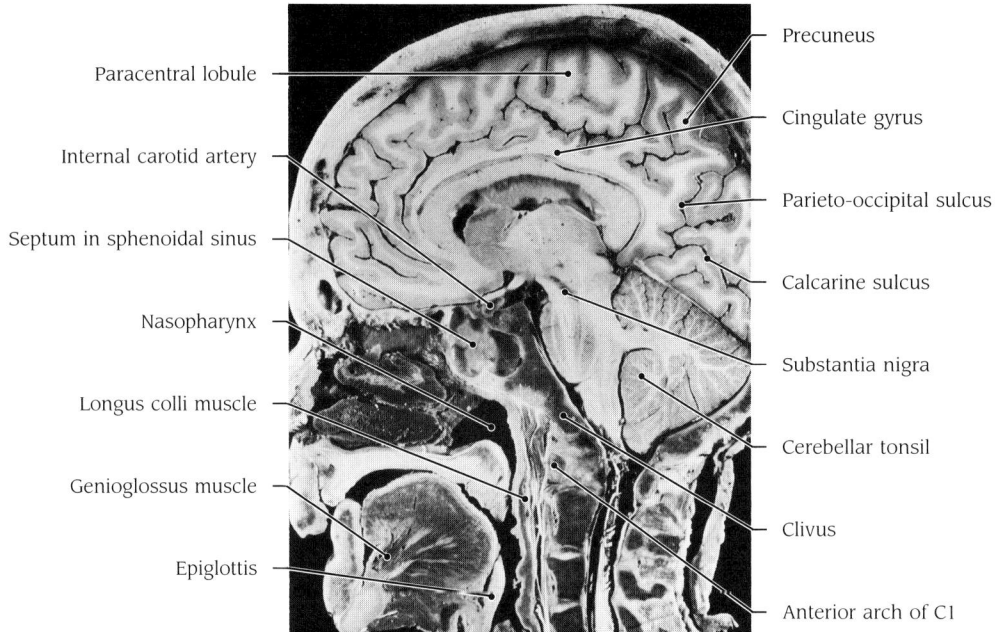
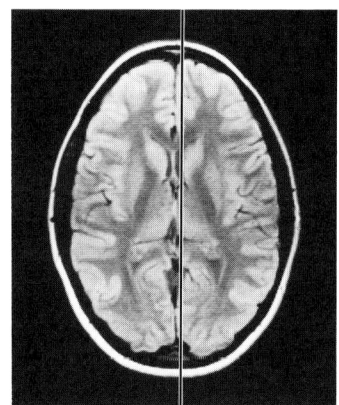

FIG. 4.6.

- The thalamus is divided into several major portions, each of which is further subdivided into several nuclei. The metathalamus is composed of the medial and lateral geniculate bodies and their named nuclei. The epithalamus includes the habenular nuclei and their commissure, the posterior commissure, and the pineal. The hypothalamus is comprised of the mamillary bodies, the tuber cinereum, the infundibulum, and the tissue adjacent to the optic chiasm. The preoptic region, although a telencephalic structure, is generally included in descriptions of the hypothalamus for functional purposes. The ventral thalamus, or subthalamus, includes the superior extensions of the red nucleus and substantia nigra, the prerubral field, the zona incerta, the subthalamic nucleus, and their associated nuclei and fiber tracts.

- The parieto-occipital and calcarine sulci are two deep sulci located in the posterior aspect of the medial hemisphere. These sulci converge anteriorly just posterior to the splenium of the corpus callosum. The anatomic variation in the angle between the parieto-occipital and calcarine sulci is considerable, although in this group of figures, little variability is shown. These sulci are separated by the cuneate gyrus.

- The precuneus, or quadrilateral area, is delimited anteriorly by the cingulate sulcus, posteriorly by the parieto-occipital sulcus, and inferiorly by the suprasplenial sulcus. The precuneus and the paracentral lobule form the medial surface of the parietal lobe.

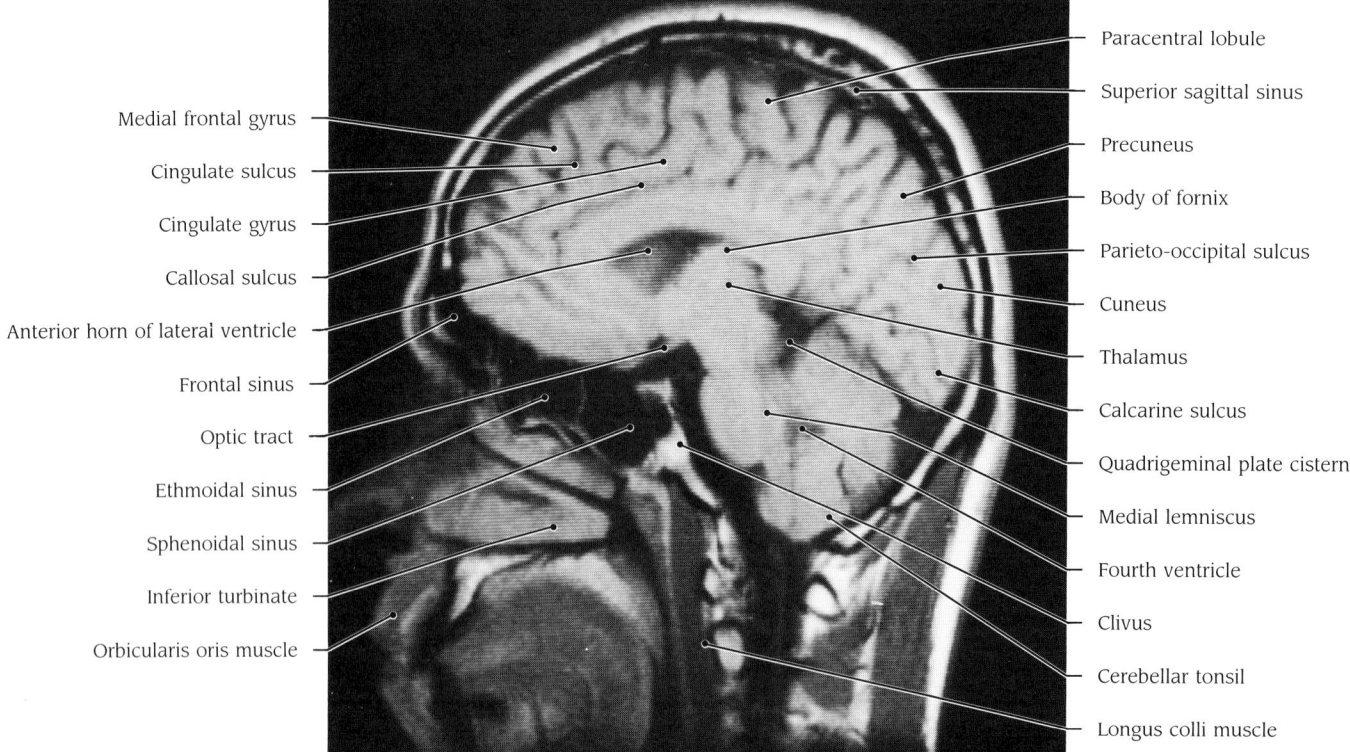

FIG. 4.7. TR = 500 msec, TE = 28 msec.

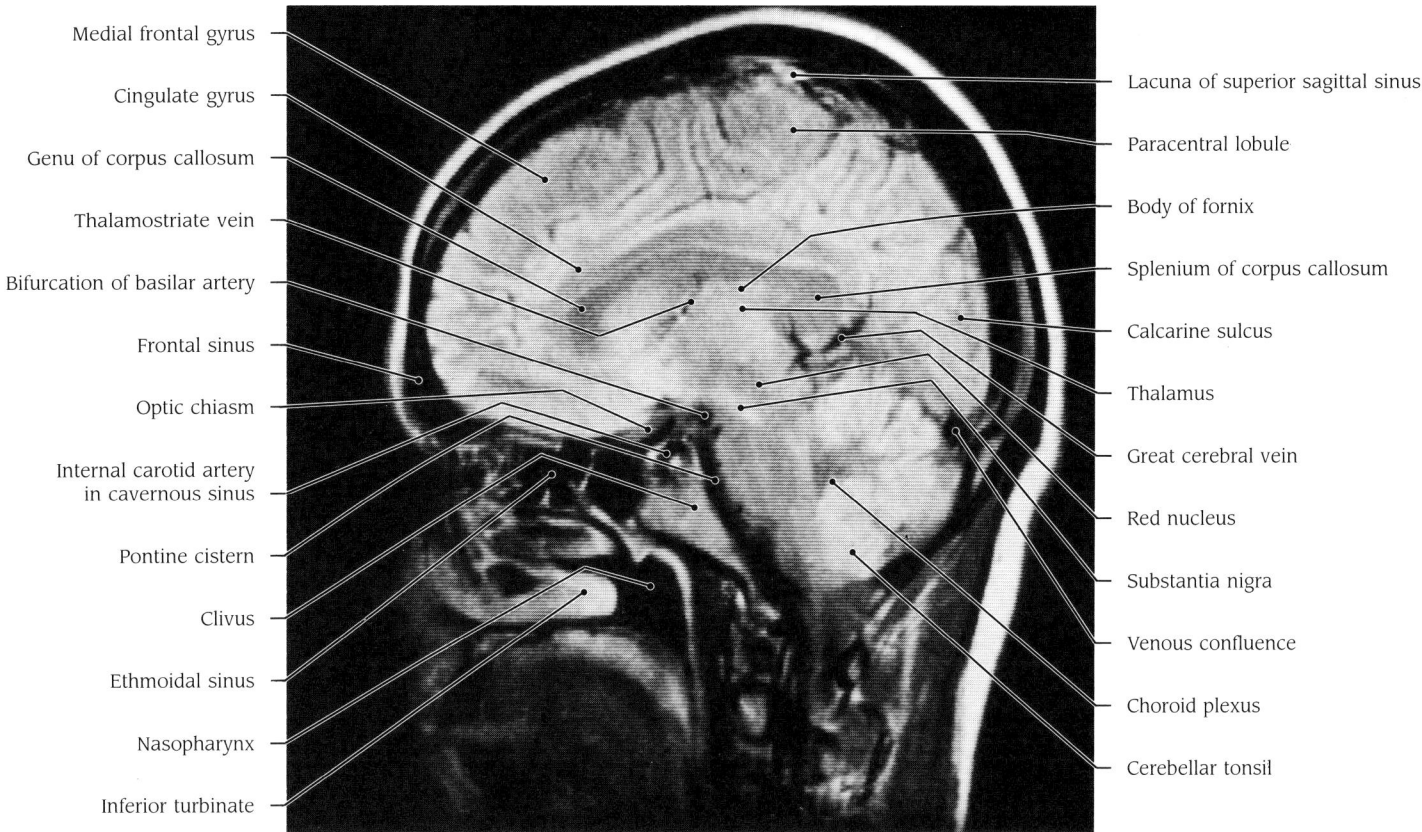

FIG. 4.8. TR = 2000 msec, TE = 28 msec.

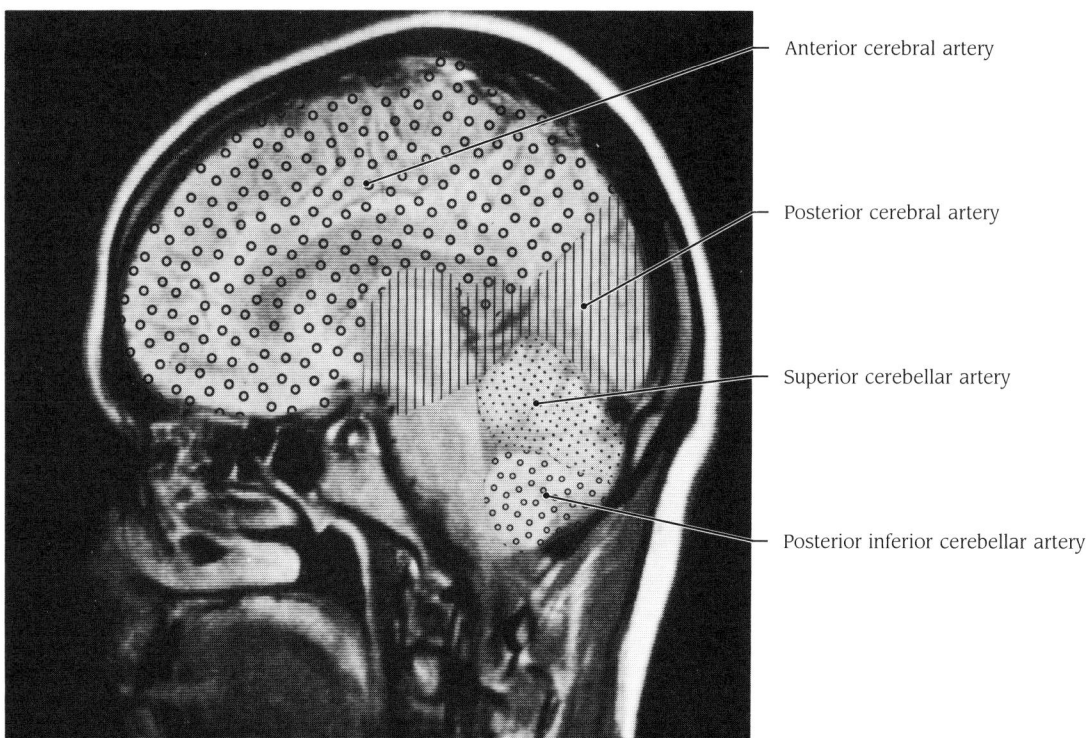

FIG. 4.9. TR = 2000 msec, TE = 28 msec. The splenium of the corpus callosum is supplied by branches of both the anterior and the posterior cerebral arteries.

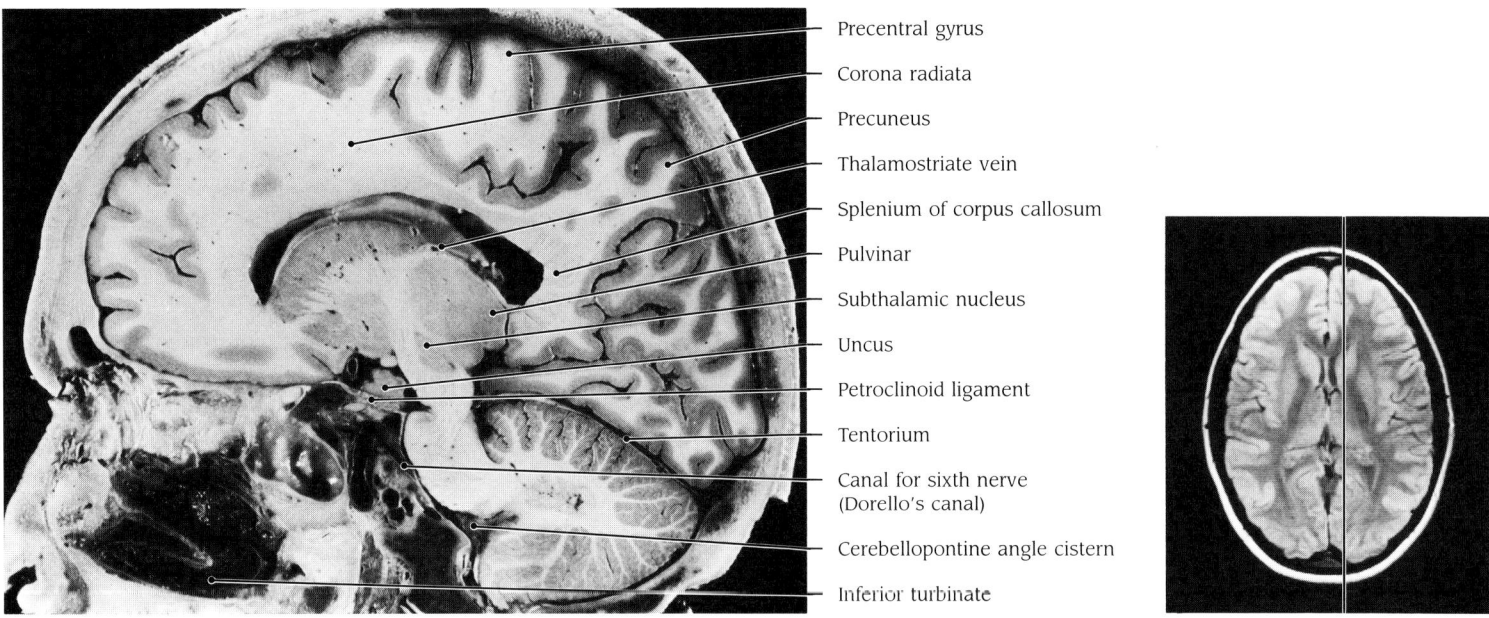

FIG. 4.10.

- The lingual gyrus is located between the calcarine and collateral sulci. It extends anteriorly and becomes the parahippocampal gyrus at the isthmus, which connects the cingulate gyrus with the parahippocampal gyrus. Anteriorly, the parahippocampal gyrus is continuous with the uncus. The uncus forms a portion of the piriform lobe, part of the olfactory system.

- The piriform lobe is composed of: (1) the prepiriform cortex, which is formed by the lateral olfactory gyrus and its continuation, the gyrus ambiens; (2) the uncus hippocampi, which includes the uncinate gyrus, the tail of the dentate gyrus or band of Giacomini, and the intralimbic gyrus; (3) the periamygdaloid area, which is comprised of the lateral olfactory stria and the gyrus semilunaris; and (4) the entorhinal area, a part of the parahippocampal gyrus.

- The nerve fibers composing the corpus callosum extend bilaterally into the white matter of the hemispheres. The fibers from the rostrum extend laterally, coursing inferior to the anterior horns of the lateral ventricles to join the orbital portions of the frontal lobes. The fibers from the genu extend anteriorly as the forceps minor to connect the medial and lateral parts of the frontal lobes. The fibers of the body of the corpus callosum extend laterally into the projection fibers of the corona radiata to join cortical areas of both hemispheres. Some of the fibers of the body and splenium of the corpus callosum form the tapetum, which borders portions of the posterior and inferior horns of the lateral ventricle. The forceps major is formed by the posterior and medial extension of the remaining fibers from the splenium into the occipital lobes.

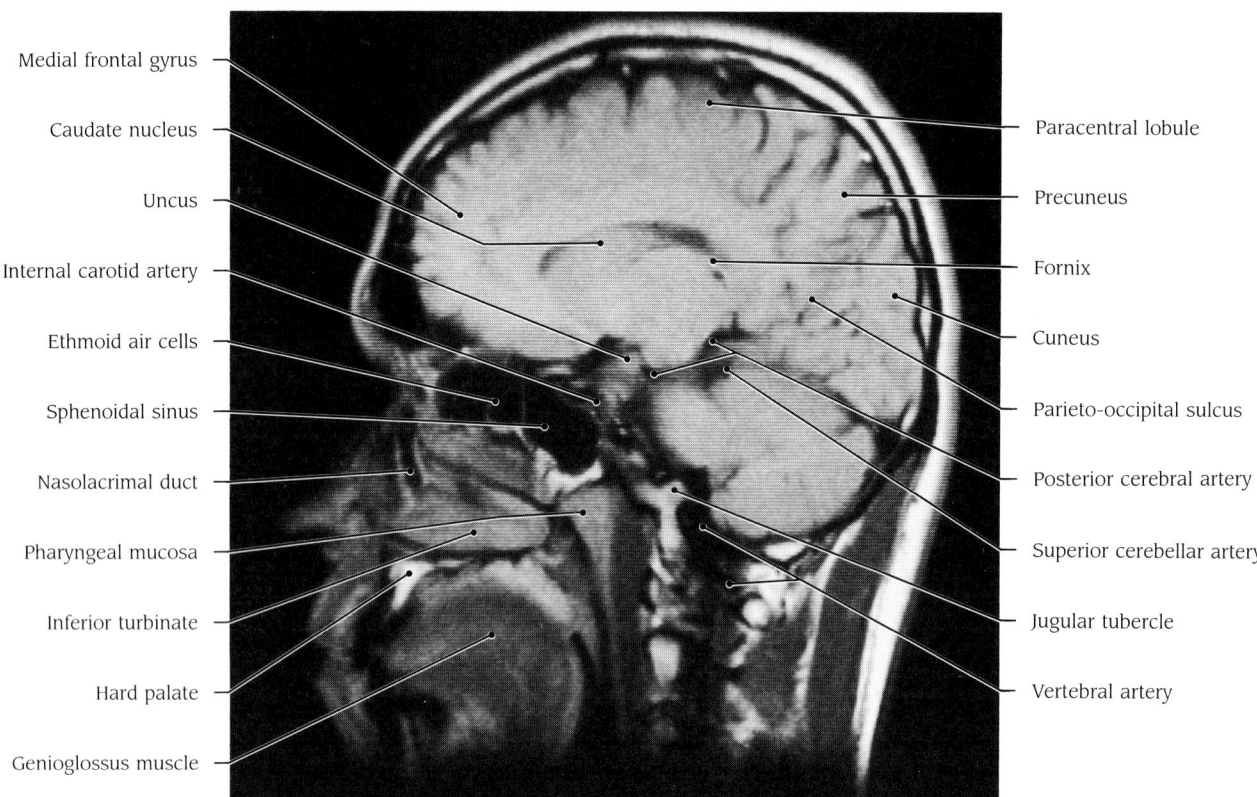

FIG. 4.11. TR = 500 msec, TE = 28 msec.

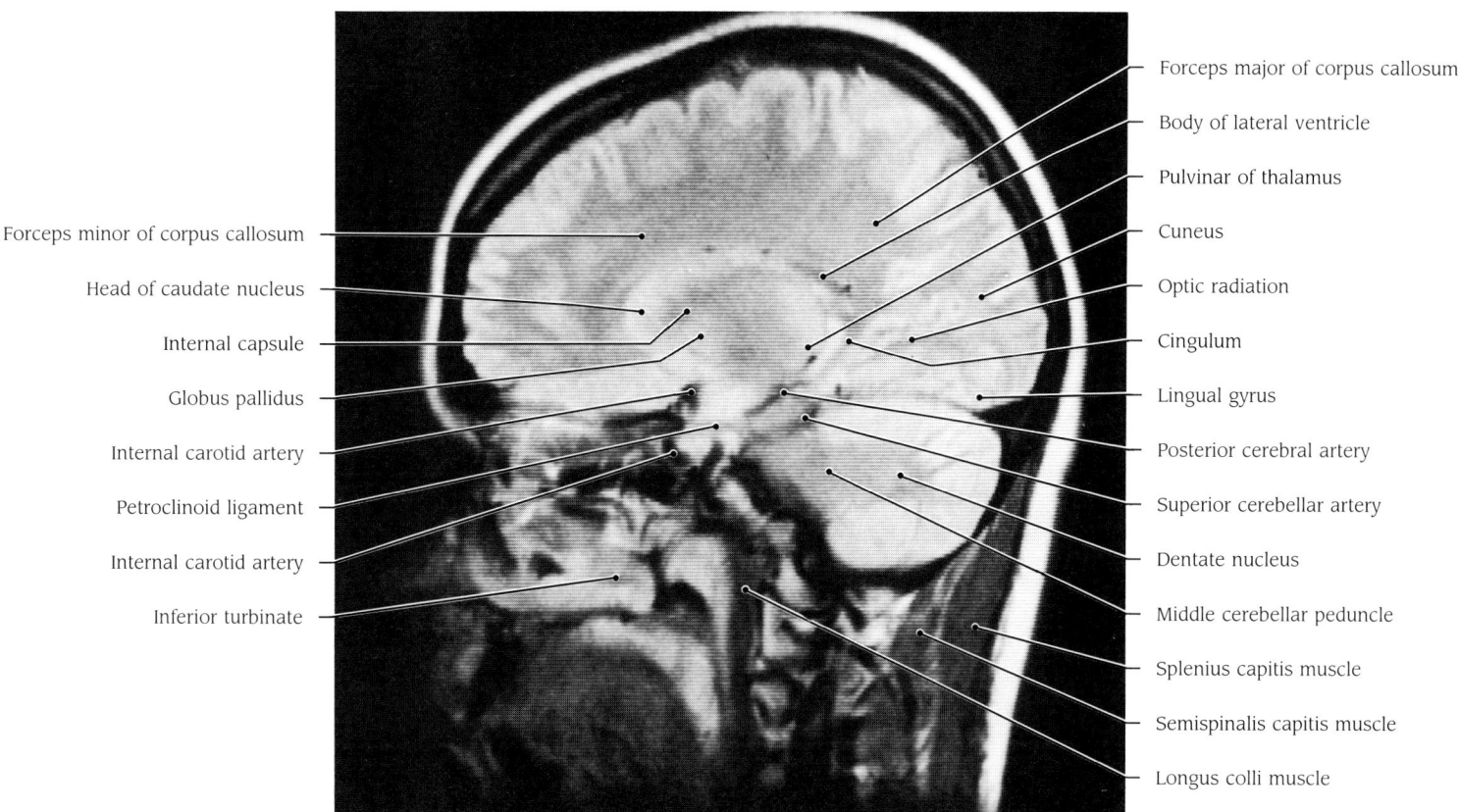

FIG. 4.12. TR = 2000 msec, TE = 28 msec.

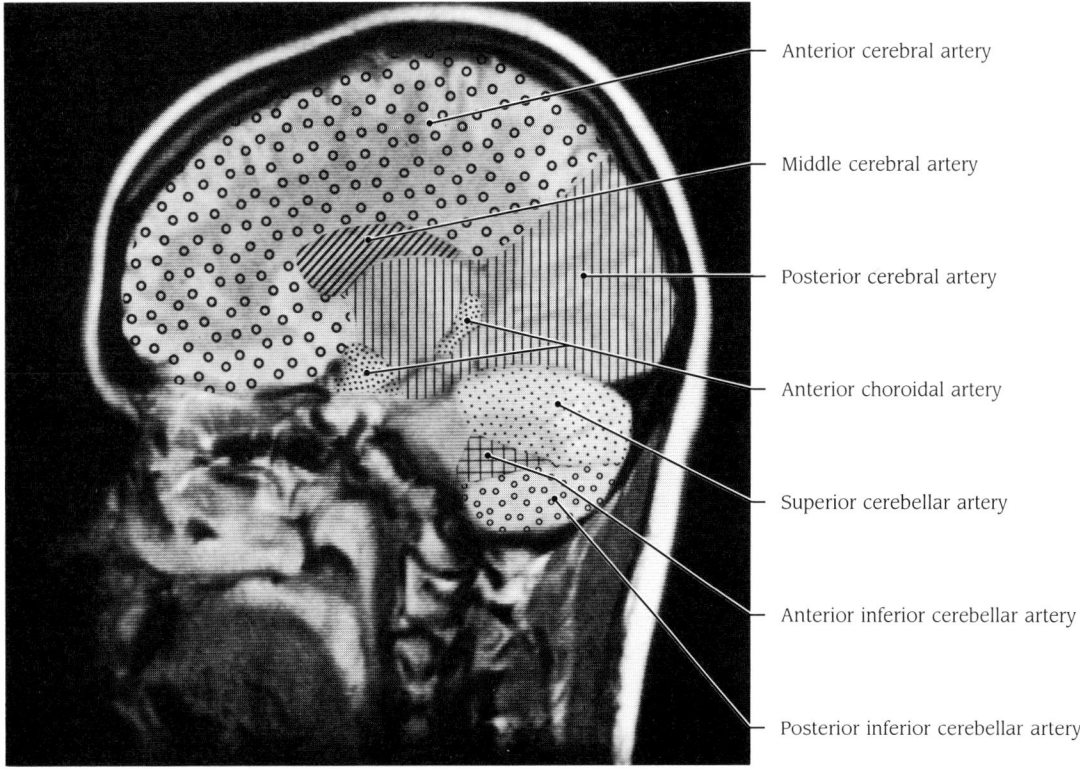

FIG. 4.13. TR = 2000 msec, TE = 28 msec.

93

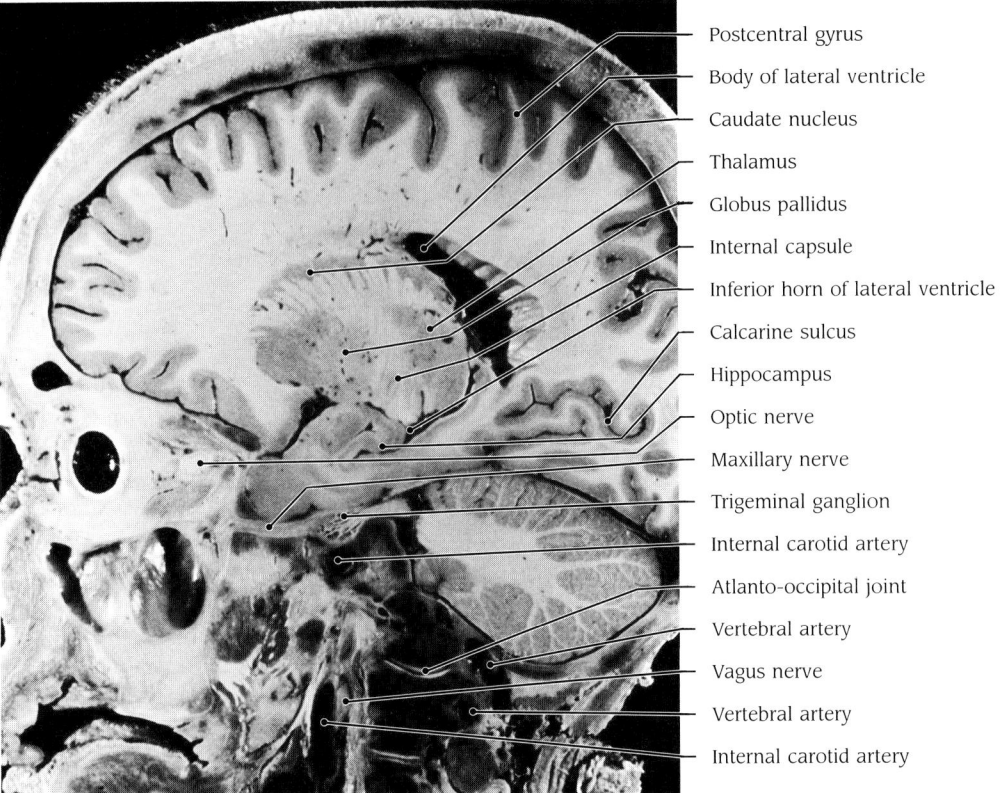
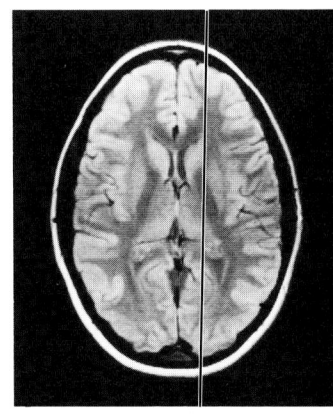

FIG. 4.14.

- The basal nuclei, often referred to as the basal ganglia, are a series of subcortical nuclear masses of gray matter. The structures included in the term, basal nuclei, vary between investigators; however, most commonly, the amygdaloid complex, the claustrum, the caudate nucleus, and the lentiform nucleus are considered to be components. The corpus striatum refers to the caudate nucleus and the lentiform nucleus. The striatum, or neostriatum, refers to the caudate nucleus and putamen; the name reflects the striations made by strands of gray matter that connect these two nuclei, which are separated by fiber bundles of the internal capsule.

- The fibers comprising the optic radiation arise in the lateral geniculate body. These fibers continue posteriorly adjacent to the superior and lateral aspects of the inferior horn and the lateral surface of the posterior horn of the lateral ventricle. The tapetum is interposed between the optic radiation and the posterior horn of the lateral ventricle.

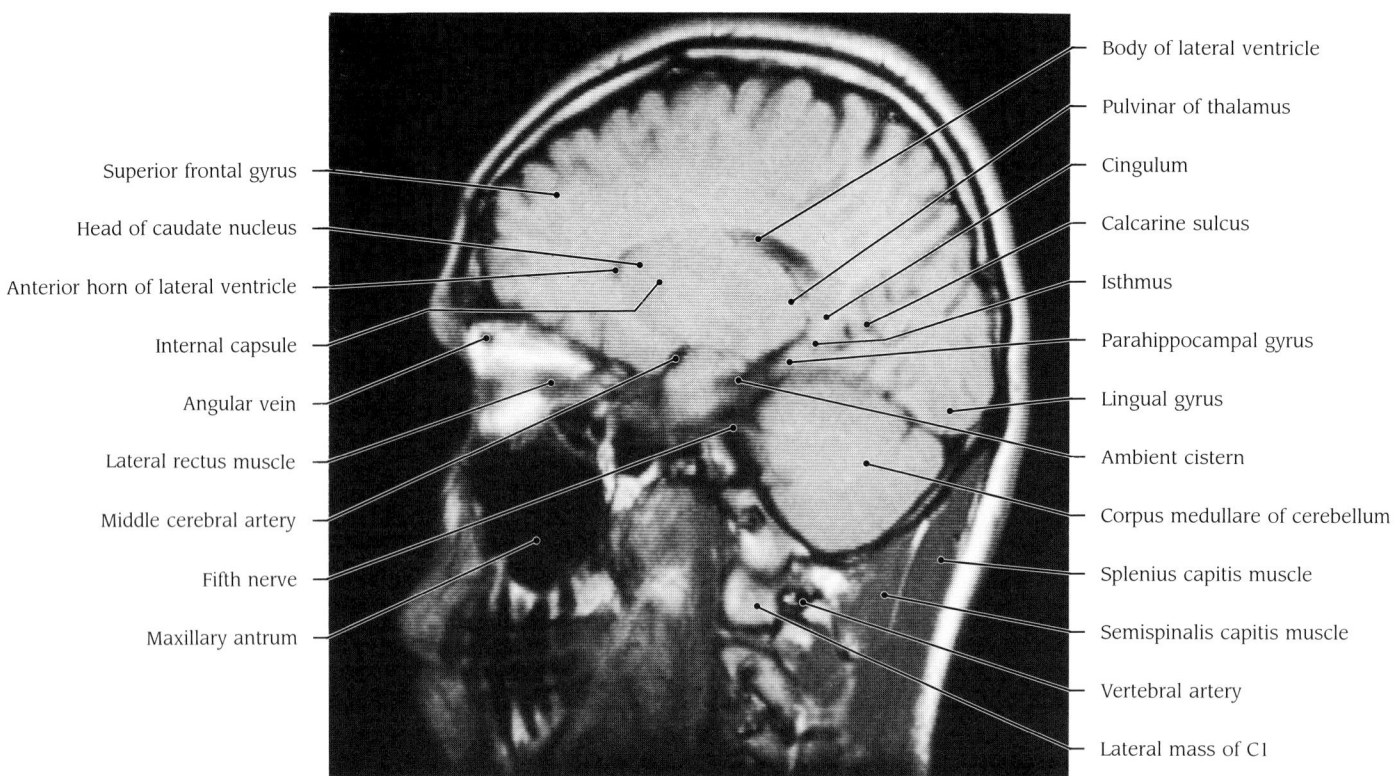

FIG. 4.15. TR = 500 msec, TE = 28 msec.

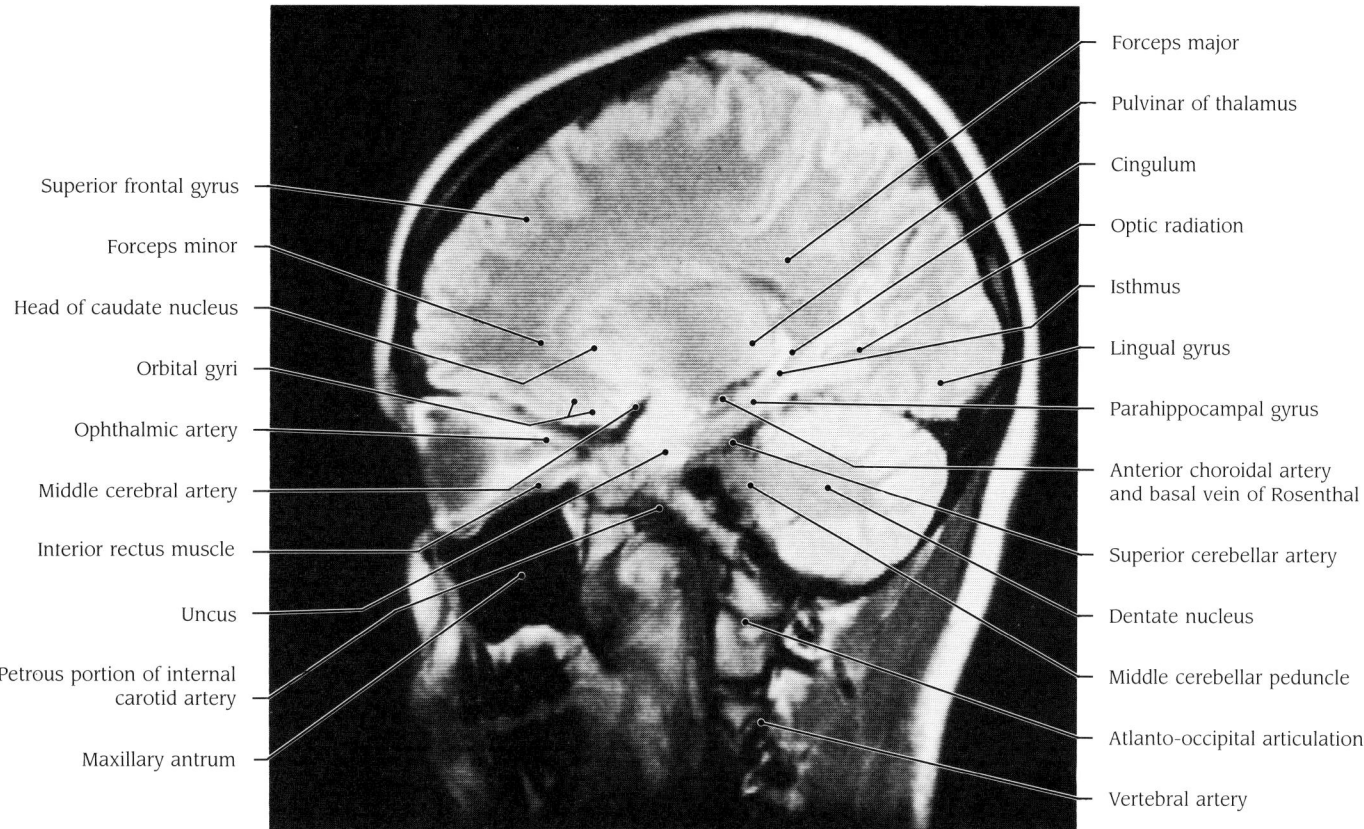

FIG. 4.16. TR = 2000 msec, TE = 28 msec.

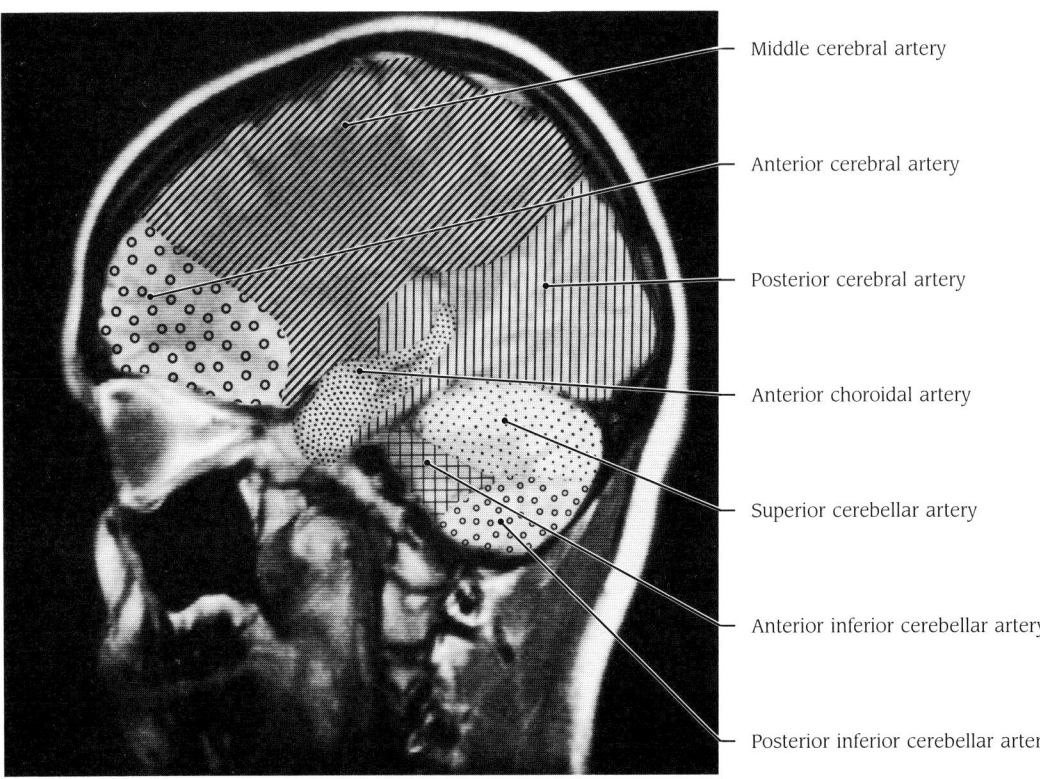

FIG. 4.17. TR = 2000 msec, TE = 28 msec.

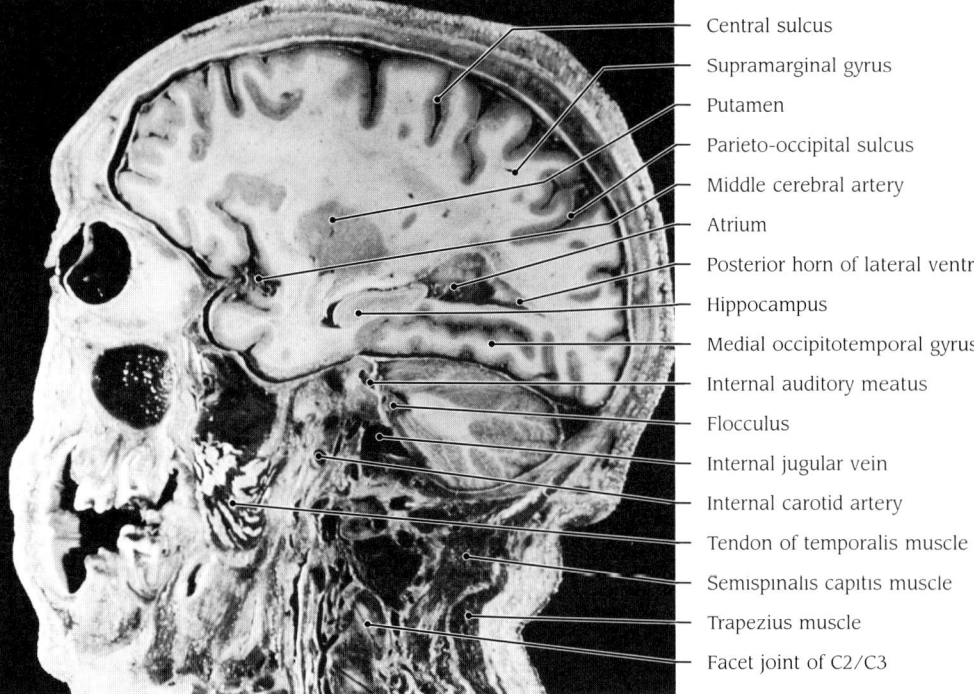
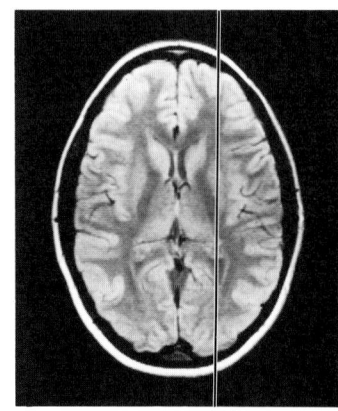

FIG. 4.18.

- The hippocampal formation develops adjacent to the outer convex portion of the choroidal fissure. It extends in an arch from the interventricular foramen to the anterior extent of the inferior horn of the lateral ventricle. The components of the hippocampal formation are generally considered to include: (1) the indusium griseum and the longitudinal striae and their extensions; (2) the gyrus fasciolaris (splenial gyrus); (3) the dentate gyrus, cornu ammonis, and subiculum; and (4) parts of the uncus.
- The indusium griseum, or supracallosal gyrus, is a thin layer of gray matter that covers the superior surface of the corpus callosum. The medial and lateral longitudinal striae are slender bundles of white matter embedded in the indusium.
- The gyrus fasciolaris, or splenial gyrus, is the thin gray-matter extension of the indusium griseum. The gyrus fasciolaris curves inferiorly, laterally, and anteriorly to become continuous with the posterior portion of the dentate gyrus.
- The hippocampus is composed of the complex layers of the dentate gyrus and cornu ammonis. It is approximately 5 cm in length and extends the length of the floor of the inferior horn of the lateral ventricle. The dentate gyrus is a strip of gray matter located superior to the subiculum and medial and inferior to the cornu ammonis. These complex infoldings may be understood by considering a line that extends medially in the coronal plane from the collateral sulcus, where the parahippocampal gyrus merges with the subiculum. The subiculum extends superomedially to the inferior aspect of the dentate gyrus and then continues and turns laterally, becoming the cornu ammonis. The cornu ammonis curves superiorly and then laterally to point inferiorly into the dentate gyrus.

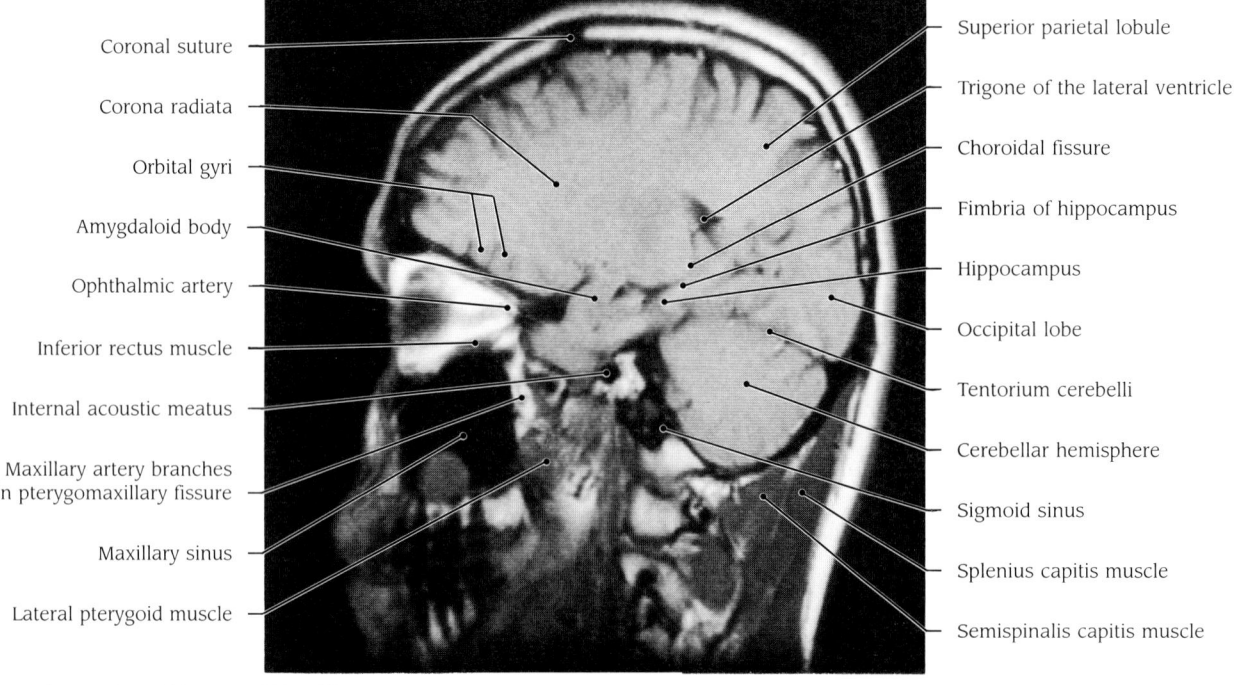

FIG. 4.19. TR = 500 msec, TE = 28 msec.

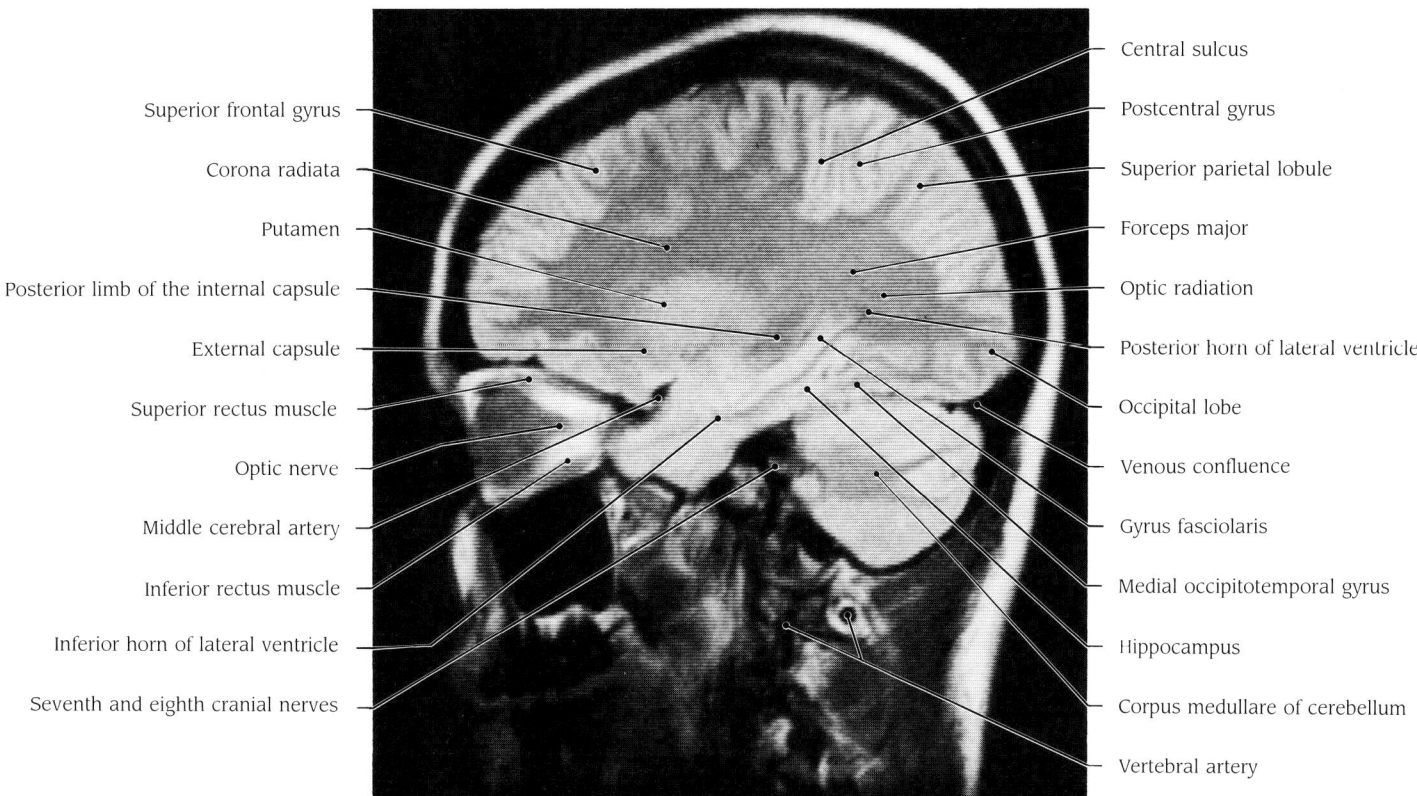

FIG. 4.20. TR = 2000 msec, TE = 28 msec.

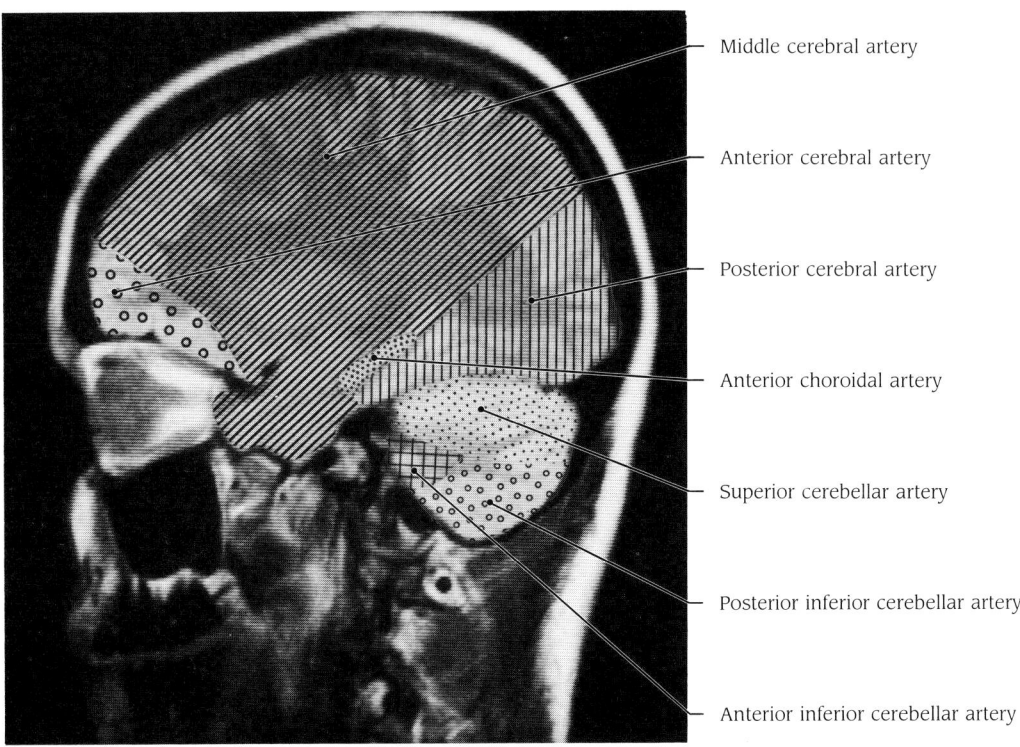

FIG. 4.21. TR = 2000 msec, TE = 28 msec.

97

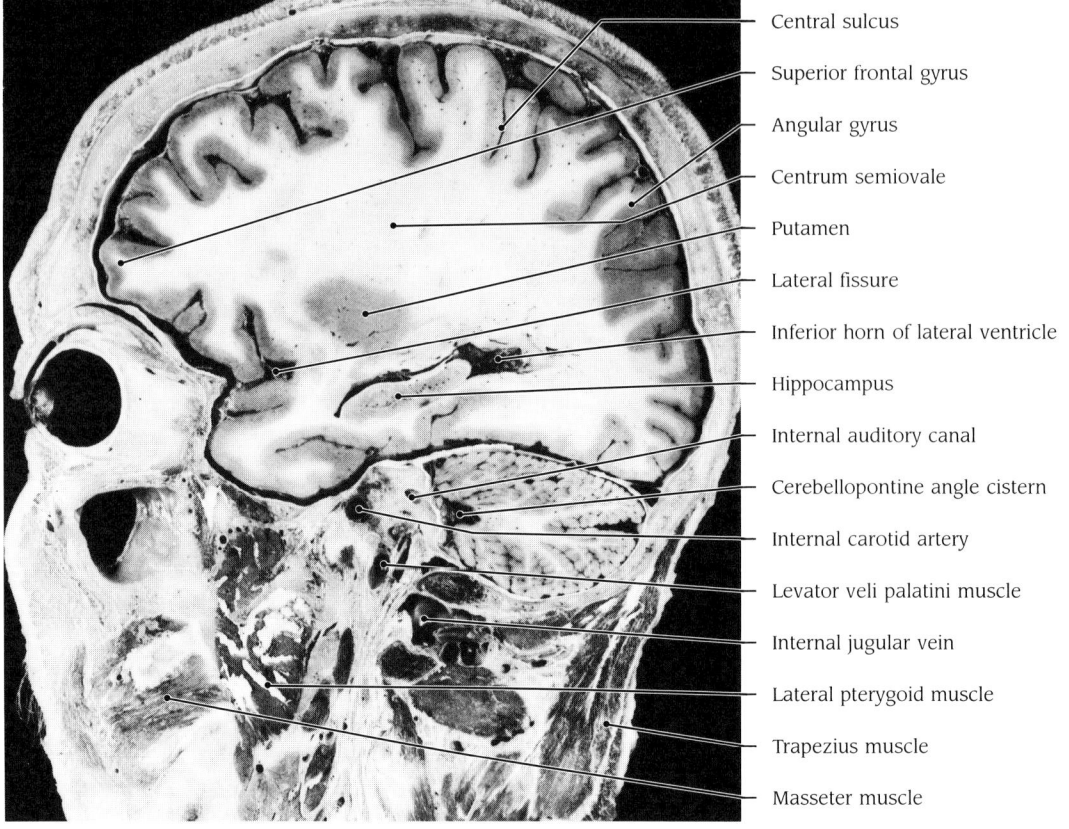

FIG. 4.22.

- The superior parietal lobule is located between the intraparietal sulcus and the superior and medial margin of the hemisphere. It is continuous anteriorly with the postcentral gyrus and posteriorly with the arcus parieto-occipitalis. The arcus parieto-occipitalis is located adjacent to the lateral part of the parieto-occipital sulcus.

- The calcar avis is an elevation on the medial wall of the posterior horn of the lateral ventricle. This eminence is formed by the cortex bordering the anterior portion of the calcarine sulcus.

- This oblique section through the petrous pyramid shows the proximity of several important structures, including the internal carotid artery, the internal jugular vein, and components of the middle and inner ear.

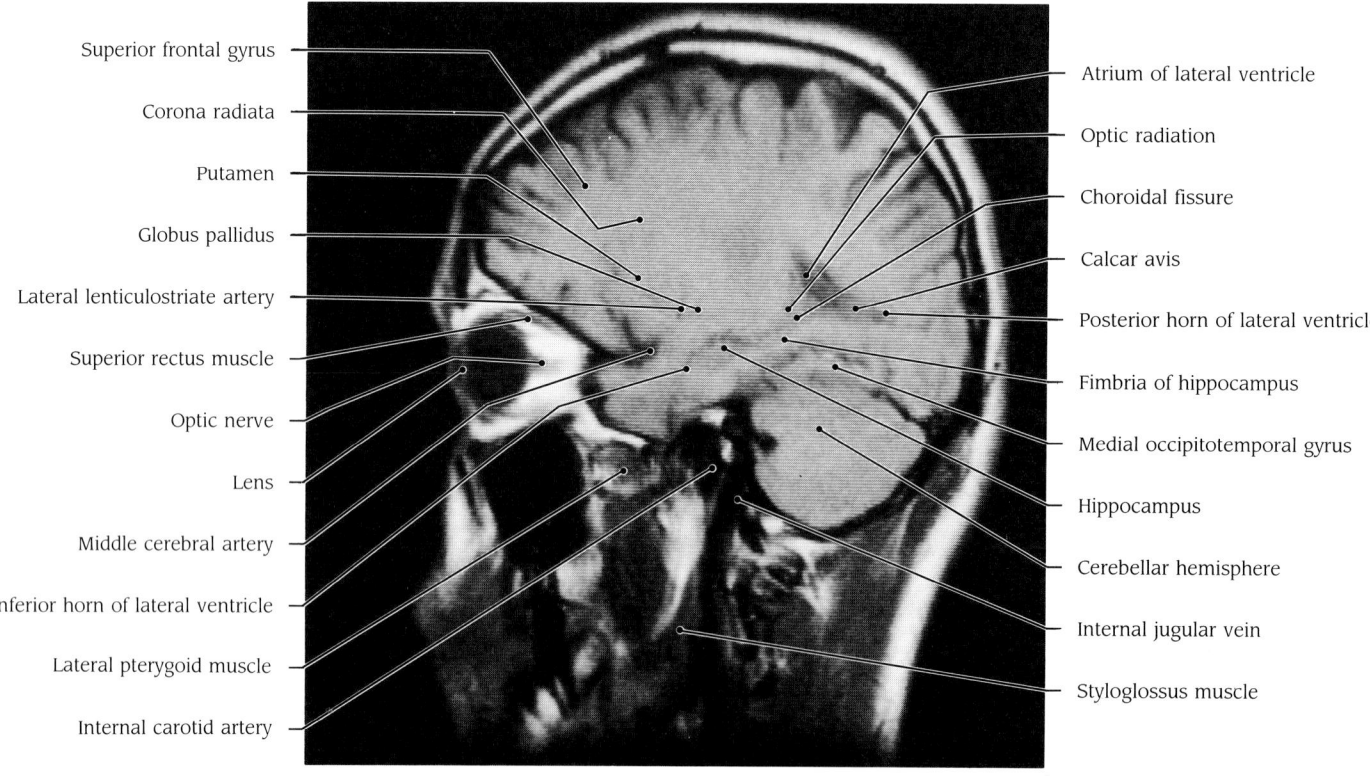

FIG. 4.23. TR = 500 msec, TE = 28 msec.

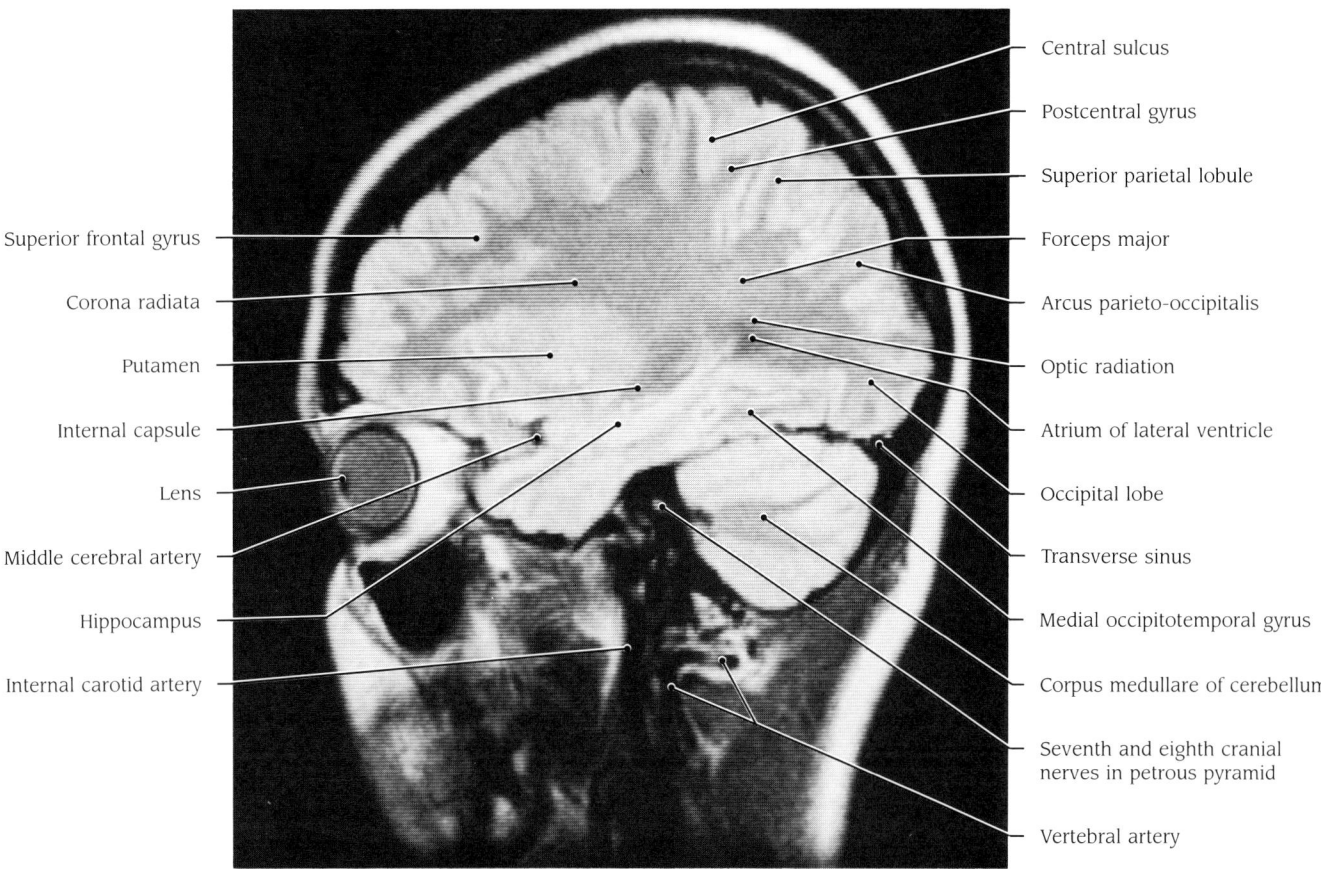

FIG. 4.24. TR = 2000 msec, TE = 28 msec.

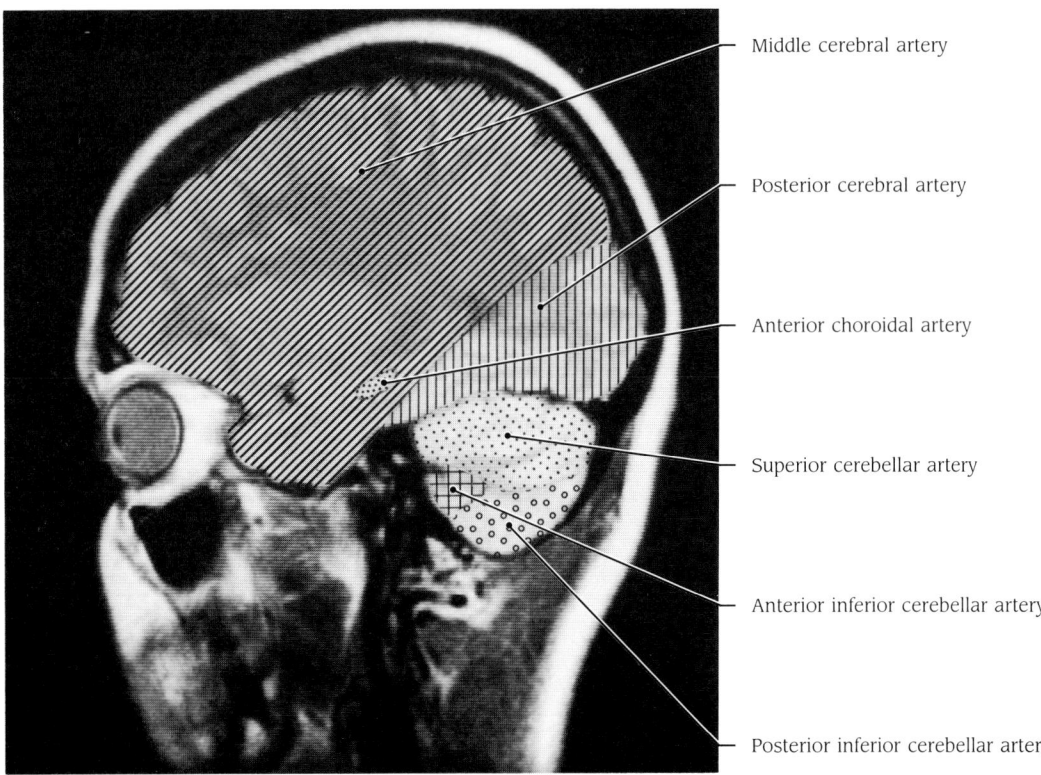

FIG. 4.25. TR = 2000 msec, TE = 28 msec.

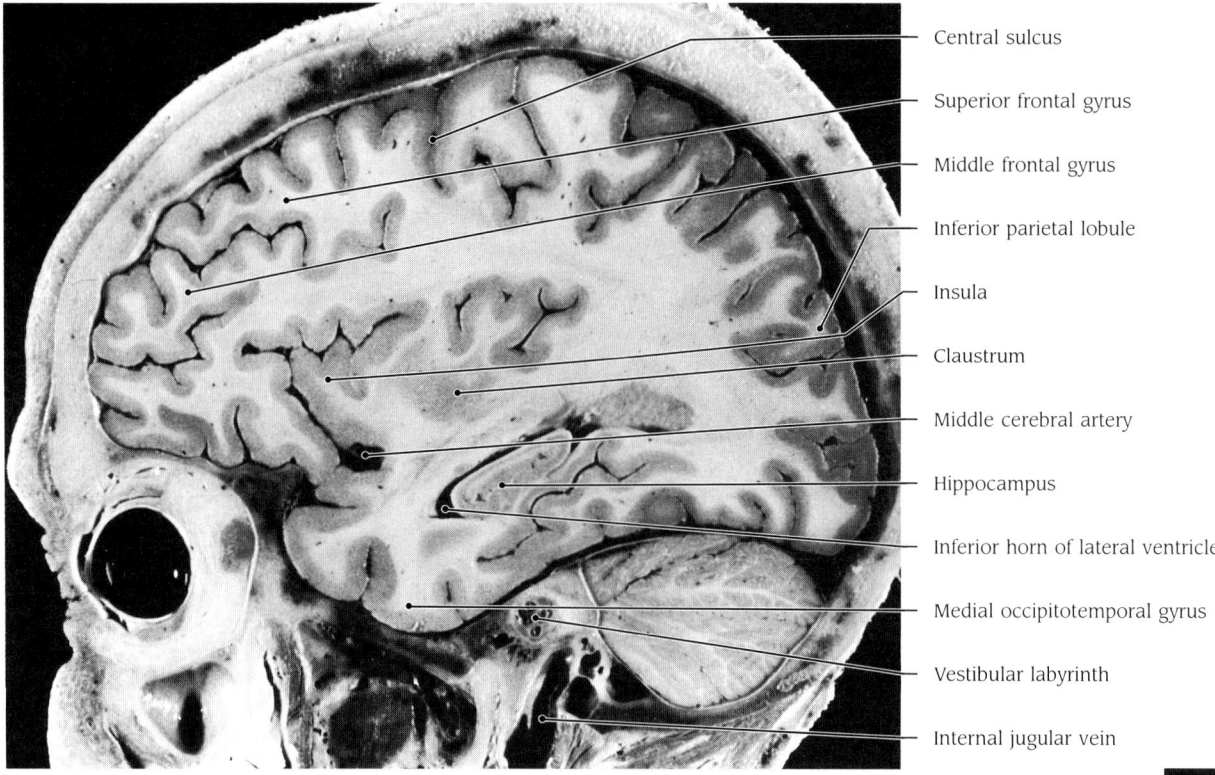

FIG. 4.26.

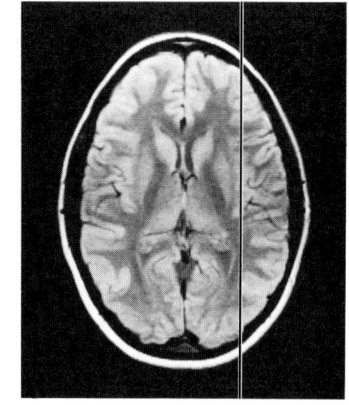

- The lateral cerebral fissure, or sulcus, is positioned on the inferior and lateral aspects of the cerebral hemisphere and is composed of a short stem and three rami. The stem begins at the anterior perforated substance and extends from the orbital surface of the frontal lobe to the anterior aspect of the temporal lobe. At the lateral surface, the stem divides into three rami: the anterior horizontal, the anterior ascending, and the posterior rami. The anterior horizontal ramus continues anteriorly into the inferior frontal gyrus, whereas the anterior ascending ramus continues superiorly into the inferior frontal gyrus. The posterior ramus runs posteriorly and superiorly and ends in the parietal lobe.

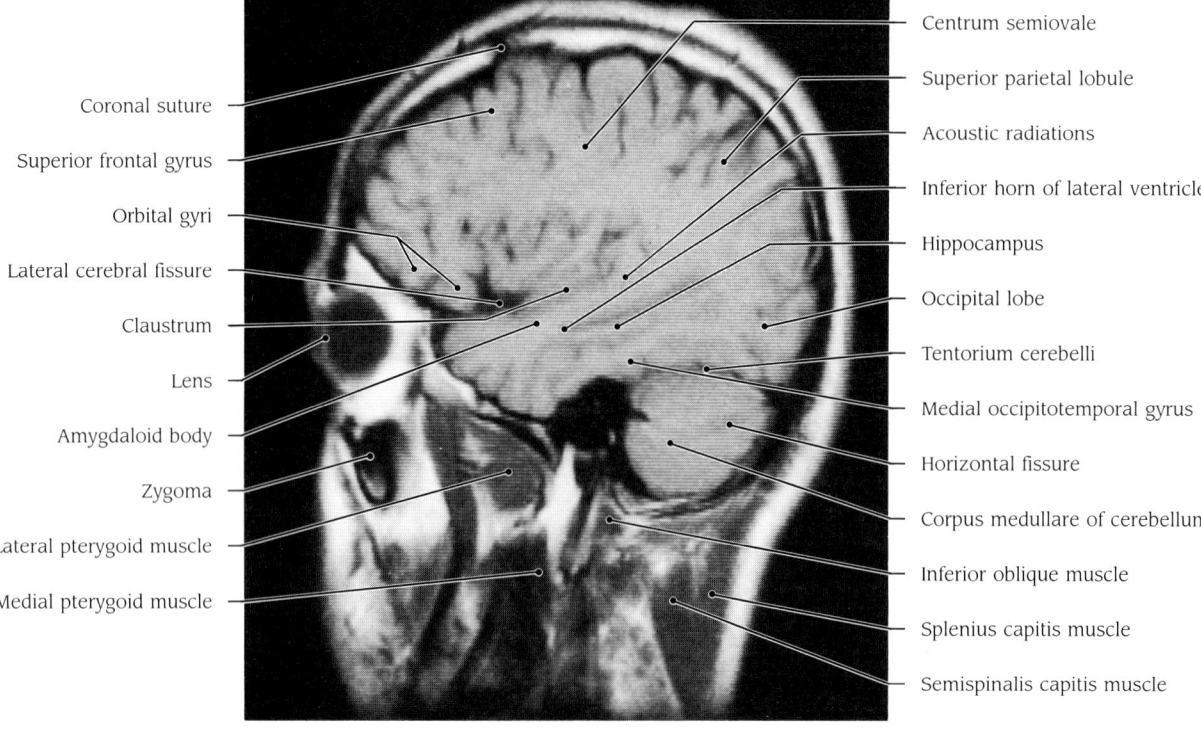

FIG. 4.27. TR = 500 msec, TE = 28 msec.

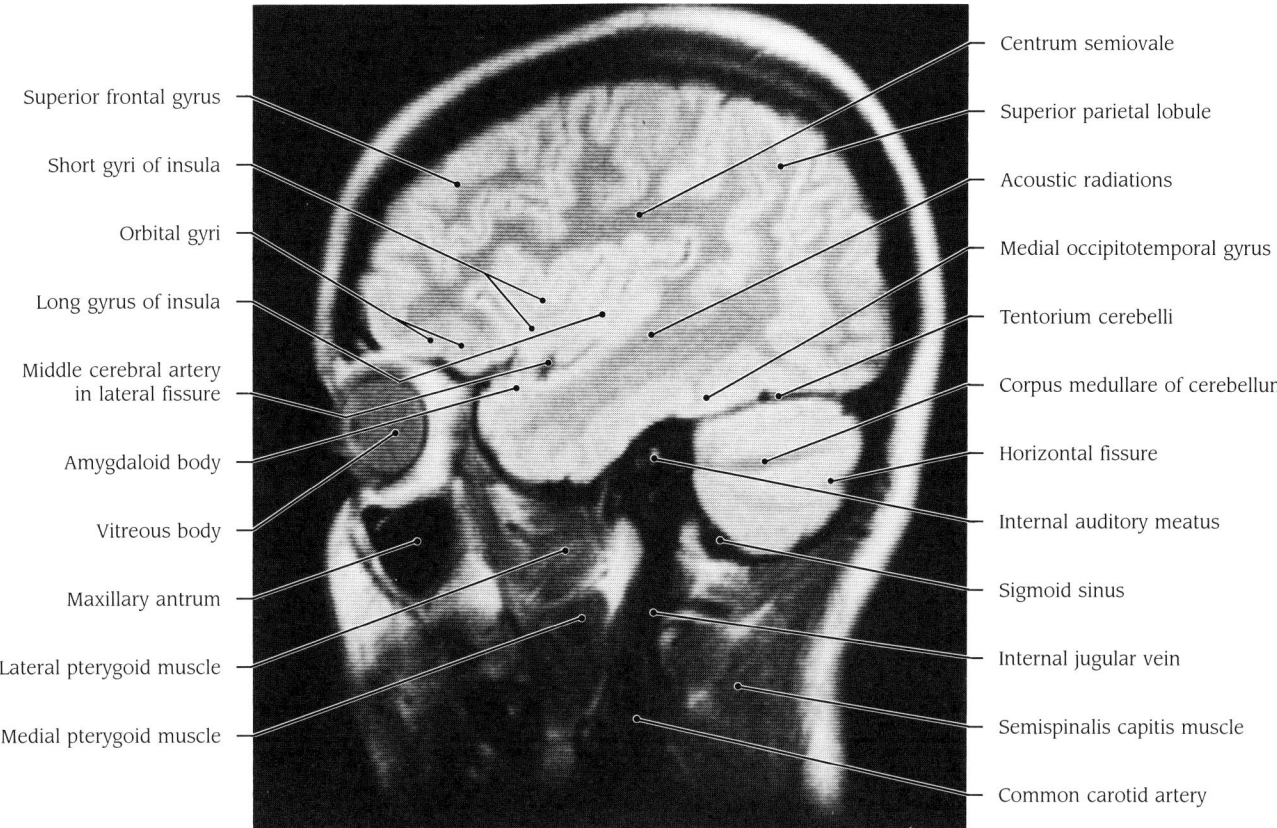

FIG. 4.28. TR = 2000 msec, TE = 28 msec.

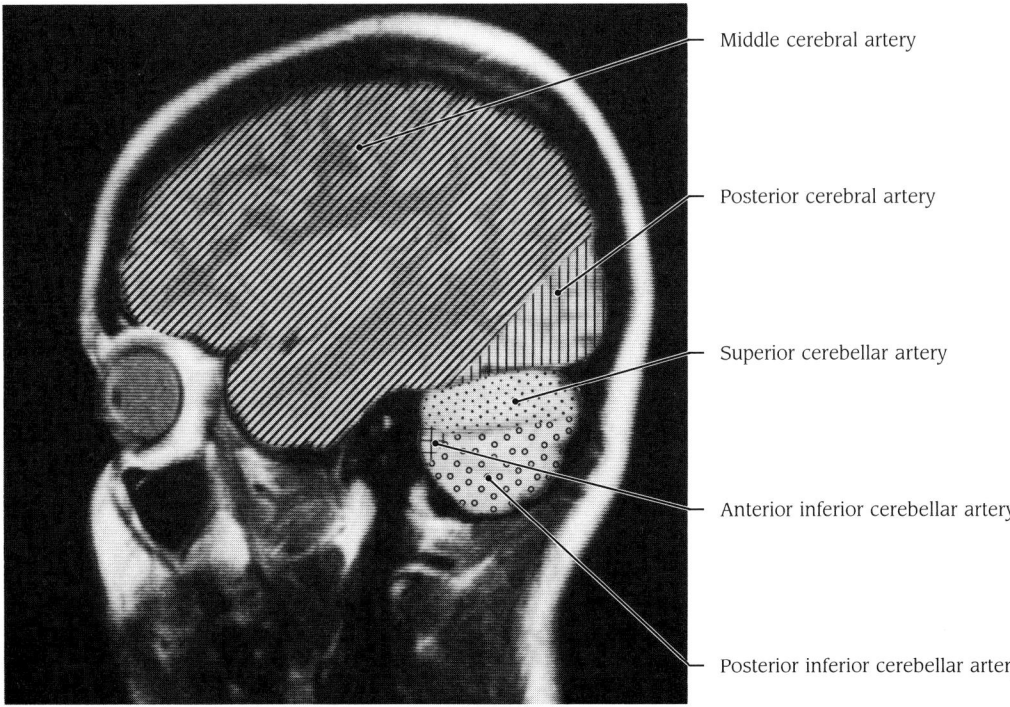

FIG. 4.29. TR = 2000 msec, TE = 28 msec.

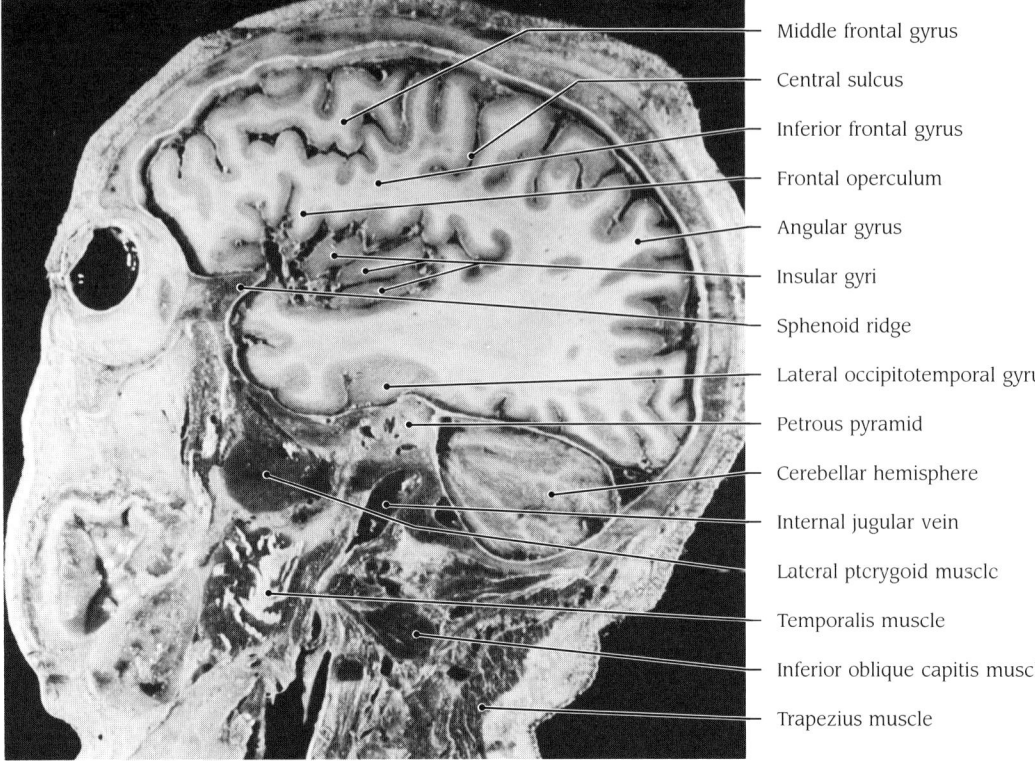
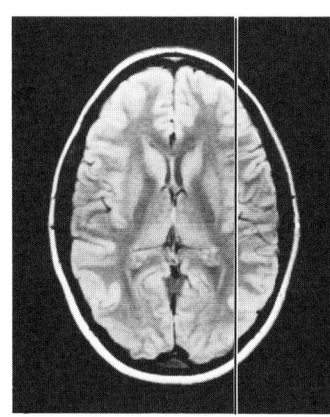

FIG. 4.30.

- The insula refers to the gray matter in the floor of the lateral sulcus, which is surrounded by the circular sulcus. The insular surface is composed of three or four short, anteriorly placed gyri, and one long posterior gyrus, separated by the central sulcus of the insula. The cortical gray matter that forms the insula is continuous with the opercula around the circular sulcus.

- The opercula are the cortical areas that overlie the insula and are divided into the frontal, parietal, and temporal opercula by the ascending and posterior rami of the lateral sulcus. The frontal operculum, which is located between the anterior and ascending rami of the lateral sulcus, is formed by the pars triangularis of the inferior frontal gyrus. The frontoparietal operculum is formed by the pars posterior of the inferior frontal gyrus, the inferior aspects of the precentral and postcentral gyri, and the inferior portion of the anterior segment of the inferior parietal lobule. The frontoparietal operculum is delimited by the ascending and posterior rami of the lateral sulcus. The temporal operculum, which is inferior to the posterior ramus, is formed by the transverse temporal gyri and the superior temporal gyrus.

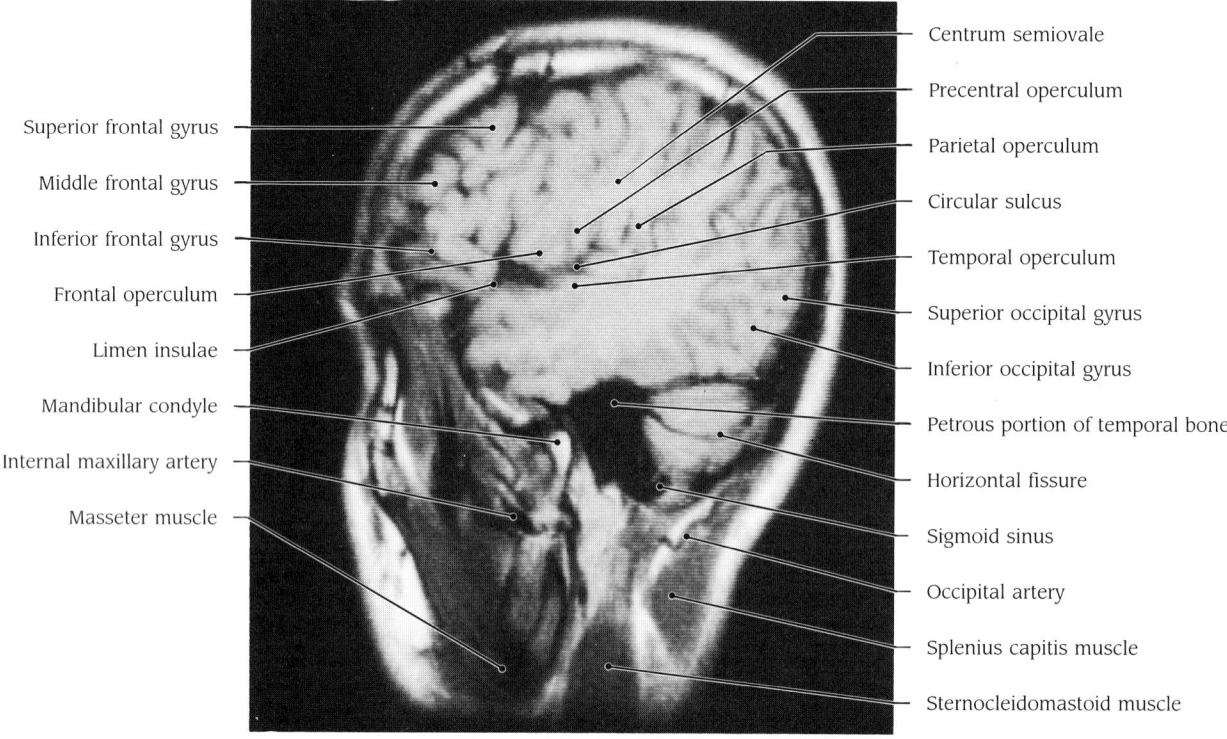

FIG. 4.31. TR = 500 msec, TE = 28 msec.

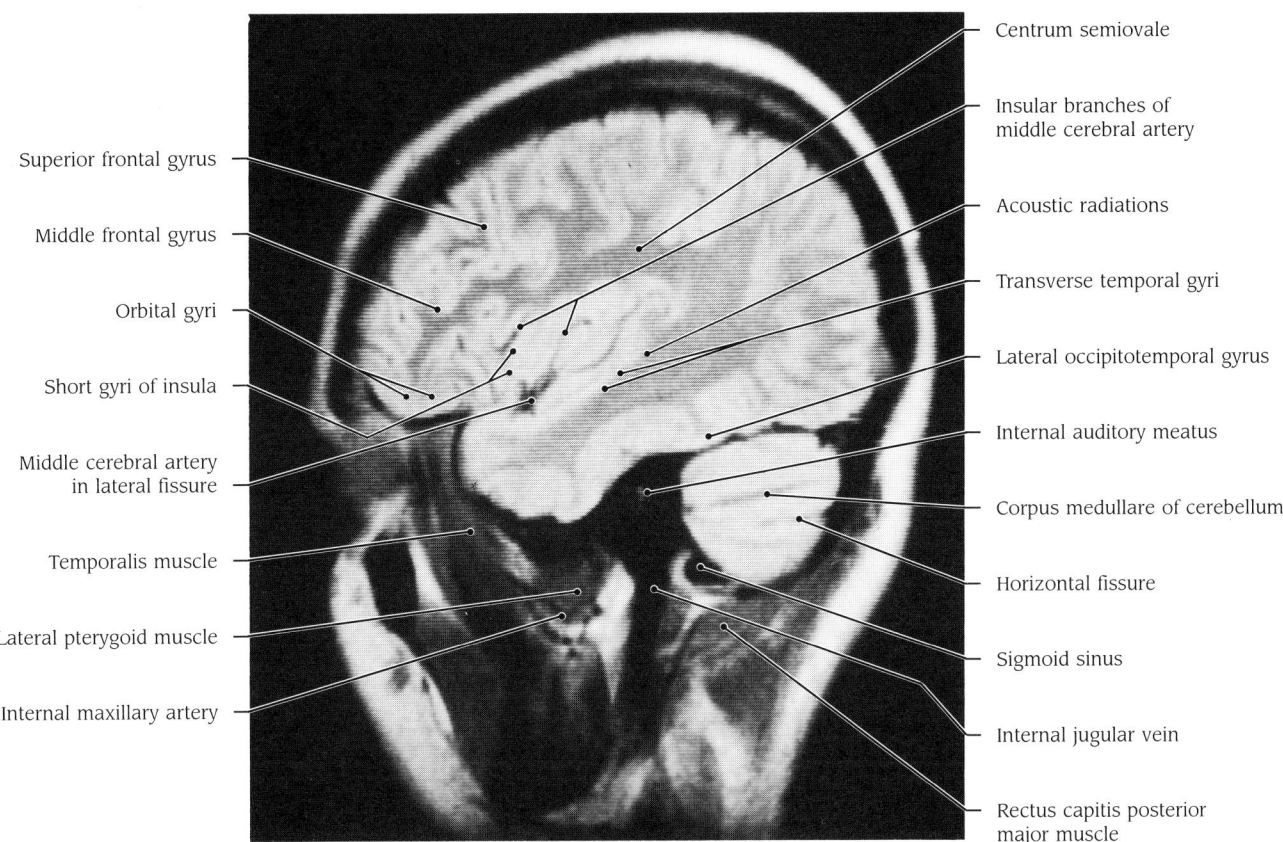

FIG. 4.32. TR = 2000 msec, TE = 28 msec.

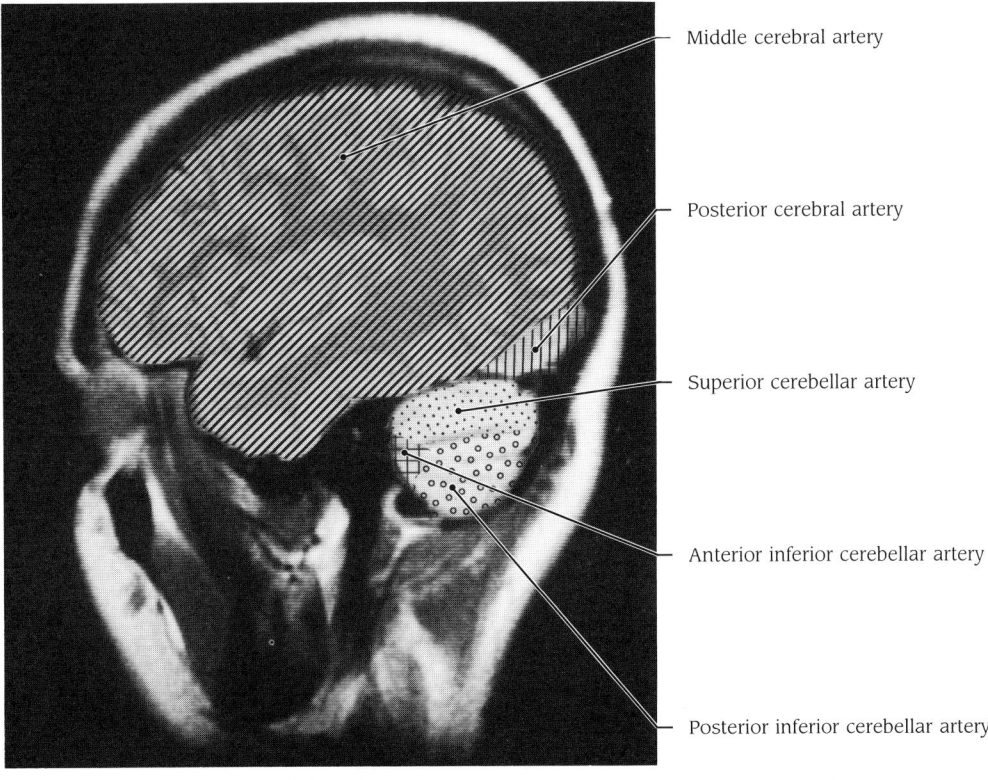

FIG. 4.33. TR = 2000 msec, TE = 28 msec.

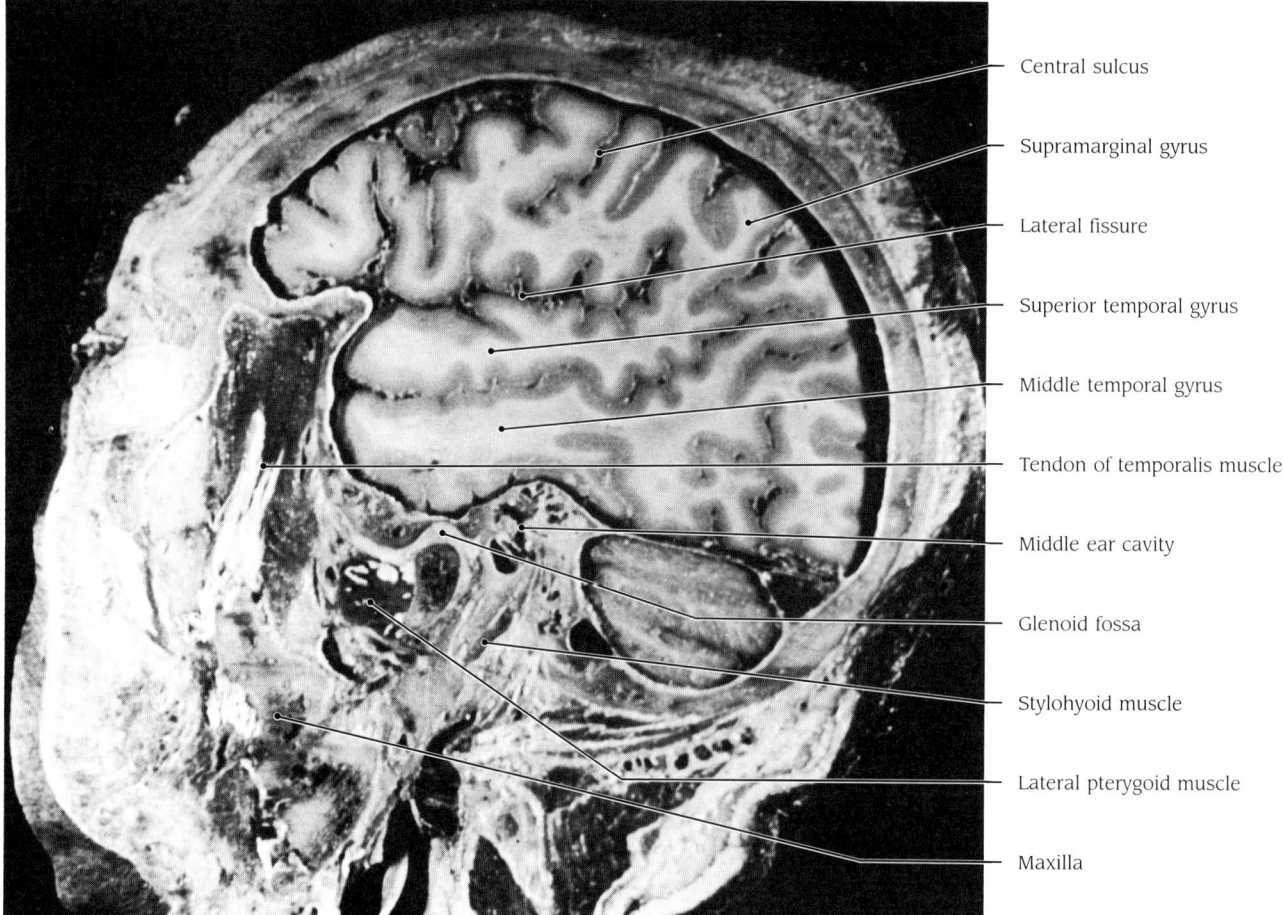

FIG. 4.34.

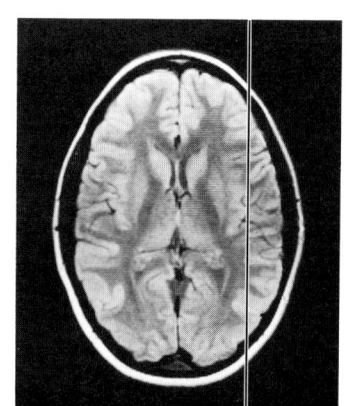

- The inferior parietal lobule is delimited superiorly by the intraparietal sulcus and anteriorly by the postcentral sulcus. It may be divided into three portions. The anterior portion is the supramarginal gyrus, which surrounds the posterior upturned portion of the posterior ramus of the lateral sulcus. The middle portion is the angular gyrus, which surrounds the posterior upturned portion of the superior temporal gyrus. The posterior portion surrounds the upturned end of the inferior temporal sulcus and extends to the occipital lobe.

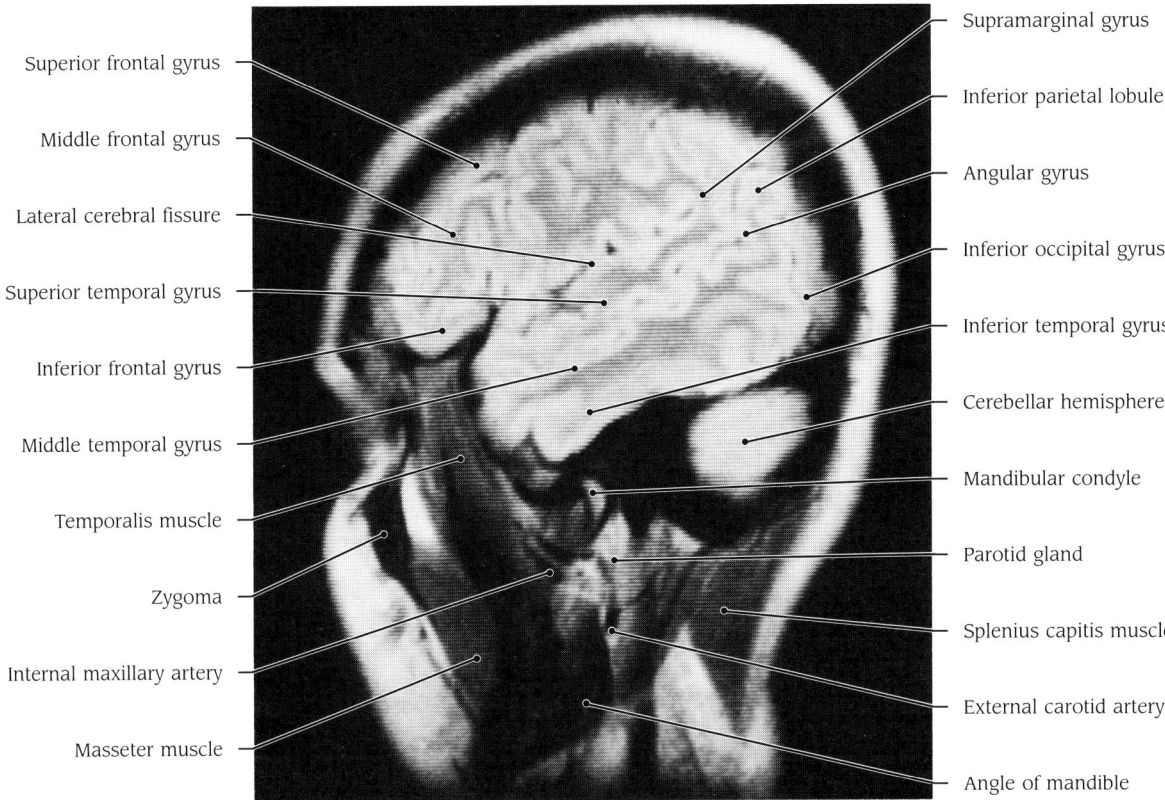

FIG. 4.35. TR = 2000 msec, TE = 28 msec.

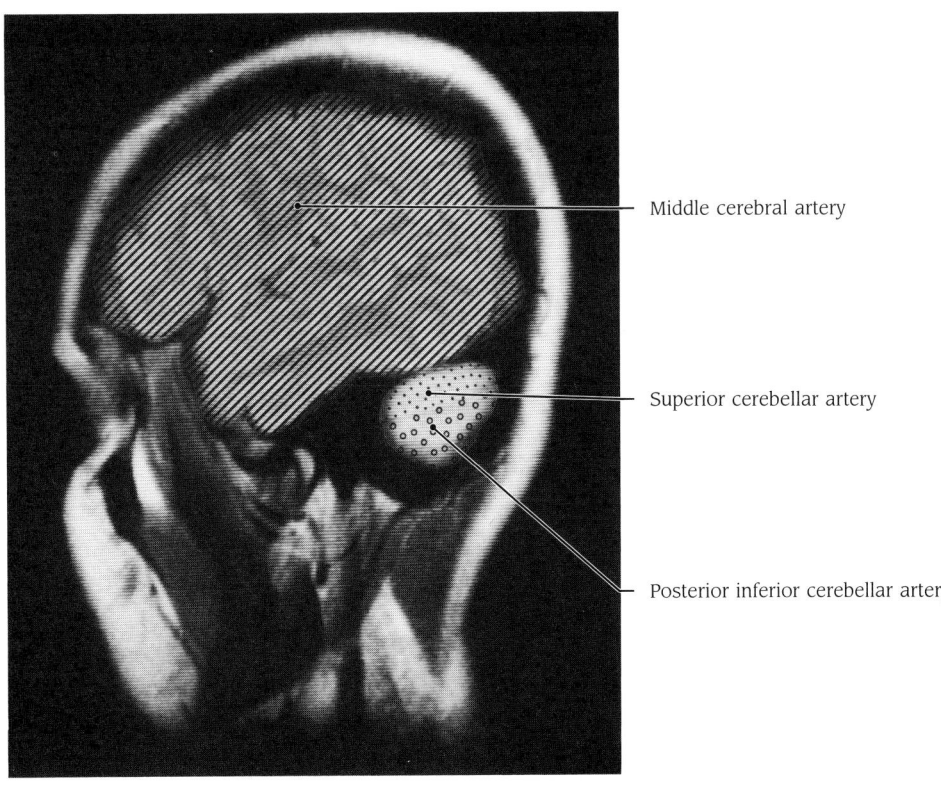

FIG. 4.36. TR = 2000 msec, TE = 28 msec.

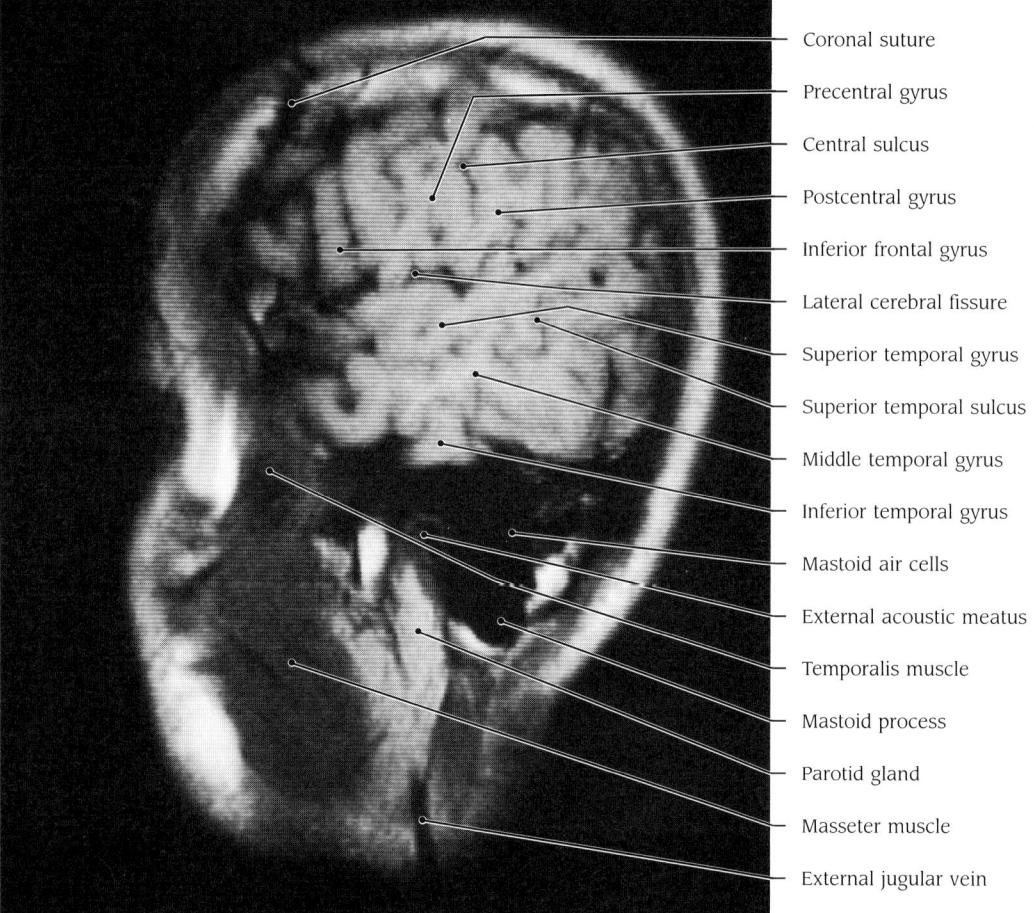

FIG. 4.37. TR = 500 msec, TE = 28 msec.

- The temporal lobe is positioned inferior to the lateral sulcus. It is delimited posteriorly by a line from the preoccipital notch to the parieto-occipital sulcus. The lateral surface of the temporal lobe is divided into the superior, middle, and inferior temporal gyri by the superior and inferior temporal sulci. The superior temporal sulcus originates near the temporal pole and extends posteriorly into the parietal lobe, running parallel to the posterior ramus of the lateral sulcus. The inferior temporal sulcus is parallel to the superior temporal sulcus and also extends posteriorly into the parietal lobe.

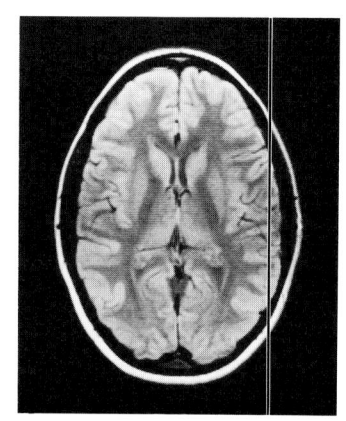

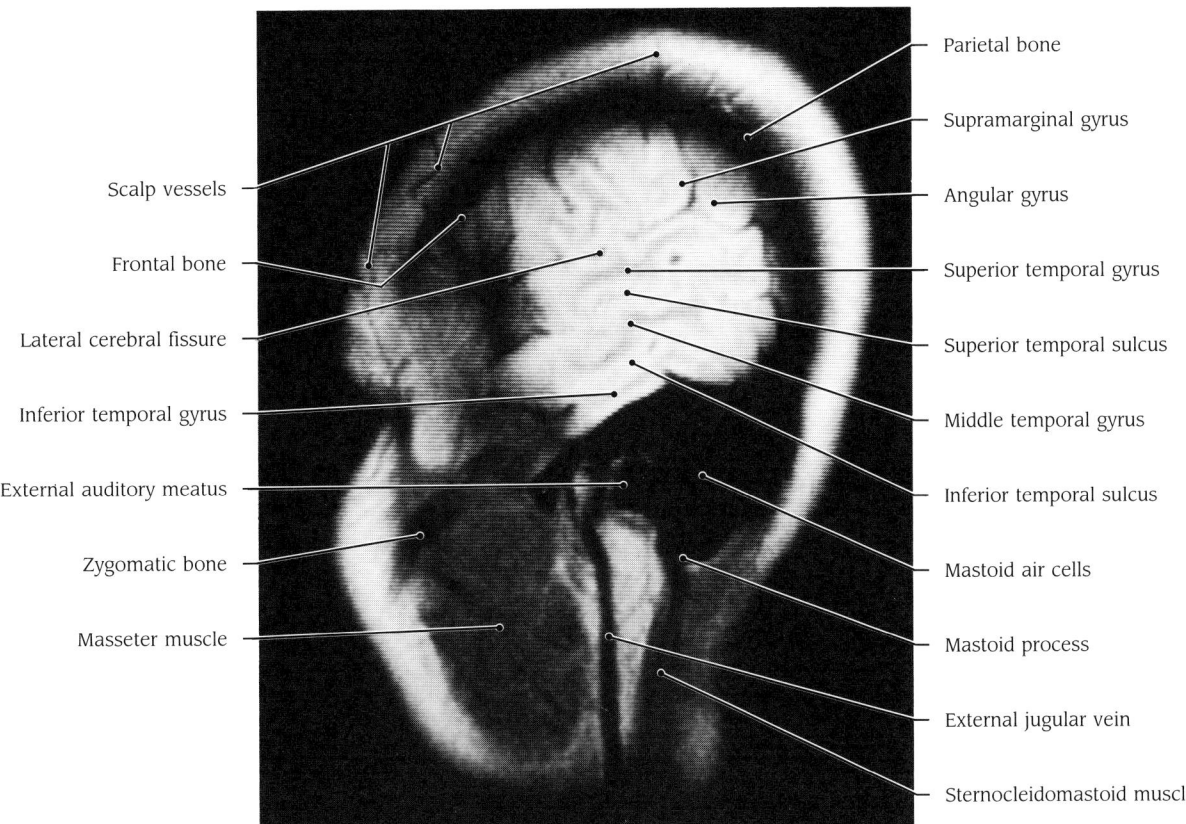

FIG. 4.38. TR = 2000 msec, TE = 28 msec.

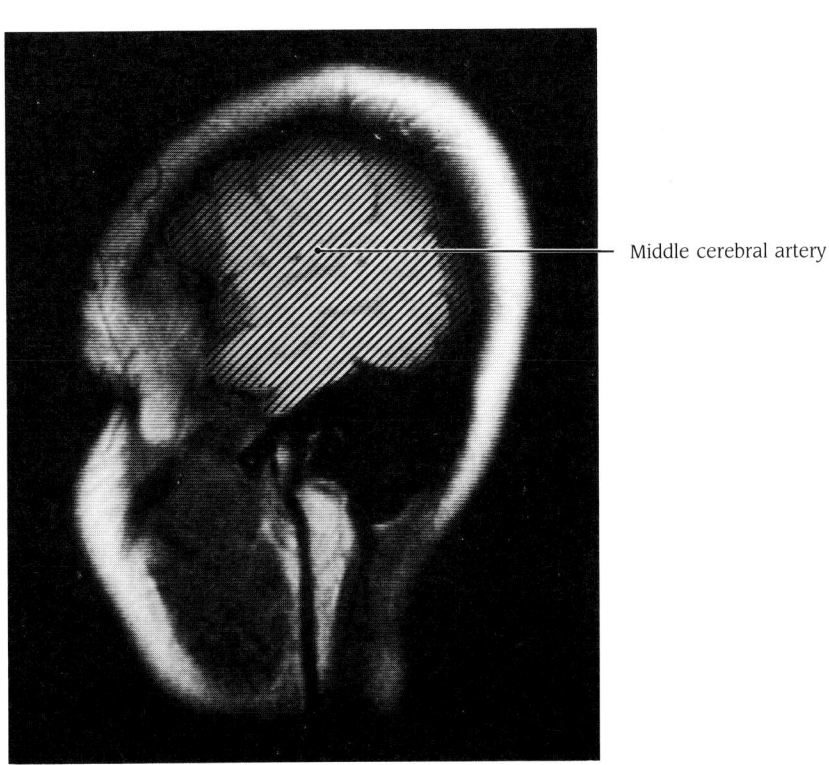

FIG. 4.39. TR = 2000 msec, TE = 28 msec.

5

Orbit

Anatomic Level	Figures
Axial Orbit	5.1–5.16
Coronal Orbit	5.17–5.27
Sagittal Orbit	5.28–5.36
Oblique Orbit	5.37–5.45

A series of cadaveric sections that extend through the orbit in the axial, coronal, sagittal, and oblique planes are shown. These sections are matched with MR images of a volunteer. The difference in the section planes between the anatomic and the magnetic resonance images reflects the variability resulting from both angulation and positioning.

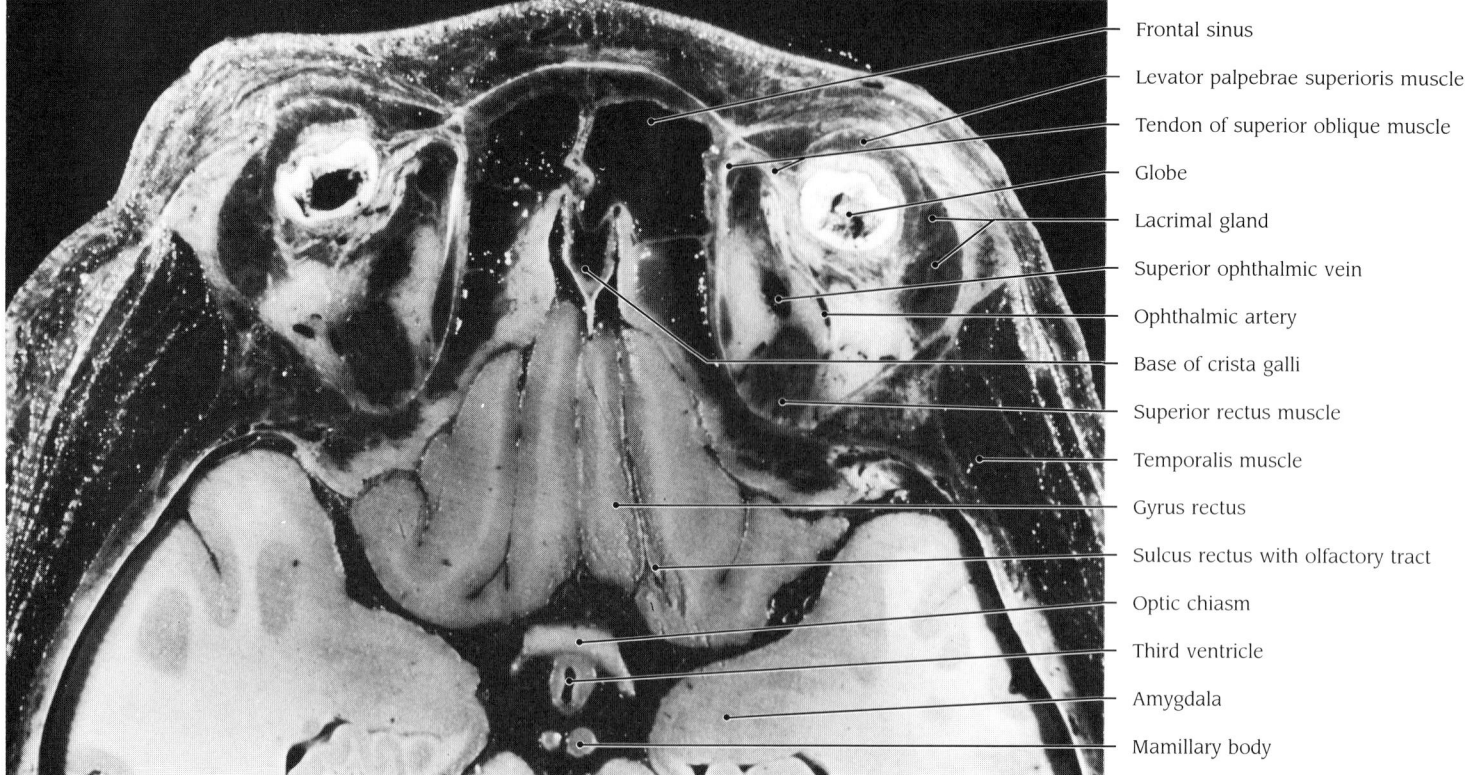

FIG. 5.1.

- The extraocular muscles include the levator palpebrae superioris, the superior rectus, the inferior rectus, the medial rectus, the lateral rectus, the superior oblique, and the inferior oblique muscles.

- The levator palpebrae superioris functions as an elevator of the upper eyelid. It originates from the inferior surface of the lesser wing of the sphenoid bone and continues anteriorly to end in a wide aponeurosis. The aponeurosis divides into superficial and deep lamellae. The fibers of the superficial lamella extend through the orbicularis oculi muscle to the skin and also attach to the anterior aspect of the superior tarsus. The inferior lamella contains nonstriated muscle fibers that form the superior tarsal muscle.

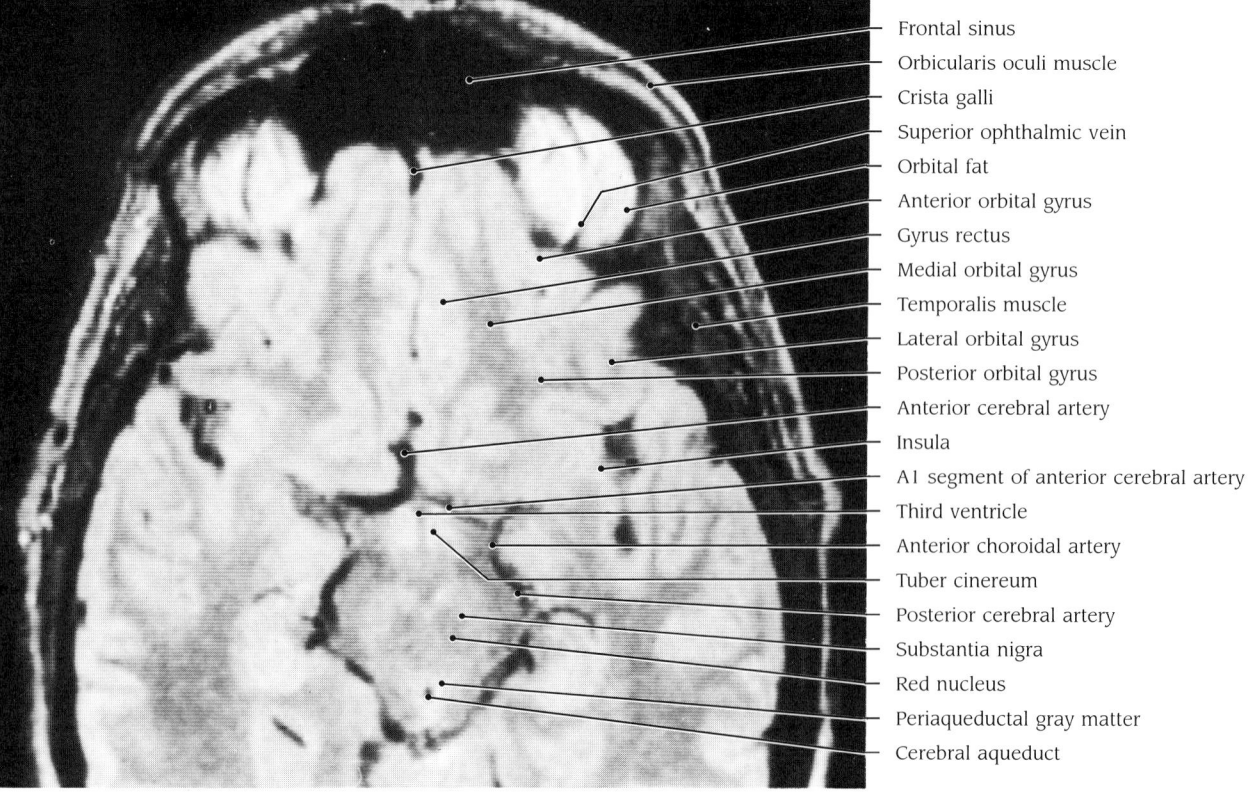

FIG. 5.2. TR = 2000 msec, TE = 50 msec.

110

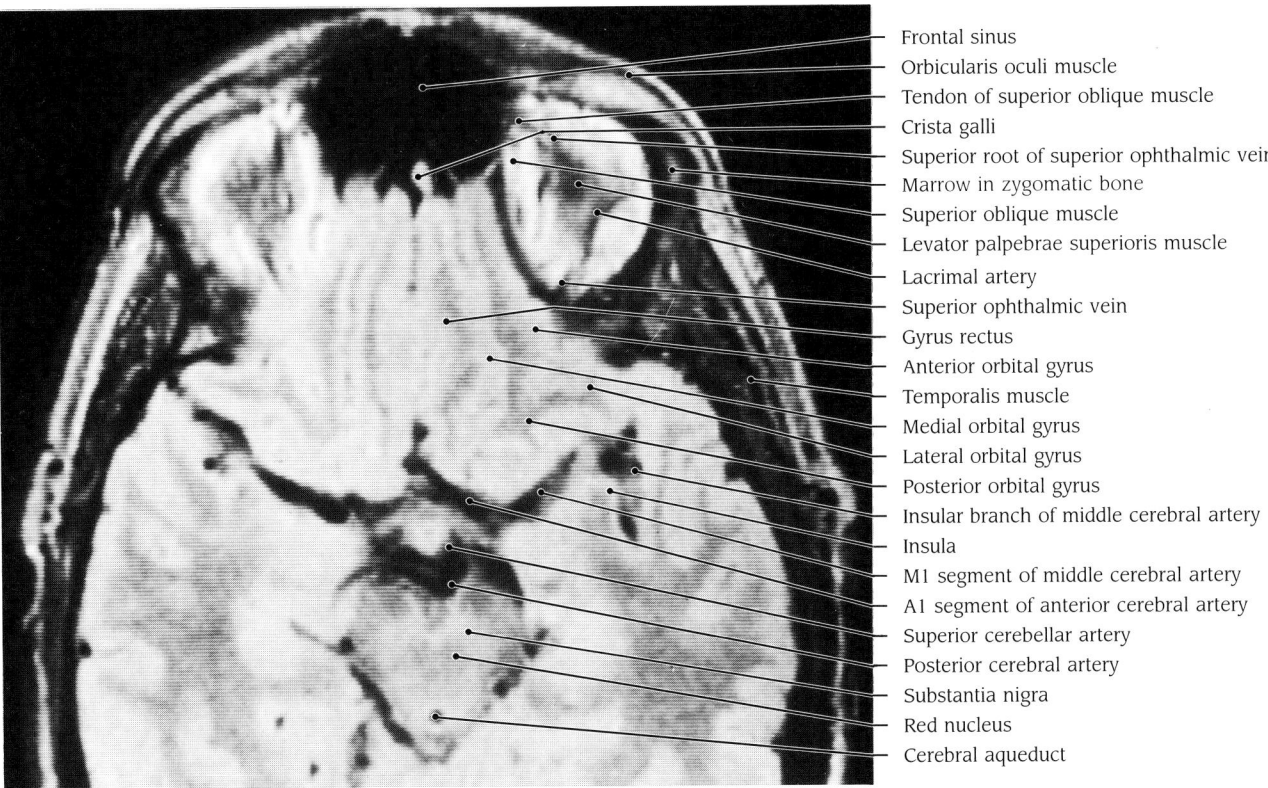

FIG. 5.3. TR = 2000 msec, TE = 50 msec.

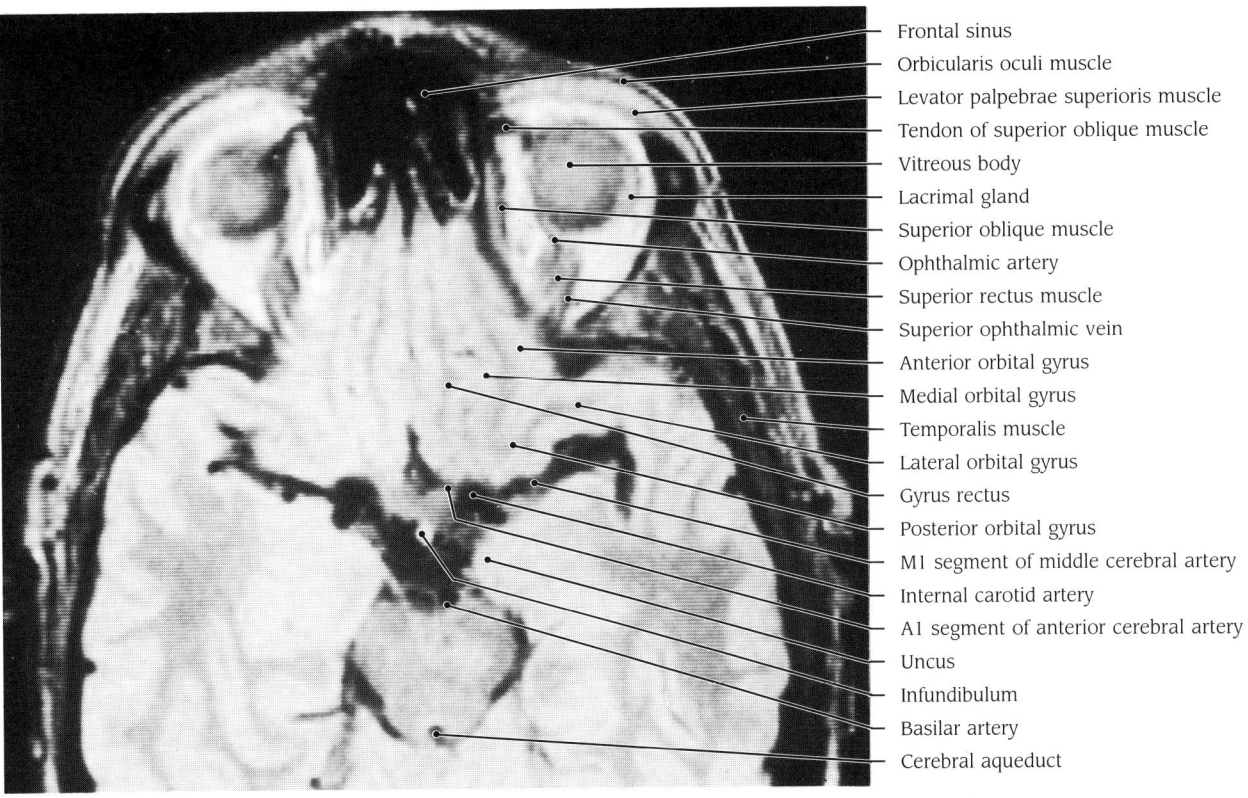

FIG. 5.4. TR = 2000 msec, TE = 50 msec.

111

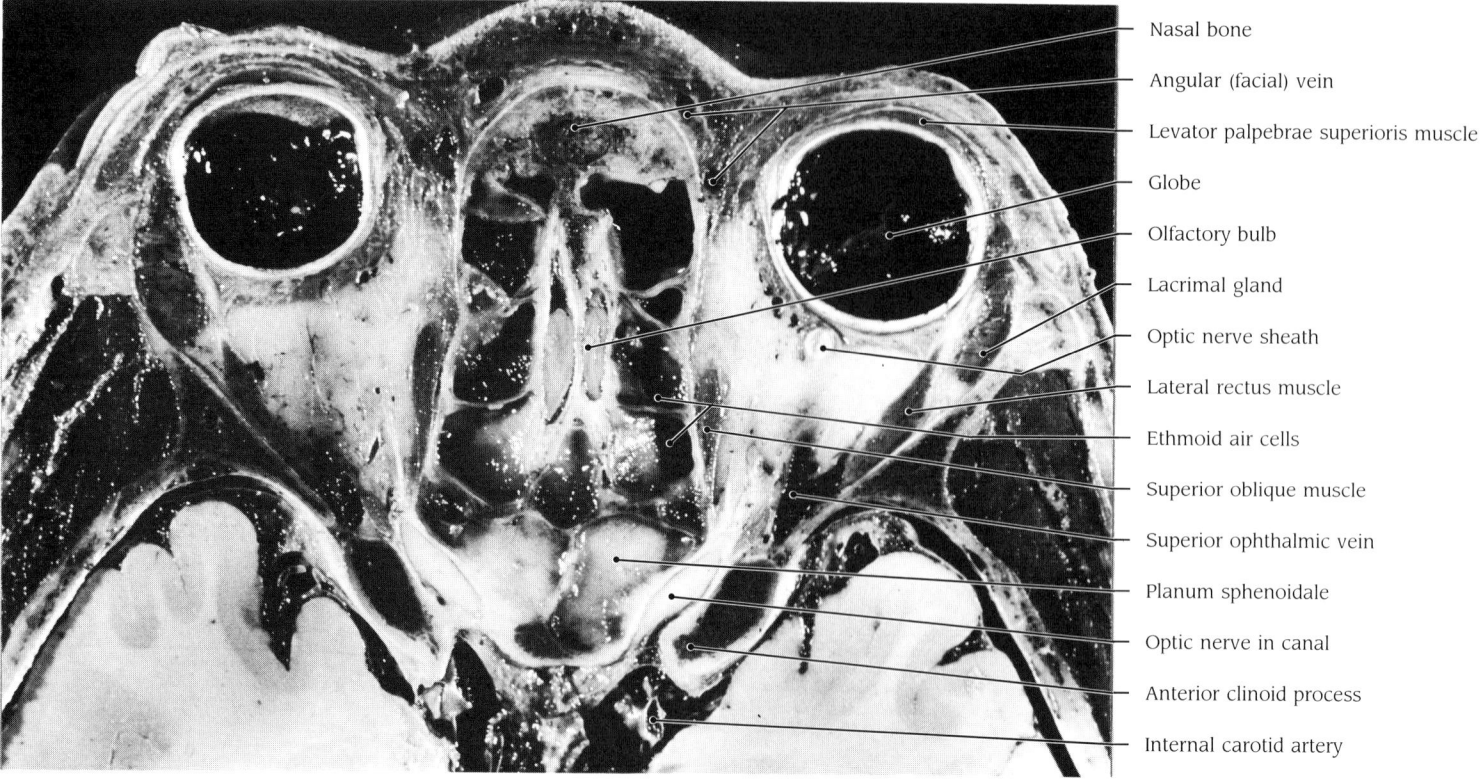

FIG. 5.5.

- The lacrimal apparatus includes (1) the lacrimal gland and its excretory ducts, which convey tears to the surface of the eye, and (2) the lacrimal canaliculi, lacrimal sac, and nasolacrimal duct, which convey tears into the nasal cavity.

- The lacrimal gland is composed of two parts: a larger, more superior orbital part, and a smaller inferior palpebral part. The orbital portion is similar to an almond in size and shape, and lies in the lacrimal fossa, just medial to the zygomatic process of the frontal bone. The palpebral portion is approximately one-third the size of the orbital portion. The palpebral portion is continuous with the orbital portion around the aponeurosis of the levator palpebrae superioris and extends into the upper eyelid to attach to the superior fornix of the conjunctiva.

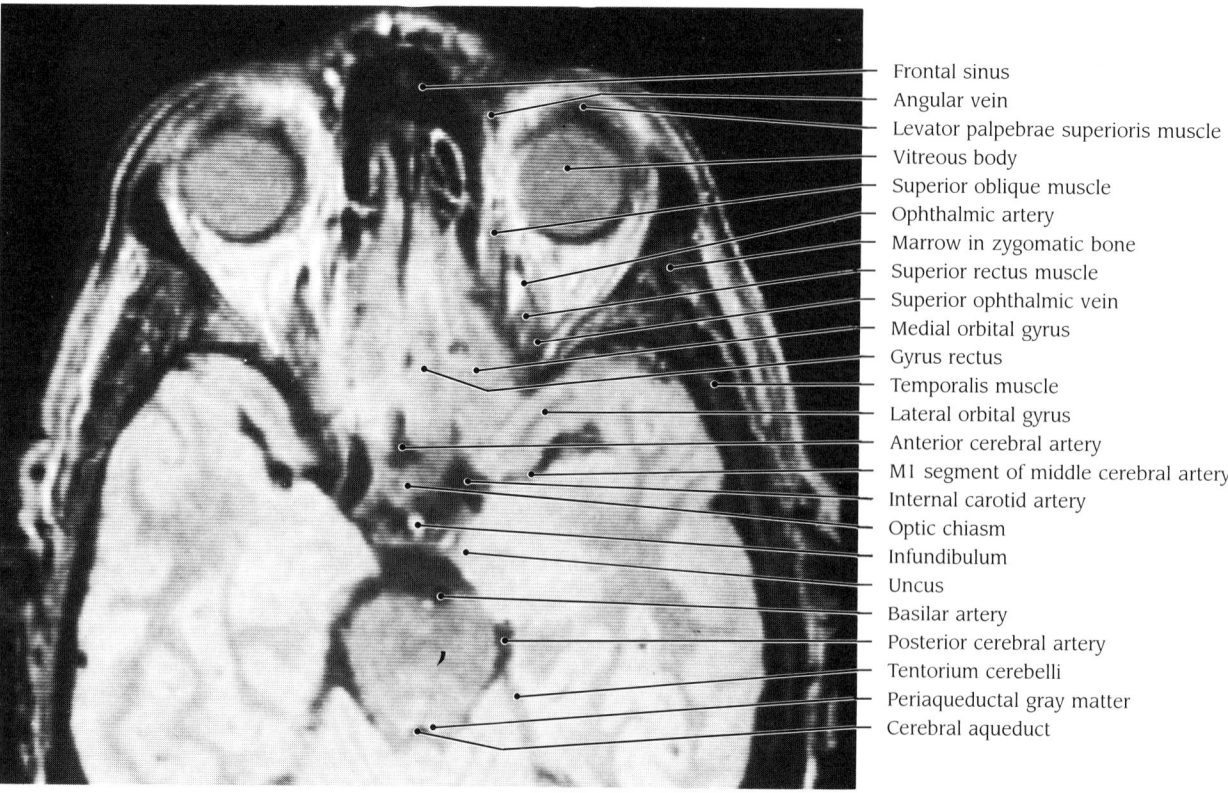

FIG. 5.6. TR = 2000 msec, TE = 50 msec.

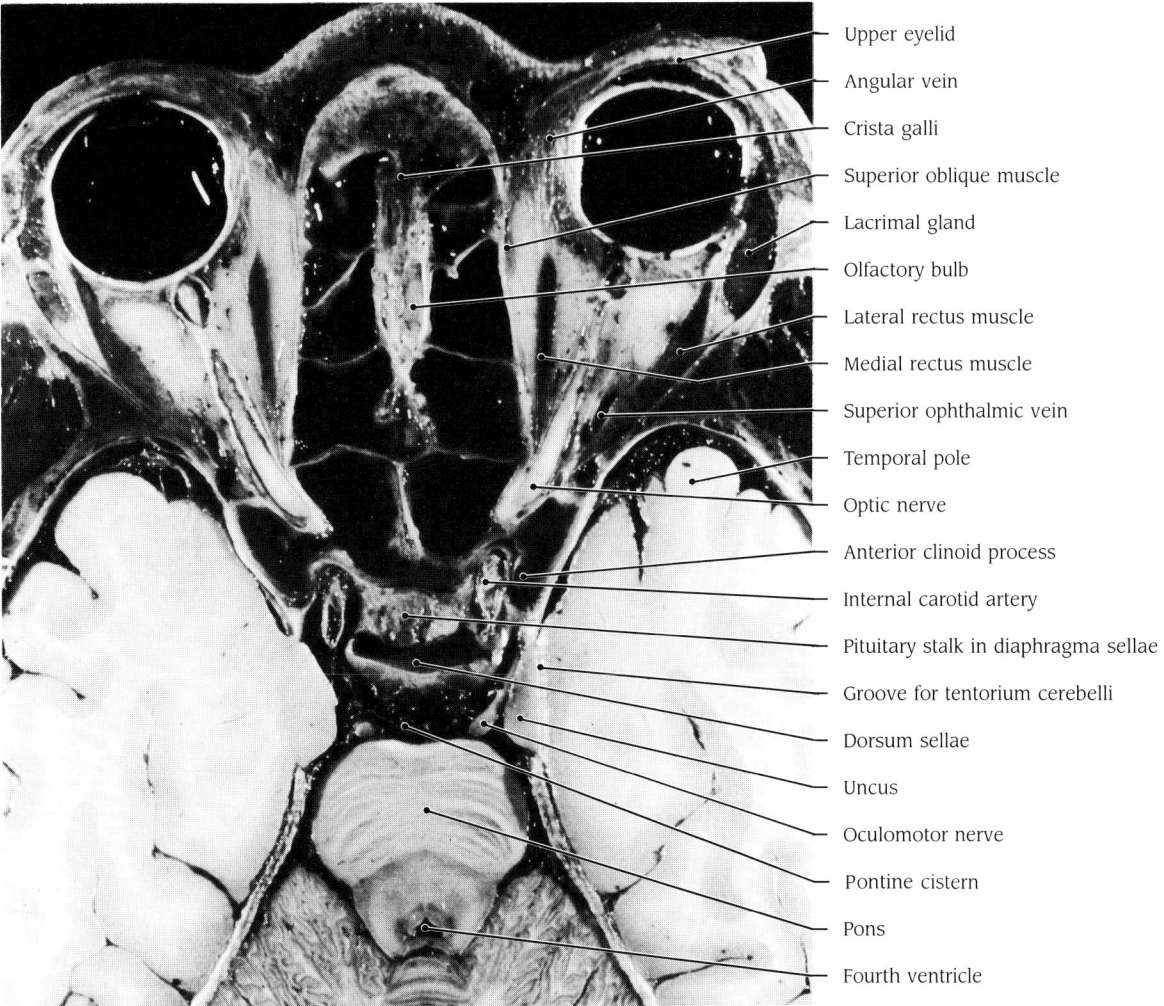

FIG. 5.7.

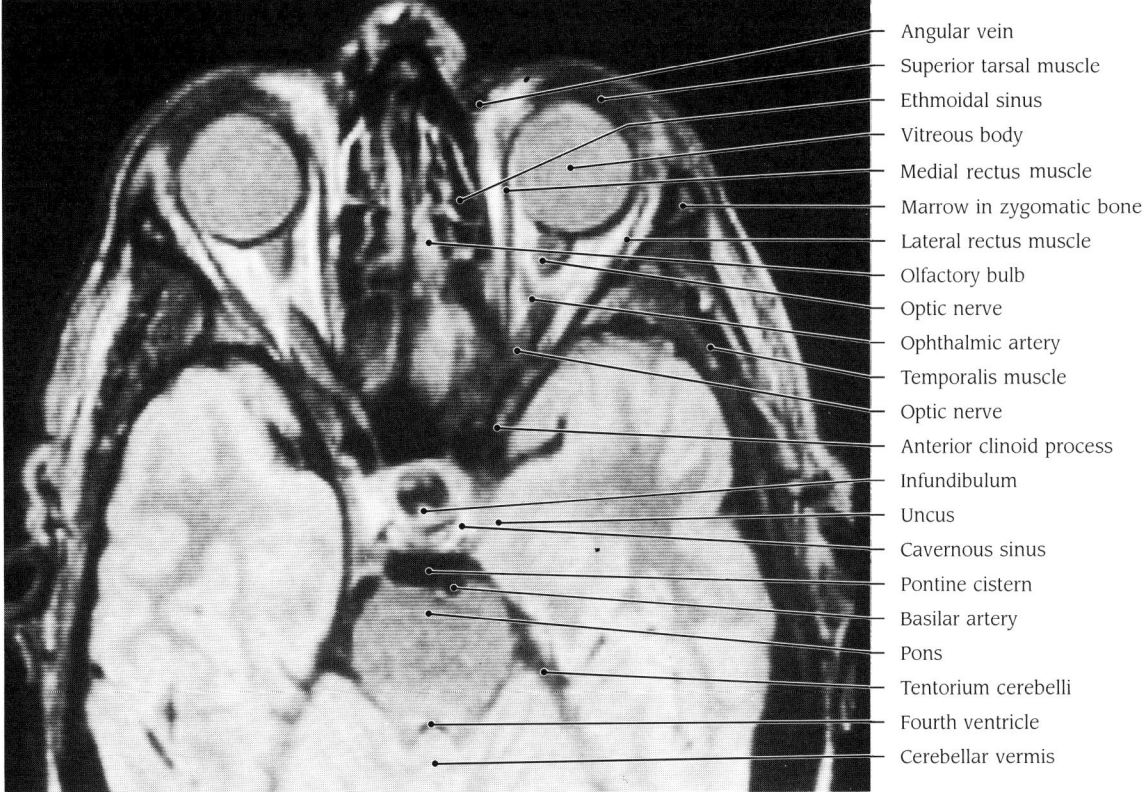

FIG. 5.8. TR = 2000 msec, TE = 50 msec.

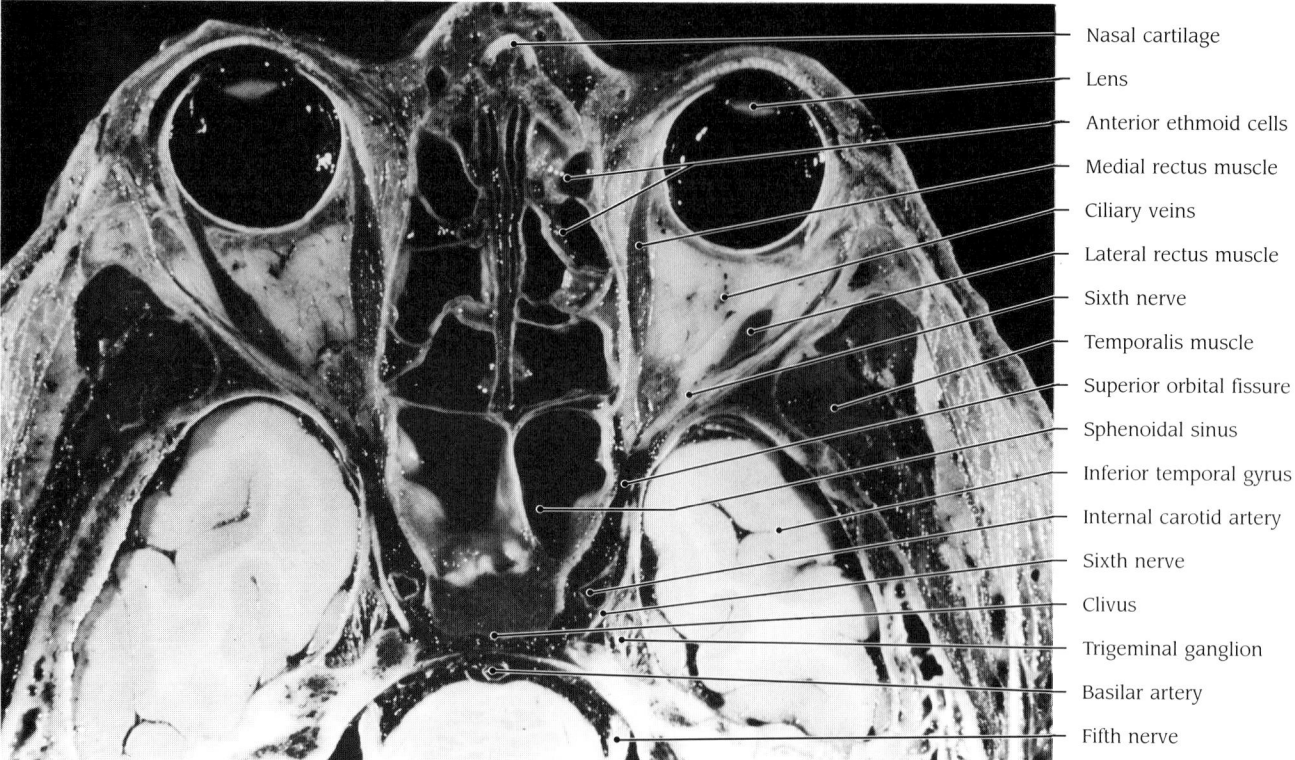

FIG. 5.9.

- The uveal tract, or vascular tunic of the eye, is a continuous structure composed of the choroid, the ciliary body, and the iris. The choroid lies adjacent to the inner surface of the sclera and extends anteriorly to the ora serrata of the retina. The ciliary body is a ventral extension of the choroid and continues from the anterior edge of the choroid into the circumference of the iris. The functions of the ciliary body include suspension of the lens, accommodation, and the production of both aqueous humor and some components of the vitreous humor.

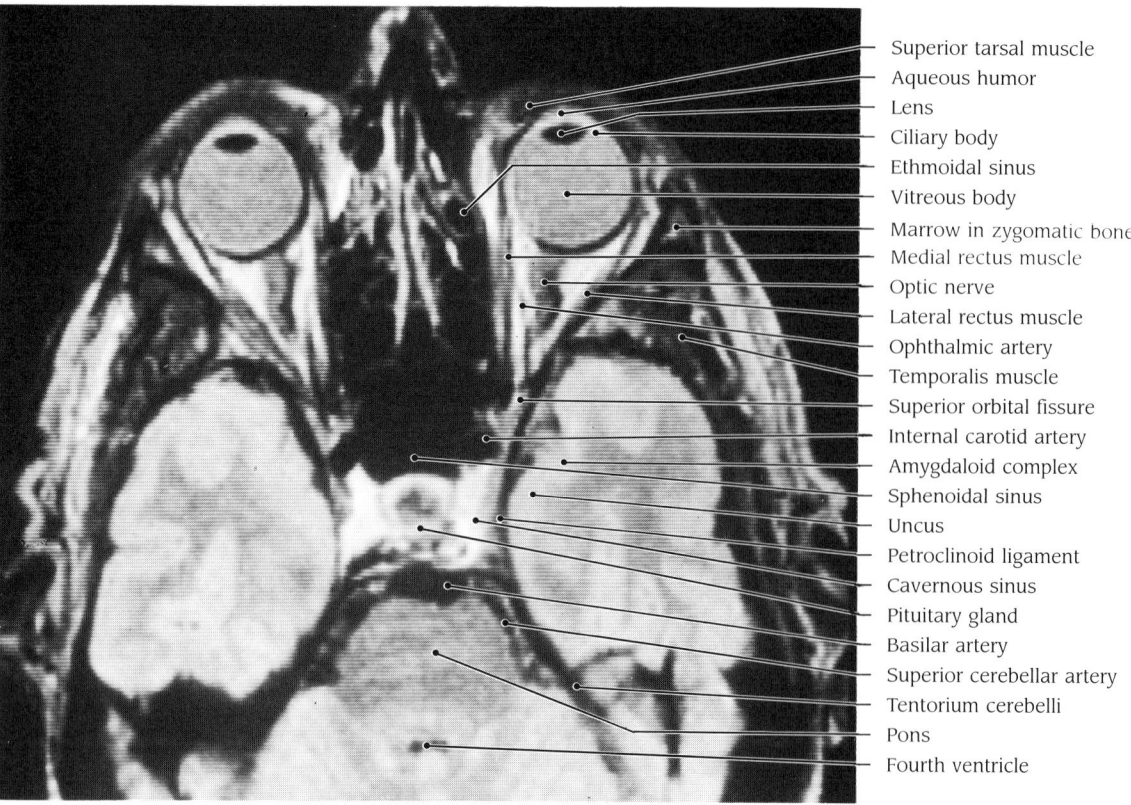

FIG. 5.10. TR = 2000 msec, TE = 50 msec.

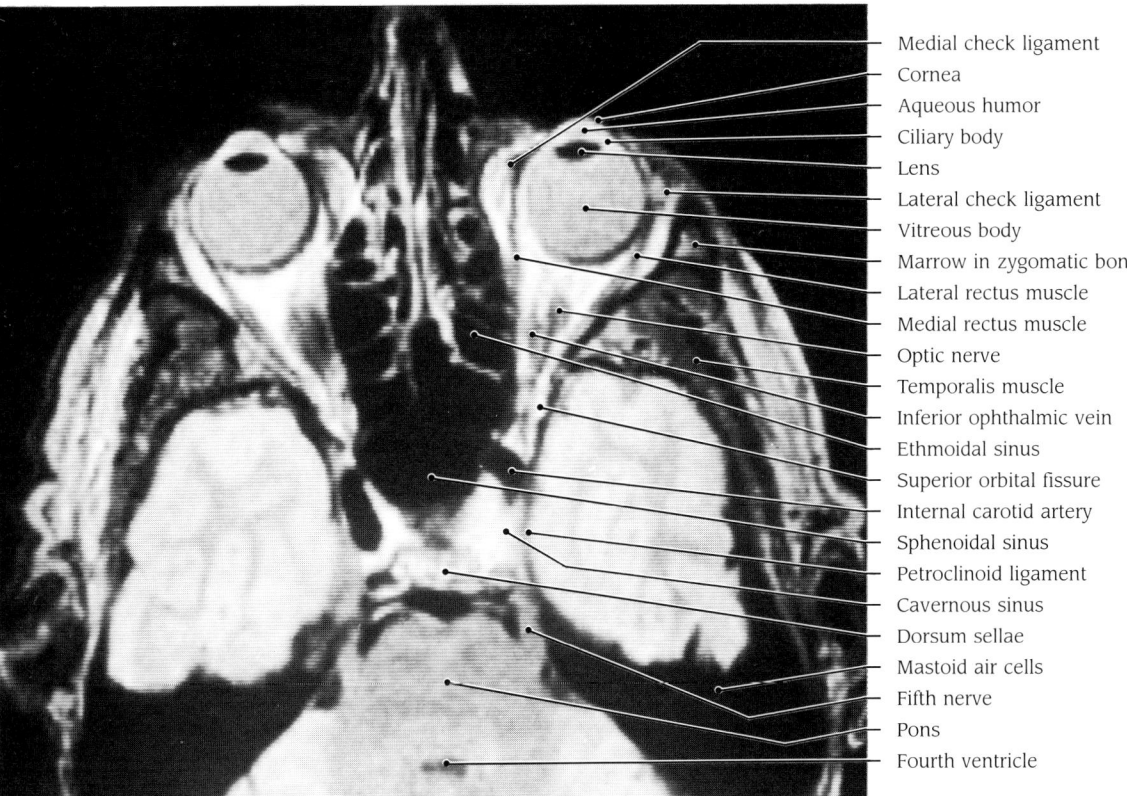

FIG. 5.11. TR = 2000 msec, TE = 50 msec.

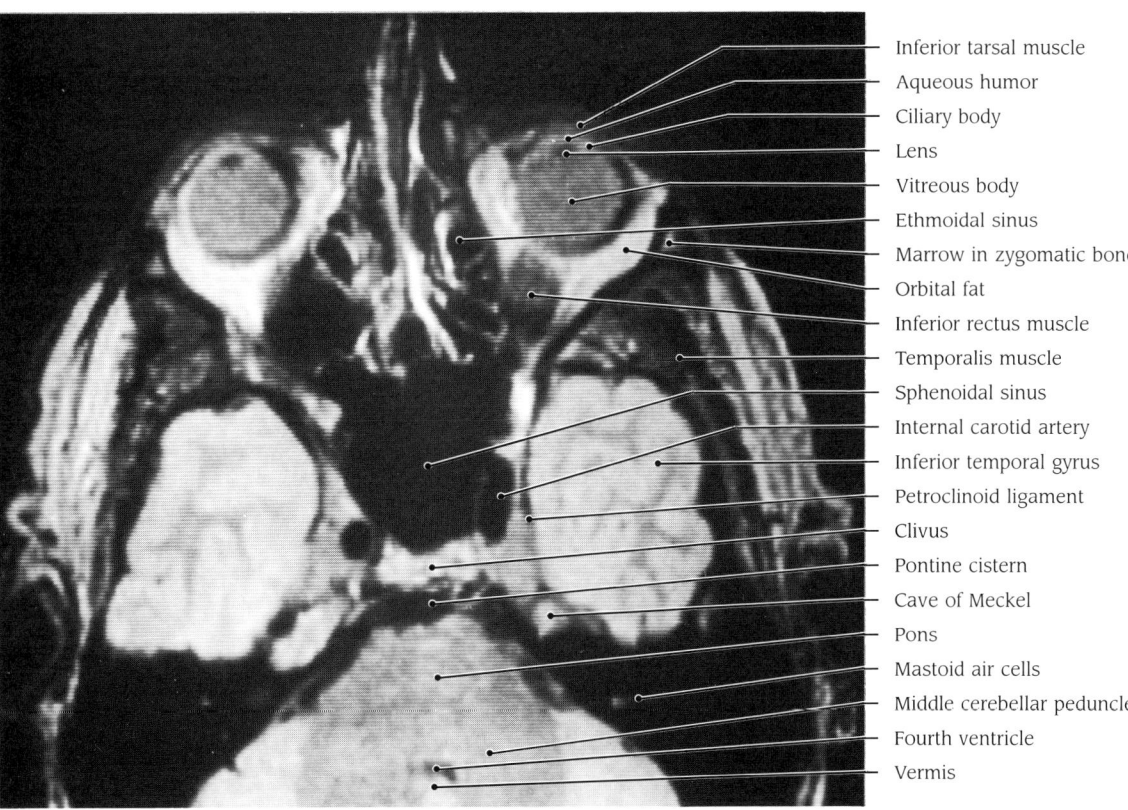

FIG. 5.12. TR = 2000 msec, TE = 50 msec.

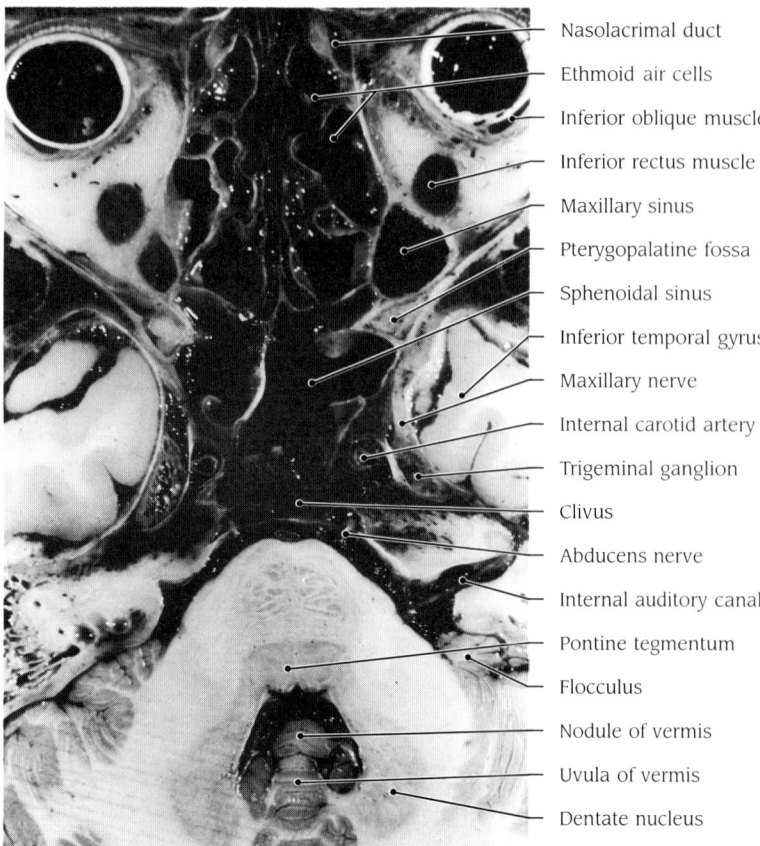

FIG. 5.13.

- The orbicularis oculi is a broad muscle located within the eyelids and around the orbit, that extends onto the temporal region and cheek. It is divided into orbital, palpebral, and lacrimal portions. The palpebral portion gently closes the lids, and acts either voluntarily or reflexly. The orbital portion usually is controlled voluntarily. With contraction of the entire muscle, the skin of the forehead, cheek, and temple approaches the medial angle of the orbit, and the eyelids are closed tightly. The lacrimal portion moves the eyelid and lacrimal papillae medially and concomitantly pulls on the lacrimal fascia and dilates the lacrimal sac.

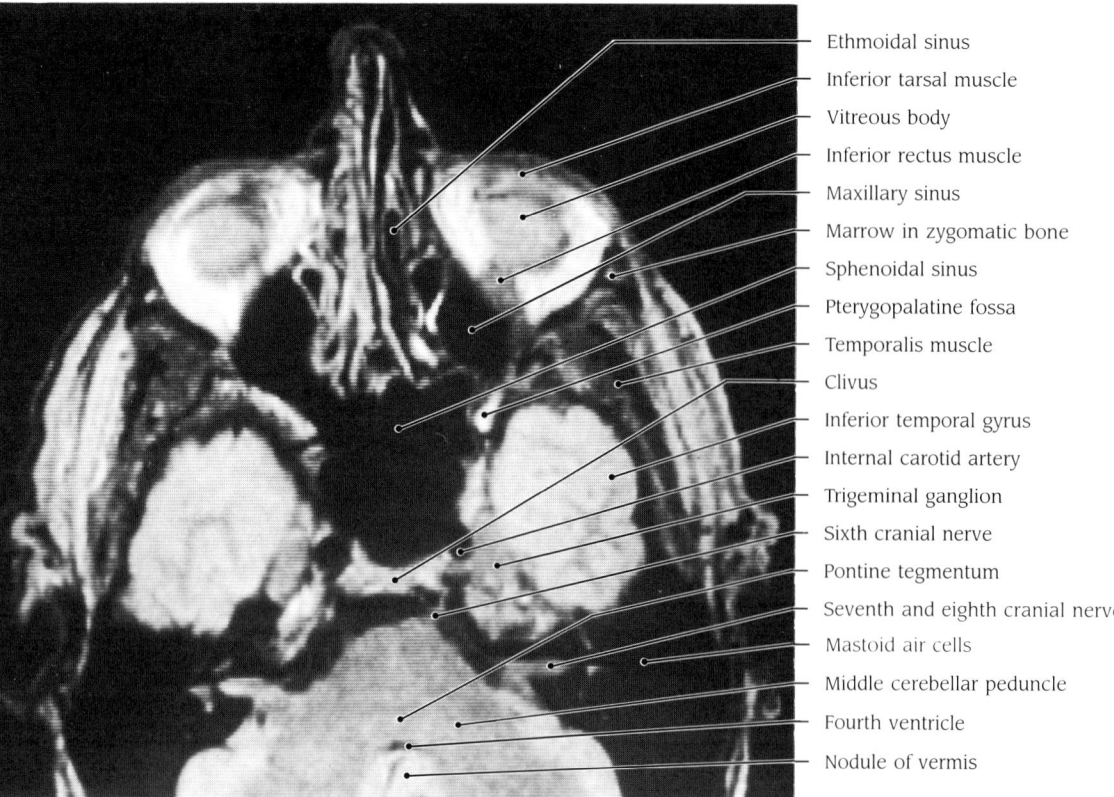

FIG. 5.14. TR = 2000 msec, TE = 50 msec.

116

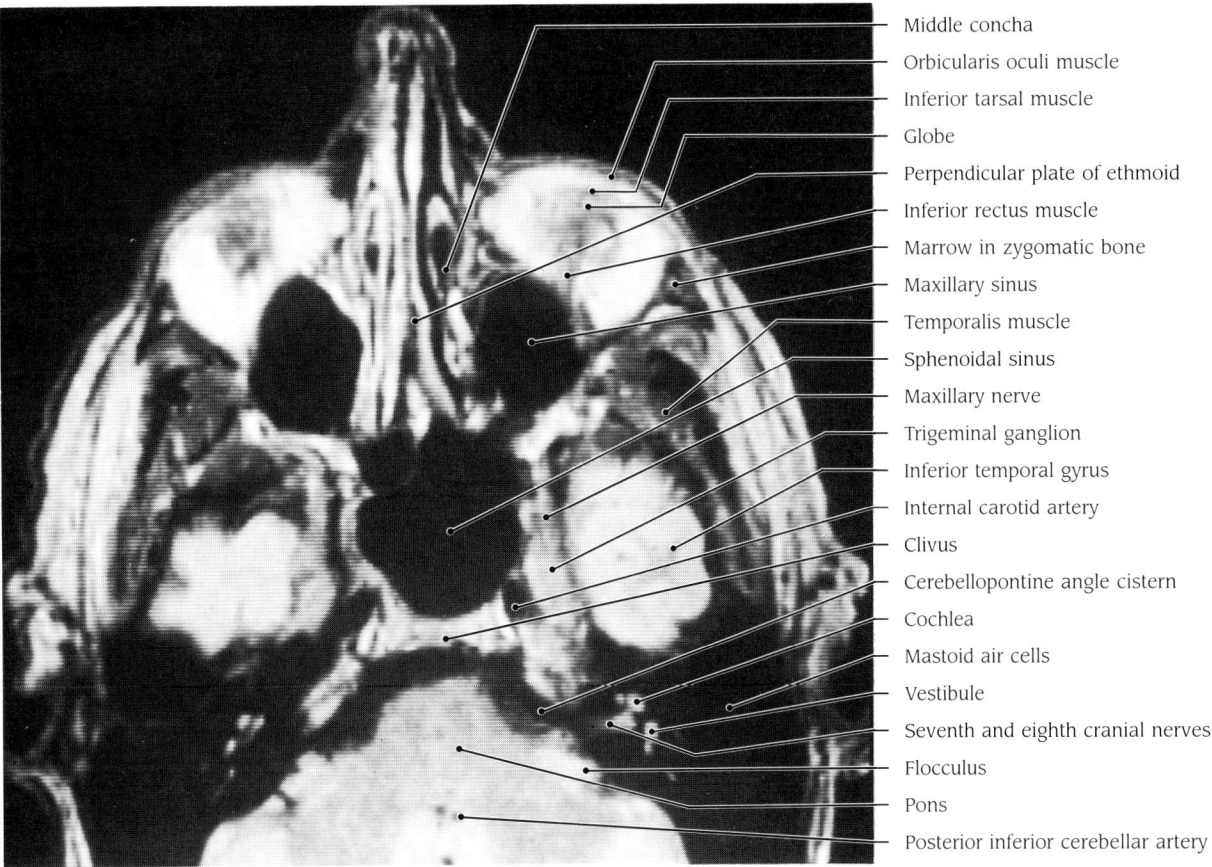

FIG. 5.15. TR = 2000 msec, TE = 50 msec.

- Middle concha
- Orbicularis oculi muscle
- Inferior tarsal muscle
- Globe
- Perpendicular plate of ethmoid
- Inferior rectus muscle
- Marrow in zygomatic bone
- Maxillary sinus
- Temporalis muscle
- Sphenoidal sinus
- Maxillary nerve
- Trigeminal ganglion
- Inferior temporal gyrus
- Internal carotid artery
- Clivus
- Cerebellopontine angle cistern
- Cochlea
- Mastoid air cells
- Vestibule
- Seventh and eighth cranial nerves
- Flocculus
- Pons
- Posterior inferior cerebellar artery

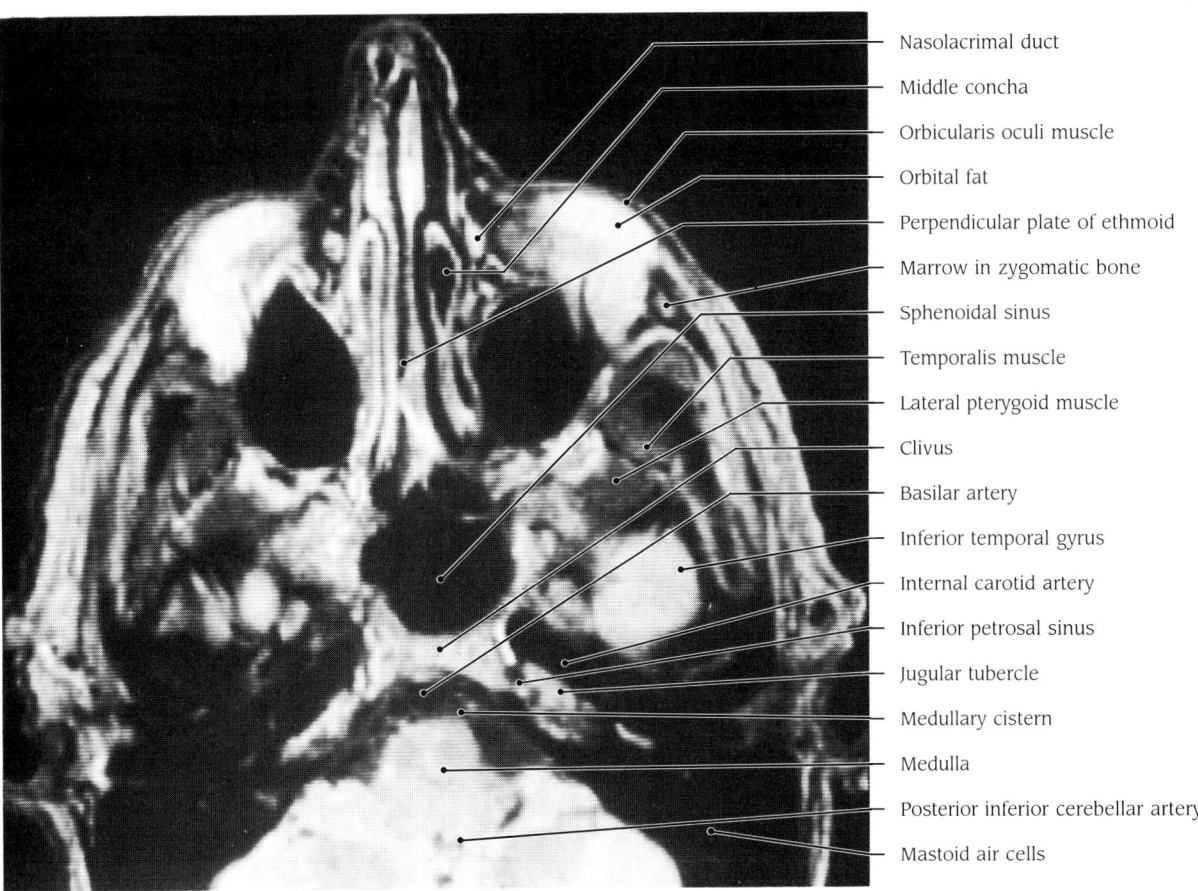

FIG. 5.16. TR = 2000 msec, TE = 50 msec.

- Nasolacrimal duct
- Middle concha
- Orbicularis oculi muscle
- Orbital fat
- Perpendicular plate of ethmoid
- Marrow in zygomatic bone
- Sphenoidal sinus
- Temporalis muscle
- Lateral pterygoid muscle
- Clivus
- Basilar artery
- Inferior temporal gyrus
- Internal carotid artery
- Inferior petrosal sinus
- Jugular tubercle
- Medullary cistern
- Medulla
- Posterior inferior cerebellar artery
- Mastoid air cells

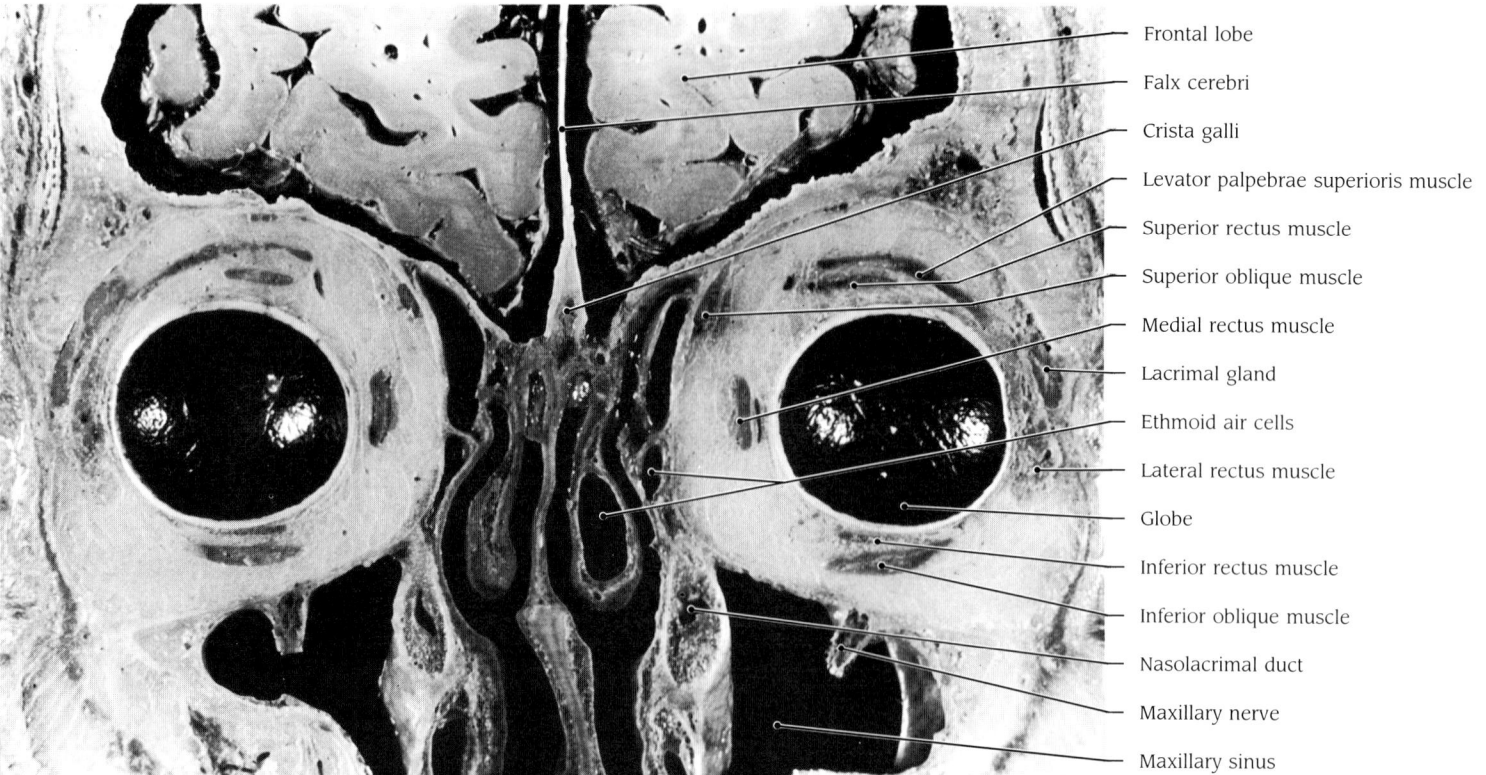

FIG. 5.17.

- The aqueous humor fills the anterior and posterior chambers. It is produced by active transport and diffusion from the capillaries of the ciliary processes. The aqueous humor enters the posterior chamber from these capillaries. It then passes through the pupillary aperture and enters the anterior chamber. The aqueous humor leaves the anterior chamber through the spaces of the iridocorneal angle and the sinus venosus sclerae and passes into the anterior ciliary veins. Increased intraocular pressure, or glaucoma, results when the resorption of the aqueous humor into the sinus venosus sclerae is impeded.

- The vitreous body is a transparent, colorless, structureless gel that fills the vitreous chamber. This gel is approximately 99% water. Other constituents include salts, mucoprotein (vitrein), and hyaluronic acid. Electron microscopy has identified fibrils and an interfibrillary substance, known as vitreous humor, in the vitreous body.

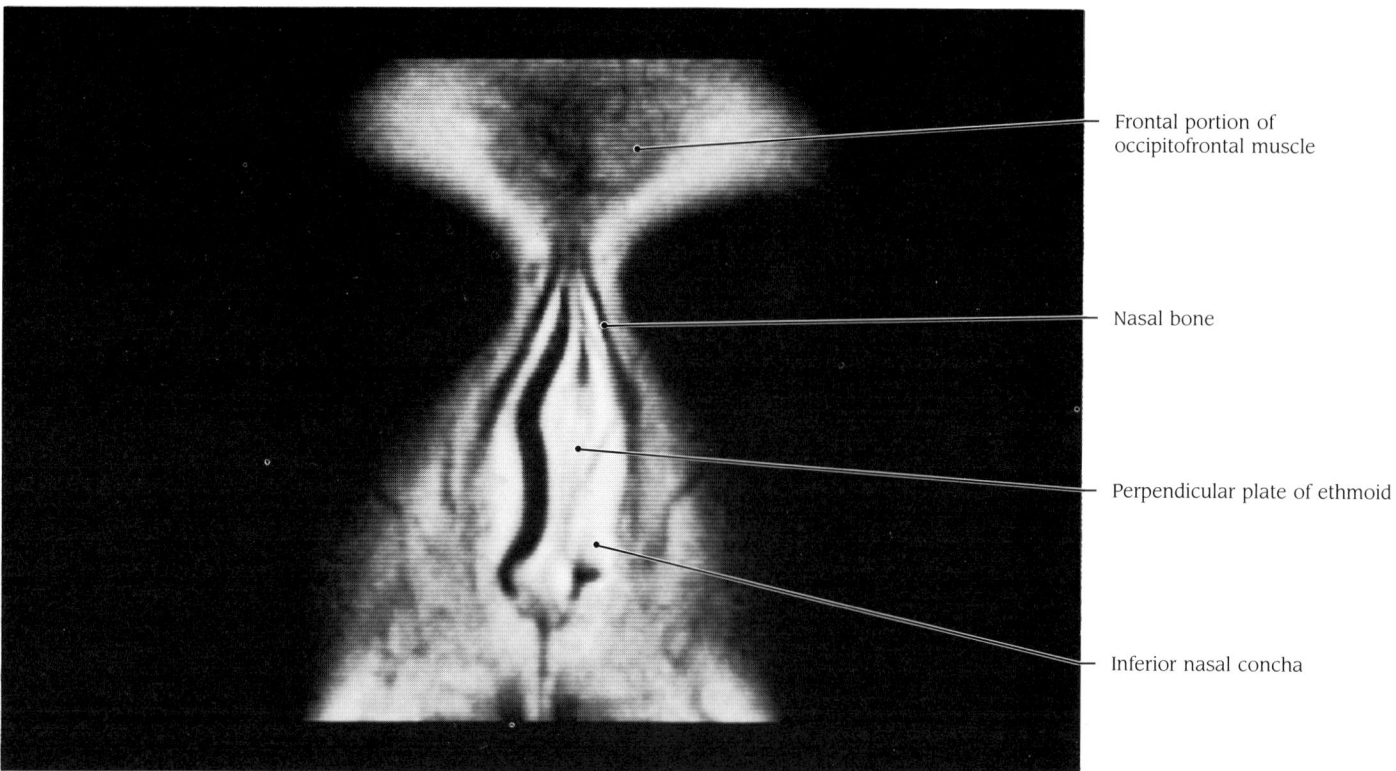

FIG. 5.18. TR = 2000 msec, TE = 28 msec.

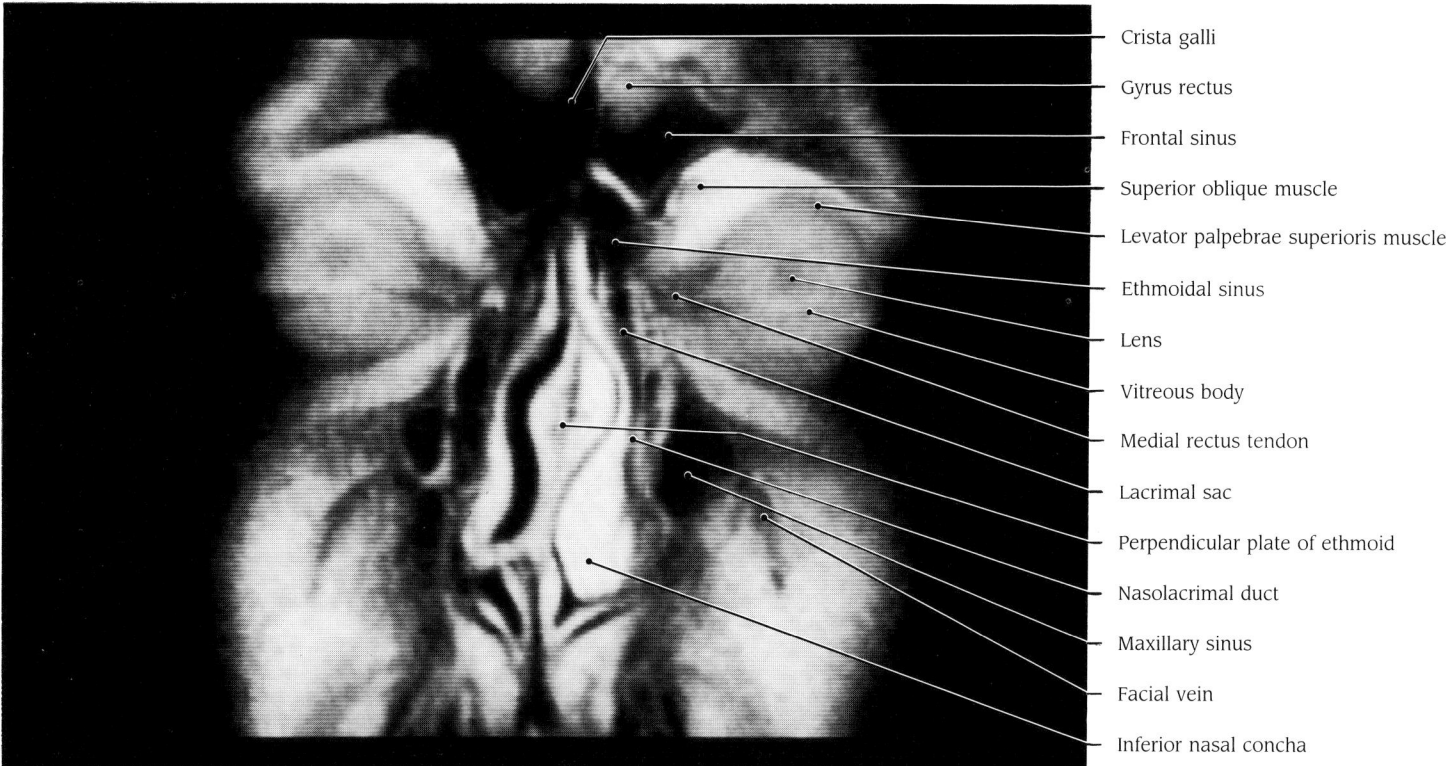

FIG. 5.19. TR = 2000 msec, TE = 28 msec.

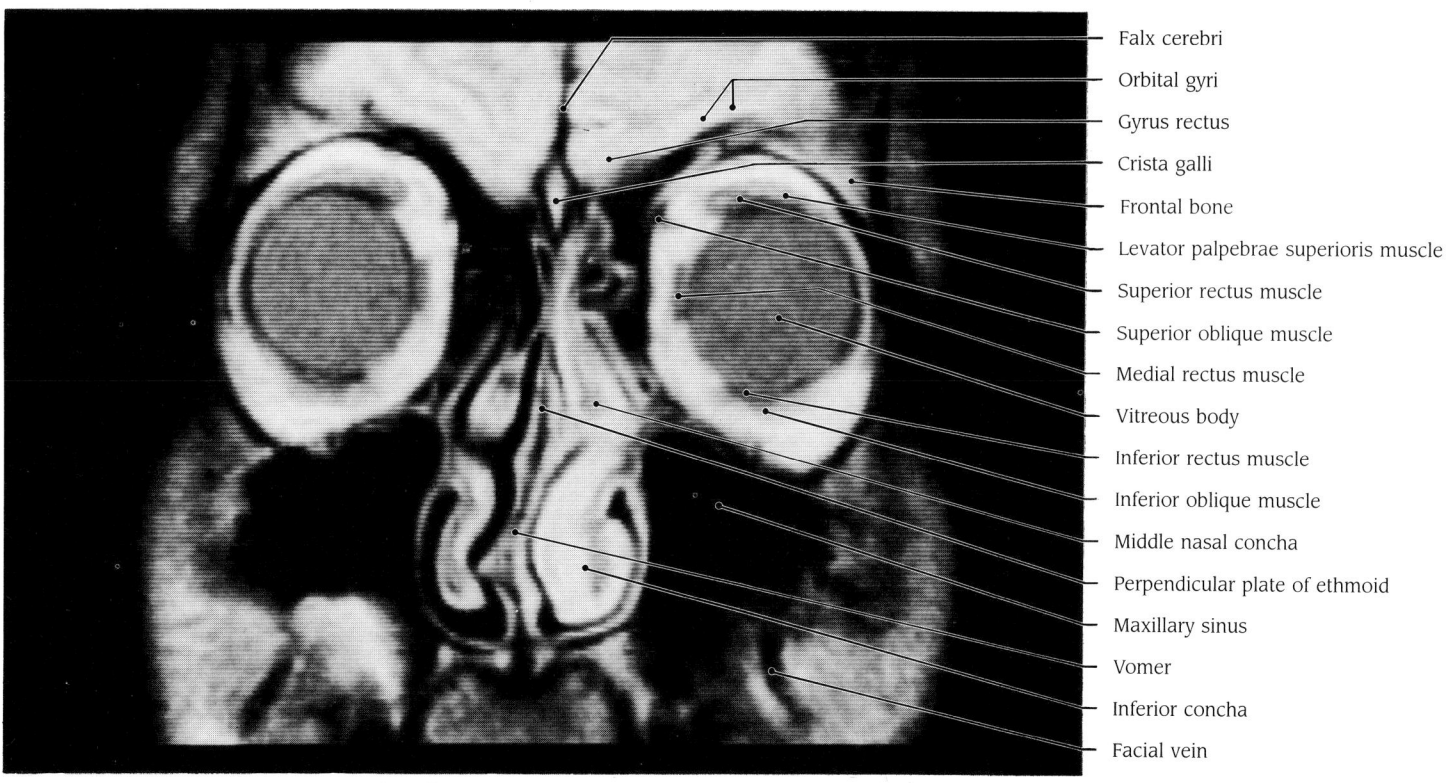

FIG. 5.20. TR = 2000 msec, TE = 28 msec.

119

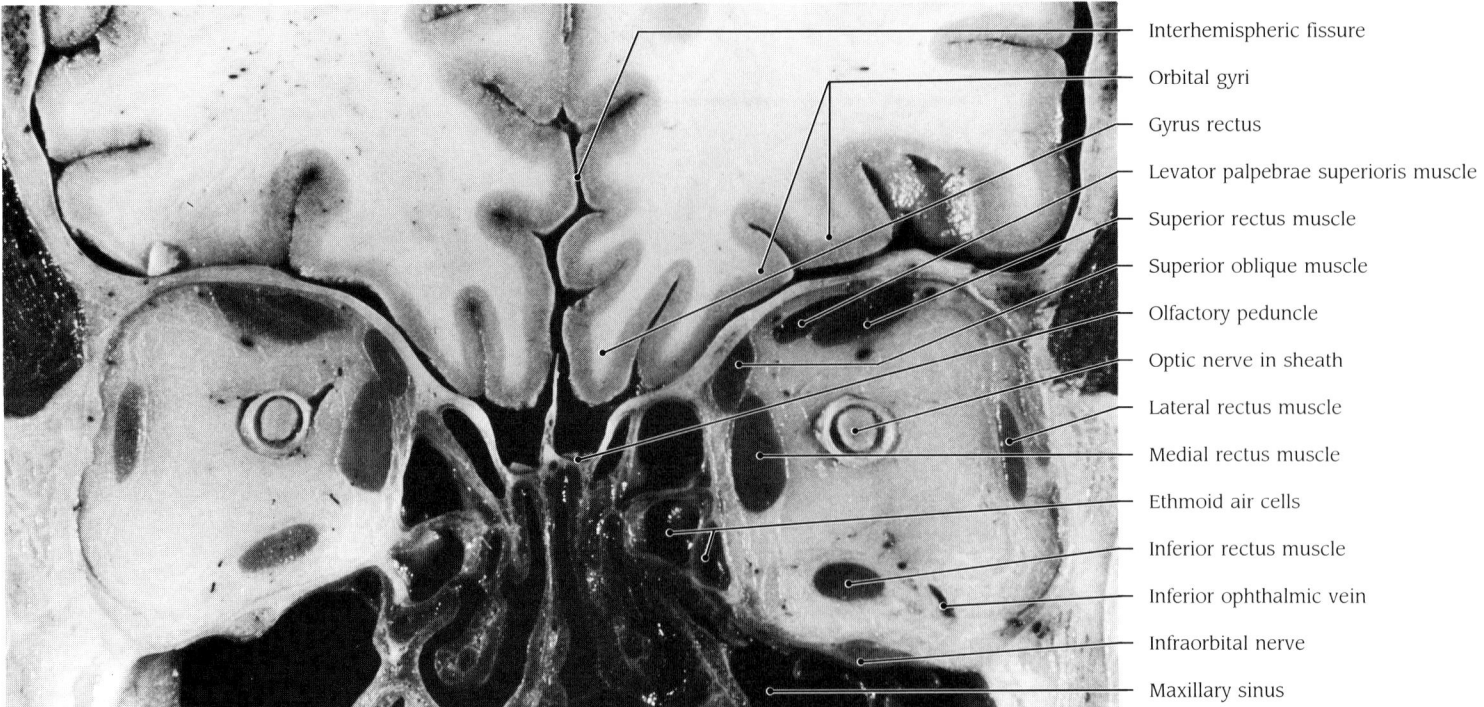

FIG. 5.21.

- The superior ophthalmic vein originates at the junction of its superior and inferior tributaries, approximately 5 mm posterior to the point where the superior oblique tendon passes through the trochlea. The superior tributary is an inferior continuation of the frontal veins. The inferior tributary is a continuation of the angular vein.

- The superior ophthalmic vein can be divided into three segments. The first segment extends from the trochlea of the superior oblique muscle to the orbital roof. This portion lies outside the muscle cone, above the superior oblique muscle. The second segment enters the muscle cone and courses along the inferior surface of the superior rectus muscle. It is closely related to the posterior pole of the globe and then crosses the optic nerve and ophthalmic artery. The third segment of the superior ophthalmic vein changes direction and courses posteriorly, medially, and slightly inferiorly. Posteriorly, the superior ophthalmic vein leaves the muscle cone and passes between the superior rectus and levator muscles medially and the lateral rectus muscle inferiorly. It leaves the orbit while passing between the lateral rectus and superior rectus muscles, continues through the superior orbital fissure, and ends at the anteroinferior portion of the cavernous sinus.

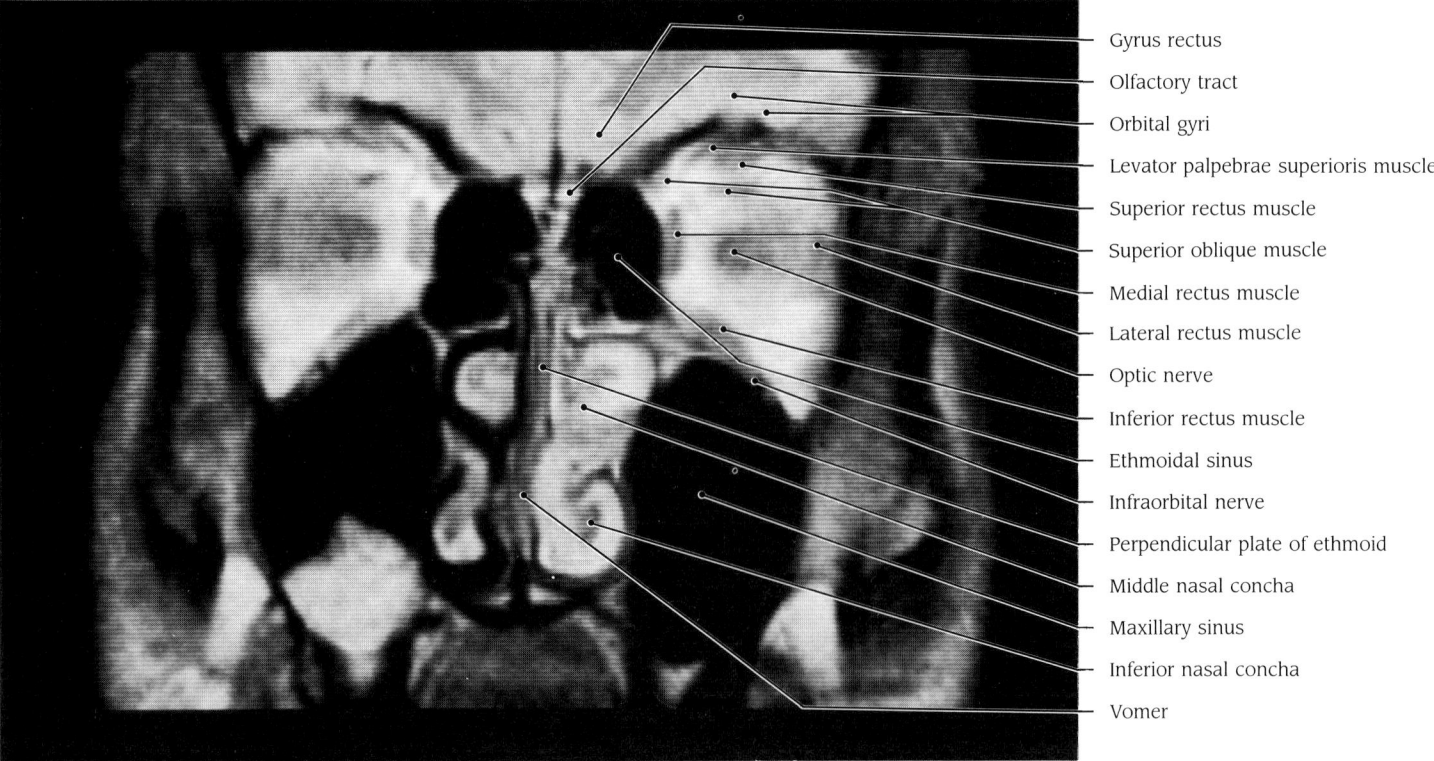

FIG. 5.22. TR = 2000 msec, TE = 28 msec.

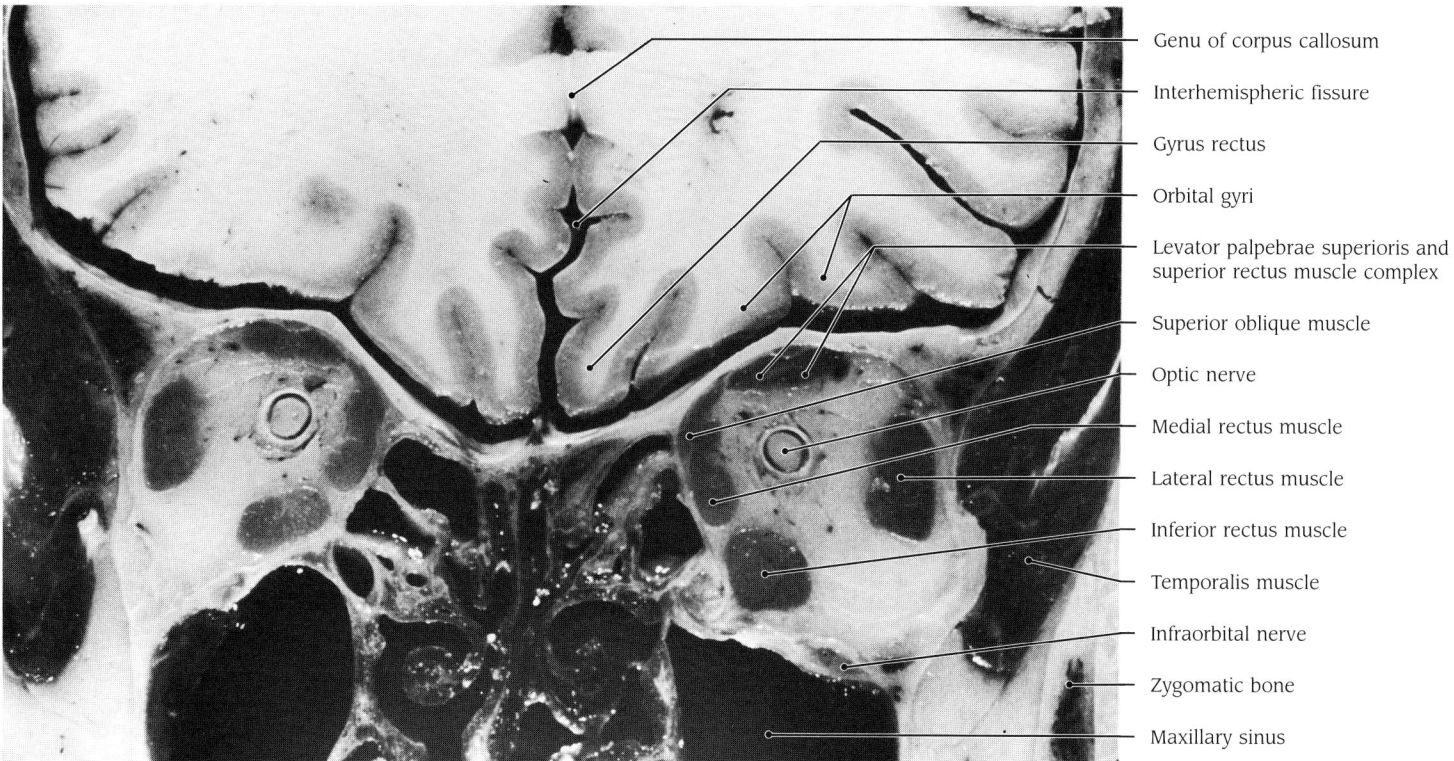

FIG. 5.23.

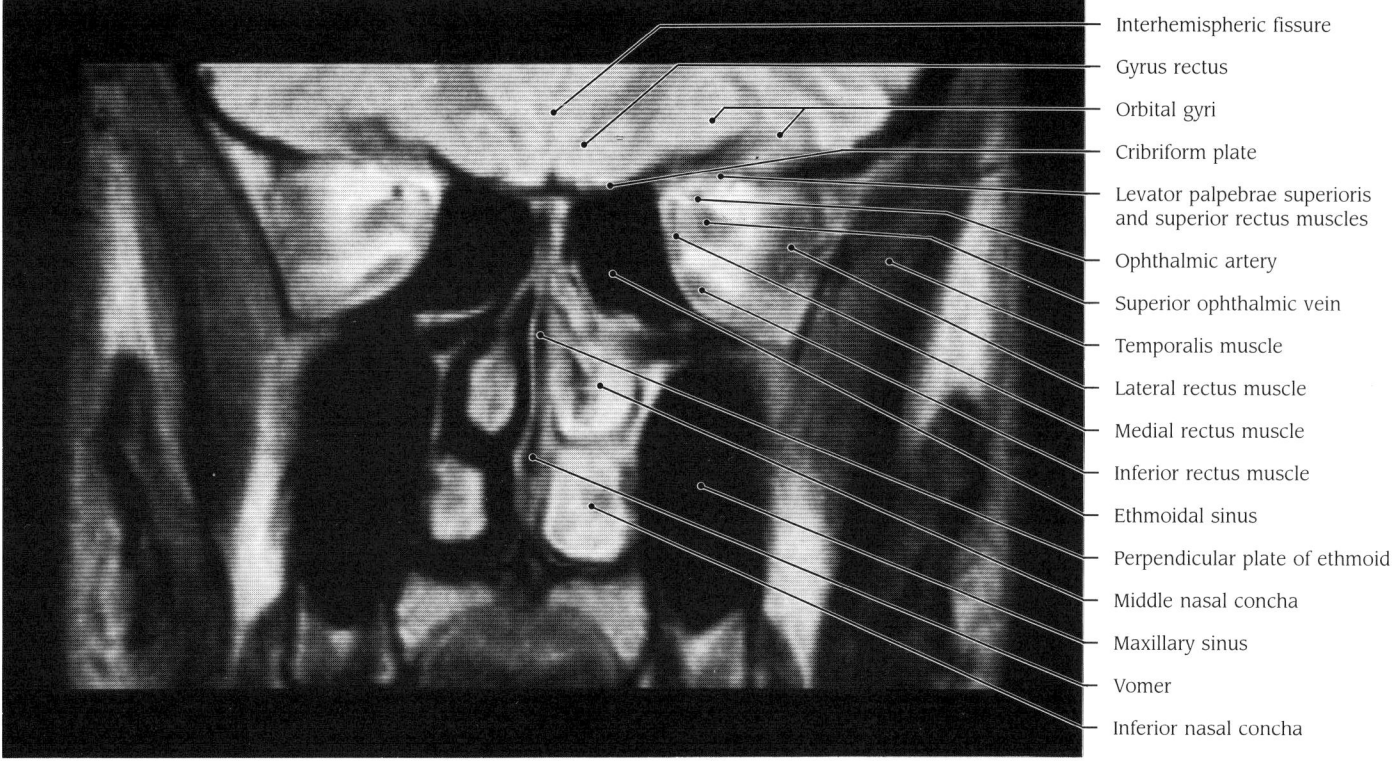

FIG. 5.24. TR = 2000 msec, TE = 28 msec.

121

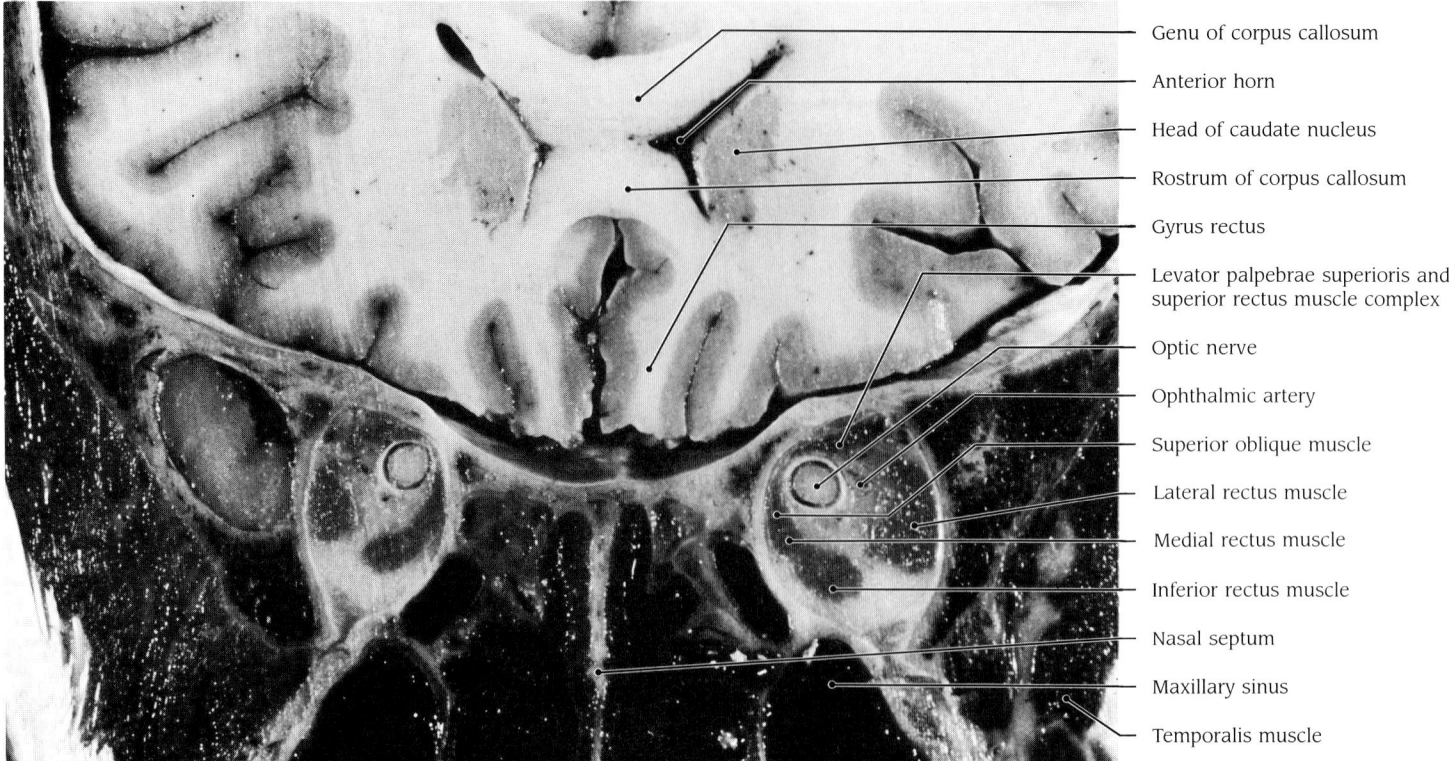

FIG. 5.25.

- The superior orbital fissure connects the middle cranial fossa and the orbit. Its boundaries are the body of the sphenoid bone, medially; the lesser wing of the sphenoid bone, superiorly; the medial aspect of the orbital surface of the greater wing, inferiorly; and the frontal bone, laterally. The fissure is triangular and widest medially; its long axis is directed superiorly, laterally, and anteriorly. The structures within the superior orbital fissure include the oculomotor, trochlear, and abducent nerves; the three branches of the ophthalmic division of the trigeminal nerve; the recurrent meningeal branch of the lacrimal artery; the orbital branch of the middle meningeal artery; and the ophthalmic veins.

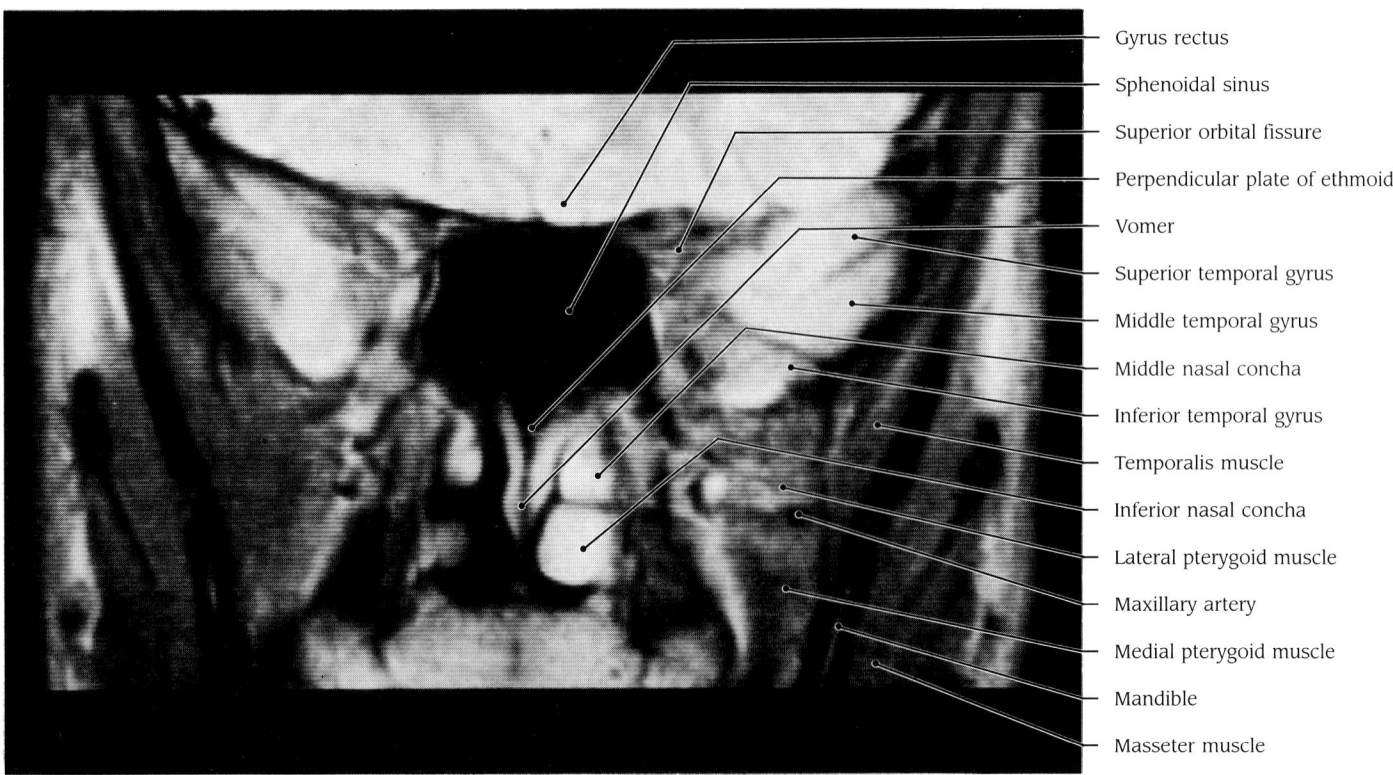

FIG. 5.26. TR = 2000 msec, TE = 28 msec.

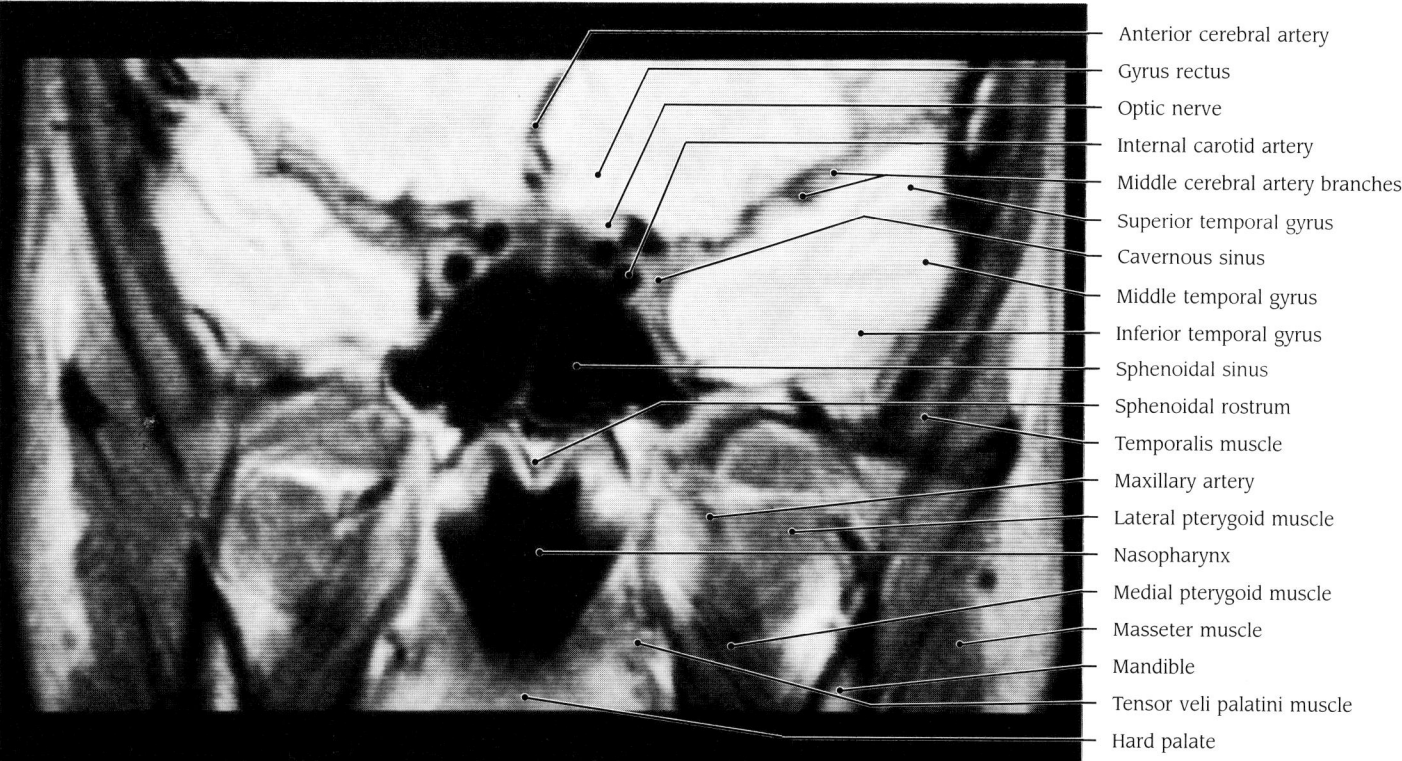

FIG. 5.27. TR = 2000 msec, TE = 28 msec.

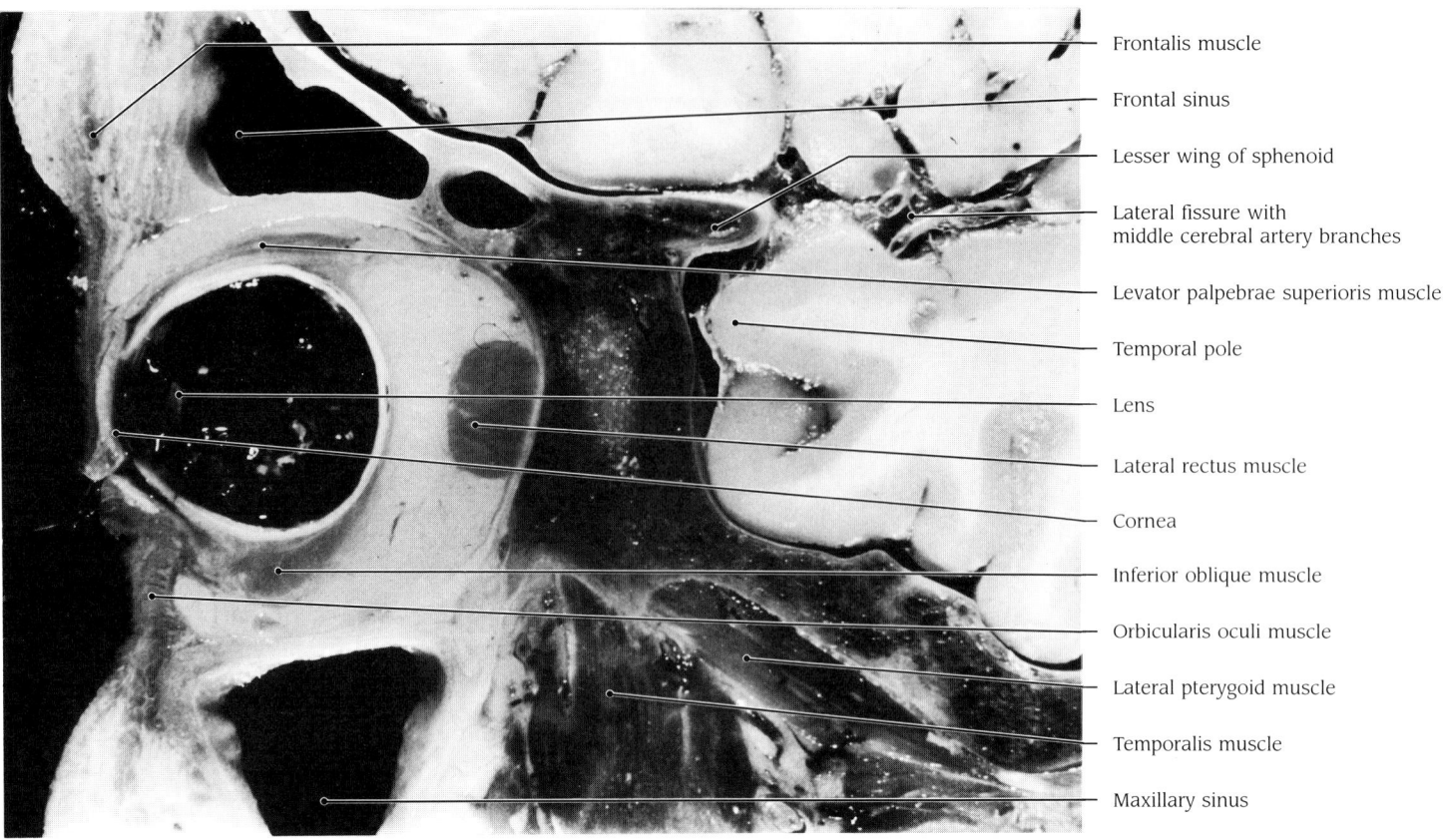

FIG. 5.28.

- The lens is a transparent, biconvex structure surrounded by a transparent, elastic capsule. It is situated posterior to the iris and anterior to the vitreous body in the hyaloid fossa. The suspensory ligament retains the lens in position.

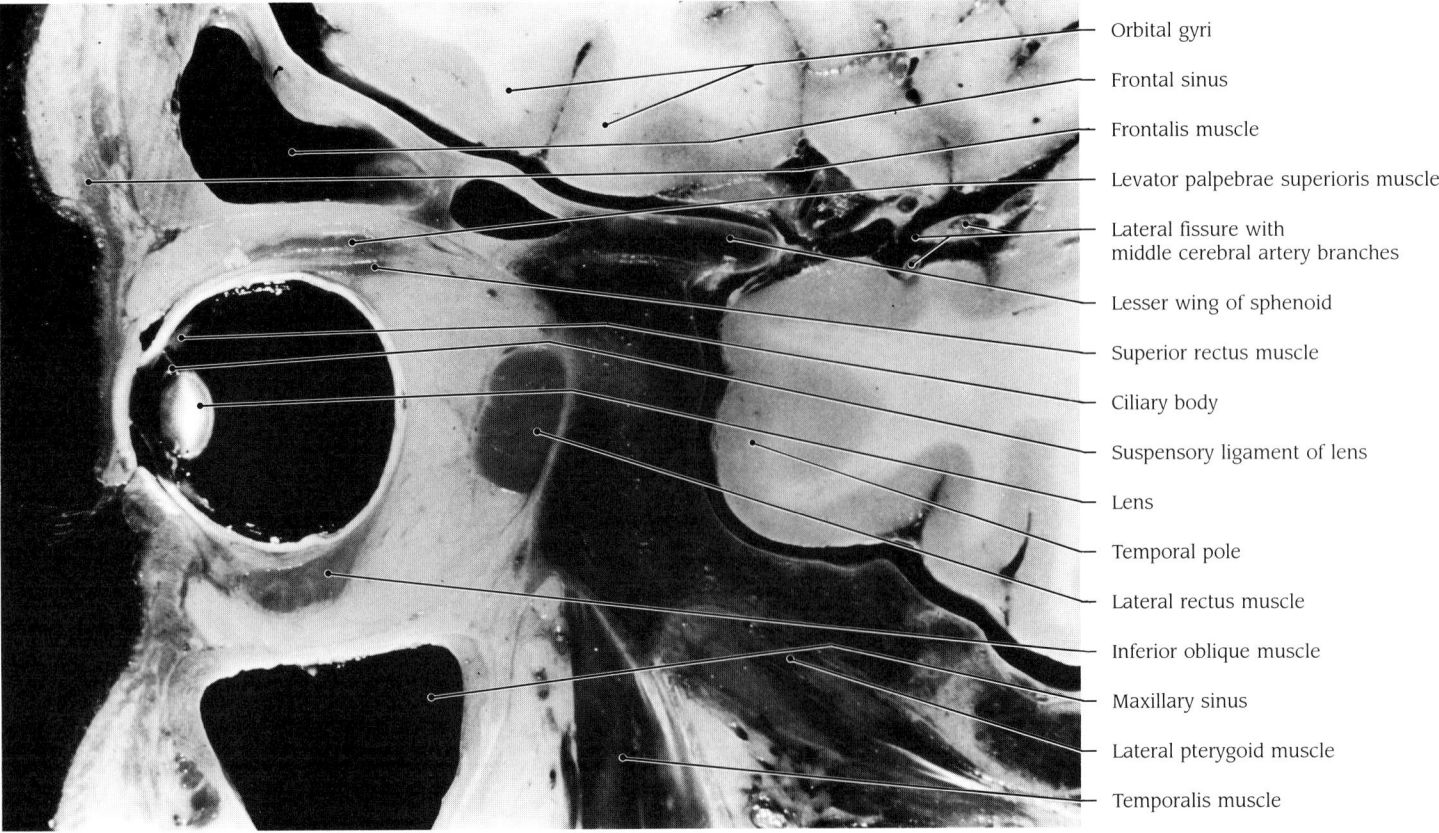

FIG. 5.29.

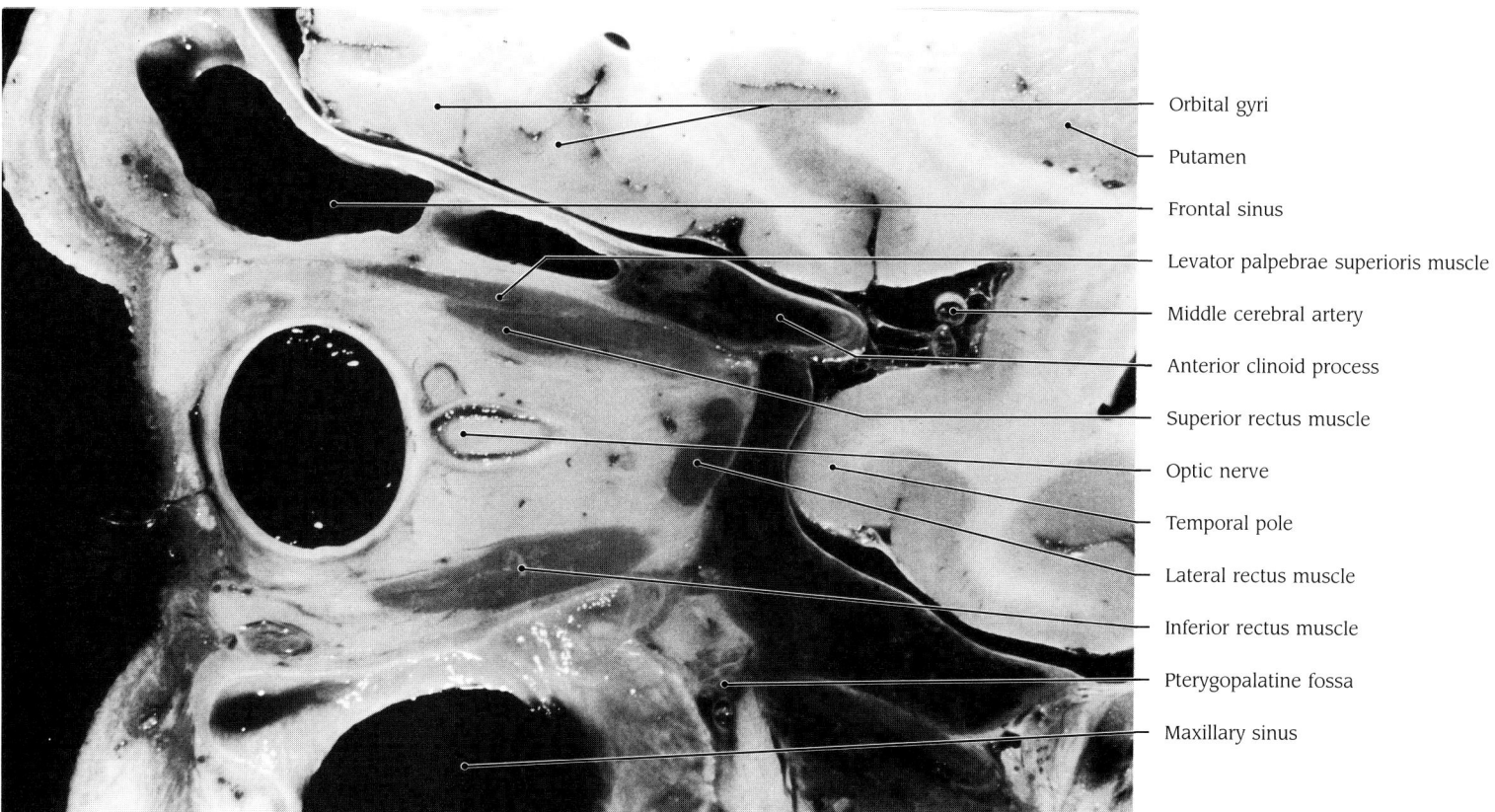

FIG. 5.30.

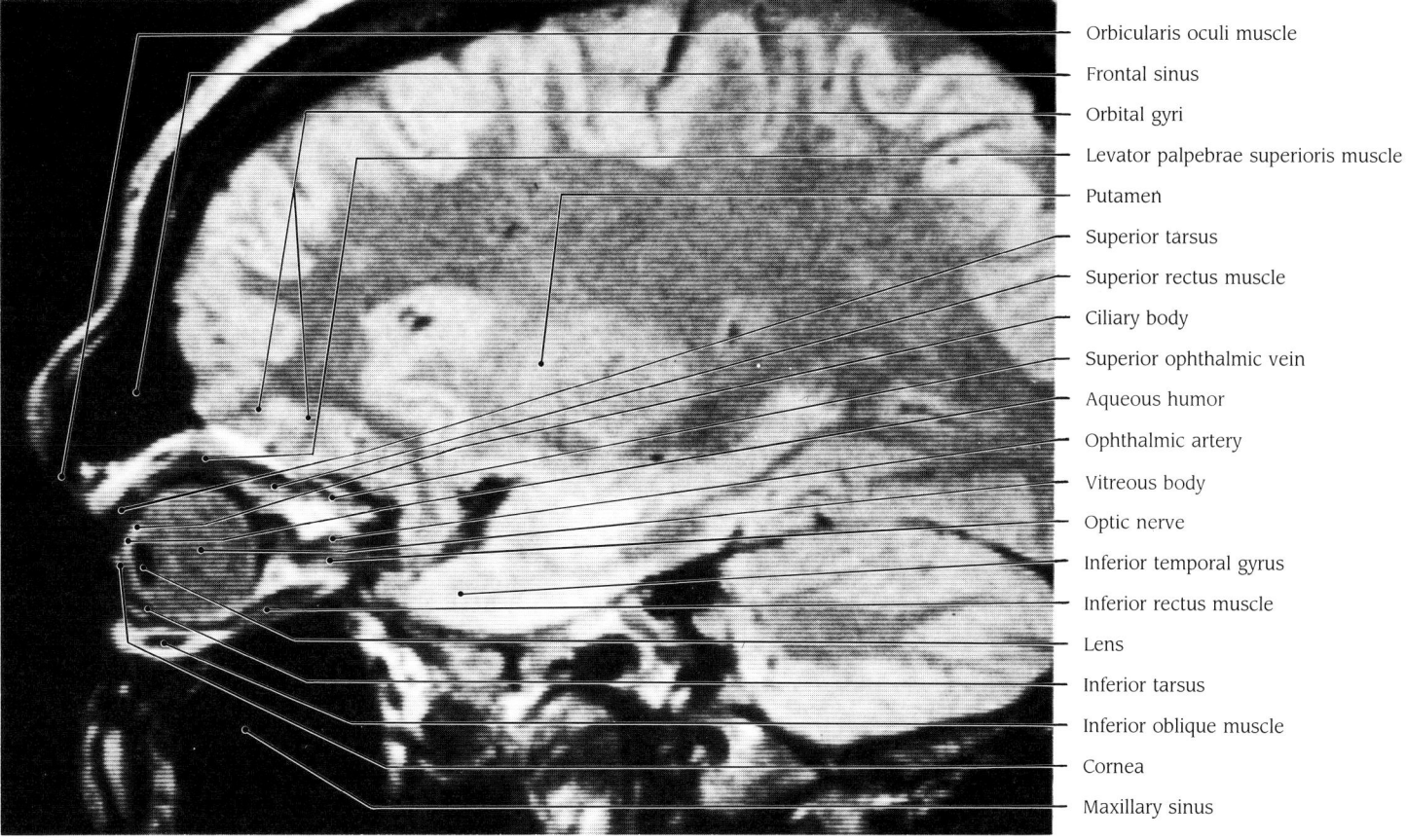

FIG. 5.31. TR = 2000 msec, TE = 50 msec.

125

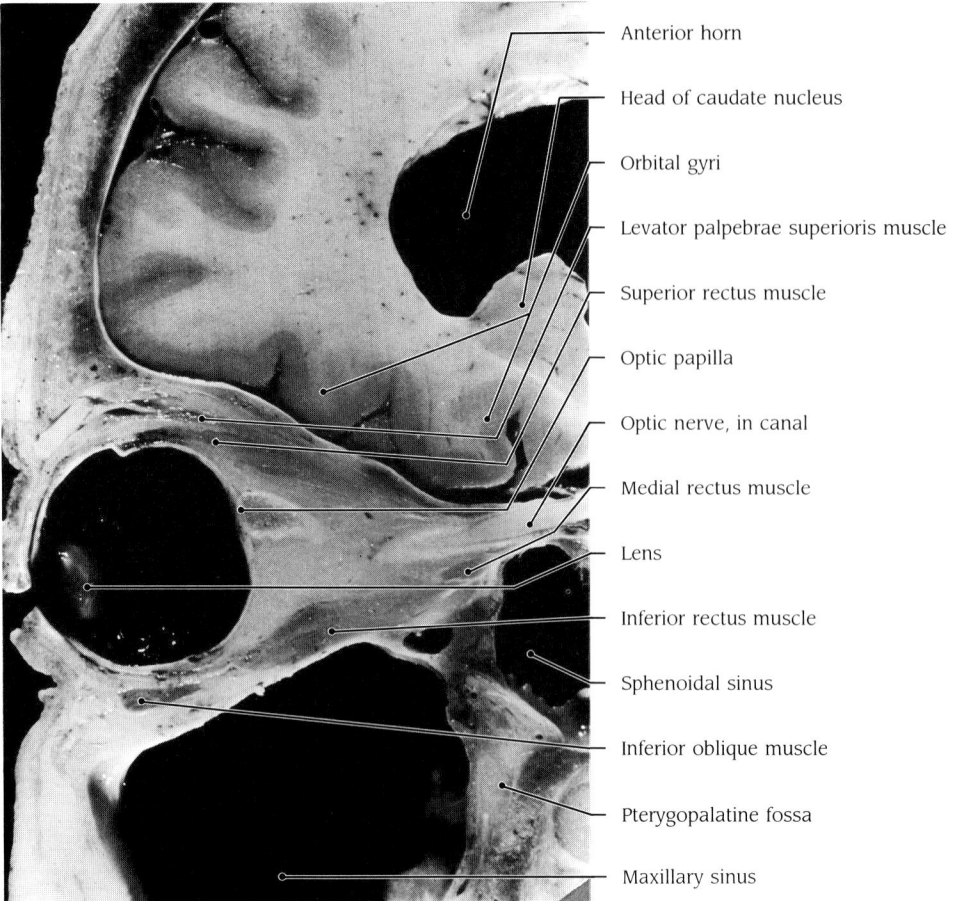

FIG. 5.32.

- The pterygopalatine fossa is a small triangular compartment that lies inferior to the apex of the orbit, posterior to the maxillary sinus, and anterior to the pterygoid plates. It is bounded anteriorly by the corpus maxillae and posteriorly by the root of the pterygoid process and by the adjoining portion of the greater wing of the sphenoid bone. The medial margin is formed by the orbital and sphenoidal processes of the palatine bone. The superior border is the body of the sphenoid bone and the inferior border is located where the perpendicular plate of the palatine bone meets the maxilla.

- The pterygopalatine fossa communicates with the infratemporal fossa, the nasal and oral cavities, the orbit, the pharynx, and the middle cranial fossa through eight passageways. The most important structures within the fossa are the maxillary nerve, the pterygopalatine ganglion, and the terminal part of the maxillary artery.

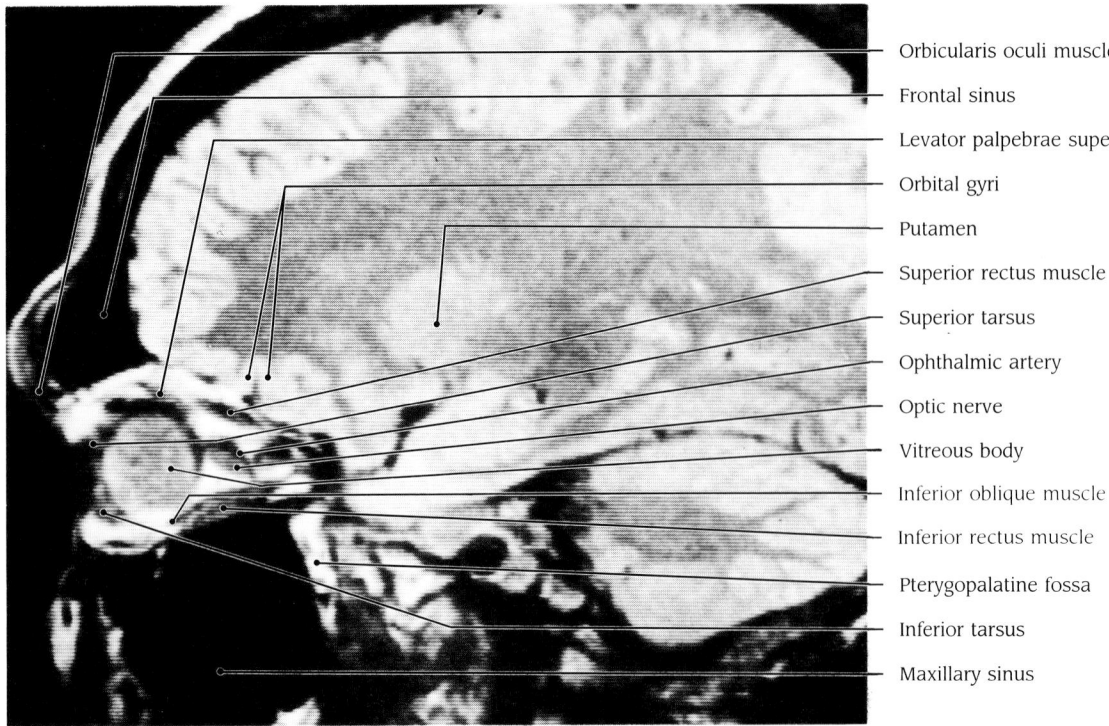

FIG. 5.33. TR = 2000 msec, TE = 50 msec.

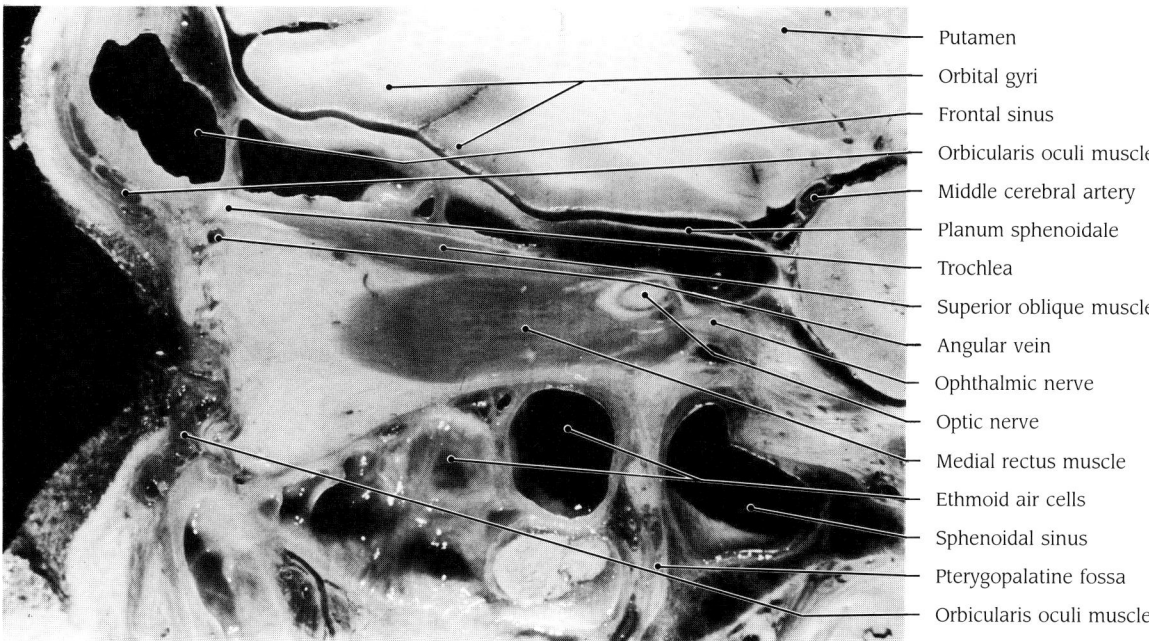

FIG. 5.34.

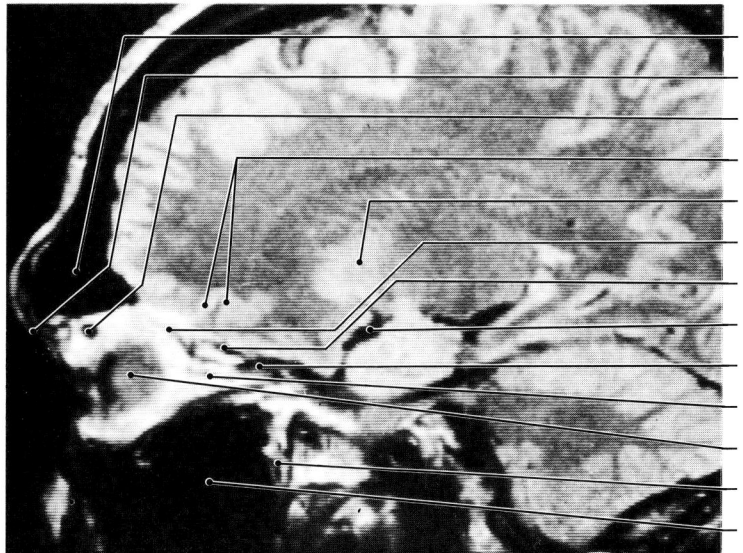

FIG. 5.35. TR = 2000 msec, TE = 50 msec.

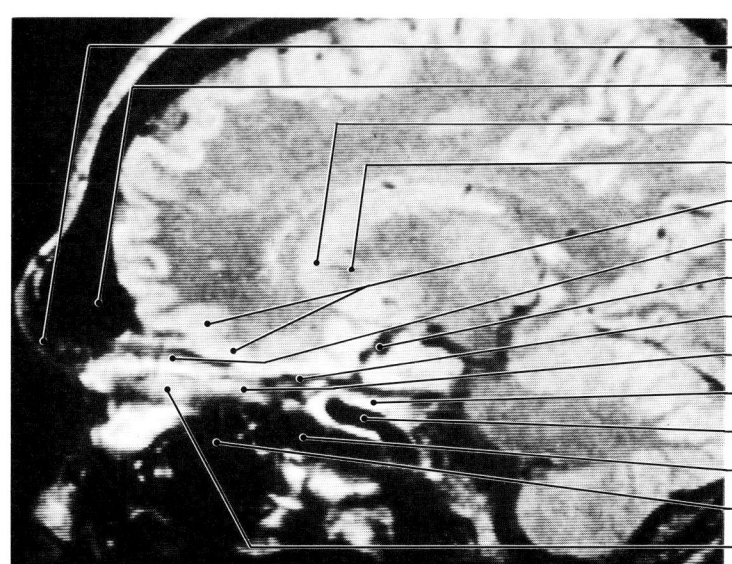

FIG. 5.36. TR = 2000 msec, TE = 50 msec.

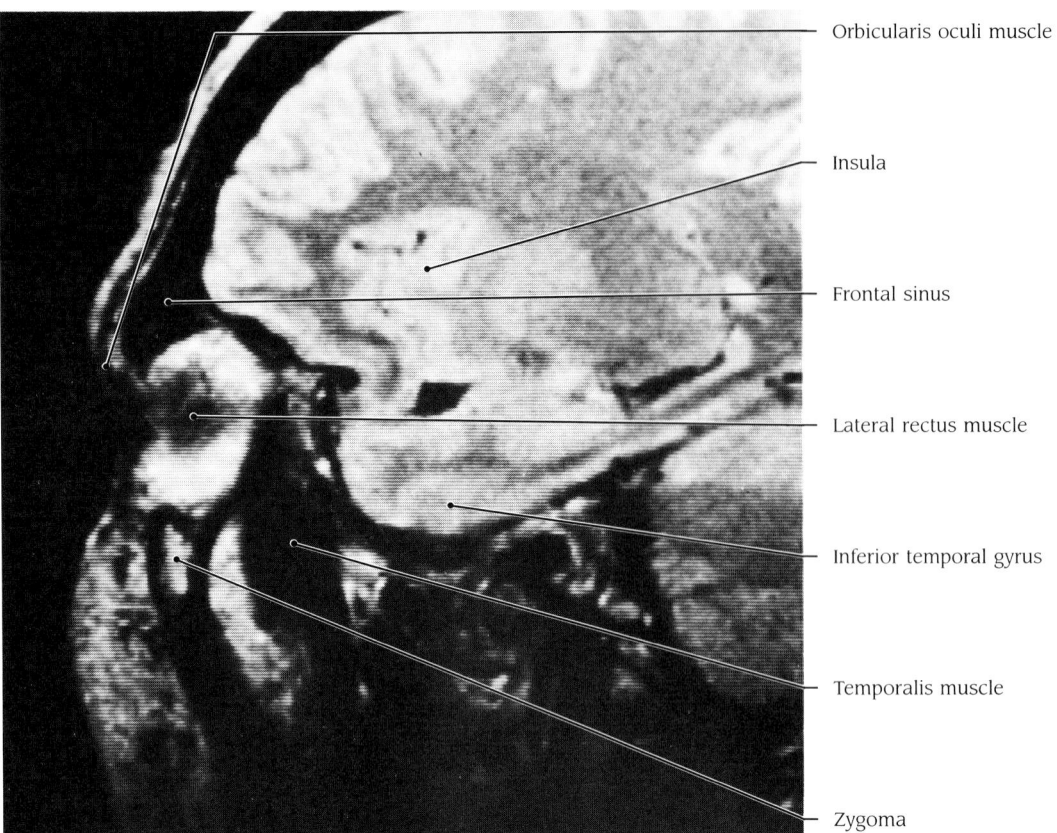

FIG. 5.37. TR = 2000 msec, TE = 50 msec.

- The superior and inferior tarsi are elongated plates of dense fibrous tissue located in the eyelids. They provide shape and support to the eyelids. The lateral palpebral ligament attaches the lateral aspect of the tarsi to the zygomatic bone. The medial palpebral ligament attaches the medial aspect of the tarsi to the lacrimal crest and the frontal process of the maxilla.

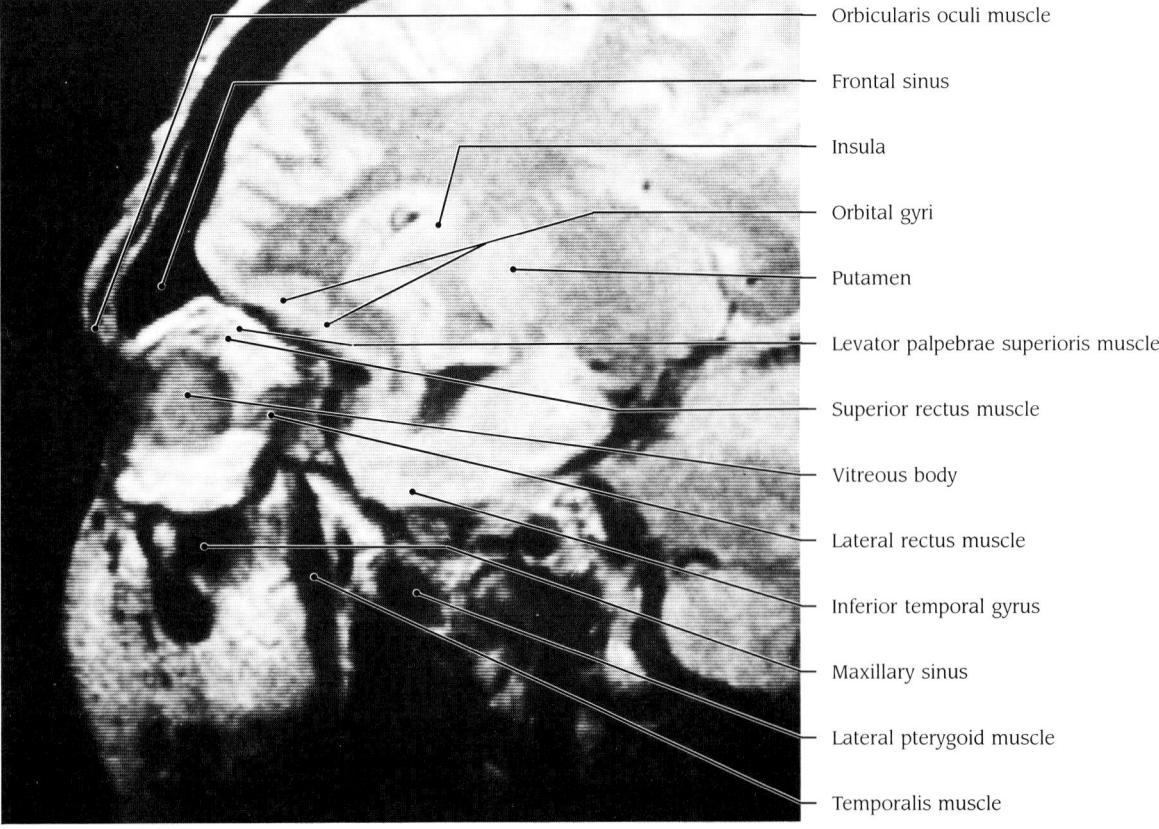

FIG. 5.38. TR = 2000 msec, TE = 50 msec.

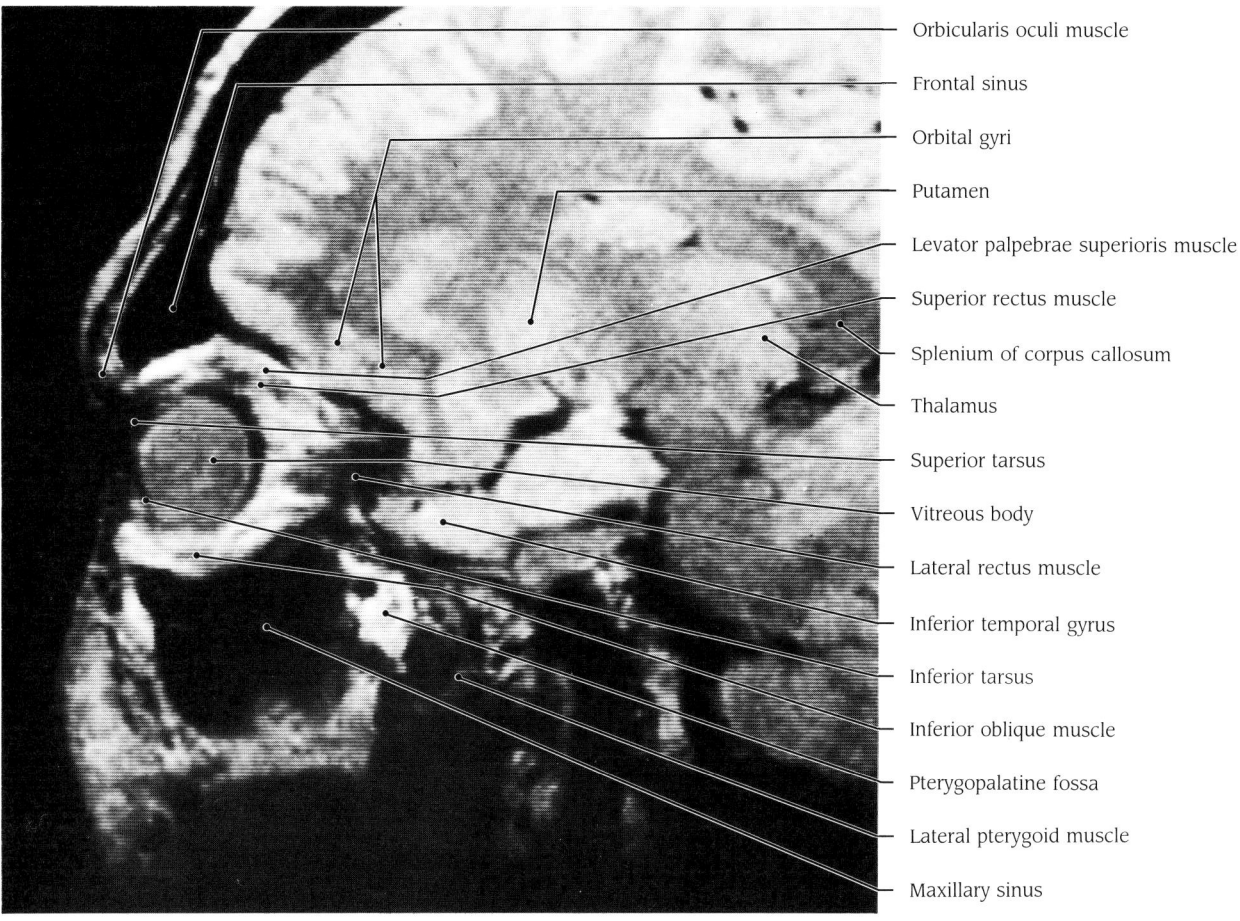

FIG. 5.39. TR = 2000 msec, TE = 50 msec.

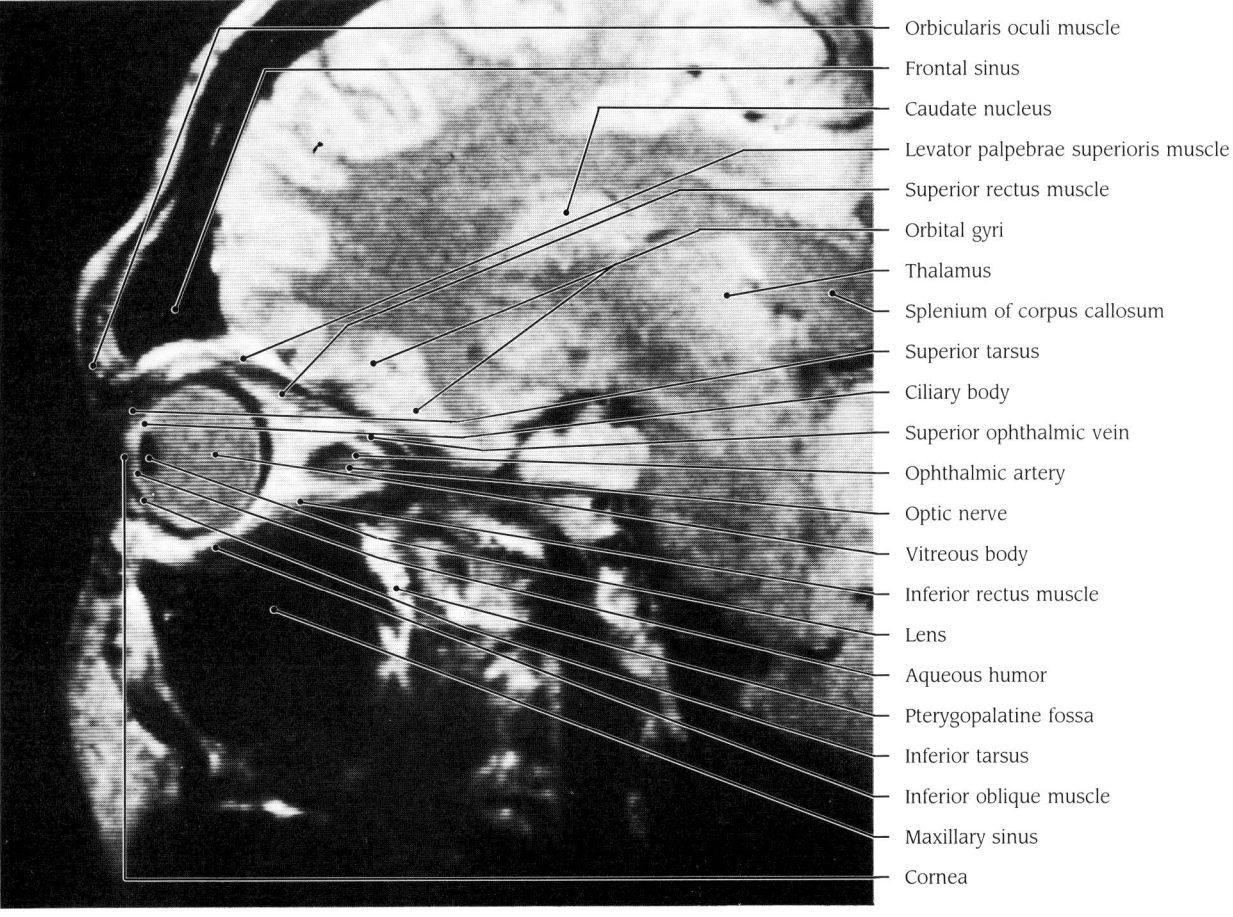

FIG. 5.40. TR = 2000 msec, TE = 50 msec.

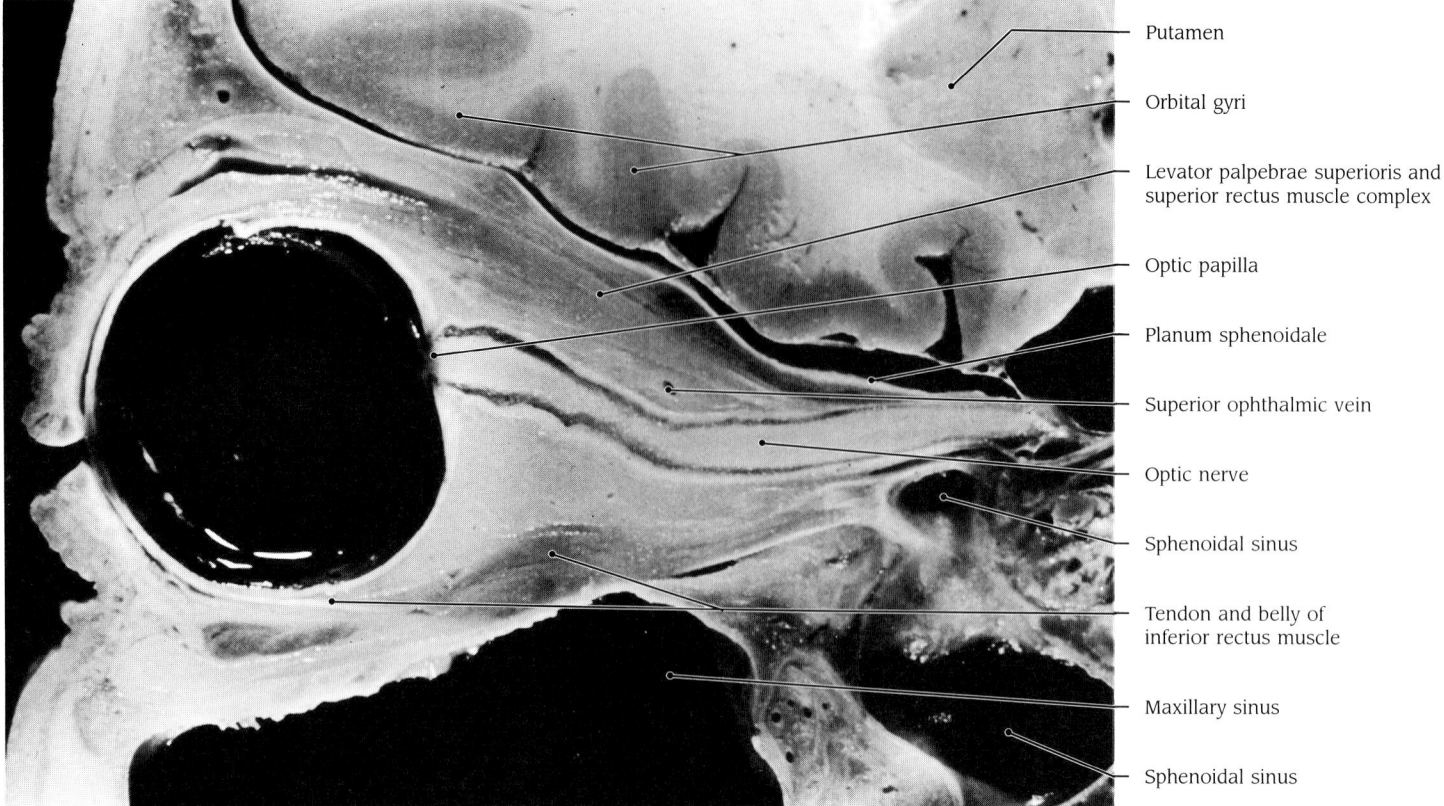

FIG. 5.41.

- The ophthalmic artery is a branch of the internal carotid artery as it leaves the cavernous sinus medial to the anterior clinoid process. The ophthalmic artery enters the orbit through the optic canal, where it is inferolateral to the optic nerve. In the orbital cavity, the ophthalmic artery runs lateral to the optic nerve and medial to the oculomotor and abducens nerves. It then crosses above the optic nerve and below the superior rectus muscle and runs toward the medial wall of the orbit. It continues anteriorly between the superior oblique and the medial rectus muscles and divides into two branches, the supratrochlear and dorsal nasal arteries, at the medial end of the upper eyelid.

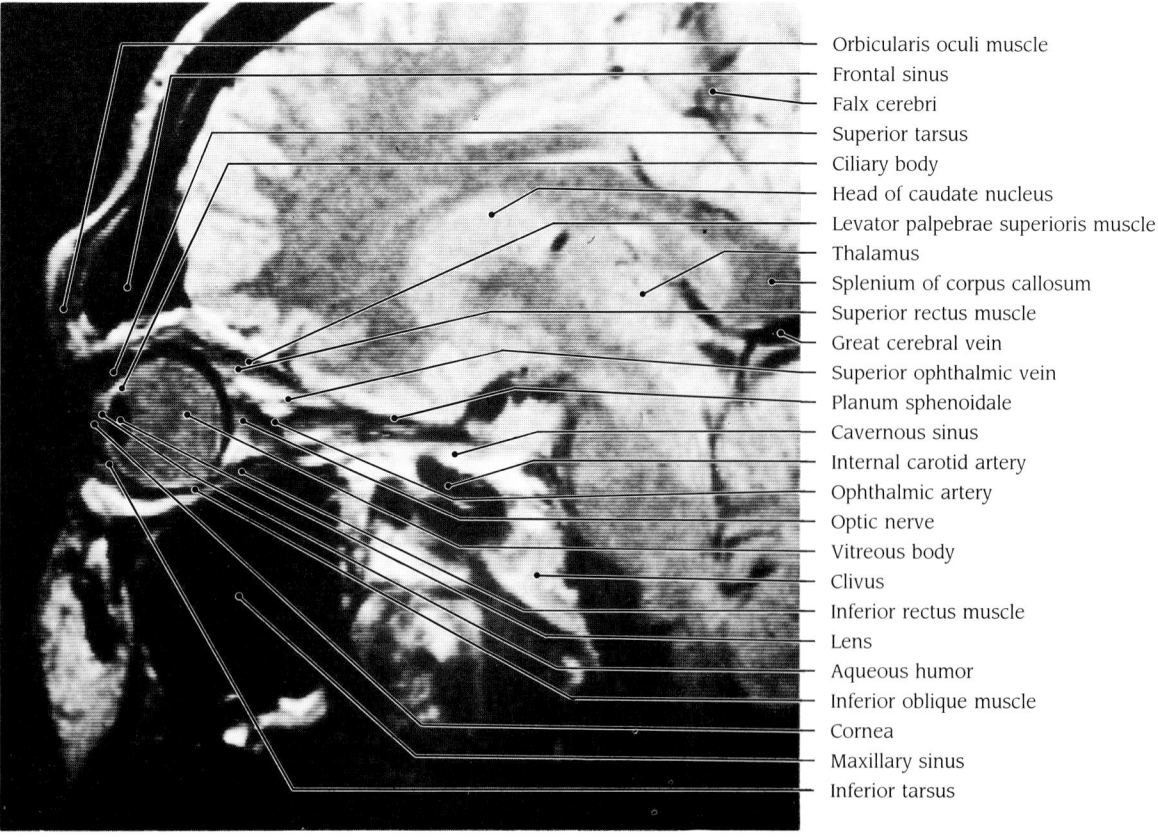

FIG. 5.42. TR = 2000 msec, TE = 50 msec.

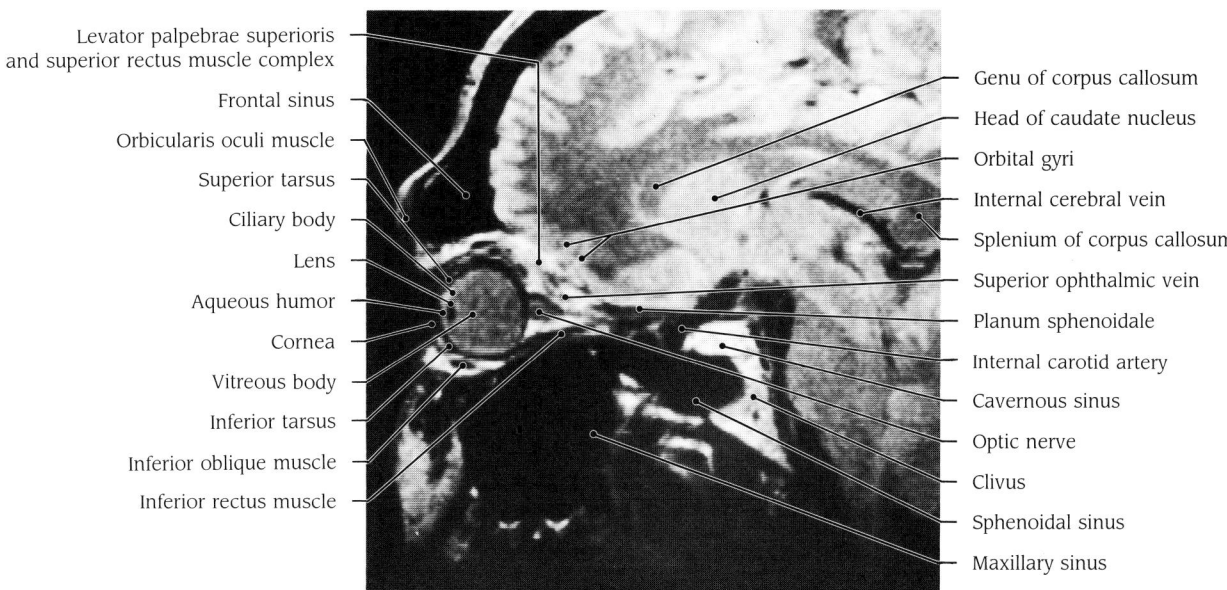

FIG. 5.43. TR = 2000 msec, TE = 50 msec.

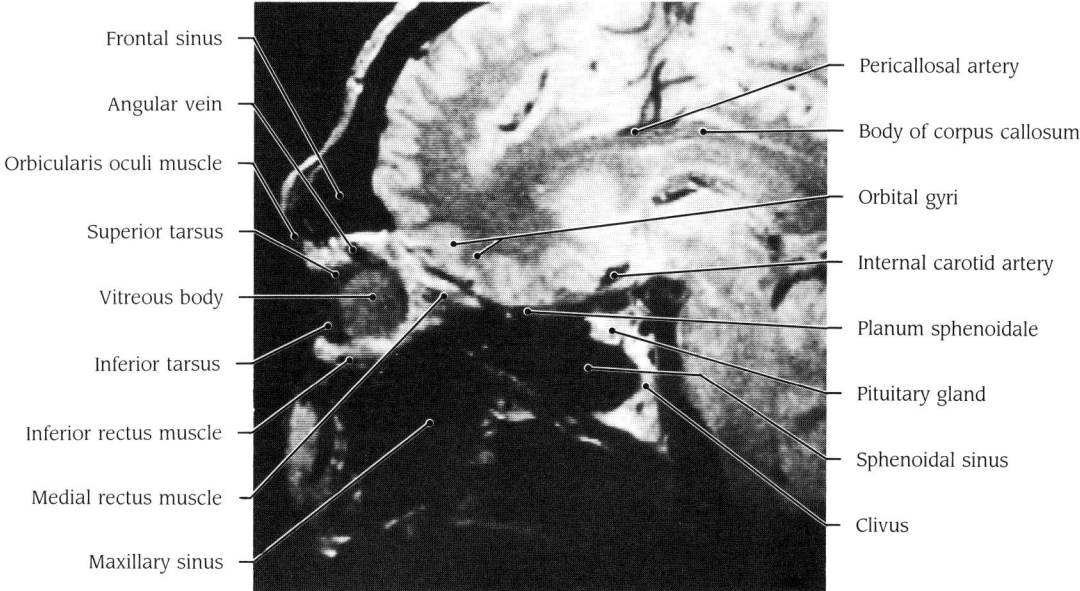

FIG. 5.44. TR = 2000 msec, TE = 50 msec.

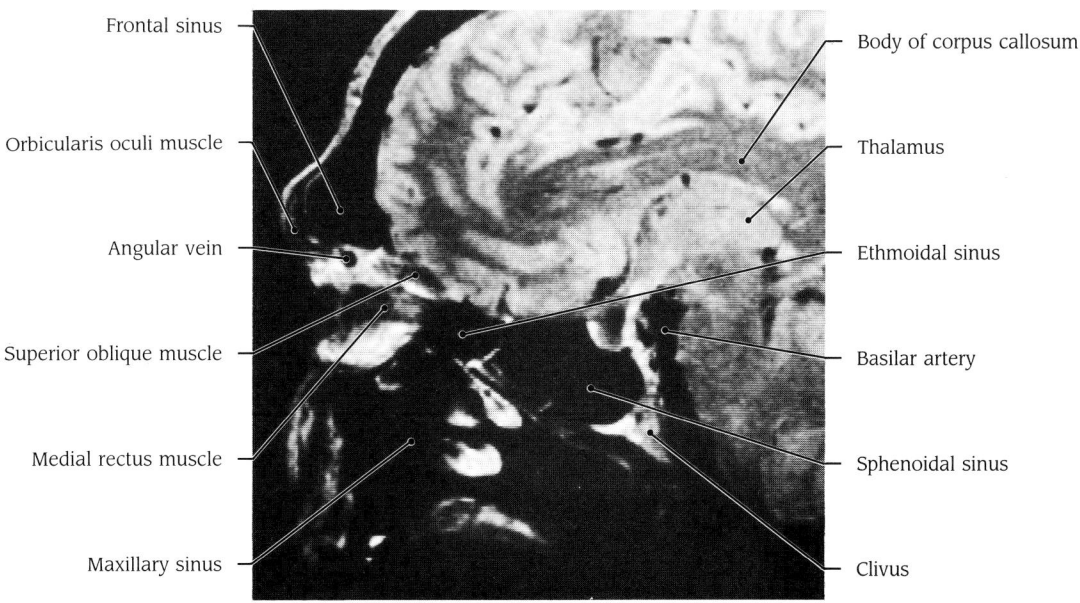

FIG. 5.45. TR = 2000 msec, TE = 50 msec.

6

Functional Systems

Functional Systems	Figures
MOTOR (efferent) PATHWAYS	
Pyramidal systems (corticospinal and corticobulbar tracts)	6.1–6.17
Basal ganglia (extrapyramidal system)	6.18–6.26
Oculomotor system	6.27–6.34
Cerebellar tracts and functions	6.35–6.41
SENSORY (afferent) PATHWAYS	
Lemniscal and anterolateral systems	6.42–6.54
Trigeminal system	6.55–6.61
Acoustic system	6.62–6.66
Vestibular system	6.67–6.70
Visual system	6.71–6.76
OLFACTION AND LIMBIC SYSTEM	6.77–6.80
SPEECH AREAS AND CONNECTIONS	6.81–6.83

Several important functional systems, with their principal pathways, cortical regions, and deep collections of gray matter, are represented here in 13 series of MR images. Most systems are displayed in the more familiar axial plane. Two systems of motor pathways, the corticospinal and the basal ganglia, are represented in axial as well as coronal images, whereas the limbic and speech systems are shown in sagittal images only.

For the sake of clarity, the pertinent areas in each section have been labeled and emphasized by stippling or cross-hatching. Many such areas have been shown larger than warranted; moreover, several functional systems share areas. The result is a schematic localization of important systems, rather than an accurately detailed microscopic atlas.

MOTOR (EFFERENT) PATHWAYS

Pyramidal system (corticospinal and corticobulbar tracts)

The pyramidal system begins in the frontoparietal region of the cerebral cortex around the central sulcus (CS). The precentral gyrus (area 4), the premotor gyrus (area 6), and the postcentral gyrus (areas 1, 2, and 3) all contribute to the formation of the descending corticospinal (CST) and corticobulbar systems.

These tracts arise from a somatotopic organization of the cortical areas: leg muscles are represented at the top of the hemisphere, head muscles are near the lateral fissure, and other body regions are represented in between. This somatotopic organization is maintained throughout, from cortex to corona radiata (CR), posterior limb of the internal capsule (IC), cerebral peduncle (CP), pons, medulla, and into the spinal cord for the corticospinal (CST) or pyramidal tract. The corticobulbar fibers end in the motor nuclei of the brain stem.

Most fibers of the corticospinal tract decussate just before descending into the lateral column (LC) of the spinal cord; the remaining fibers stay ipsilateral until they reach the segment of destination, where they decussate. Most corticobulbar fibers supply the contralateral, as well as the ipsilateral, motor nuclei of the cranial nerves; exceptions are the fibers to the facial nucleus for the lower face and the fibers to the hypoglossal nucleus, all of which are purely contralateral.

Lesions of the corticospinal tract itself may lead to a flaccid paralysis with reduced deep tendon reflexes. Spinal cord lesions, however, usually involve, in addition, the rubrospinal and reticulospinal tracts. The result is a spastic paralysis with increased or abnormal reflexes.

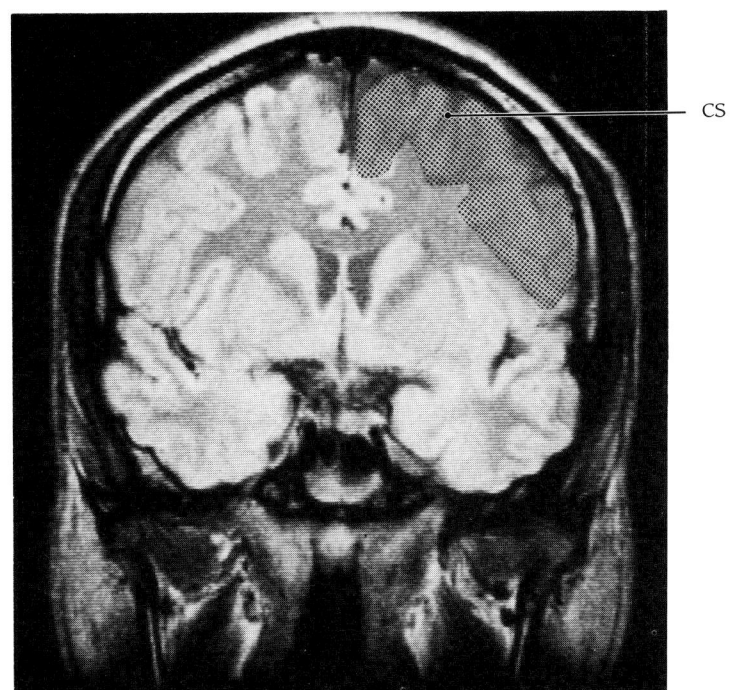

FIG. 6.1.

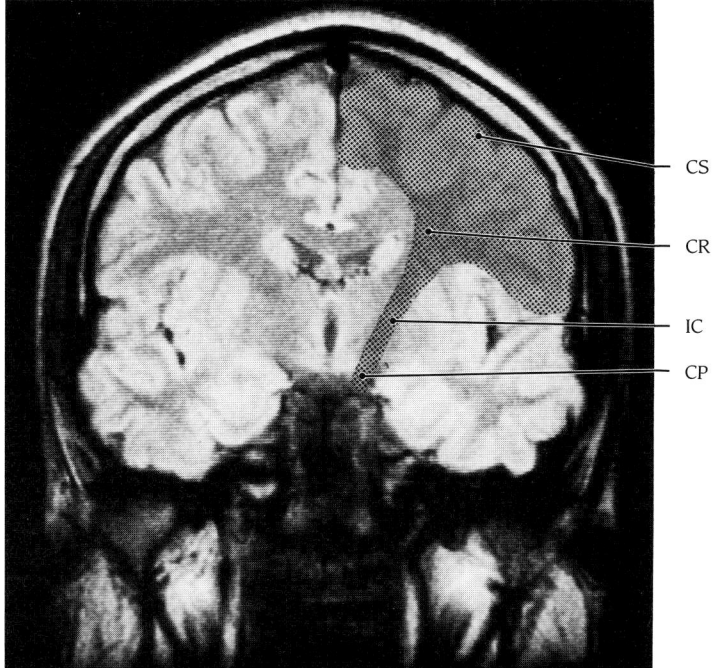

FIG. 6.2.

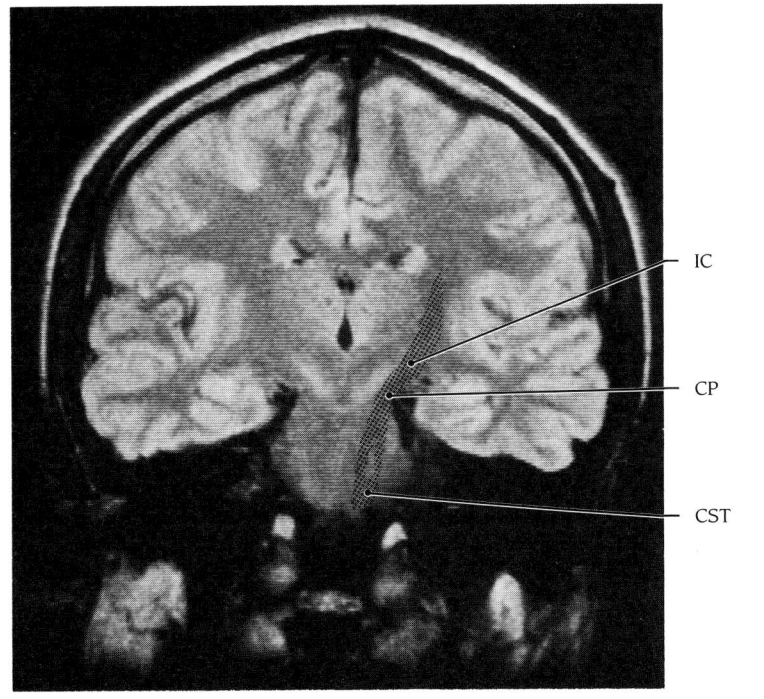

FIG. 6.3.

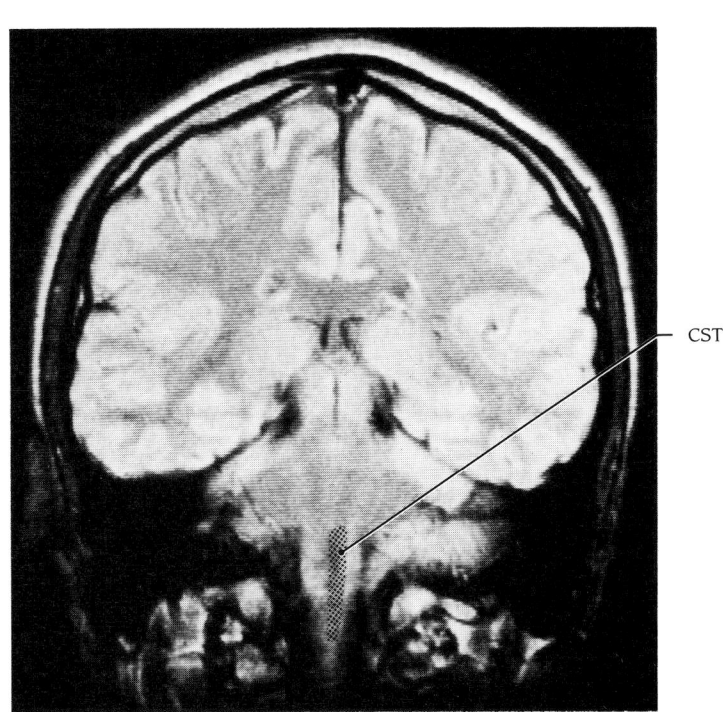

FIG. 6.4.

CP: cerebral peduncle; CR: corona radiata; CS: central sulcus; CST: corticospinal tract; IC: internal capsule.

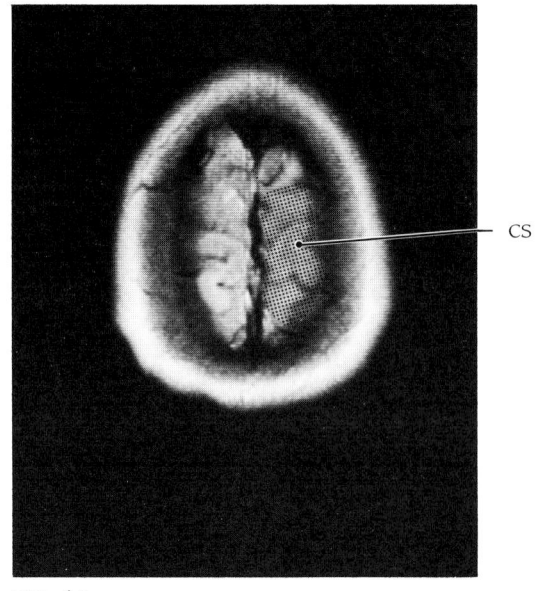

FIG. 6.5.

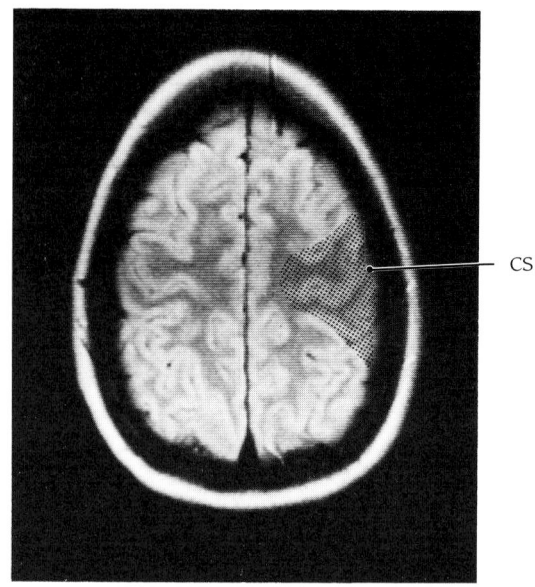

FIG. 6.6.

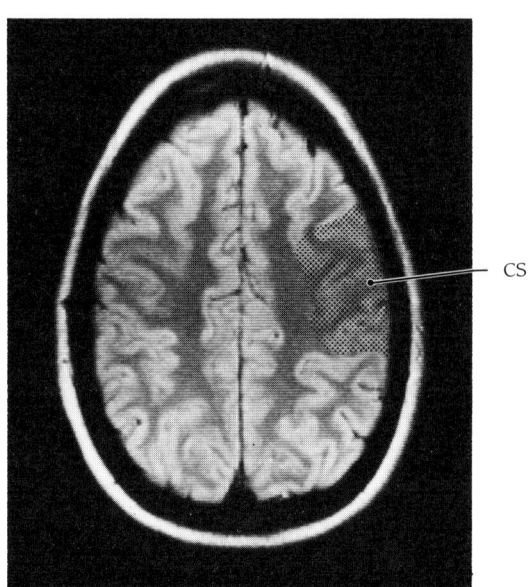

FIG. 6.7.

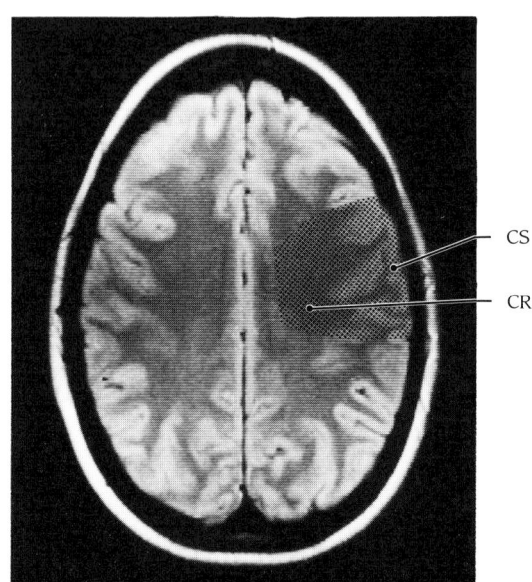

FIG. 6.8.

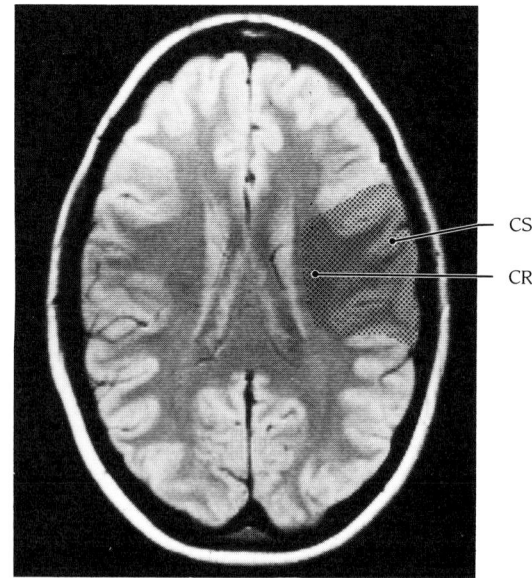

FIG. 6.9.

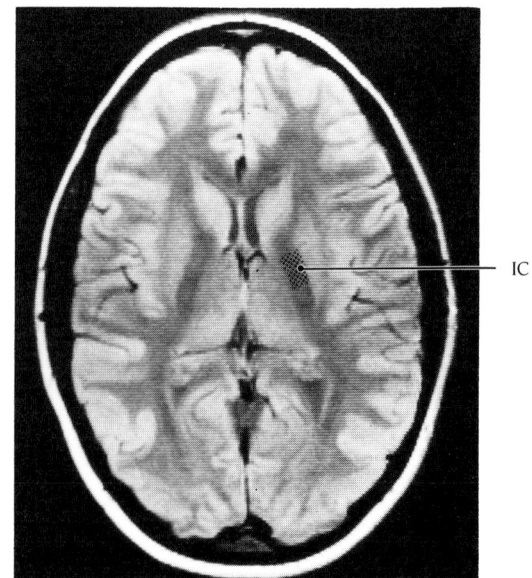

FIG. 6.10.

CR: corona radiata; CS: central sulcus; IC: internal capsule.

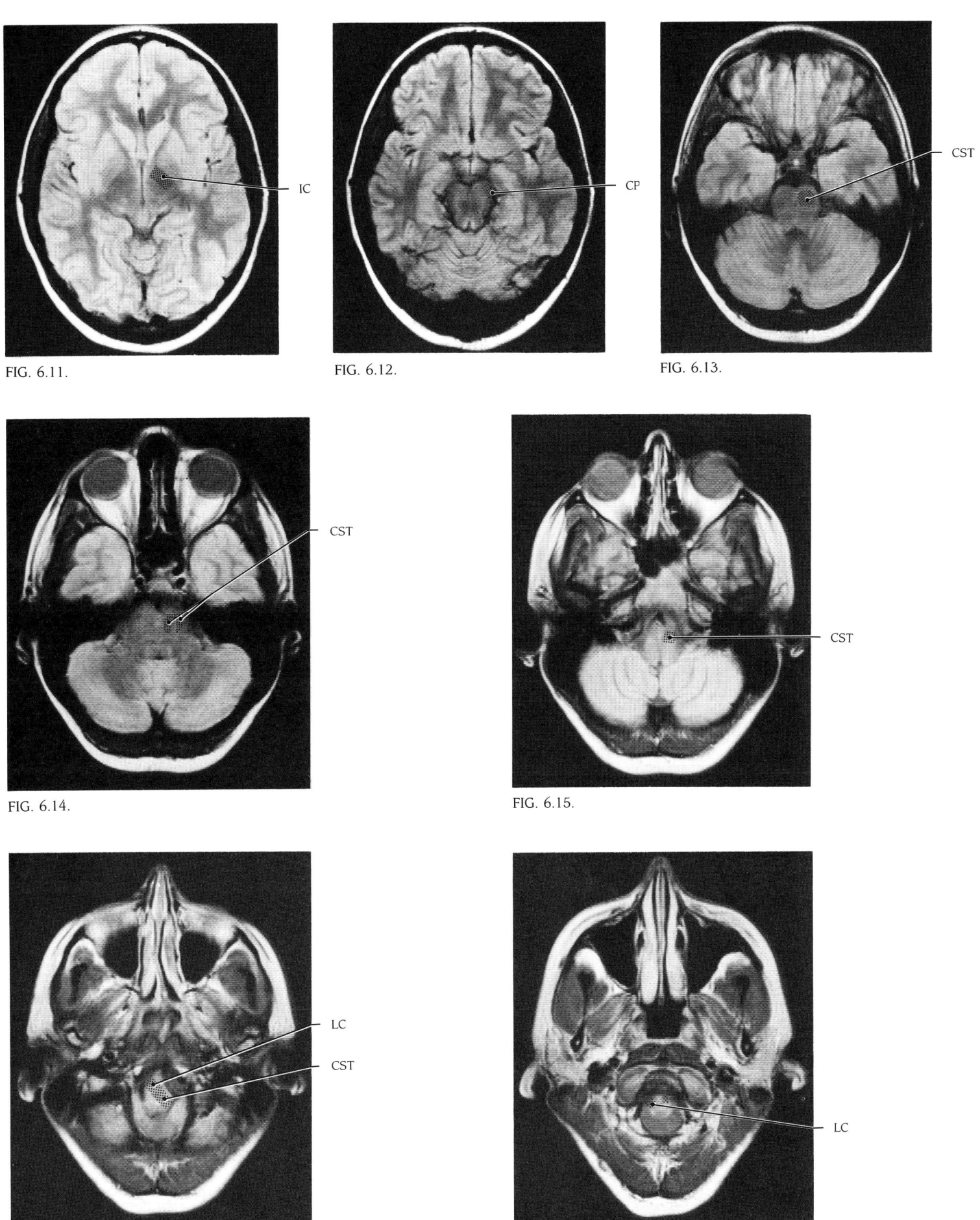

FIG. 6.11.

FIG. 6.12.

FIG. 6.13.

FIG. 6.14.

FIG. 6.15.

FIG. 6.16.

FIG. 6.17.

CP: cerebral peduncle; CST: corticospinal tract; IC: internal capsule; LC: lateral columns.

Basal ganglia (extrapyramidal system)

The basal ganglia are subcortical gray matter nuclei that are interconnected with extensive cortical regions, as well as with parts of the thalamus. This system of so-called extrapyramidal fiber tracts and gray matter areas exerts an influence on the motor cells of the spinal cord, which are not under volitional control, in contrast to the corticospinal system.

The basal ganglia consist of the caudate nucleus (CA) and putamen (PU) (together referred to as the corpus striatum), the globus pallidus (GP), the subthalamic nucleus, the red nucleus (RN), and the substantia nigra (SN). Other gray matter areas may be included, e.g., claustrum, lateral vestibular nucleus, etc. The putamen and globus pallidus together are referred to as the lentiform nucleus.

The interconnections between many individual components of this system are extensive. From the cerebral cortex, fibers descend to the caudate nucleus, from which connections are made to the putamen and the globus pallidus. Some fibers then loop back to the ventral thalamus (VT) and, hence, to the cerebral cortex, whereas others descend to the subthalamic and red nuclei and to the substantia nigra. The latter give rise to descending pathways to the anterior horn cells of the spinal cord. The cerebellar outflow reaches the red nucleus and the ventral thalamus similarly, so that the extrapyramidal system is influenced by cerebellar function (see section entitled, Cerebellum).

Characteristic forms of dyskinesia are associated with lesions in individual nuclei of the basal ganglia system: the caudate nucleus is related to chorea, the subthalamic nucleus to ballismus, and the substantia nigra to parkinsonism. Athetosis may be caused by lesions in several areas.

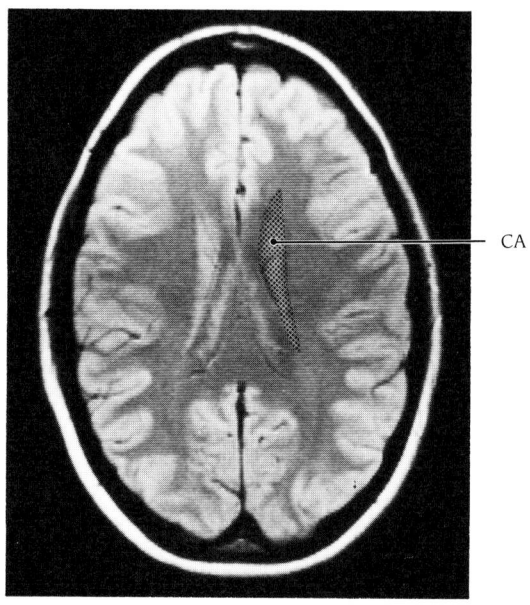

FIG. 6.18.

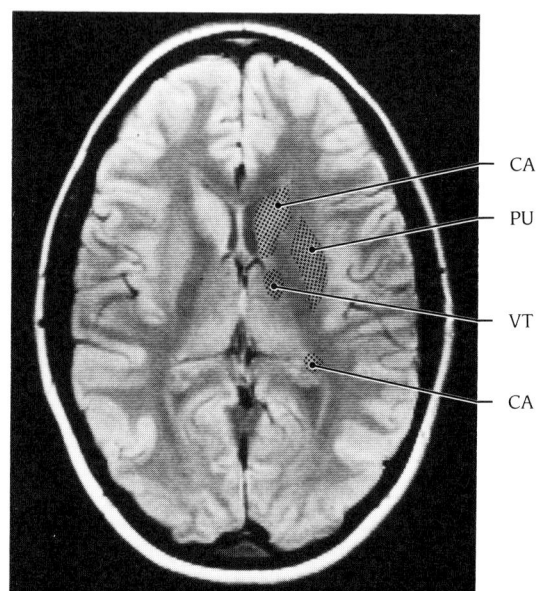

FIG. 6.19.

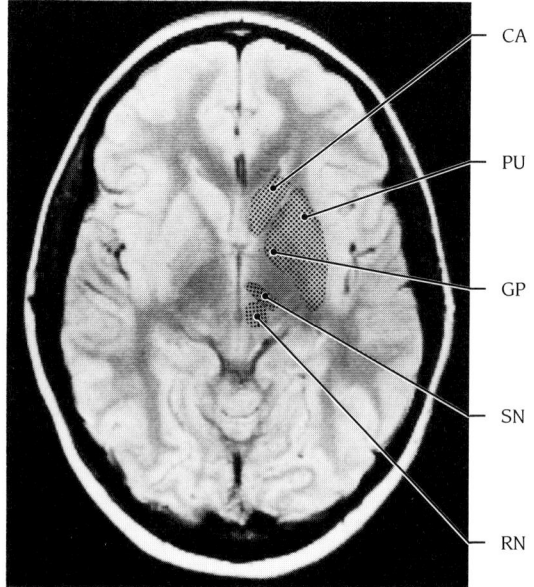

FIG. 6.20.

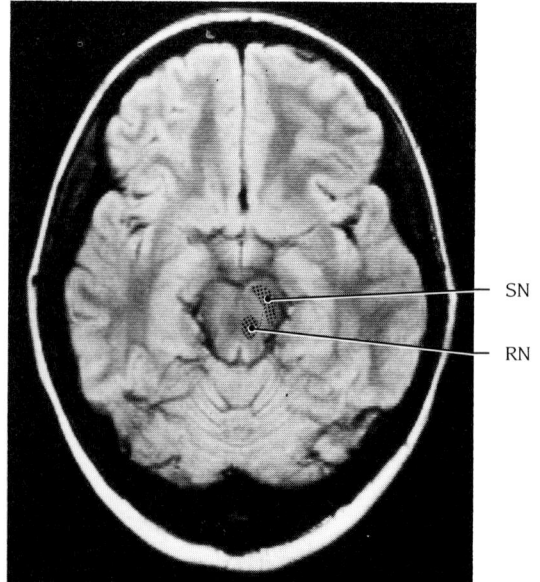

FIG. 6.21.

CA: caudate nucleus; GP: globus pallidus; PU: putamen; RN: red nucleus; SN: substantia nigra; VT: ventral thalamus.

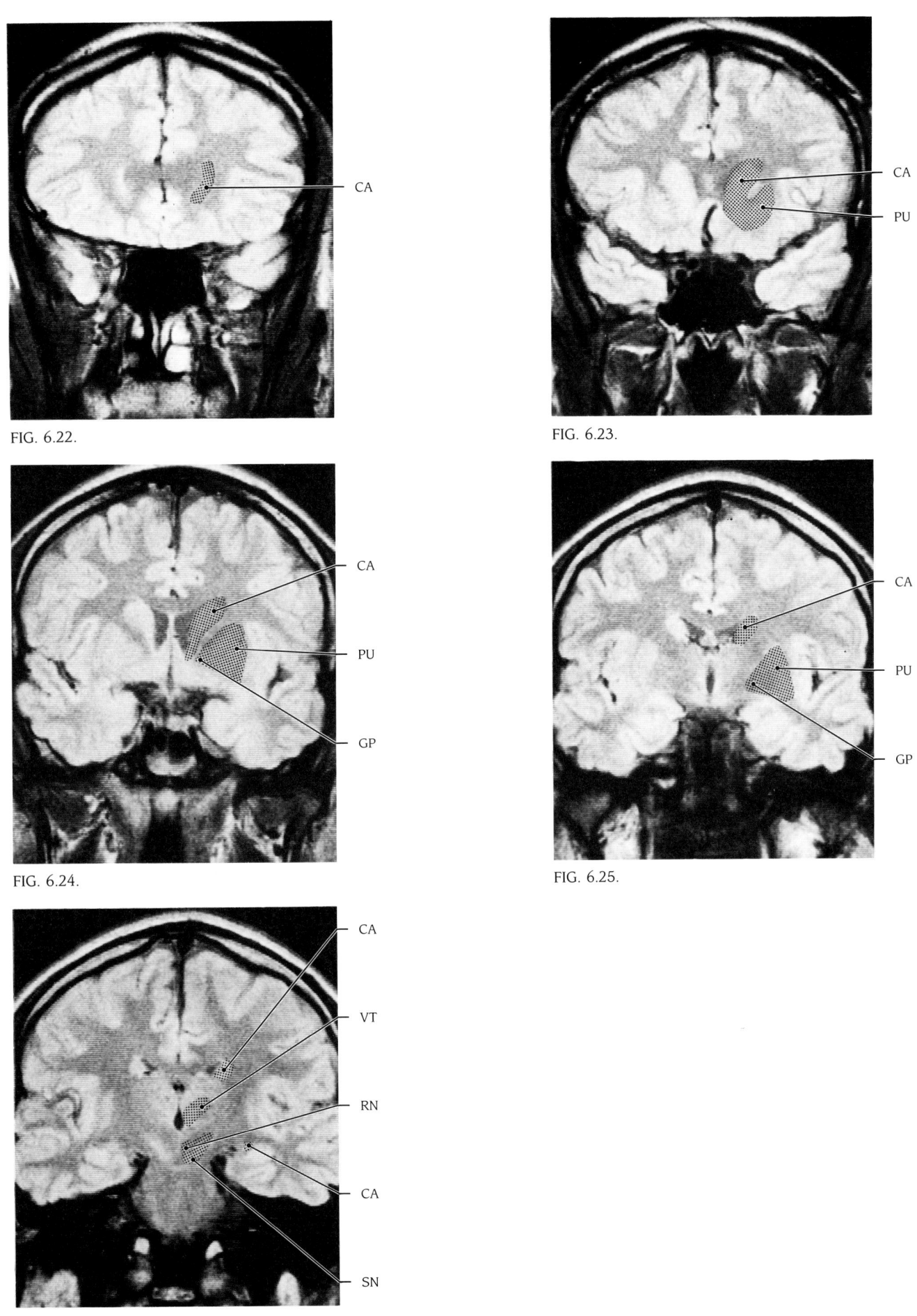

FIG. 6.22.

FIG. 6.23.

FIG. 6.24.

FIG. 6.25.

FIG. 6.26.

CA: caudate nucleus; GP: globus pallidus; PU: putamen; RN: red nucleus; SN: substantia nigra; VT: ventral thalamus.

Oculomotor system

The cerebral cortical eye field (CF; area 8) is concerned with coordination of movement between both eyes, independent of visual stimuli; it is located in the middle frontal gyrus. The occipital, visual projection cortex (VC; area 17), as well as adjacent gyri, are involved in the pursuit of visual stimuli. Both cortical regions connect to the pretectal area (PA), the superior colliculus (SC), and other midbrain regions. Whereas the nuclei of the oculomotor and trochlear nerves lie in the midbrain tegmentum below the aqueduct, the abducens nuclei are found in the pons, below the fourth ventricle. The medial longitudinal fasciculus (MLF) interconnects these cranial nerve nuclei with the vestibular complex (see section entitled, Vestibular System).

Lesions in the region just lateral to the abducens nucleus (paramedian pontine reticular formation [PRF]) disrupt contralateral conjugate lateral gaze movements, as do lesions in the cortical eye field. Vertical conjugate gaze movements are impaired by lesions in the region of the superior colliculi; tumors in the pineal region may cause such impairment (Parinaud's syndrome). Interruption of the medial longitudinal fasciculus (e.g., by a multiple sclerosis plaque) leads to so-called internuclear ophthalmoplegia, in which lateral gaze movements are disrupted while abduction is still possible. Lesions in individual nerve nuclei or, more frequently, in the third, fourth, or sixth cranial nerves themselves, lead to a characteristic unilateral paralysis of certain eye muscles associated with diplopia and/or strabismus. Nystagmus may be related to vestibular stimulation or dysfunction caused by cerebellar lesions or by visual stimuli (opticokinetic nystagmus).

The size of the pupil is governed by the interplay of its constrictor muscle, which is innervated by the oculomotor nerve and parasympathetic fibers, with its dilator muscle, which is innervated by sympathetic fibers. A lesion in a third nerve or associated nucleus leads to mydriasis, whereas a small pupil (miosis) may result from interruption of the sympathetic innervation of the eye (Horner's syndrome).

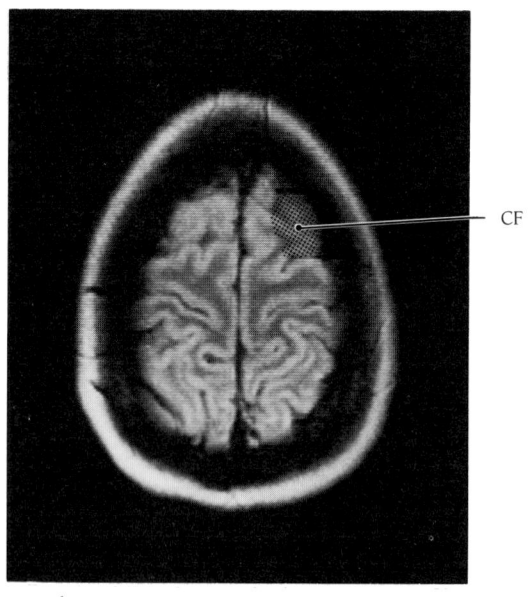

FIG. 6.27.

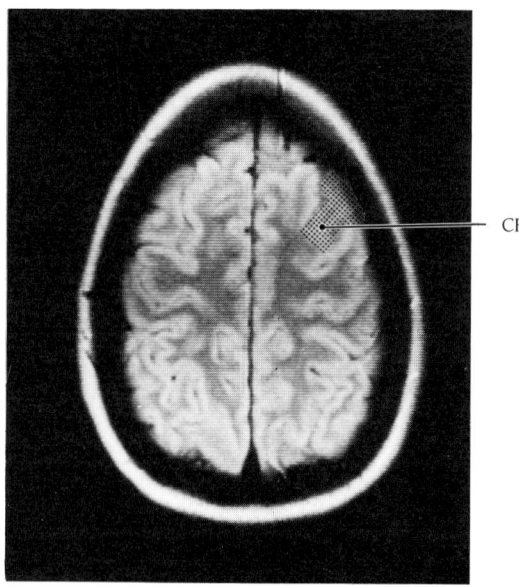

FIG. 6.28.

CF: cortical eye field.

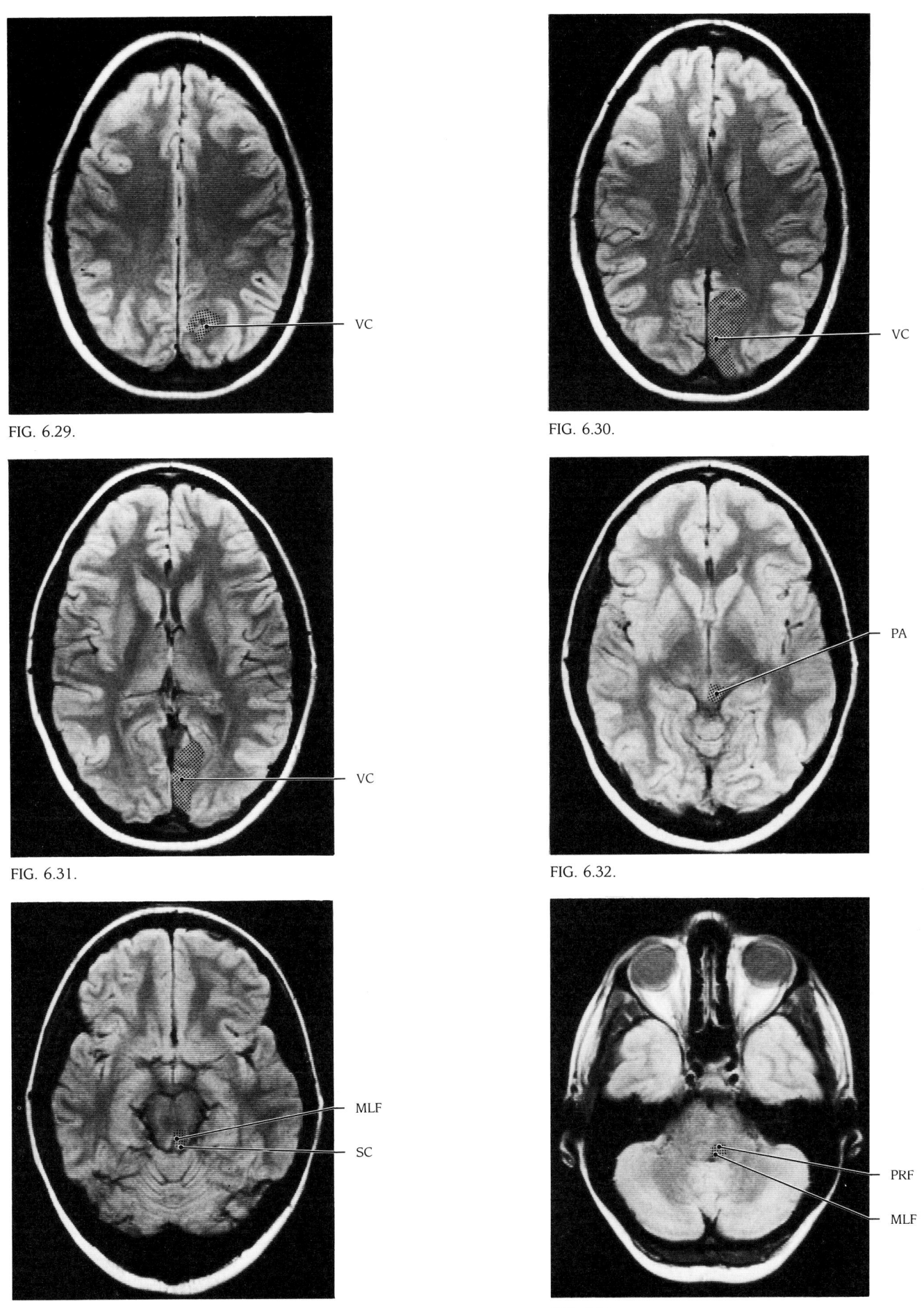

FIG. 6.29.

FIG. 6.30.

FIG. 6.31.

FIG. 6.32.

FIG. 6.33.

FIG. 6.34.

MLF: medial longitudinal fasciculus; PA: pretectal area; PRF: paramedian reticular formation; SC: superior colliculus; VC: visual cortex.

Cerebellar tracts and functions

The cerebellum is involved in the coordination of fine movements, especially in the extremities (neocerebellum [NC]); of propulsive, automatic movements, such as walking, running, or swimming (paleocerebellum [PC]); and of primitive movements concerned with maintenance of position (archicerebellum or flocculonodular lobes [FN]). The cerebellar cortex thus can be divided into three regions; the flocculus and nodule of the vermis are the "oldest" part, whereas the anterior and posterior vermis and anterior lobe are considered to be the paleocerebellar cortex. The neocerebellar cortex extends over all other cerebellar regions.

These different functions of the cerebellum are reflected by their afferent connections; the archicerebellum receives connections from the vestibular nerves and nuclei (via the inferior cerebellar peduncles [IP]), whereas spinocerebellar tracts and olivocerebellar fibers project to the paleocerebellar cortex, mainly by way of the inferior cerebellar peduncle. Extensive cerebral cortical regions in the frontal and temporal lobes project to the pontine nuclei, from which fibers emanate and cross via the large middle cerebellar peduncle (MP) to the neocerebellar cortex. The outflow from the cerebellum is mainly from the dentate nucleus by way of the superior cerebellar peduncles (SP), which end in the contralateral red nuclei (RN) and ventral thalamus (VT). From these relay stations, fibers descend to the contralateral spinal cord or to the cerebral cortex and extrapyramidal system.

Lesions in the archicerebellum or the paleocerebellum, or in their afferent pathways, may lead to disturbances of position, as well as to truncal ataxia, which resembles drunkenness. Neocerebellar lesions result in loss of coordination of muscle movements: repetitive opposite movements can no longer be executed quickly or correctly (dysdiadochokinesia), target-directed movements are performed poorly (resulting in dysmetria and/or intention tremor), and general hypotonia of the muscles occurs.

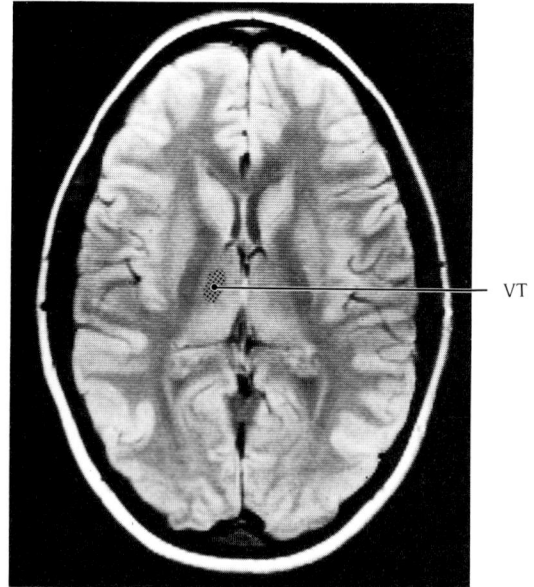

FIG. 6.35.

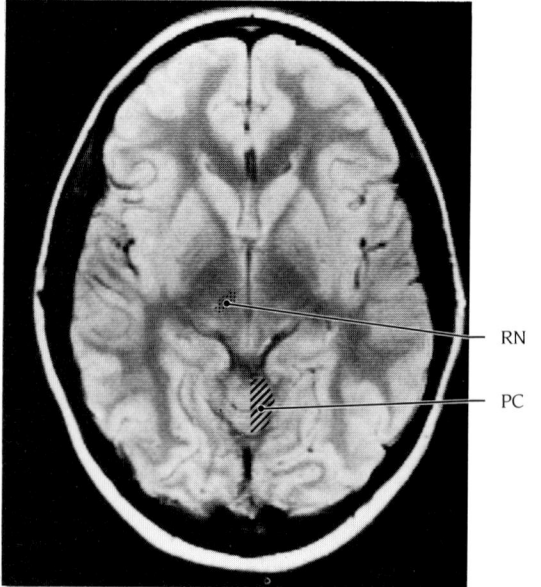

FIG. 6.36.

PC: paleocerebellum; RN: red nucleus; VT: ventral thalamus.

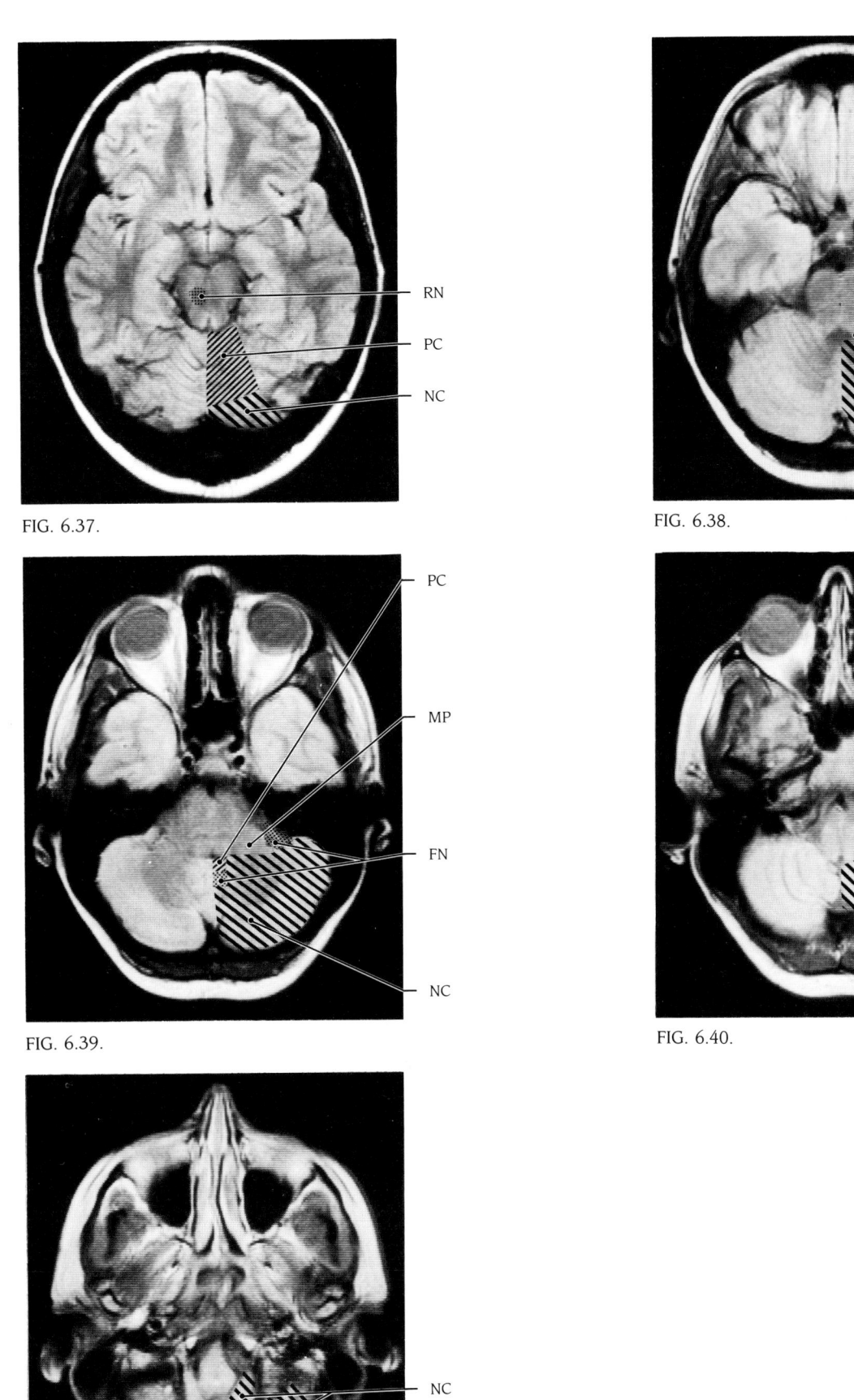

FIG. 6.37.

FIG. 6.38.

FIG. 6.39.

FIG. 6.40.

FIG. 6.41.

FN: flocculonodular lobe; IP: inferior cerebellar peduncle; MP: middle cerebellar peduncle; NC: neocerebellum; PC: paleocerebellum; RN: red nucleus; SP: superior cerebellar peduncle.

SENSORY (AFFERENT) PATHWAYS

Lemniscal and anterolateral systems

The lemniscal or dorsal column system (DC) of ascending fibers conveys impulses of fine and discriminative touch, as well as of proprioception or position sense, from the peripheral sense organs in the skin and tendons to the cerebral cortex. In the spinal cord, the fibers of this system course in the dorsal columns, where the upper extremity is represented in the tractus cuneatus and the lower regions of the body in the tractus gracilis. These tracts synapse in the lower medulla; the fibers of the nucleus gracilis and the nucleus cuneatus then ascend in the contralateral medial lemniscus (ML) to end in the posterolateral thalamus. The pathway then projects by way of the posterior limb of the internal capsule (IC) and the posterior corona radiata (CR) to the primary projection area in the postcentral gyrus (PG) of the parietal lobe, as well as adjacent secondary areas. Somatotopic organization is maintained throughout the lemniscal system so that the lower body is represented at the top of the hemisphere and the upper extremity at the middle of the postcentral gyrus.

Discrete lesions in this system may result in loss of position and tactile sense in well-defined areas of the body.

The anterolateral (ventrolateral) system, or spinothalamic tract (ST), relays sensory impulses of pain, temperature, and gross mechanical distortion from the periphery to the thalamus and cerebral cortex.

Afferent fibers synapse in the dorsal gray matter of the spinal cord, slightly above the segmental level of entry, then cross to course upward in the anterolateral region of the white matter as the spinothalamic tract (ST). This tract continues upward through the lateral brainstem and ends in the posterolateral thalamus (PL). Collateral fibers are given off in the spinal cord as well as in the brainstem, to form a polysynaptic spinoreticular tract, which ascends to the pontine reticular formation and the intralaminar nuclei of the thalamus.

Because the spinothalamic tract lies so close to the medial lemniscus at the level of the midbrain, it cannot be distinguished in these images. From the posterolateral thalamus, much of the anterolateral system projects by way of the posterior limb of the internal capsule (IC) to the postcentral gyrus (PG) of the parietal lobe; some fibers terminate at the thalamus. The spinoreticular tract projects extensively to the cerebral cortex.

A somatotopic organization exists within the spinothalamic system; thus, the lower extremity is represented laterally in the cord and at the top of the hemisphere. The upper extremity and neck are localized more medially in the cord and lower in the postcentral gyrus. Pain in the face is not conveyed by the spinothalamic system (see section entitled, Trigeminal System).

Discrete lesions in the spinothalamic system may result in the loss of pain (sharp) and temperature sensation. Disturbances in the spinoreticular system, as well as in its thalamic area, may lead to a sensation of deep, burning, or chronic pain.

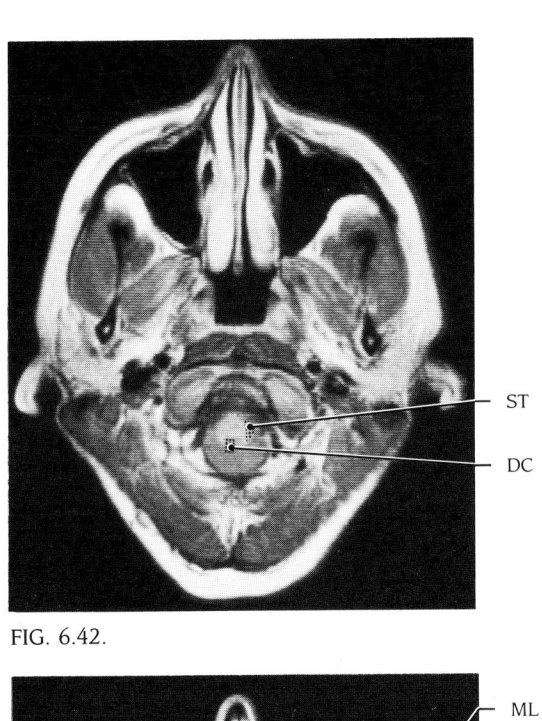

FIG. 6.42.

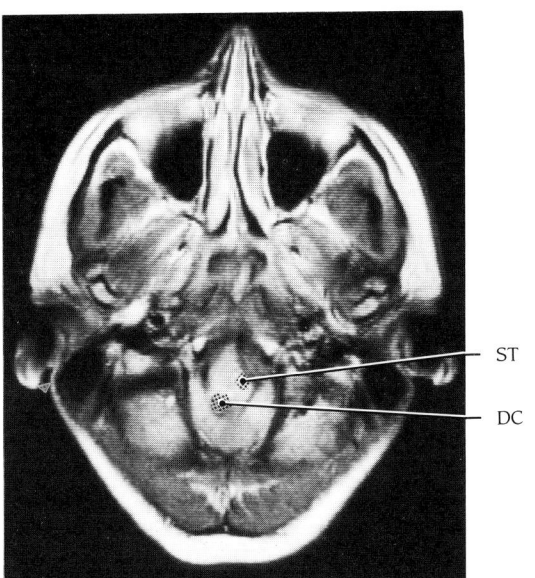

FIG. 6.43.

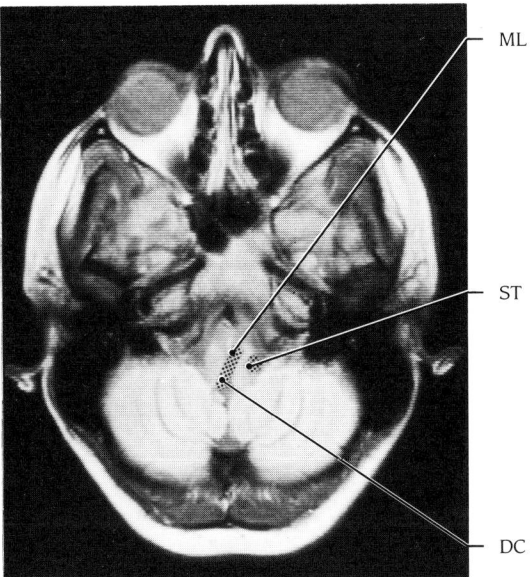

FIG. 6.44.

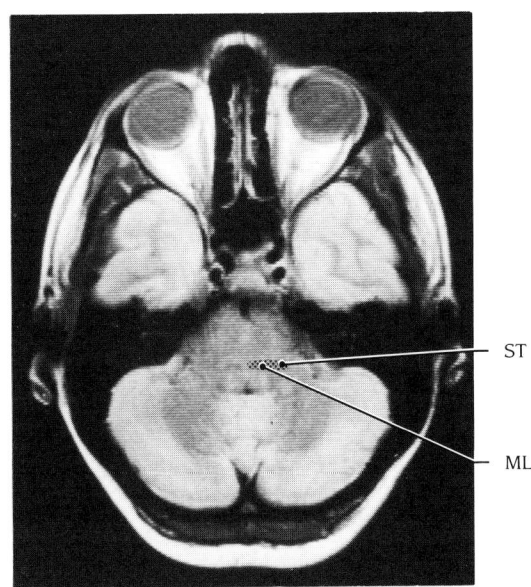

FIG. 6.45.

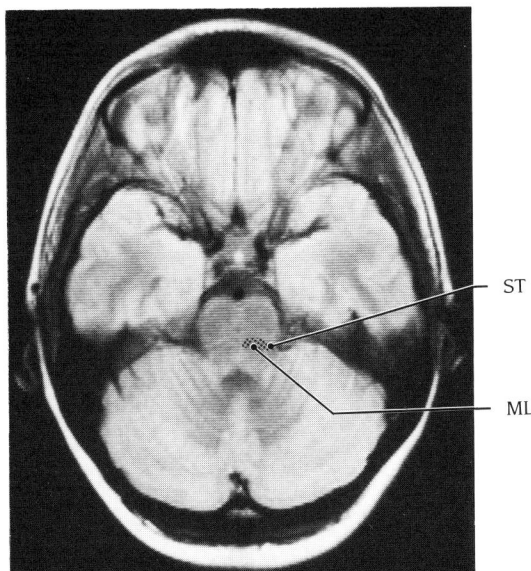

FIG. 6.46.

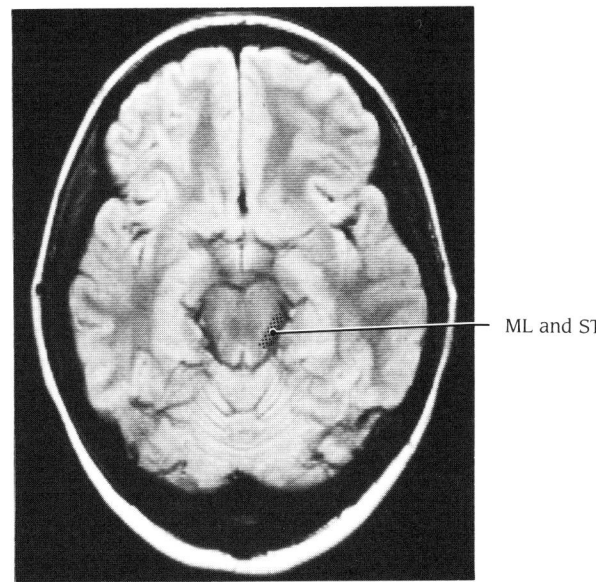

FIG. 6.47.

DC: dorsal columns; ML: medial lemniscus; ST: spinothalamic tract.

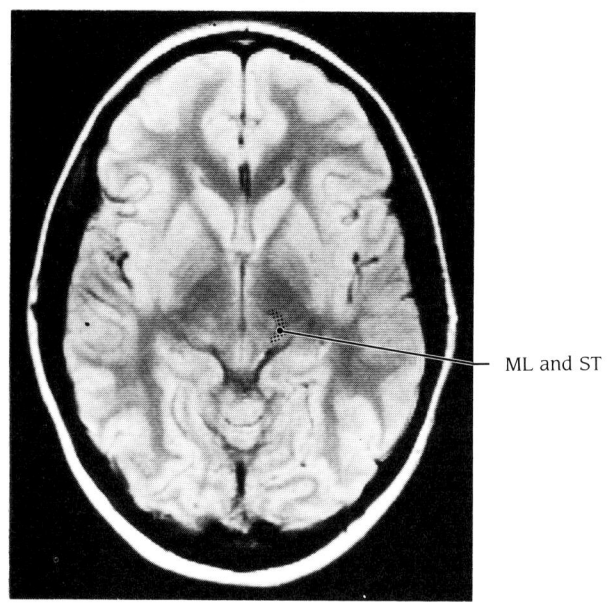

FIG. 6.48.

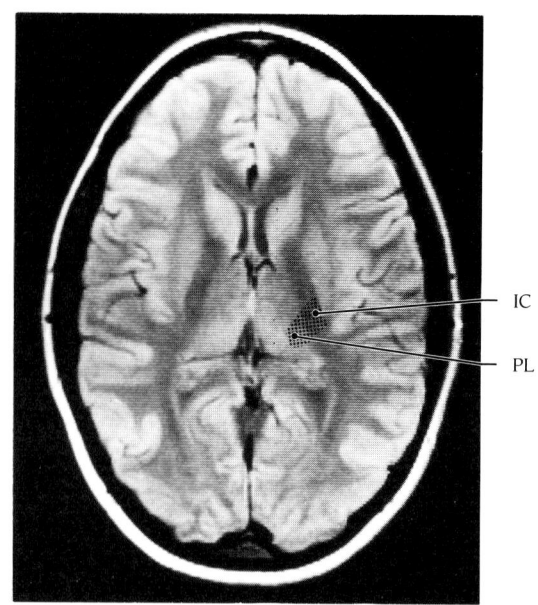

FIG. 6.49.

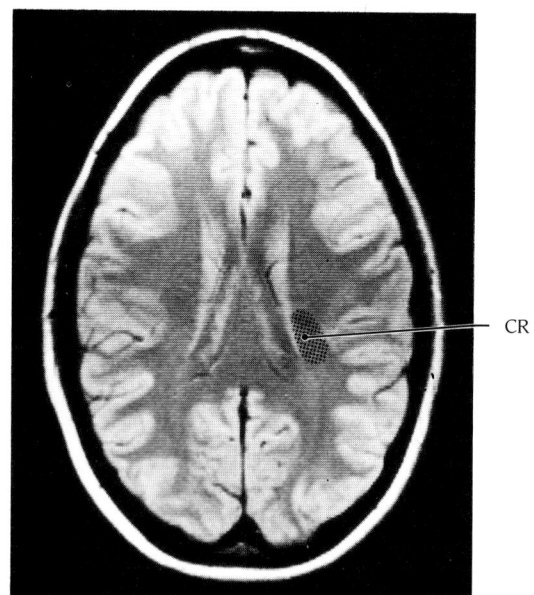

FIG. 6.50.

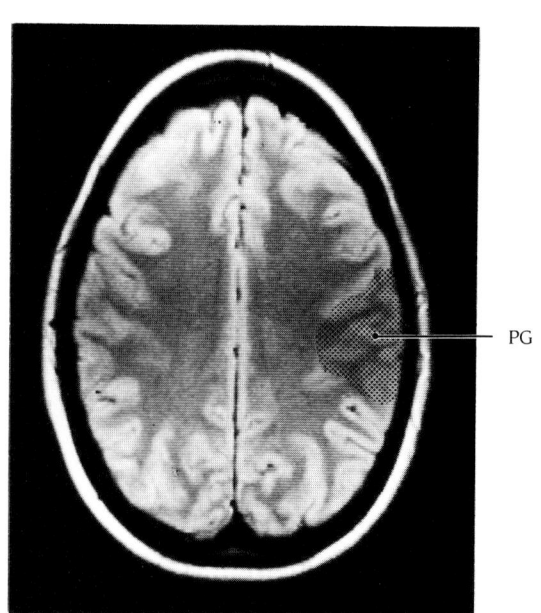

FIG. 6.51.

CR: corona radiata; IC: internal capsule; PG: postcentral gyrus; PL: posterolateral thalamus; ML: medial lemniscus; ST: spinothalamic tract.

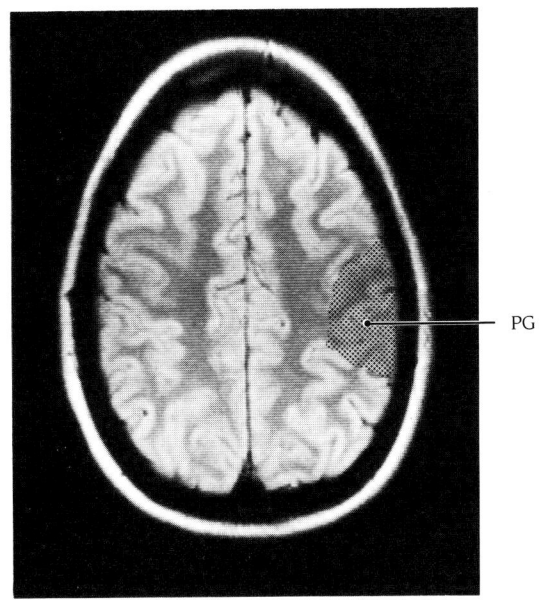

FIG. 6.52.

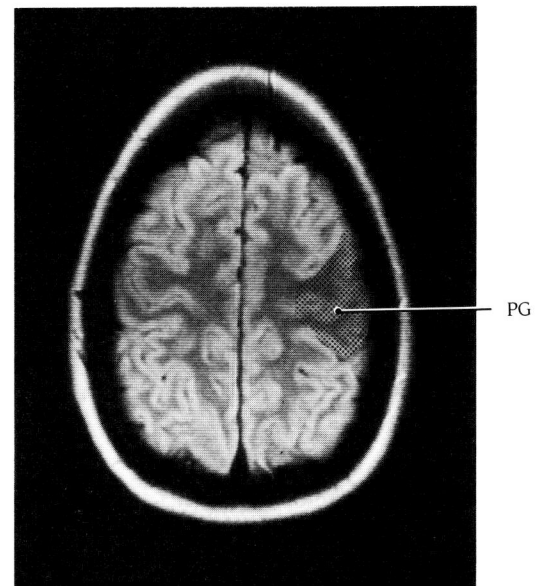

FIG. 6.53.

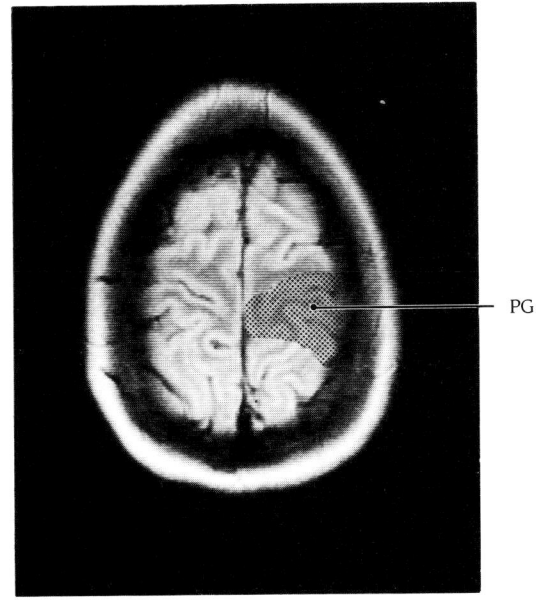

FIG. 6.54.

PG: postcentral gyrus

Trigeminal System

Sensation (touch, pain, temperature) in one half of the face is relayed to the cerebral cortex by way of the sensory fibers of the fifth cranial nerve and of a few fibers in the seventh, ninth, and tenth cranial nerves. The cell body of most of these afferent neurons is in the trigeminal ganglion (GV). All these fibers synapse either in the main sensory nucleus of the fifth cranial nerve (MSV) in the pons (touch) or in the caudal part of the spinal nucleus of the fifth cranial nerve (SV) (pain and temperature). Secondary fibers of the trigeminal system then ascend in the contralateral trigeminal lemniscus (TL) and end in the posteromedial thalamus (PM). Tertiary thalamocortical fibers course by way of the posterior limb of the internal capsule (IC) to the lower face portion of the postcentral gyrus (PG), as well as adjacent areas. A somatotopic organization is maintained throughout the system.

Discrete lesions in the trigeminal system (e.g., caused by multiple sclerosis plaques) may lead to well-defined areas of sensory loss in the face. Irritations of parts of the system may result in painful sensation (tic douloureux) of the face, usually restricted to the area innervated by one division of the fifth nerve.

The peripheral section of the motor or masticatory division of the trigeminus originates in the motor nucleus, just medial to the main sensory nucleus. Then, efferent fibers course with the third trigeminal division to innervate the muscles of mastication and the tensor tympani muscle in the middle ear.

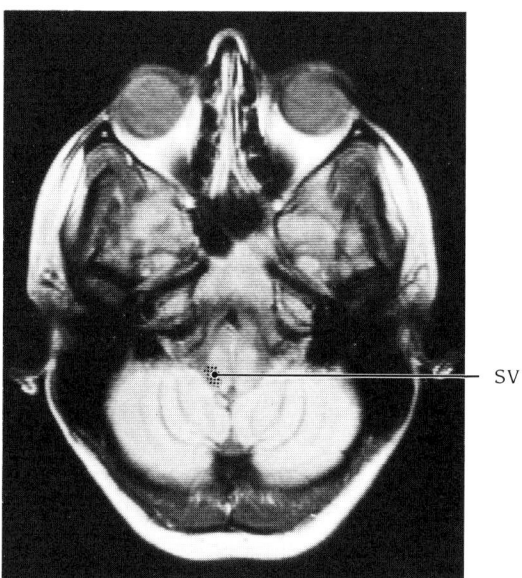

FIG. 6.55.

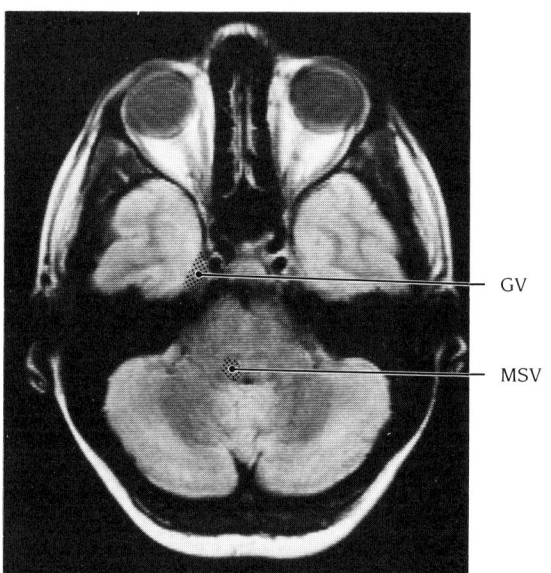

FIG. 6.56.

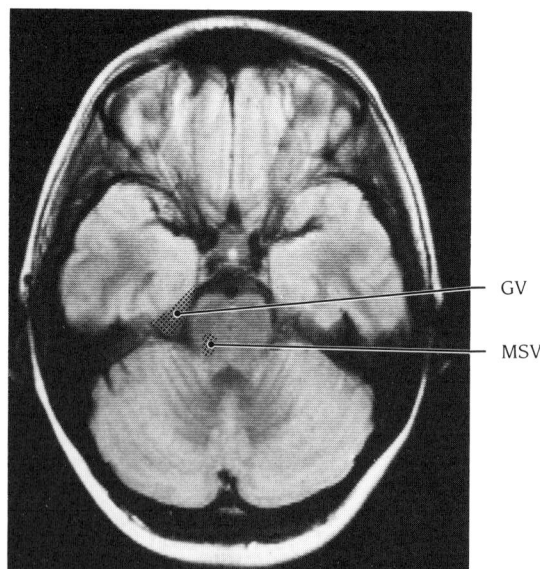

FIG. 6.57.

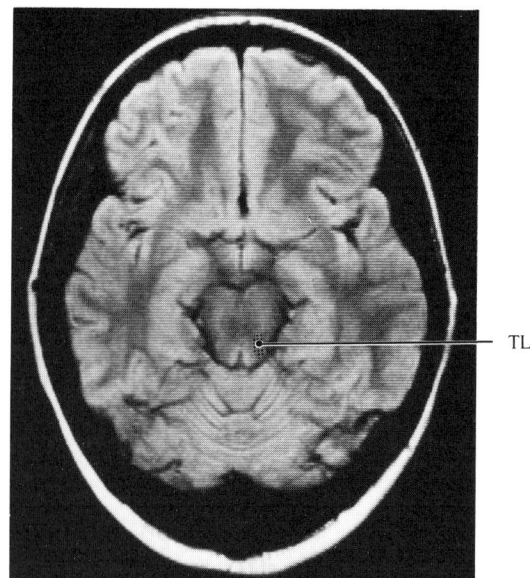

FIG. 6.58.

GV: trigeminal ganglion; MSV: main sensory nucleus of the fifth cranial nerve; SV: spinal nucleus and tract of the fifth cranial nerve; TL: trigeminal lemniscus.

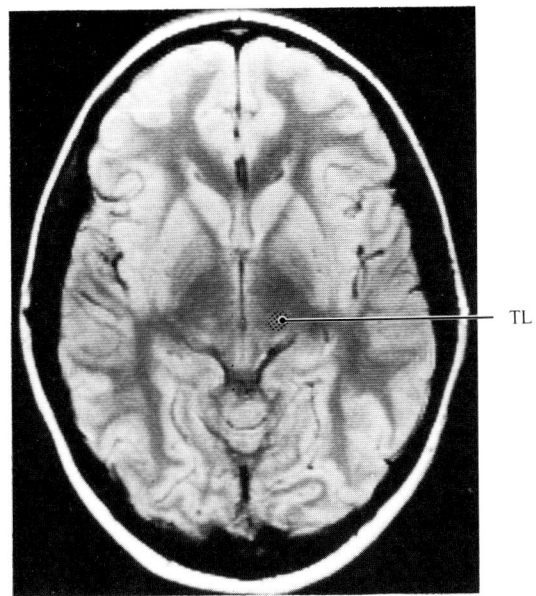

FIG. 6.59.   FIG. 6.60.

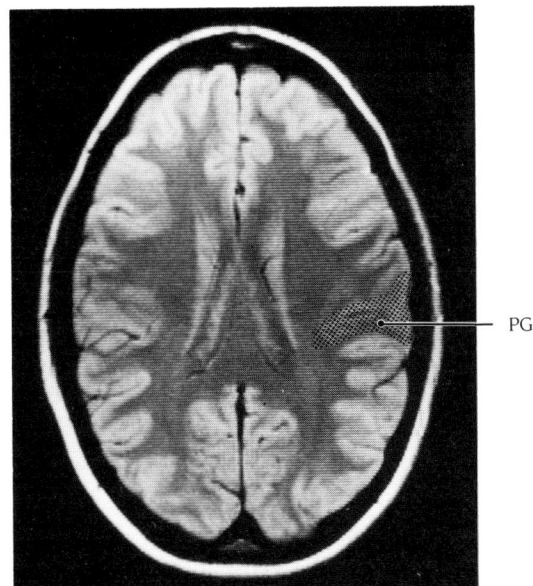

FIG. 6.61.

TL: trigeminal lemniscus; PM: posteromedial thalamus; PG: postcentral gyrus.

Acoustic system

Impulses generated in the cochlea are conducted by way of the acoustic portion of the eighth cranial nerve to the cochlear nuclei (CN) in the lower brainstem. Projections from the cochlear nuclei course upward on both sides of the brainstem in the lateral lemniscus (LL) and end in the ipsilateral, as well as contralateral, inferior colliculus (ICO) and medial geniculate body (MG, a thalamic nucleus). For clarity, only one side is shown. Localization of sound is determined at several levels of this projection pathway. From the medial geniculate body, the final projection fibers course posterior to the internal capsule and terminate in the transverse gyri of the medial superior temporal gyrus (TG). Tonotopic organization is maintained throughout the acoustic system.

Lesions in the cochlea may unilaterally affect acuity of hearing; similarly, interruption of an acoustic nerve leads to unilateral deafness. Above the level of the cochlear nuclei, however, loss of hearing is minimal because of the bilateral projection. Localization may be impaired, however.

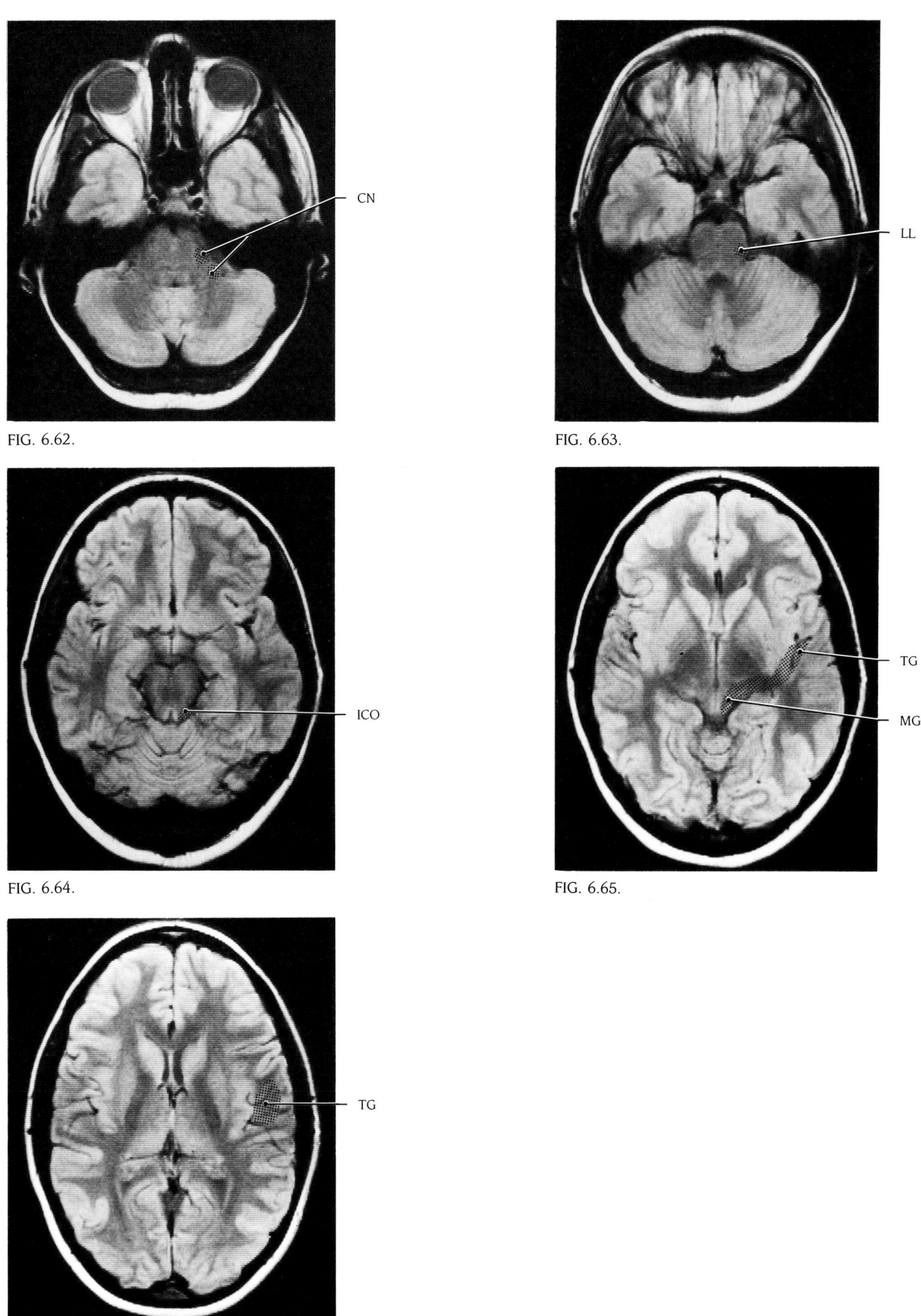

FIG. 6.62.

FIG. 6.63.

FIG. 6.64.

FIG. 6.65.

FIG. 6.66.

CN: cochlear nucleus; ICO: inferior colliculus; LL: lateral lemniscus; MG: medial geniculate body; TG: temporal gyrus.

Vestibular system

Impulses generated in the static labyrinth, for the sense of position in space, or in the semicircular canals, for the sense of directional acceleration, are conveyed to the vestibular nuclei (VN) in the brainstem, located just below the lateral extent of the floor of the fourth ventricle. Some vestibular fibers go directly to the archicerebellum, which consists of the flocculonodular lobes (FN; see section entitled, Cerebellum).

Each of the four vestibular nuclei has slightly different connections. The superior nucleus is associated with the archicerebellum, whereas the lateral nucleus sends its axons down the spinal cord to effect extension of the extremities in the event of a sudden loss of equilibrium.

The remaining two nuclei (medial and inferior), as well as the superior nucleus, contribute fibers to the medial longitudinal fasciculus (MLF) and the nuclei of the third, fourth, and sixth cranial nerves. Thus, ocular movements are affected by vestibular function. In addition, fibers course to the central thalamus (CT) and then to the projection area for the sense of position and position change located in the parietal lobe near the face region of the postcentral gyrus (PG).

Lesions in the vestibular system may lead to transient spontaneous nystagmus, loss of evoked nystagmus, loss of equilibrium, and various sensations of dizziness.

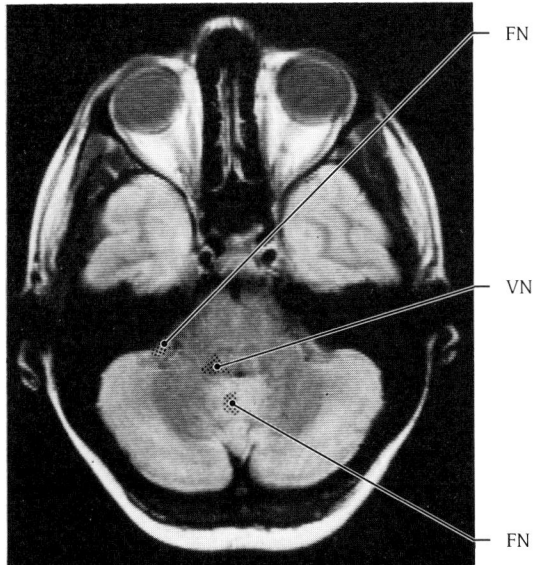

FIG. 6.67.

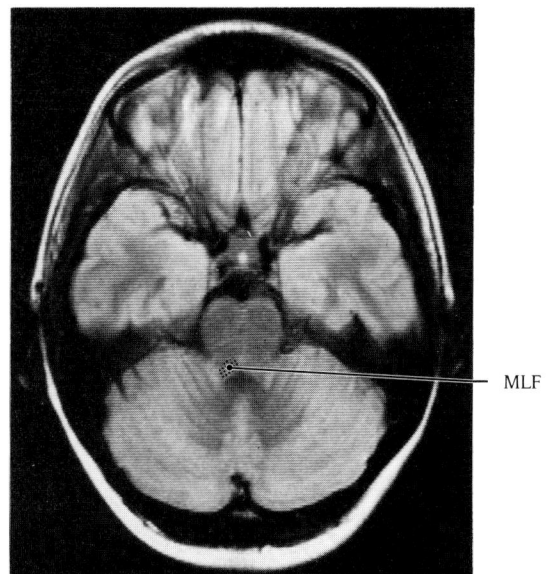

FIG. 6.68.

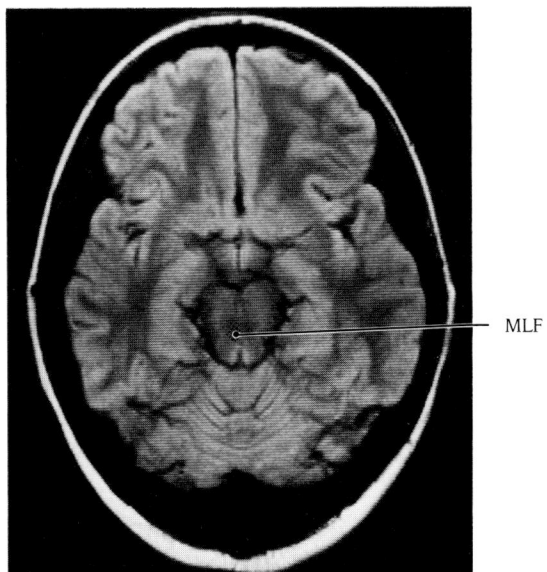

FIG. 6.69.

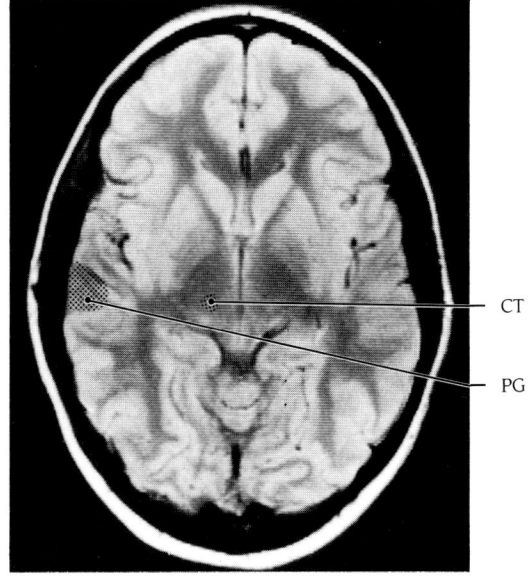

FIG. 6.70.

CT: central thalamus; FN: flocculonodular lobe; MLF: medial longitudinal fasciculus; PG: postcentral gyrus; VN: vestibular nuclei.

Visual system

The axons of the ganglion cell layer of the retinae give rise to the optic nerves (ON), which partially cross in the optic chiasm to become the optic tracts (OT). These tracts, containing visual impulses from a temporal or nasal half of each retina, end in the lateral geniculate bodies (LG) of the thalamus. The final projection pathway is by way of the optic, or geniculocalcarine, radiation (OR), which terminates in the visual cortex (VC, area 17) above and below the calcarine fissure.

The lower part of the optic radiation loops around the inferior horn of the lateral ventricle, far forward into the temporal lobe. This Meyer's loop, which carries impulses from the lower half of both retinae, may be destroyed by a temporal lobe lesion, resulting in a contralateral upper quadrantanopsia.

A lesion of an entire geniculate body, or transection of an optic tract, may lead to contralateral homonymous hemianopsia. Total destruction of the visual cortex of one side, e.g., with posterior cerebral artery occlusion, results in a similar visual deficit. A lesion in the middle of the chiasm, such as may occur with a pituitary tumor with suprasellar extension, may cause a partial or complete bitemporal hemianopsia because it affects fibers from the nasal half of each retina located there.

Some of the fibers (or their collateral processes) in the optic tract terminate in the pretectal region of the posterior dorsal right and left diencephalon. From this ill-defined area, connections course to both third nerve nuclei as part of the circuit for the pupillary light reflex.

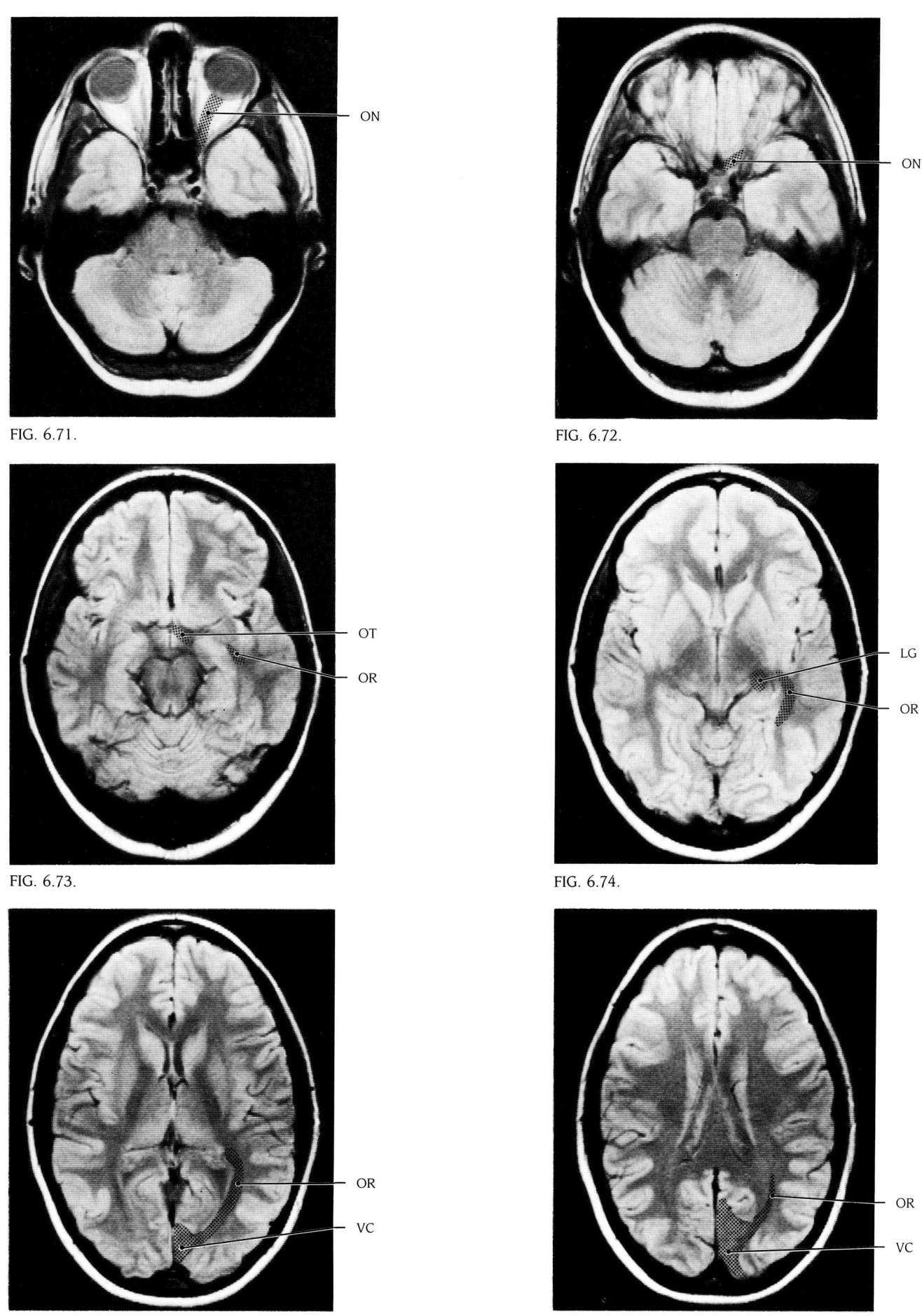

FIG. 6.71.

FIG. 6.72.

FIG. 6.73.

FIG. 6.74.

FIG. 6.75.

FIG. 6.76.

LG: lateral geniculate body; ON: optic nerve; OR: optic radiation; OT: optic tract; VC: visual cortex.

OLFACTION AND LIMBIC SYSTEM

The structures subserving the sense of smell are limited in extent, according to modern views. From the upper nasal mucosa, some two dozen fine olfactory nerves pass through the lamina cribrosa to synapse in the olfactory bulbs (OB). From here, olfactory peduncles (OP), or tracts, course back at the base of the frontal lobe and end in the cortical projection areas near the uncus (gyrus semilunaris and gyrus ambiens). Two other terminations are found in the gray matter underlying the anterior perforated space and in the gray matter between the anterior commissure and the septum (AS). The latter two regions are probably involved in hypothalamic reflexes that are triggered by olfactory stimuli.

The limbic system is a system of primitive cortical areas with interconnections and outflow into the hypothalamus (HT) and the anterior thalamus (AT), both directly and indirectly. Anatomically, this system is situated along the "hilus" of the cerebral hemisphere, where a transition, or limbus, to the diencephalon exists. The hippocampal formation, consisting of hippocampus (HP), dentate gyrus, and other primitive gray cortex, and its fimbria-fornix (FX), in addition to the amygdaloid complex (AM) and its stria terminalis, jointly influence hypothalamic and thalamic functions. A third input comes from the olfactory terminations in the basal forebrain. Surrounding most of these three subsystems (and the corpus callosum) is the "great limbic lobe of Broca" (GL), which consists of a transition cortex between the modern neocortex and the primitive limbic system cortex. This great limbic convolution is composed of the subcallosal, cingulate, retrosplenial, and parahippocampal gyri.

Several interrelated functions have been associated with part or all of the limbic system. The limbic system has been considered a regulatory system superimposed on autonomic centers of the hypothalamus, brainstem, and spinal cord. Similarly, structures of the limbic system influence hypothalamic and pituitary endocrine functions. Certain basic drives, or patterns of behavior important for the individual or for the species, have their substrate in limbic-hypothalamic interaction: e.g., feeding, drinking, aggression, and propagation. Autonomic and endocrine aspects of these drives are well established. The role of olfactory stimuli and reflexes is likewise well-known.

The traditional view, however, that most limbic system structures are essentially tertiary olfactory centers ("rhinencephalon") has long since been refuted.

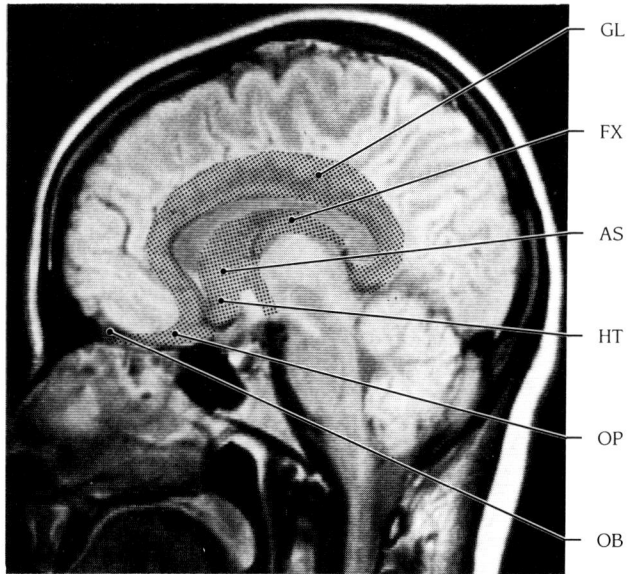

FIG. 6.77.

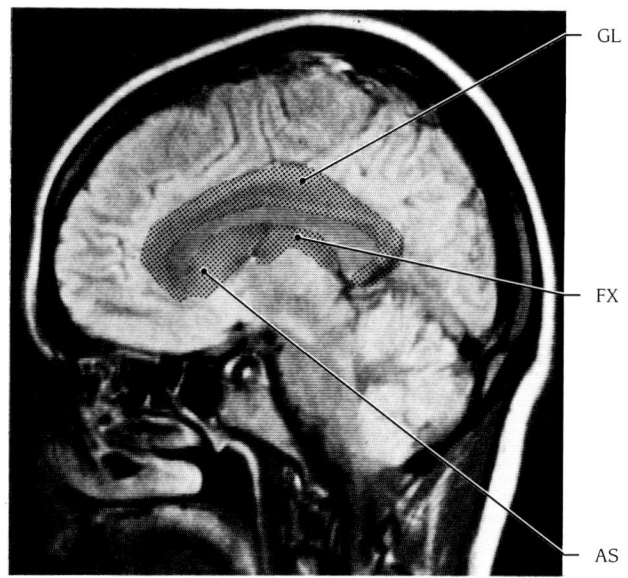

FIG. 6.78.

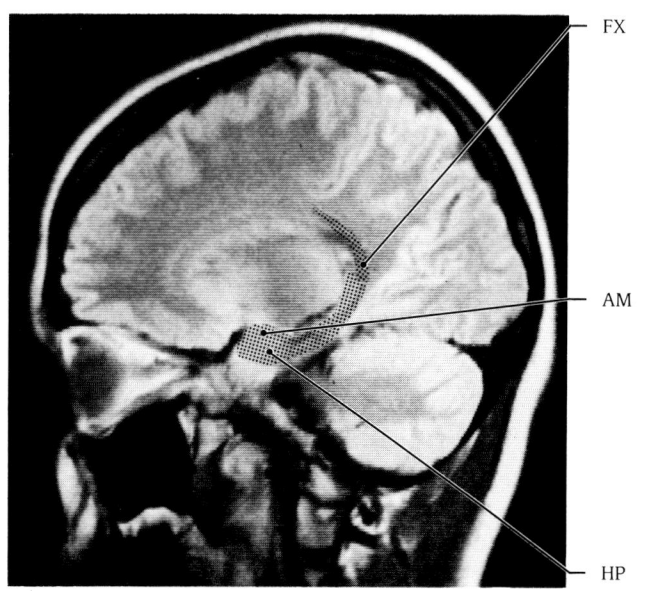

FIG. 6.79.

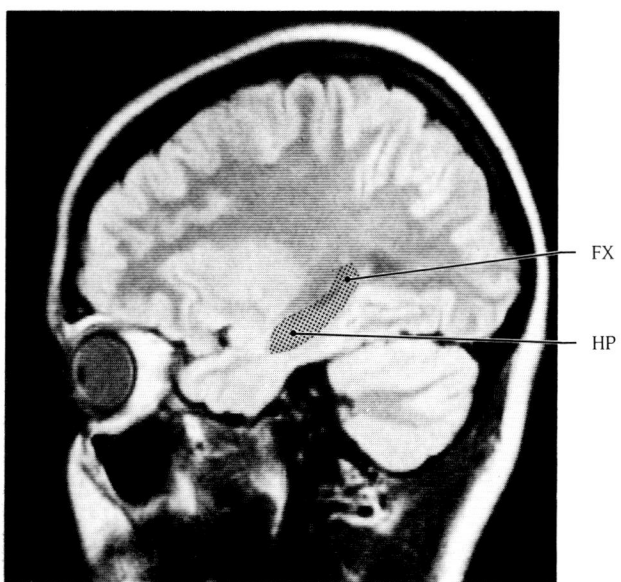

FIG. 6.80.

AM: amygdaloid complex; AS: septum and anterior commissure area; FX: fornix; GL: great limbic lobe; HP: hippocampus; HT: hypothalamus; OB: olfactory bulb; OP: olfactory peduncle.

SPEECH AREAS AND CONNECTIONS

Traditionally, several regions in the dominant hemisphere have been designated as speech areas. The motor speech area of Broca (MS) lies in the frontal opercular region, whereas the sensory speech area of Wernicke (SS) is located on the medial side of the superior temporal gyrus. The frontal motor speech area (MS) is associated with the coordination of the motor aspects of speech; a lesion in this region leads to the production of unintelligible words, or no sound at all. Lesions in the sensory speech area (SS) result in the inability to understand spoken language. A subcortical fiber system, the arcuate fasciculus (AF), connects these two speech areas; lesions in this system appear to be involved in global aphasia. The angular gyrus has been associated with anomia, the inability to identify and name objects and persons. Descending pathways, in part along the corticobulbar tract, lead to the effector nuclei of the twelfth, tenth, seventh, and fifth cranial nerves, which are concerned with the formation of separate speech sounds. Destruction of these pathways, of their associated cranial nerves, or of their nuclei leads to forms of dysarthria.

Although there is considerable clinical evidence that destruction or ischemia of the cortical speech areas leads to forms of aphasia, the importance and extent of underlying fiber systems are less clear. As yet, animal models have not elucidated this functional relationship.

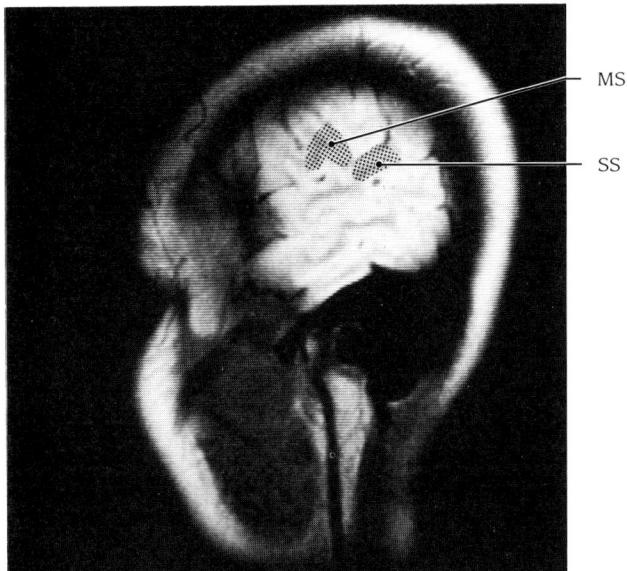

FIG. 6.81.

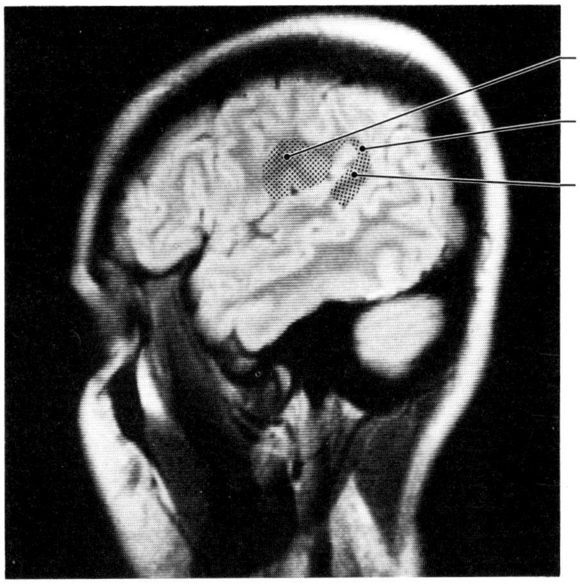

FIG. 6.82.

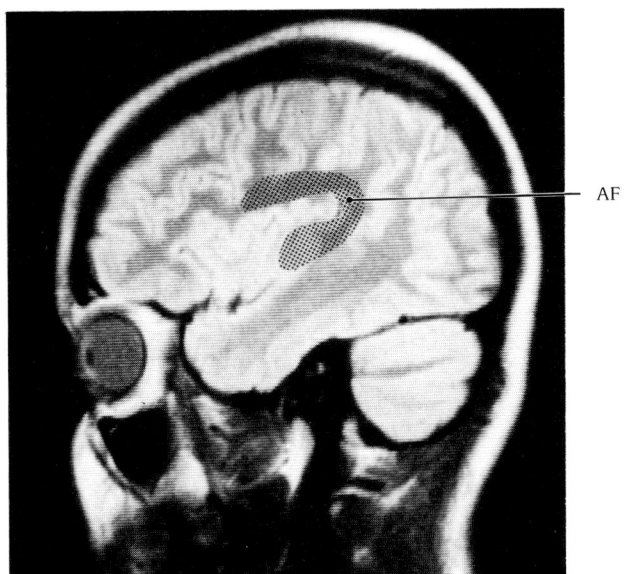

FIG. 6.83.

AF: arcuate fasciculus; MS: motor speech area; SS: sensory speech area.

7

Face, Neck, and Cervical Spine, Axial Plane

Anatomic Level	Figure
Foramen magnum and nasopharynx	7.1–7.4
C2 and C3 vertebrae and oropharynx	7.5–7.16
C4 and C5 vertebrae and laryngopharynx	7.17–7.25
Larynx	7.26–7.34

A series of cadaveric axial sections that extend from the foramen magnum through the larynx are shown. These sections are matched with transaxial magnetic resonance images of a volunteer. Additional anatomic sections and detailed views of the bony skeleton are included for clarification at some levels. The difference in the section planes between the anatomic and the magnetic resonance images reflects the variability resulting from both angulation and positioning. Motion inevitably degrades magnetic resonance images obtained in areas most susceptible to movement caused by respiration. In this series, this effect is most prominent in the images through the lower neck at the level of the larynx.

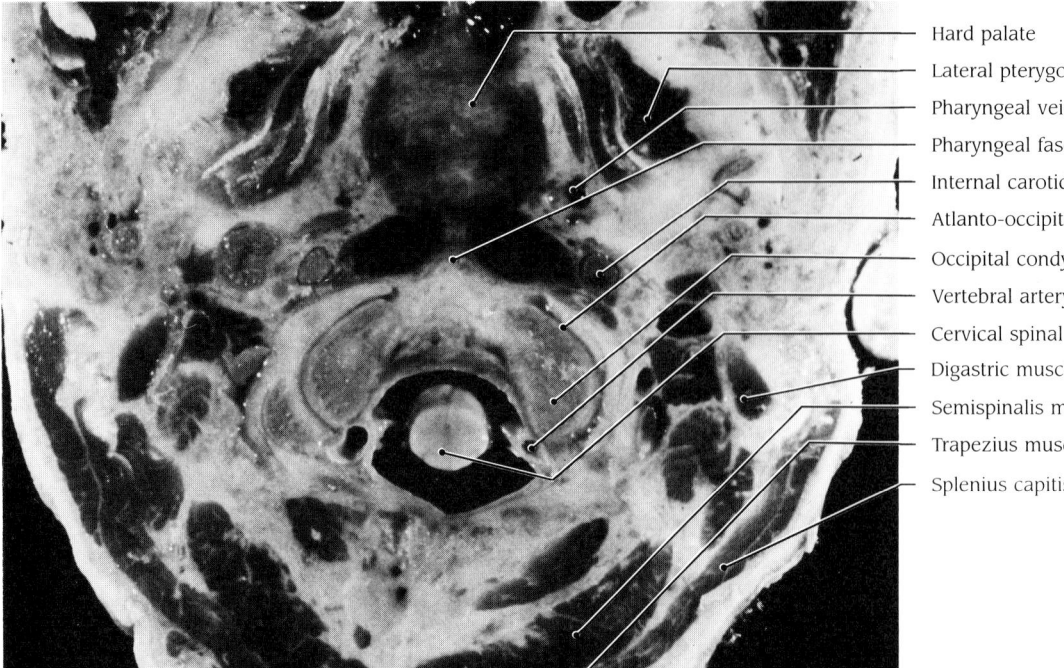

FIG. 7.1.

Hard palate
Lateral pterygoid muscle
Pharyngeal vein
Pharyngeal fascia
Internal carotid artery
Atlanto-occipital joint
Occipital condyle
Vertebral artery
Cervical spinal cord
Digastric muscle
Semispinalis muscle
Trapezius muscle
Splenius capitis muscle

- The pharynx is a musculomembranous tube that extends from the base of the skull to the level of the sixth cervical vertebra opposite the lower border of the cricoid cartilage. The pharynx is composed of three parts: the nasal, the oral, and the laryngeal (sometimes referred to as the hypopharynx). The nasal part of the pharynx, seen at this level, lies posterior to the nose and superior to the soft palate.

- The eustachian tube, or auditory tube, is the communication channel from the tympanic cavity to the nasopharynx. The auditory tube is composed of a bony portion and a cartilaginous portion. The bony segment extends from the anterior wall of the tympanic cavity to the junction of the squamous and petrous portions of the temporal bone. The cartilaginous segment attaches to the medial end of the bony portion and ends at the tubal elevation behind the pharyngeal orifice of the tube.

- The parotid gland, the largest of the salivary glands, lies between the mandible and the sternocleidomastoid muscle, below the external acoustic meatus. The medial portion extends forward along the deep aspect of the ramus to reach the medial pterygoid muscle, whereas the lateral portion projects anteriorly along the surface of the masseter muscle, where a small part of the gland, the accessory part, which is often detached, lies between the zygomatic arch above and the parotid duct below.

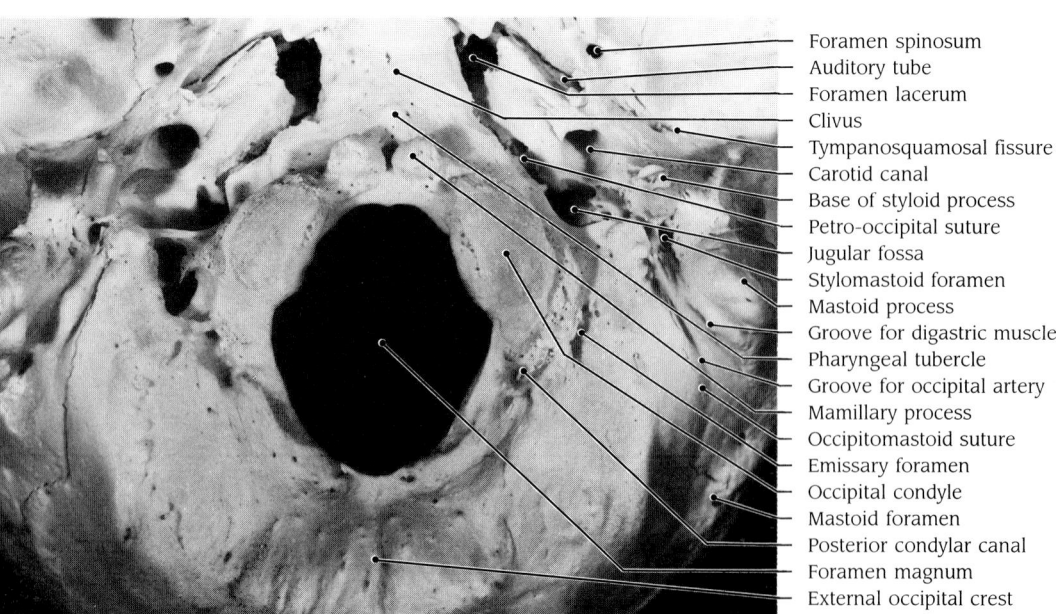

Foramen spinosum
Auditory tube
Foramen lacerum
Clivus
Tympanosquamosal fissure
Carotid canal
Base of styloid process
Petro-occipital suture
Jugular fossa
Stylomastoid foramen
Mastoid process
Groove for digastric muscle
Pharyngeal tubercle
Groove for occipital artery
Mamillary process
Occipitomastoid suture
Emissary foramen
Occipital condyle
Mastoid foramen
Posterior condylar canal
Foramen magnum
External occipital crest

FIG. 7.2. Basal view of bony structures around the foramen magnum. (From de Groot, J.: Correlative Neuroanatomy of Computed Tomography and Magnetic Resonance Imaging. Philadelphia, Lea & Febiger, 1984.)

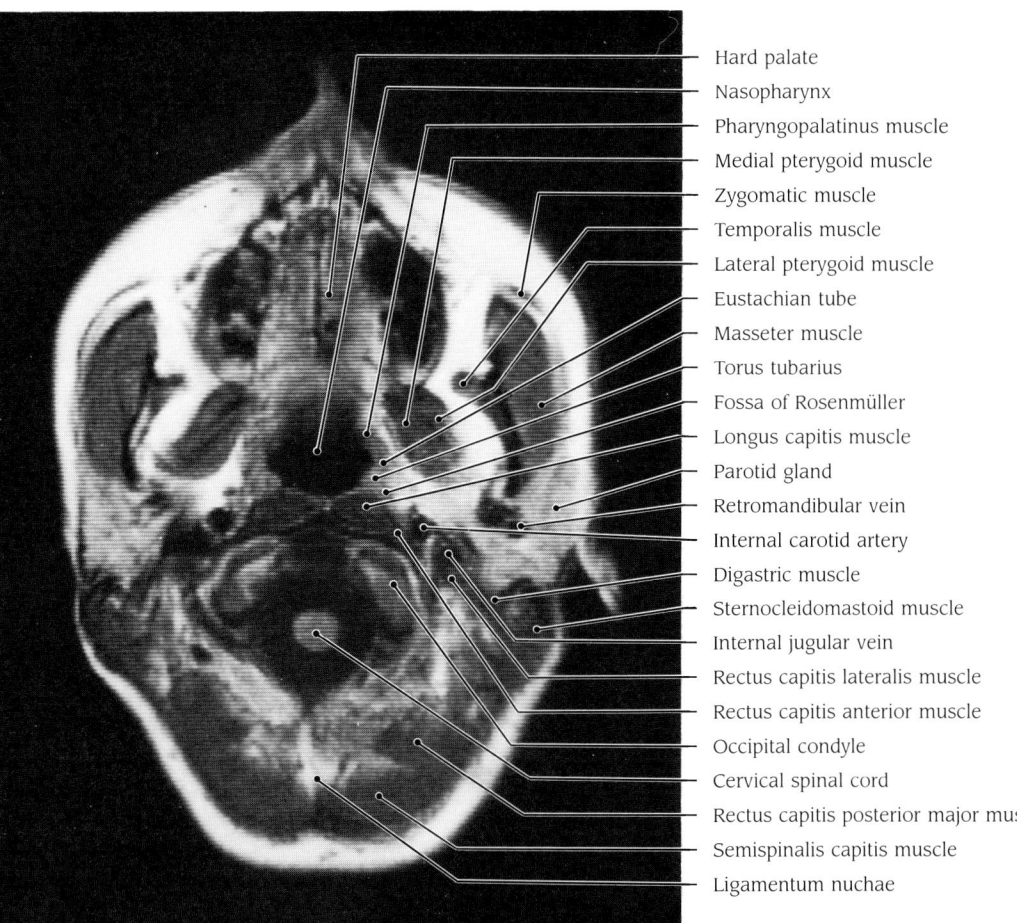

FIG. 7.3. TR = 500 msec, TE = 28 msec.

- Hard palate
- Nasopharynx
- Pharyngopalatinus muscle
- Medial pterygoid muscle
- Zygomatic muscle
- Temporalis muscle
- Lateral pterygoid muscle
- Eustachian tube
- Masseter muscle
- Torus tubarius
- Fossa of Rosenmüller
- Longus capitis muscle
- Parotid gland
- Retromandibular vein
- Internal carotid artery
- Digastric muscle
- Sternocleidomastoid muscle
- Internal jugular vein
- Rectus capitis lateralis muscle
- Rectus capitis anterior muscle
- Occipital condyle
- Cervical spinal cord
- Rectus capitis posterior major muscle
- Semispinalis capitis muscle
- Ligamentum nuchae

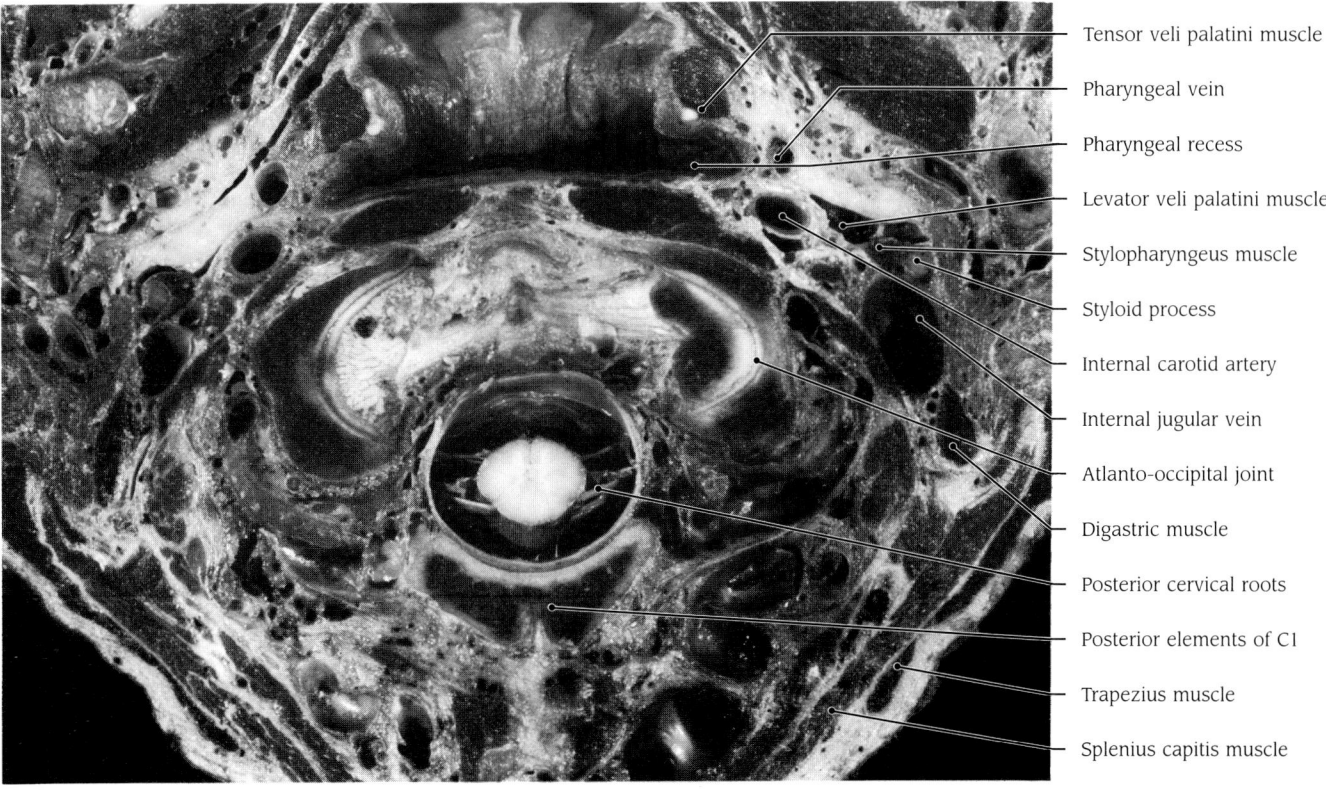

FIG. 7.4.

- Tensor veli palatini muscle
- Pharyngeal vein
- Pharyngeal recess
- Levator veli palatini muscle
- Stylopharyngeus muscle
- Styloid process
- Internal carotid artery
- Internal jugular vein
- Atlanto-occipital joint
- Digastric muscle
- Posterior cervical roots
- Posterior elements of C1
- Trapezius muscle
- Splenius capitis muscle

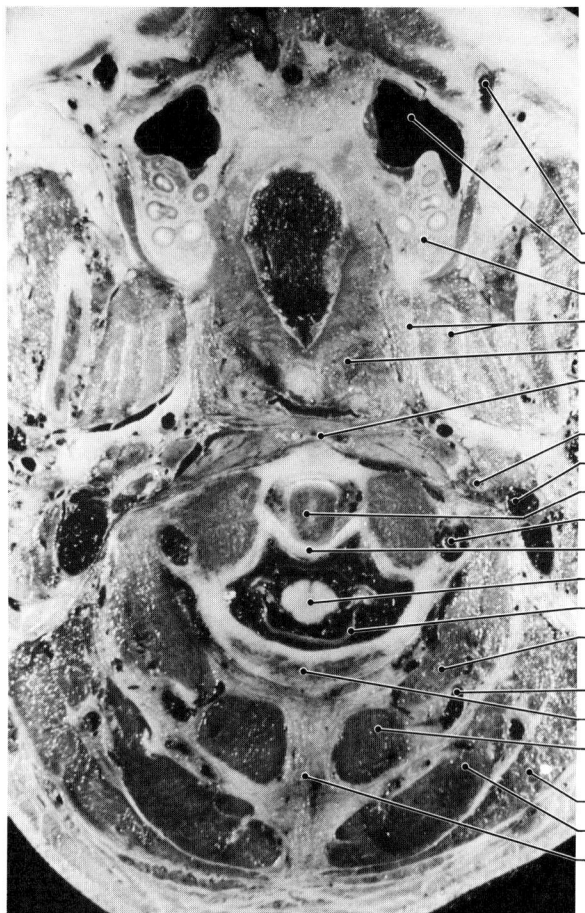
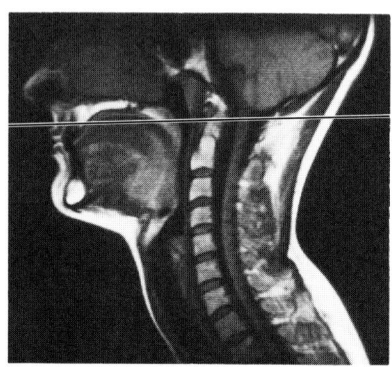

FIG. 7.5.

- The oropharynx extends from the soft palate to the upper border of the epiglottis. Anteriorly, the oropharynx opens into the mouth and faces the pharyngeal portion of the tongue. The lateral wall is bounded by the palatopharyngeal arch and the tonsil. The body of C2 and the superior portion of the body of C3 are on the level of the oropharynx posteriorly.

- The palatine tonsils are two collections of lymphoid tissue located in the lateral walls of the oral part of the pharynx. The tonsils lie in the tonsillar sinus between the palatoglossal and palatopharyngeal arches. The palatine tonsils are part of a circle of lymphoid tissue that surrounds the opening into the digestive and respiratory tubes. The lingual tonsil forms the anterior and inferior ring; the palatine tonsils and the lymphoid tissue near the auditory tubes form the lateral portions; and the pharyngeal tonsil forms the posterior, superior ring.

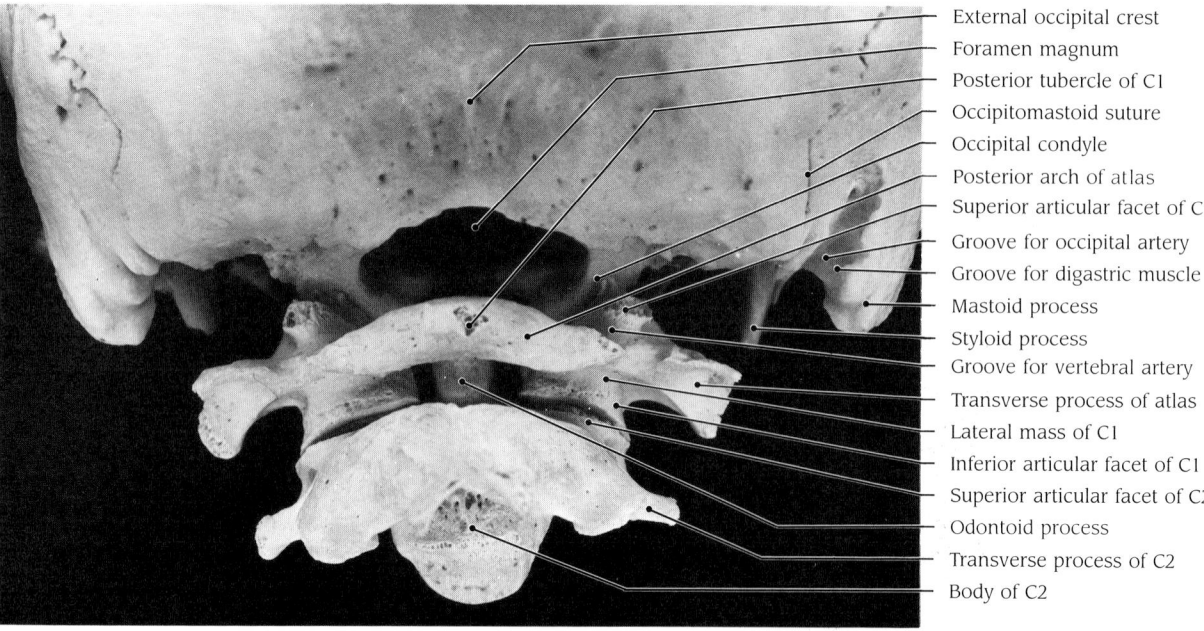

FIG. 7.6. Posterior view of the bony elements of the craniovertebral junction. (From de Groot, J.: Correlative Neuroanatomy of Computed Tomography and Magnetic Resonance Imaging. Philadelphia, Lea & Febiger, 1984.)

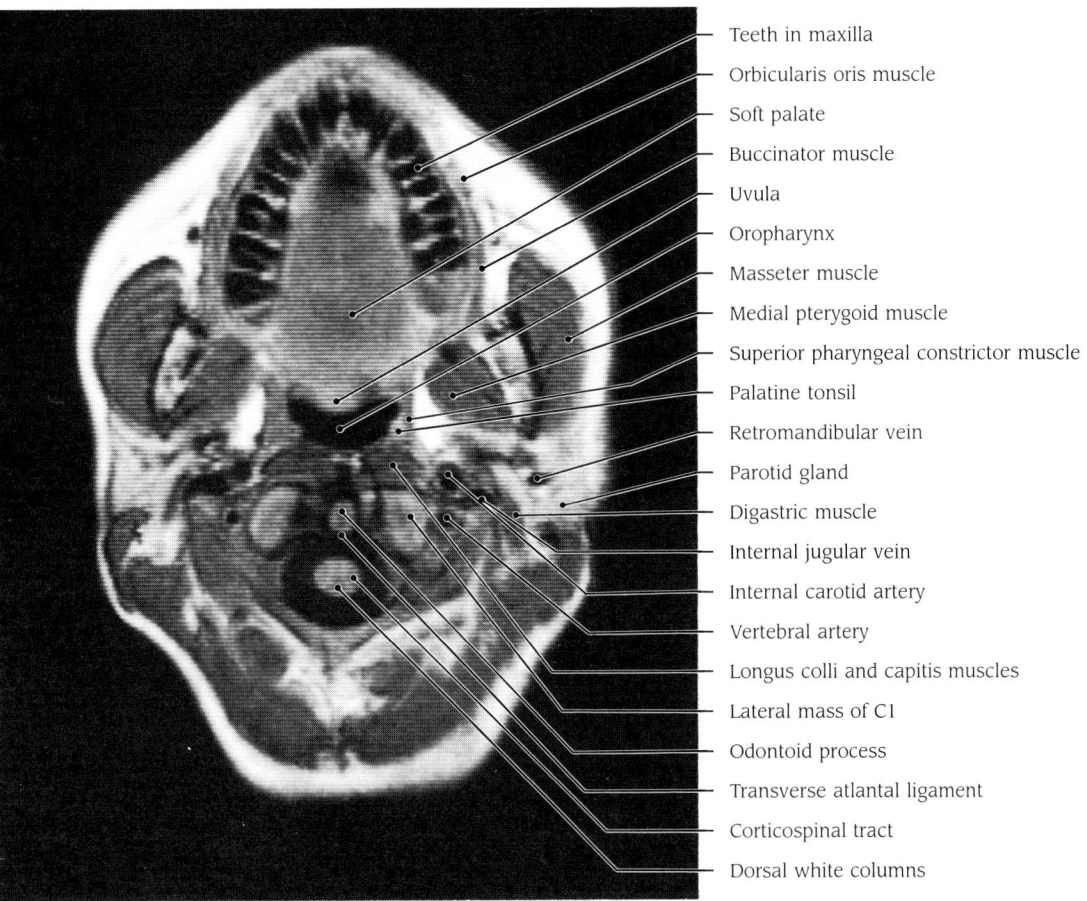

FIG. 7.7. TR = 500 msec, TE = 28 msec.

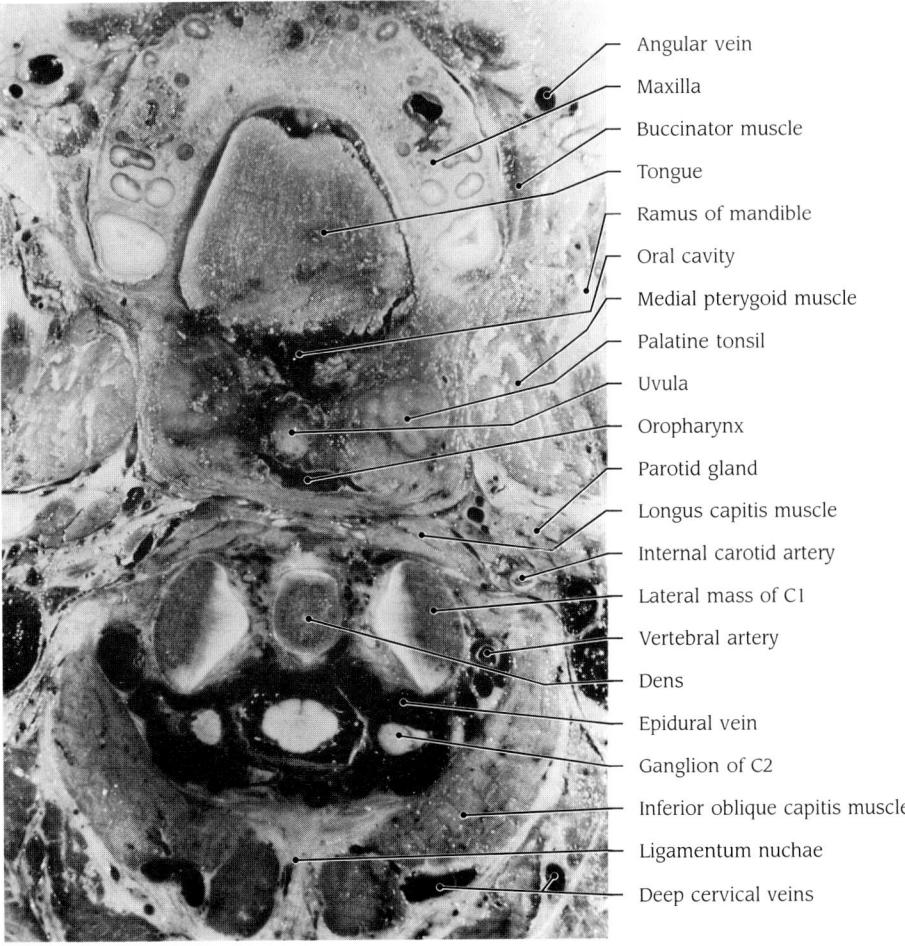

FIG. 7.8.

165

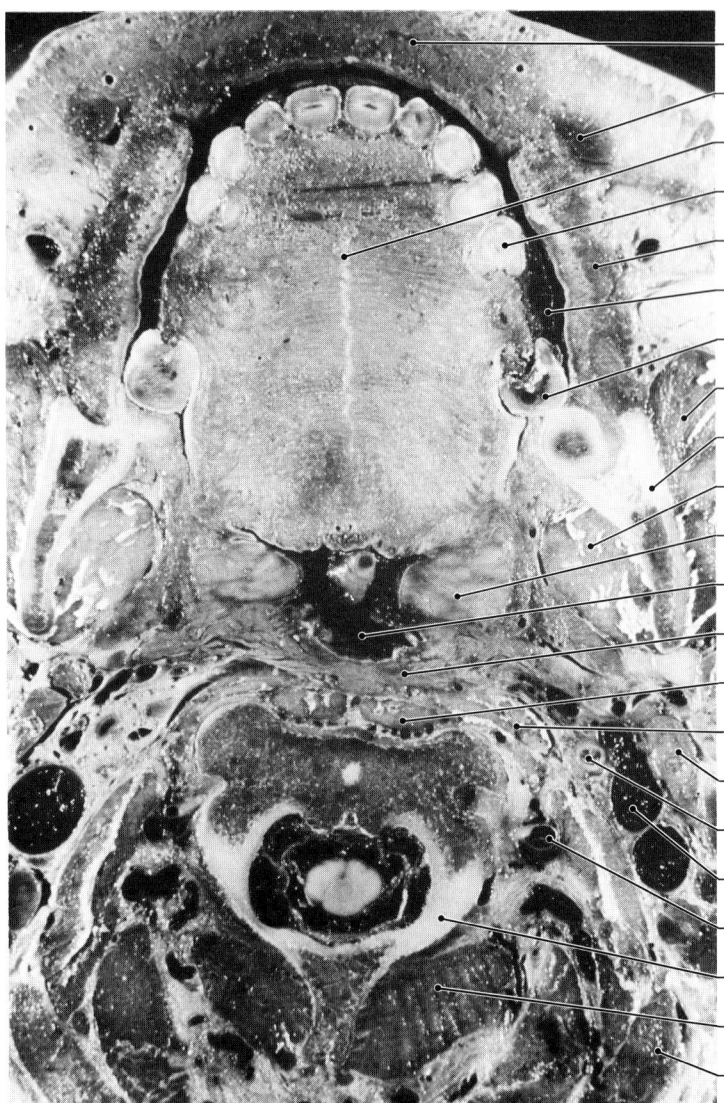
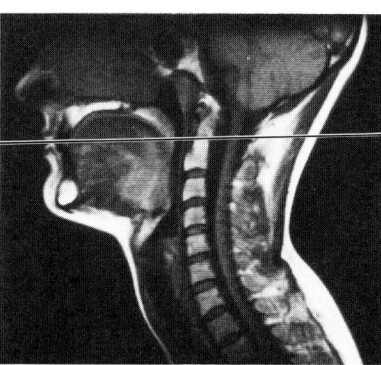

FIG. 7.9.

- The muscles of the pharynx include the superior, middle, and inferior constrictors and three additional muscles, the stylopharyngeus, the salpingopharyngeus, and the palatopharyngeus, which descend obliquely into the muscular wall of the pharynx.

- The oropharyngeal isthmus is the aperture between the mouth and the pharynx. It is bounded superiorly by the soft palate, inferiorly by the dorsum of the tongue, and laterally by the palatoglossal arches. The palatoglossal arches, formed by the palatoglossus muscles and their covering mucous membranes, appose during deglutition to separate the mouth cavity from the oropharynx.

- The muscles of mastication are the masseter, the temporalis, and the pterygoid. The masseter, temporalis, and medial pterygoid muscles function to elevate the mandible, close the mouth, and approximate the teeth. The temporalis muscle additionally serves to retract the mandible after it has been protruded. The lateral pterygoid muscles depress the mandible, thereby opening the mouth. Protrusion of the mandible is produced by the action of the medial and lateral pterygoid muscles in concert, whereas lateral movements result from the alternate action of the medial and lateral pterygoid muscles of each side. These muscles are innervated by the mandibular division of the trigeminal nerve.

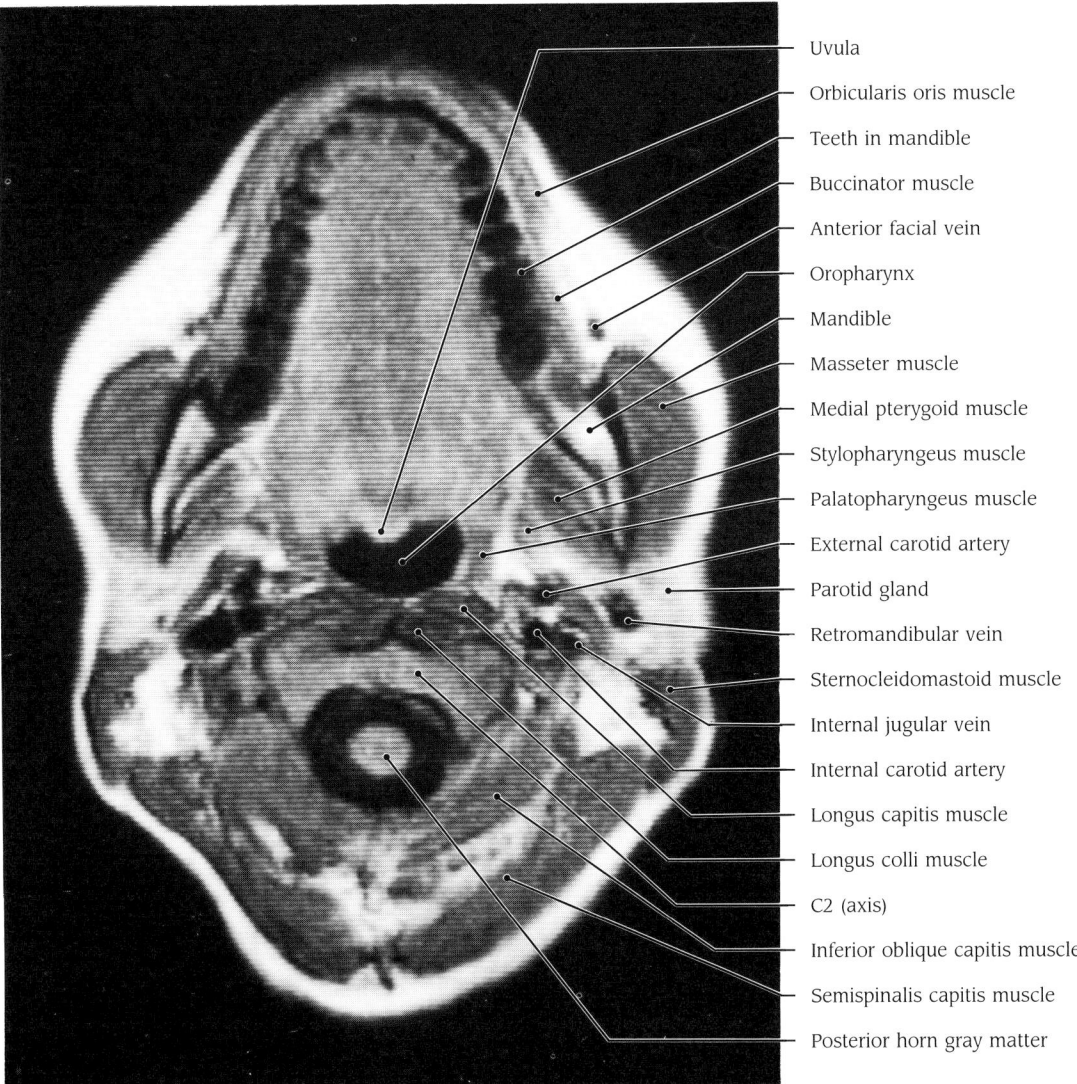

FIG. 7.10. TR = 500 msec, TE = 28 msec.

- Uvula
- Orbicularis oris muscle
- Teeth in mandible
- Buccinator muscle
- Anterior facial vein
- Oropharynx
- Mandible
- Masseter muscle
- Medial pterygoid muscle
- Stylopharyngeus muscle
- Palatopharyngeus muscle
- External carotid artery
- Parotid gland
- Retromandibular vein
- Sternocleidomastoid muscle
- Internal jugular vein
- Internal carotid artery
- Longus capitis muscle
- Longus colli muscle
- C2 (axis)
- Inferior oblique capitis muscle
- Semispinalis capitis muscle
- Posterior horn gray matter

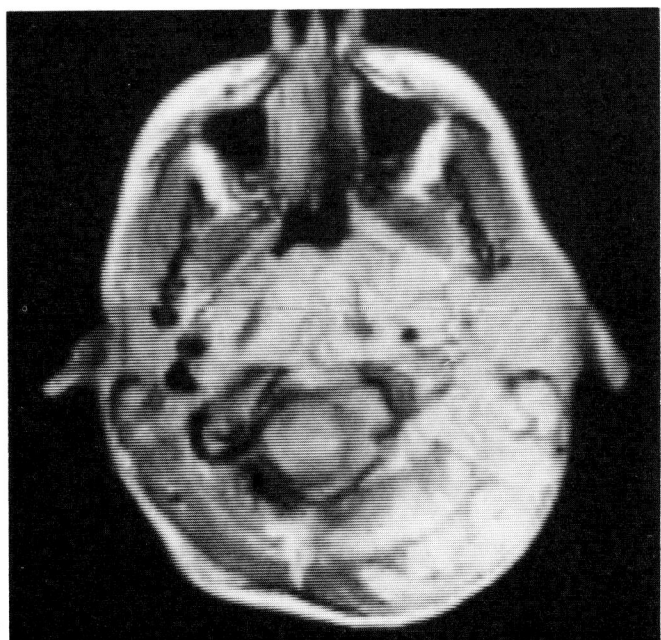

FIG. 7.11. TR = 2000 msec, TE = 28 msec. An extensive neurofibroma displaces the spinal cord to the right, occludes the left internal jugular vein, and effaces most of the oropharynx.

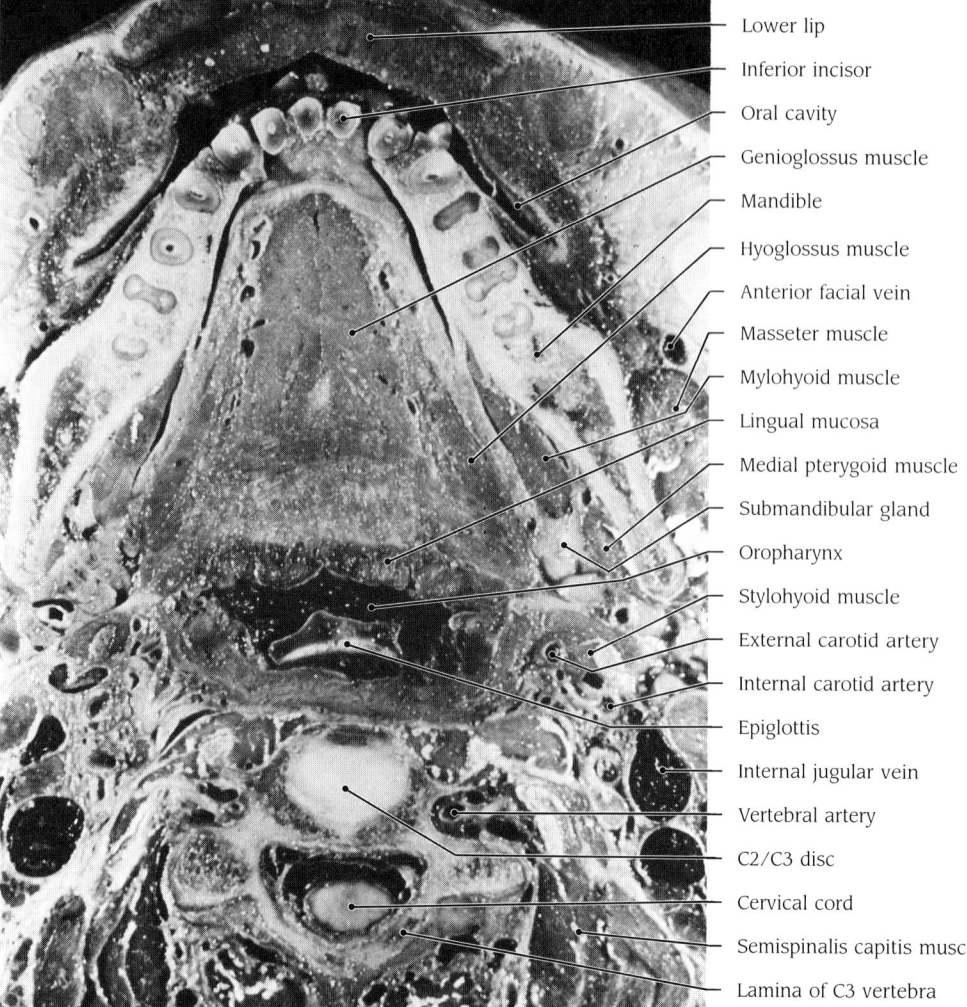
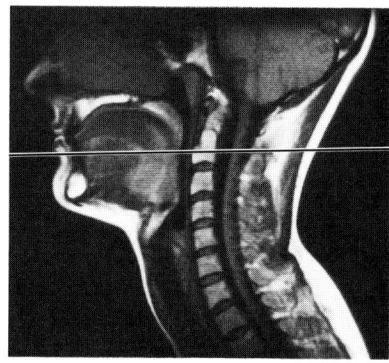

Lower lip
Inferior incisor
Oral cavity
Genioglossus muscle
Mandible
Hyoglossus muscle
Anterior facial vein
Masseter muscle
Mylohyoid muscle
Lingual mucosa
Medial pterygoid muscle
Submandibular gland
Oropharynx
Stylohyoid muscle
External carotid artery
Internal carotid artery
Epiglottis
Internal jugular vein
Vertebral artery
C2/C3 disc
Cervical cord
Semispinalis capitis muscle
Lamina of C3 vertebra

FIG. 7.12.

- The salivary glands consist of three large paired glands (the parotid, submandibular, and sublingual glands), the smaller anterior lingual glands, and the multiple small glands in the mucous membranes of the tongue, lips, cheek, and palate. The sublingual gland, the smallest of the three principal salivary glands, lies inferior to the mucous membrane of the floor of the mouth, in the sublingual fossa of the mandible, close to the symphysis mentis.

- The tongue is separated in halves by a median fibrous septum, the septum linguae, which is attached inferiorly to the body of the hyoid bone. Two varieties of muscles comprise the tongue: the extrinsic, which have attachments outside the tongue and cause gross movements, and the intrinsic, which are contained within the tongue and help to shape the tongue itself. The extrinsic muscles include the genioglossus, hyoglossus, styloglossus, and palatoglossus. The intrinsic muscles are the superior and inferior longitudinal, the transverse, and the vertical.

- The hypoglossal nerve supplies all the intrinsic and extrinsic muscles of the tongue, with the exception of the palatoglossus muscle, which is supplied by the vagus nerve.

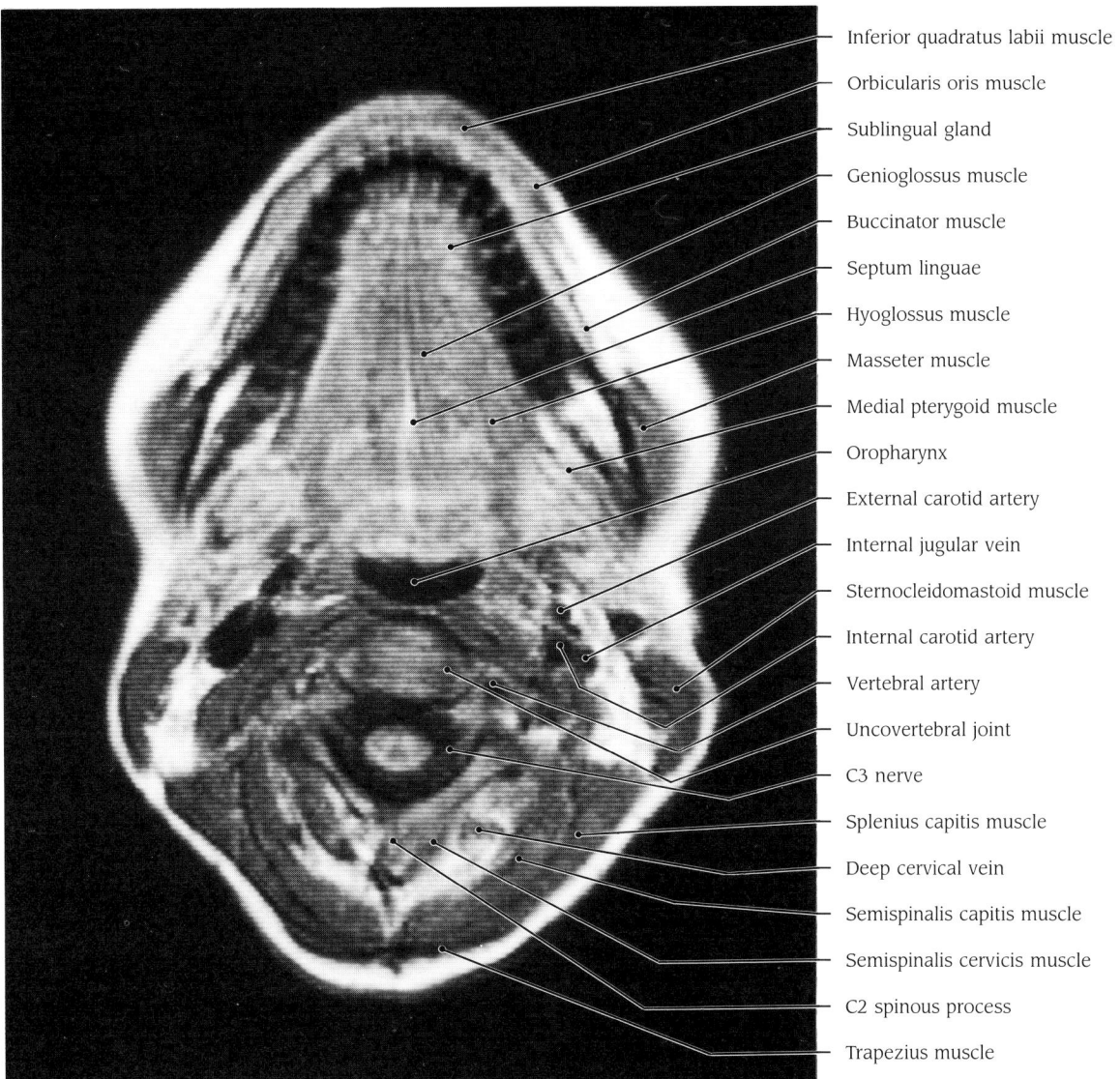

FIG. 7.13. TR = 500 msec, TE = 28 msec.

- Inferior quadratus labii muscle
- Orbicularis oris muscle
- Sublingual gland
- Genioglossus muscle
- Buccinator muscle
- Septum linguae
- Hyoglossus muscle
- Masseter muscle
- Medial pterygoid muscle
- Oropharynx
- External carotid artery
- Internal jugular vein
- Sternocleidomastoid muscle
- Internal carotid artery
- Vertebral artery
- Uncovertebral joint
- C3 nerve
- Splenius capitis muscle
- Deep cervical vein
- Semispinalis capitis muscle
- Semispinalis cervicis muscle
- C2 spinous process
- Trapezius muscle

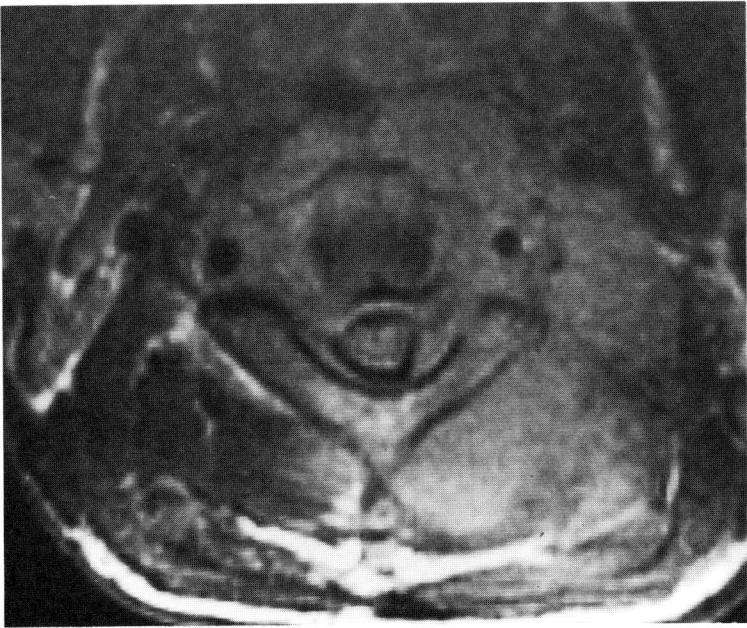

FIG. 7.14. TR = 839 msec, TE = 39 msec. An extensive lymphoma surrounds the spinal cord, displaces the left posterior neck musculature, and effaces the oropharynx.

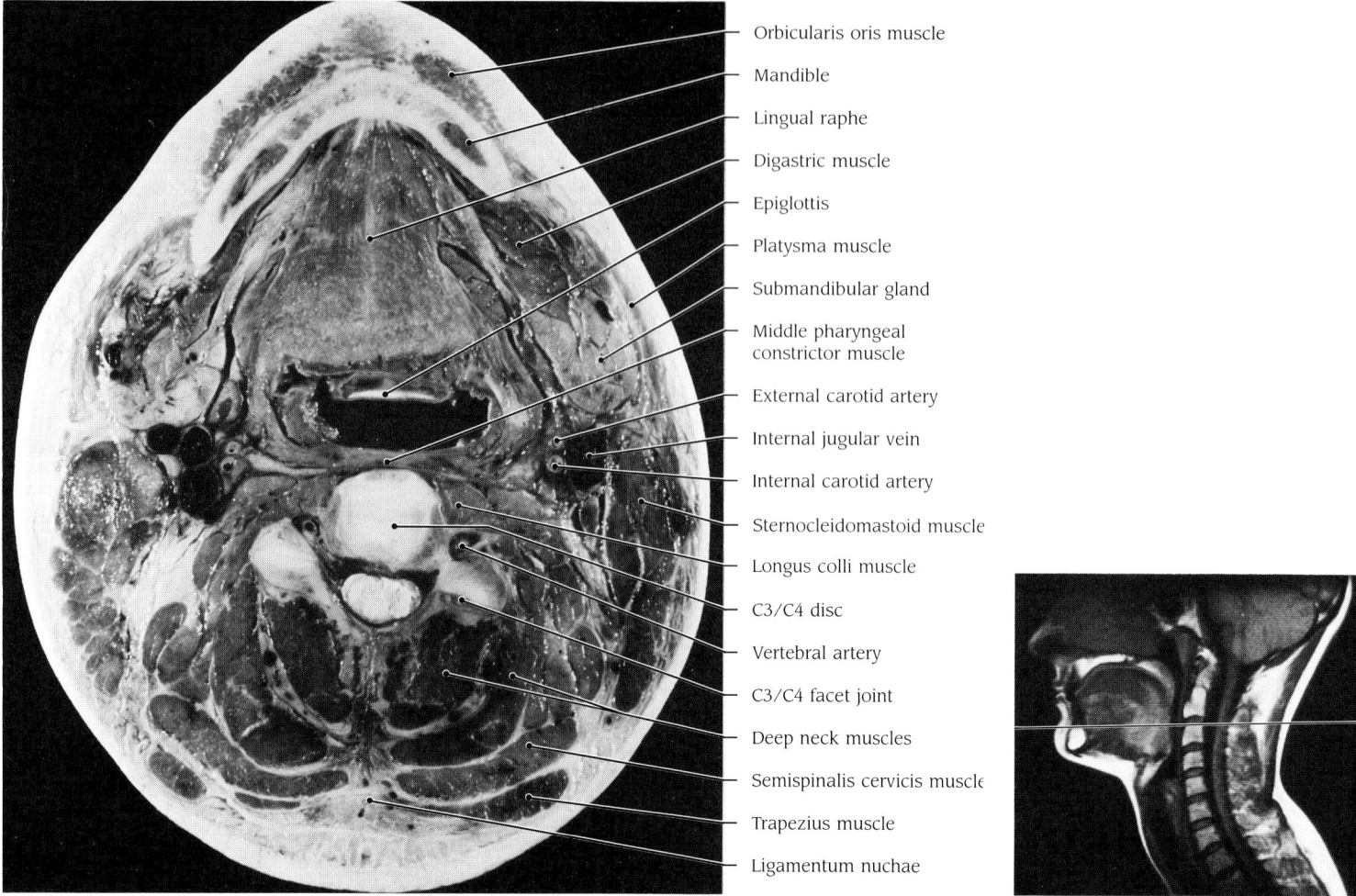

FIG. 7.15.

- The middle constrictor muscle of the pharynx is composed of two parts: the chondropharyngeal and the ceratopharyngeal.
- The superior constrictor muscle of the pharynx is the thinnest of the constrictors and is composed of four parts: the pterygopharyngeal, the buccopharyngeal, the mylopharyngeal, and the glossopharyngeal.
- The submandibular gland consists of a larger superficial part and a smaller deep part that are continuous with each other around the posterior border of the mylohyoid muscle. The submandibular gland lies in the submandibular fossa on the inner surface of the body of the mandible.

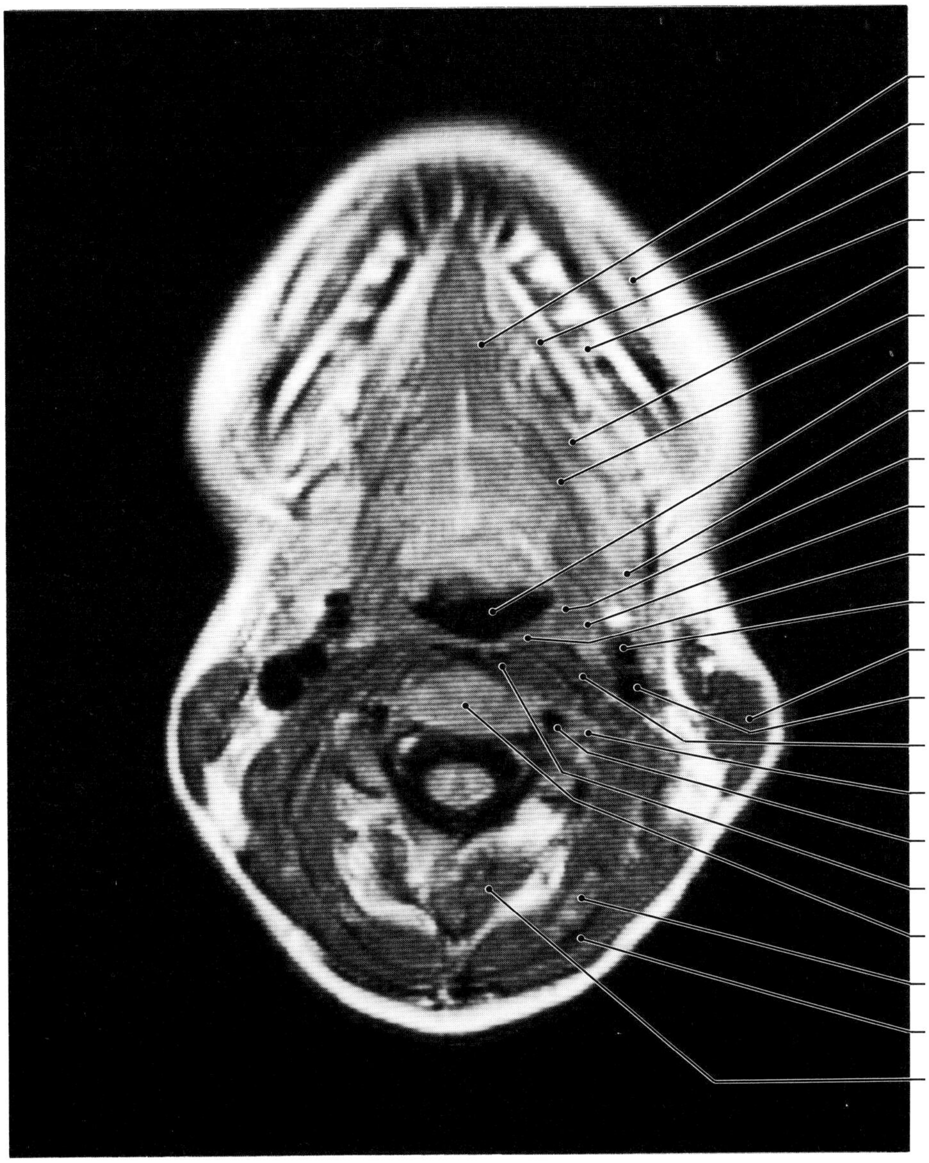

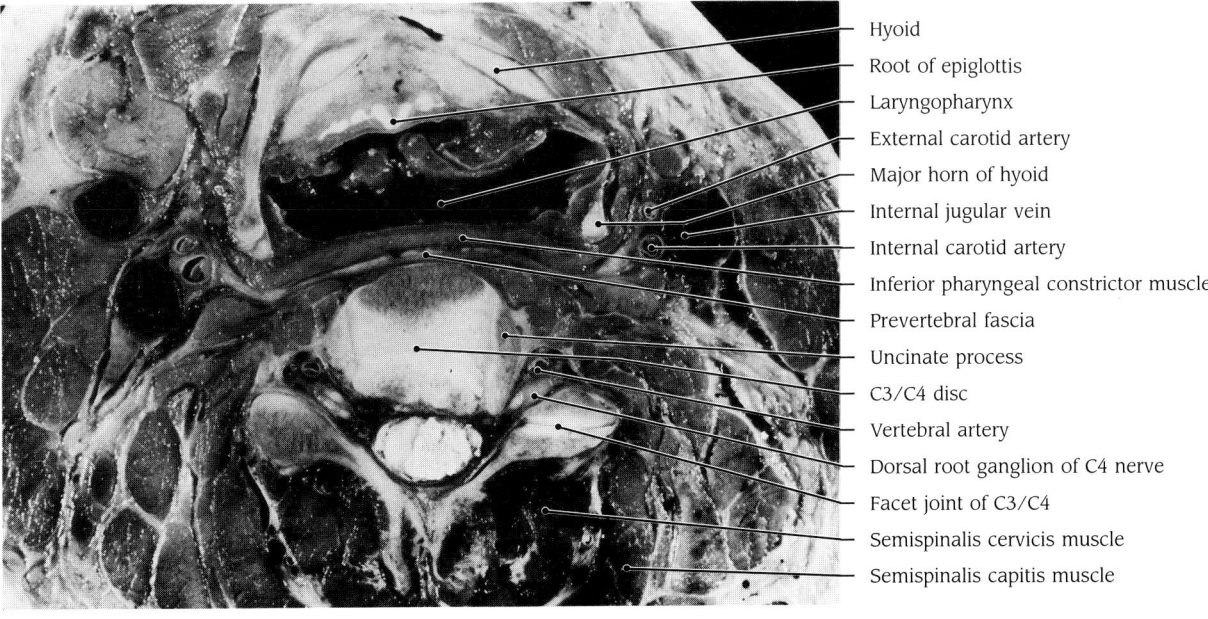

FIG. 7.16. TR = 500 msec, TE = 28 msec.

- Geniohyoid muscle
- Platysma muscle
- Digastric muscle
- Mandible
- Mylohyoid muscle
- Hyoglossus muscle
- Oropharynx
- Submandibular gland
- Pharyngopalatinus and stylopharyngeus muscles
- Stylohyoid muscle
- Pharyngeal constrictor muscles
- Internal carotid artery
- Sternocleidomastoid muscle
- Internal jugular vein
- Longus capitis muscle
- Transverse process of C3
- Vertebral artery
- Longus colli muscle
- C3 vertebral body
- Semispinalis capitis muscle
- Splenius capitis muscle
- Semispinalis cervicis and multifidus muscles

FIG. 7.17.

- Hyoid
- Root of epiglottis
- Laryngopharynx
- External carotid artery
- Major horn of hyoid
- Internal jugular vein
- Internal carotid artery
- Inferior pharyngeal constrictor muscle
- Prevertebral fascia
- Uncinate process
- C3/C4 disc
- Vertebral artery
- Dorsal root ganglion of C4 nerve
- Facet joint of C3/C4
- Semispinalis cervicis muscle
- Semispinalis capitis muscle

171

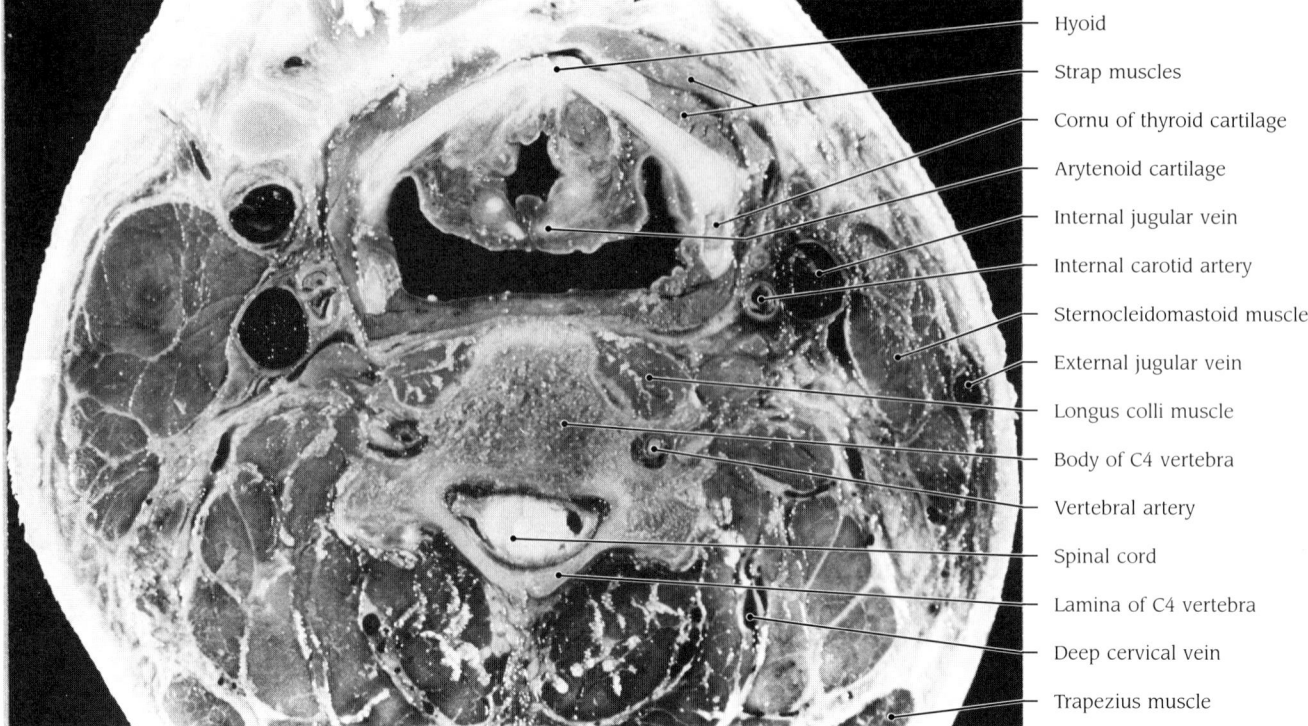

FIG. 7.18.

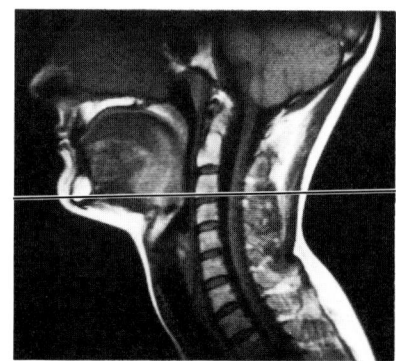

- The laryngeal part of the pharynx extends from the superior margin of the epiglottis to the inferior border of the cricoid cartilage, where it is continuous with the esophagus.
- The inferior constrictor muscle of the pharynx is the thickest of the constrictor muscles and is composed of the cricopharyngeus and the thyropharyngeus. In the process of deglutition, the sphincteric function is performed by the cricopharyngeus, whereas the propulsive function is performed by the thyropharyngeus.
- The cartilaginous skeleton of the larynx is composed of the thyroid, the cricoid, and the epiglottis, as well as of the paired arytenoid, cuneiform and corniculate cartilages.
- The epiglottis, a thin sheet of elastic fibrocartilage, projects superiorly behind the tongue and body of the hyoid bone, anterior to the opening of the larynx. The hyoepiglottic ligament connects the epiglottis to the superior border of the hyoid bone. The vallecula is the depression on either side of the median glossoepiglottic fold.

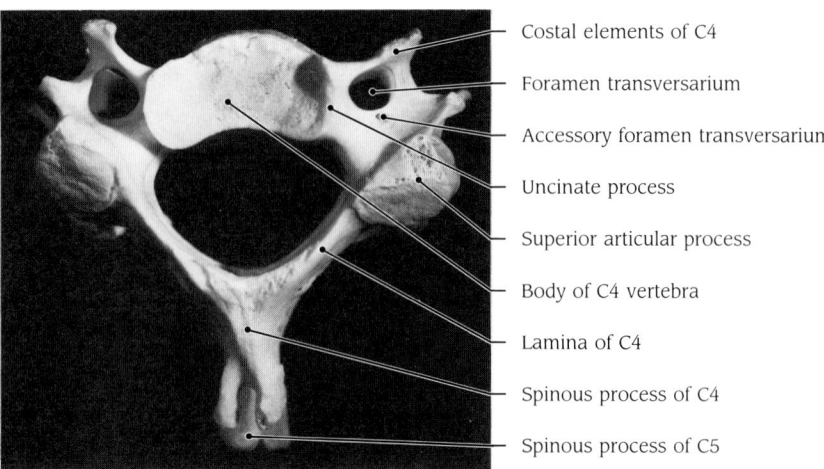

FIG. 7.19. Superior view of C4 and C5 vertebrae.

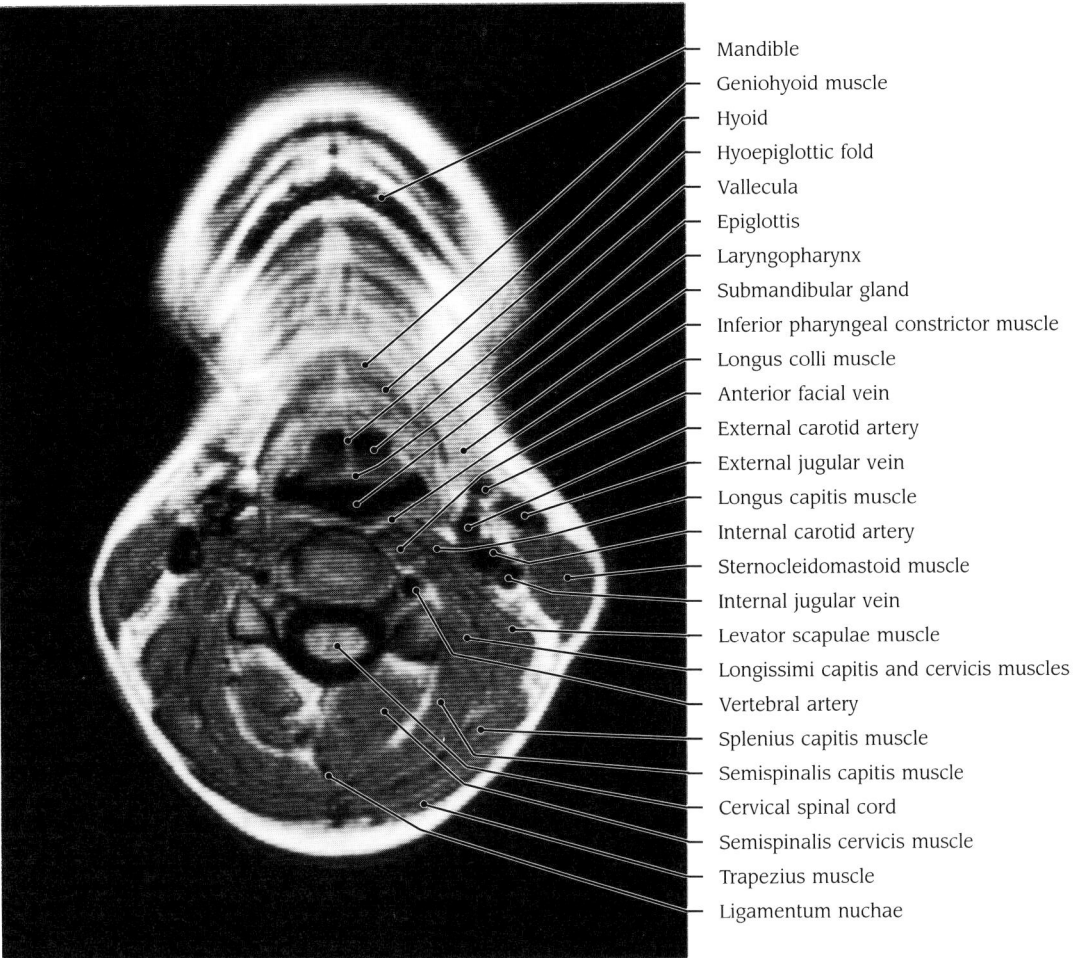

FIG. 7.20. TR = 500 msec, TE = 28 msec.

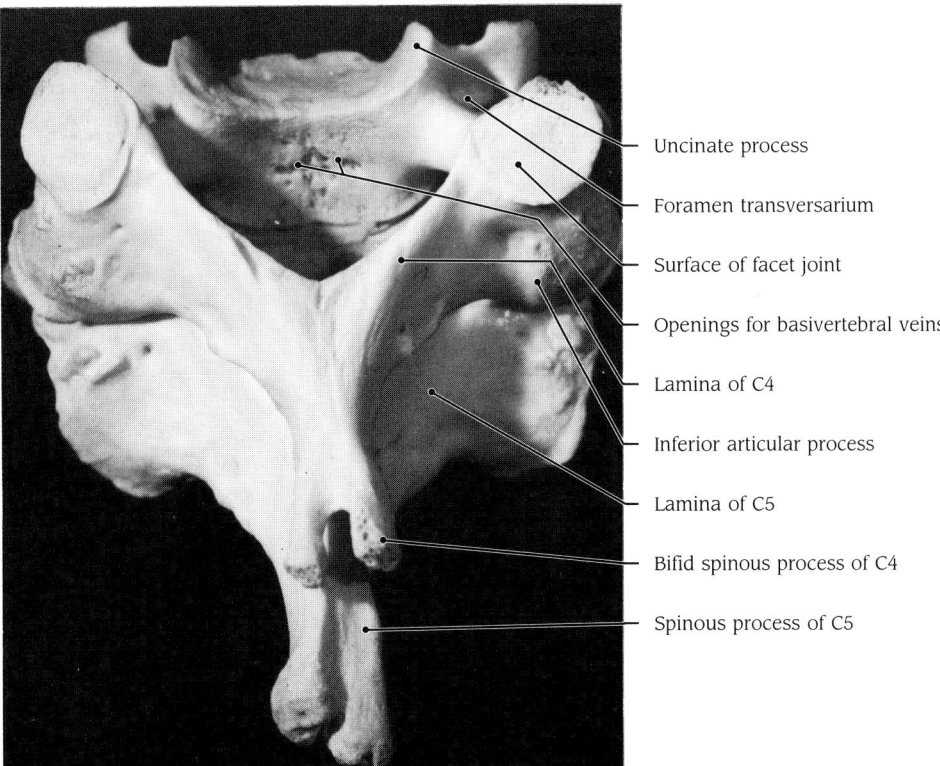

FIG. 7.21. Posterosuperior view of C4 and C5 vertebrae. (From de Groot, J.: Correlative Neuroanatomy of Computed Tomography and Magnetic Resonance Imaging. Philadelphia, Lea & Febiger, 1984.)

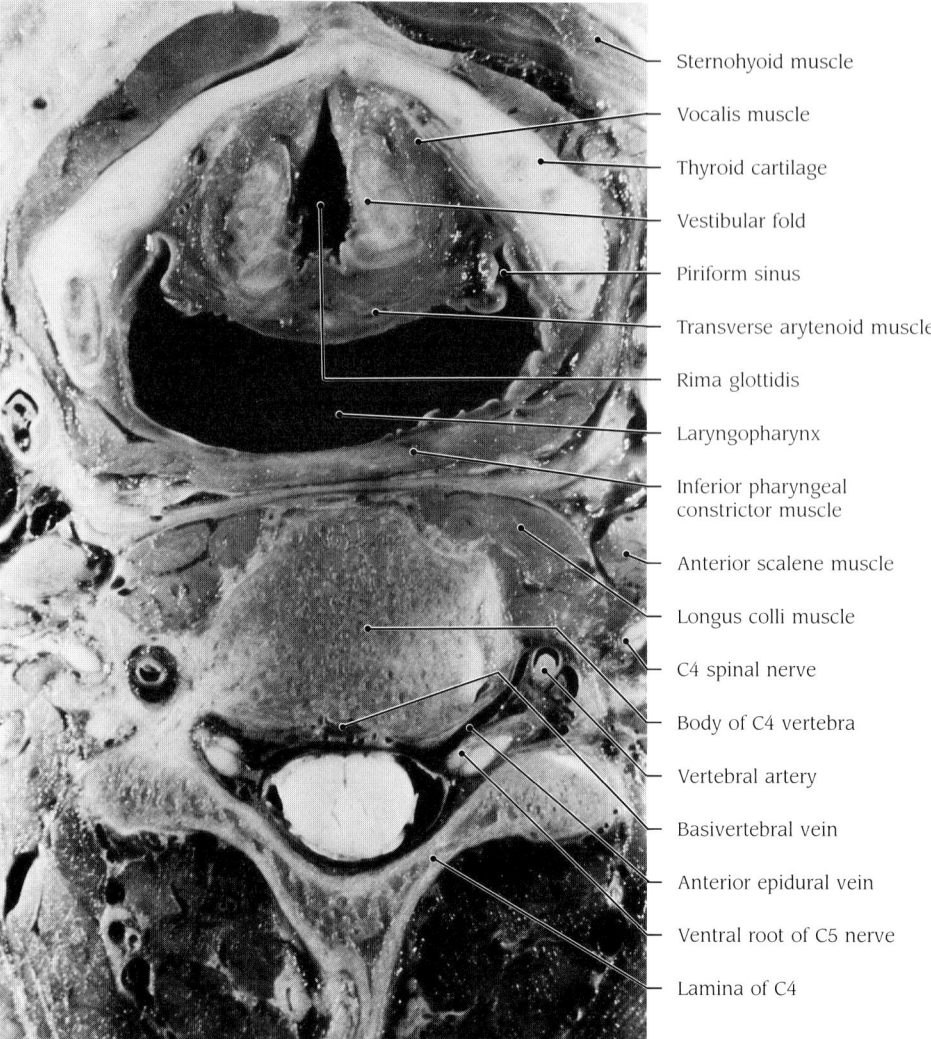

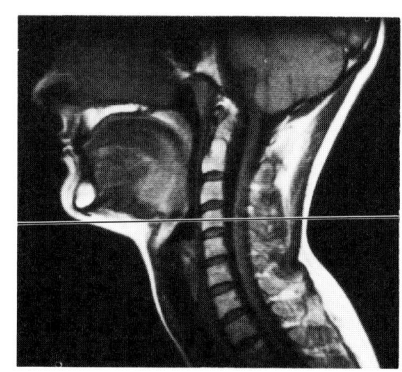

- Sternohyoid muscle
- Vocalis muscle
- Thyroid cartilage
- Vestibular fold
- Piriform sinus
- Transverse arytenoid muscle
- Rima glottidis
- Laryngopharynx
- Inferior pharyngeal constrictor muscle
- Anterior scalene muscle
- Longus colli muscle
- C4 spinal nerve
- Body of C4 vertebra
- Vertebral artery
- Basivertebral vein
- Anterior epidural vein
- Ventral root of C5 nerve
- Lamina of C4

FIG. 7.22.

- The piriform fossae, or sinuses, are small recesses that lie on each side of the laryngeal orifice. They are bordered medially by the aryepiglottic folds and laterally by the thyroid cartilage and the thyrohyoid membrane.

- The longus capitis muscle has a single broad origin at the basilar part of the occipital bone and inserts at the transverse processes of the third, fourth, fifth, and sixth cervical vertebrae. This muscle, which overlies or is lateral to the longus colli muscle, functions as a flexor of the head.

- The longus colli muscle is located anterior to the vertebral column between the atlas and the third thoracic vertebra. This complex muscle has multiple tendinous origins and insertions that are separated into the inferior oblique, the superior oblique, and the vertical parts. The inferior oblique part extends from the anterior aspect of the bodies of the first two or three thoracic vertebrae to the anterior tubercle of the transverse processes of the fifth and sixth cervical vertebrae. The superior oblique part runs from the anterior tubercles of the transverse processes of the third, fourth, and fifth cervical vertebrae to the anterolateral aspect of the tubercle on the anterior arch of the atlas. The vertical part extends from the anterior surface of the fifth, sixth, and seventh cervical vertebrae and the first, second, and third thoracic vertebrae to the anterior aspect of the second, third, and fourth cervical vertebrae. The longus colli muscle functions to flex the neck anteriorly or laterally or to rotate it to the opposite side.

- Superior articular process of C4
- Costal element
- Transverse process
- Facet joint
- Spinous process of C4
- Body of C5
- Inferior articular process of C5

FIG. 7.23. Lateral view of C4 and C5 vertebrae. (From de Groot, J.: Correlative Neuroanatomy of Computed Tomography and Magnetic Resonance Imaging. Philadelphia, Lea & Febiger, 1984.)

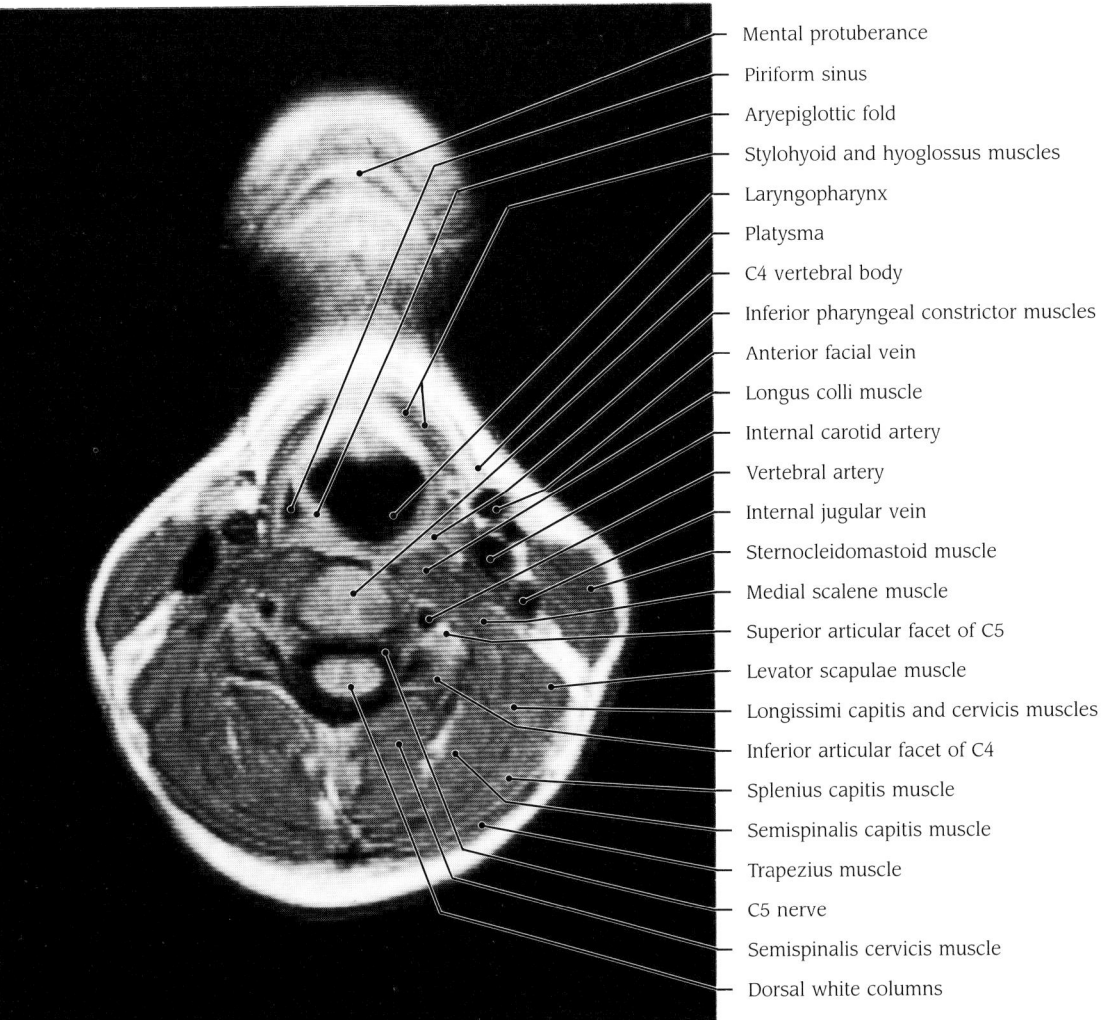

FIG. 7.24. TR = 500 msec, TE = 28 msec.

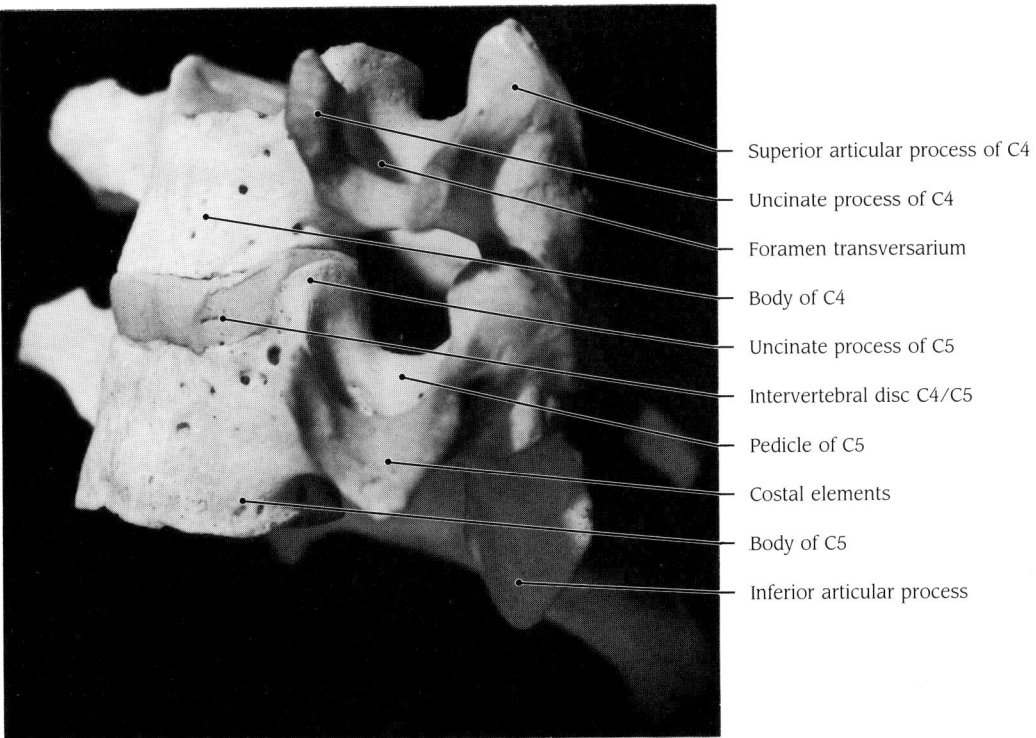

FIG. 7.25. Oblique view of C4 and C5 vertebrae. (From de Groot, J.: Correlative Neuroanatomy of Computed Tomography and Magnetic Resonance Imaging. Philadelphia, Lea & Febiger, 1984.)

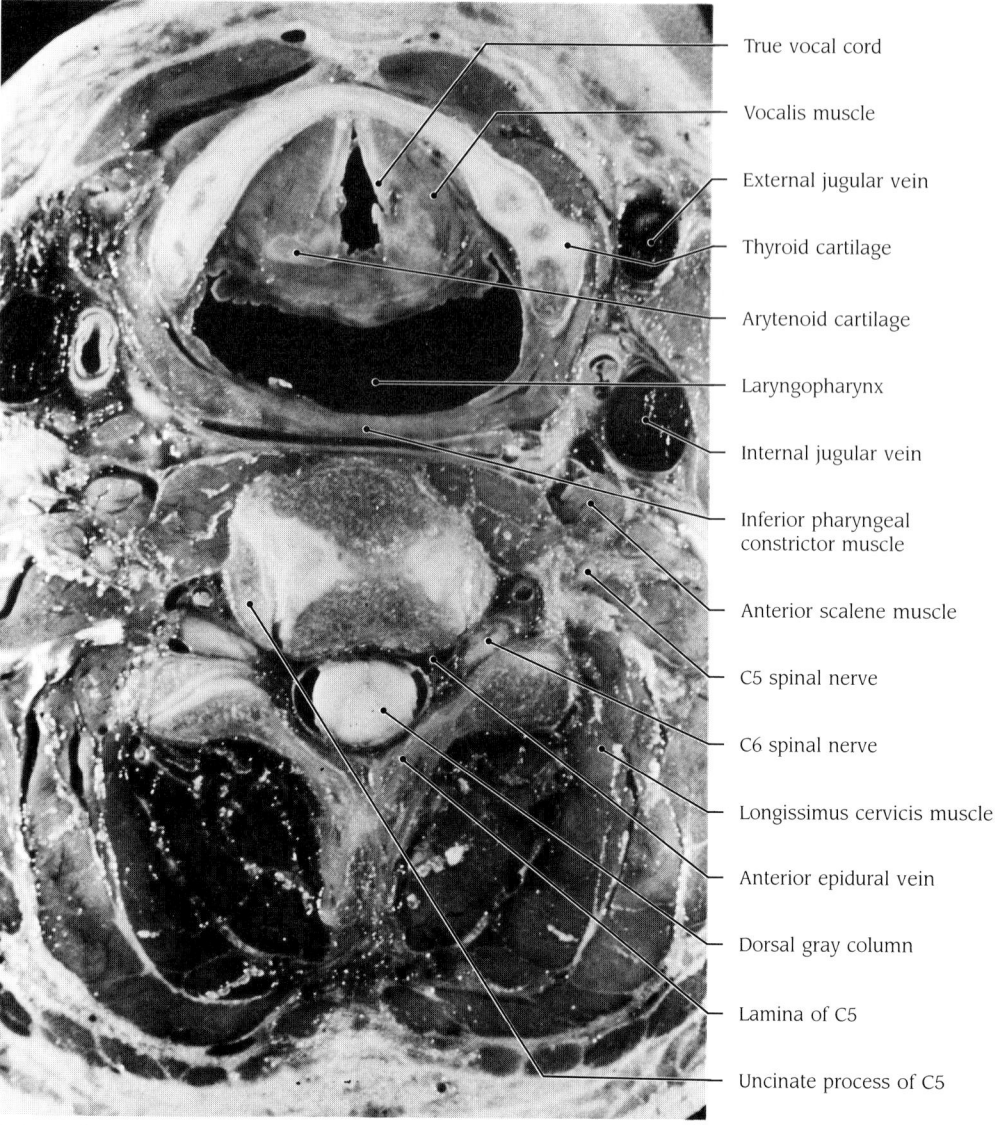

FIG. 7.26.

- The largest cartilage of the larynx is the thyroid cartilage. It is composed of two quadrilateral portions that fuse anteriorly to form the laryngeal prominence, or Adam's apple. The angle of fusion is about 90° in men and about 120° in women. The smaller size of the thyroid angle in men is associated with the larger projection of the laryngeal prominence, the longer vocal fold, and deeper pitch of the voice.
- The white substance of the spinal cord between the posterior median and posterolateral sulci on each side is the posterior funiculus. The posterointermediate sulcus divides the posterior funiculus into two large fiber tracts, the fasciculus gracilis, which is medial, and the fasciculus cuneatus, which is lateral (see Chap. 6).
- The dorsal root ganglia of the fifth, sixth, seventh, and eighth cervical nerves, as well as of the first thoracic nerves, are much larger than the ganglia of the upper cervical nerves. This increase in size reflects the region of origin of the brachial plexus. Similarly, the spinal cord is larger in diameter at the same levels.

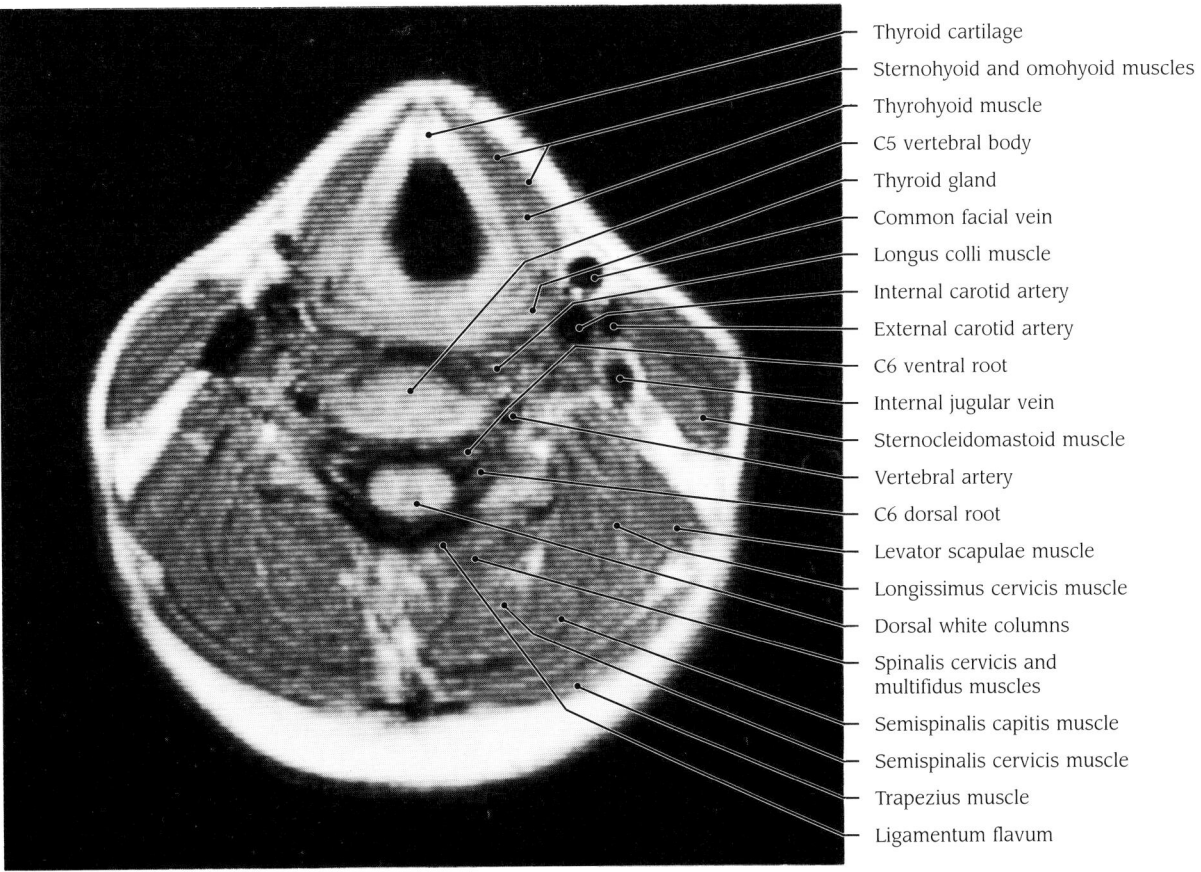

FIG. 7.27. TR = 500 msec, TE = 28 msec.

- Thyroid cartilage
- Sternohyoid and omohyoid muscles
- Thyrohyoid muscle
- C5 vertebral body
- Thyroid gland
- Common facial vein
- Longus colli muscle
- Internal carotid artery
- External carotid artery
- C6 ventral root
- Internal jugular vein
- Sternocleidomastoid muscle
- Vertebral artery
- C6 dorsal root
- Levator scapulae muscle
- Longissimus cervicis muscle
- Dorsal white columns
- Spinalis cervicis and multifidus muscles
- Semispinalis capitis muscle
- Semispinalis cervicis muscle
- Trapezius muscle
- Ligamentum flavum

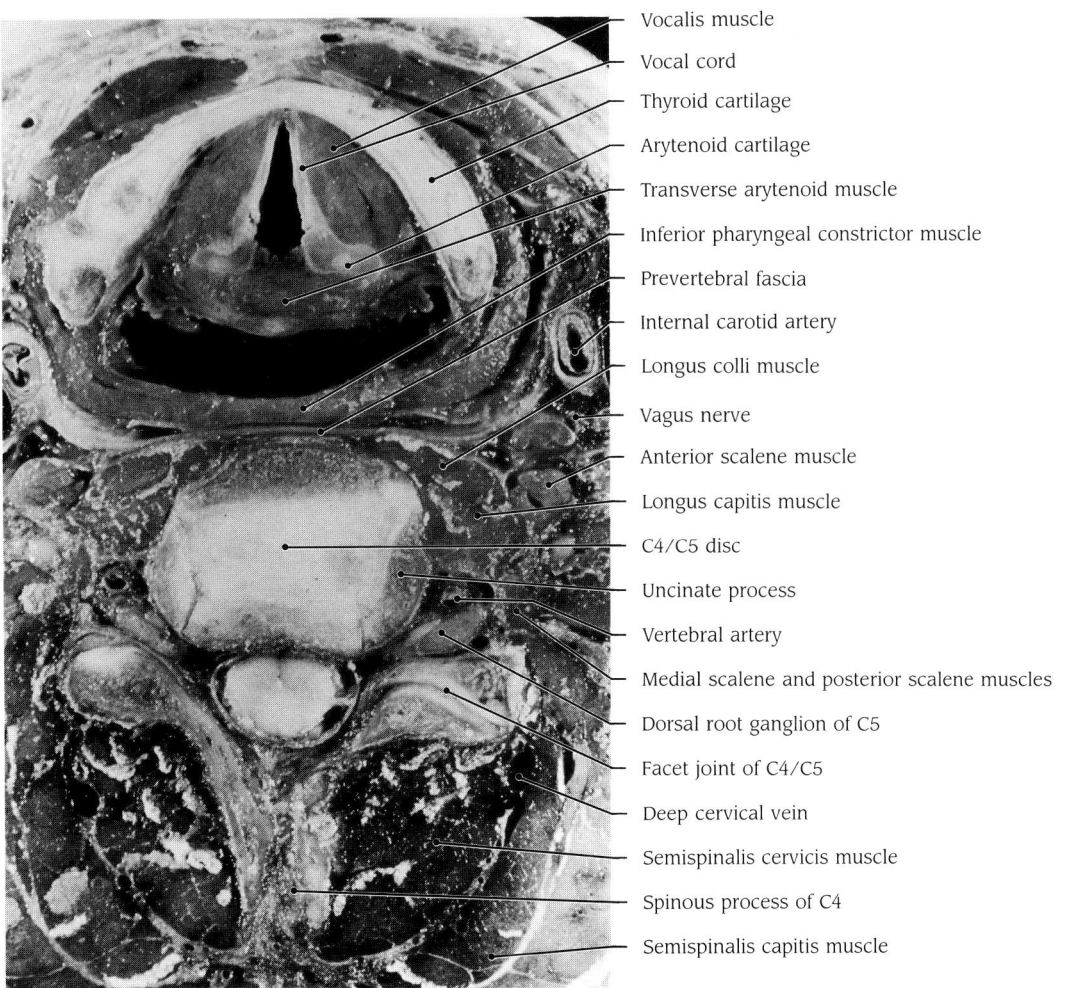

FIG. 7.28.

- Vocalis muscle
- Vocal cord
- Thyroid cartilage
- Arytenoid cartilage
- Transverse arytenoid muscle
- Inferior pharyngeal constrictor muscle
- Prevertebral fascia
- Internal carotid artery
- Longus colli muscle
- Vagus nerve
- Anterior scalene muscle
- Longus capitis muscle
- C4/C5 disc
- Uncinate process
- Vertebral artery
- Medial scalene and posterior scalene muscles
- Dorsal root ganglion of C5
- Facet joint of C4/C5
- Deep cervical vein
- Semispinalis cervicis muscle
- Spinous process of C4
- Semispinalis capitis muscle

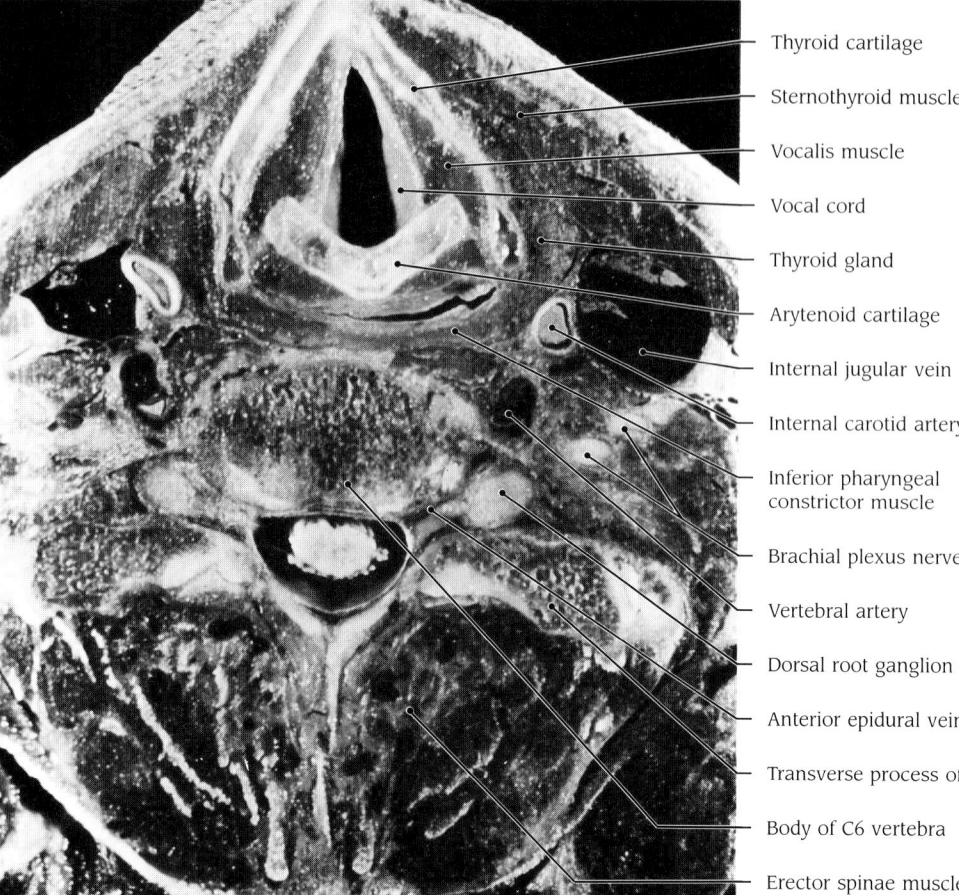

FIG. 7.29.

- The cavity of the larynx extends from the laryngeal inlet, where it communicates with the pharynx, to the inferior edge of the cricoid cartilage, where it is continuous with the trachea. The larynx is divided into three parts by two mucous membrane folds. The superior folds are called the vestibular folds, and the fissure separating them is called the rima vestibuli. The inferior folds are called the vocal folds (sometimes referred to as vocal cords), and the fissure between them is the rima glottidis.

- The upper portion of the larynx, the vestibule, extends from the laryngeal inlet to the vestibular folds.

- The middle part of the laryngeal cavity is the smallest and extends from the rima vestibuli to the rima glottidis. It opens into a fusiform recess between the vestibular and vocal folds into the sinus of the larynx, which communicates anteriorly and superiorly with the saccule of the larynx.

- The lower part of the laryngeal cavity extends from the level of the vocal folds to the inferior border of the cricoid cartilage.

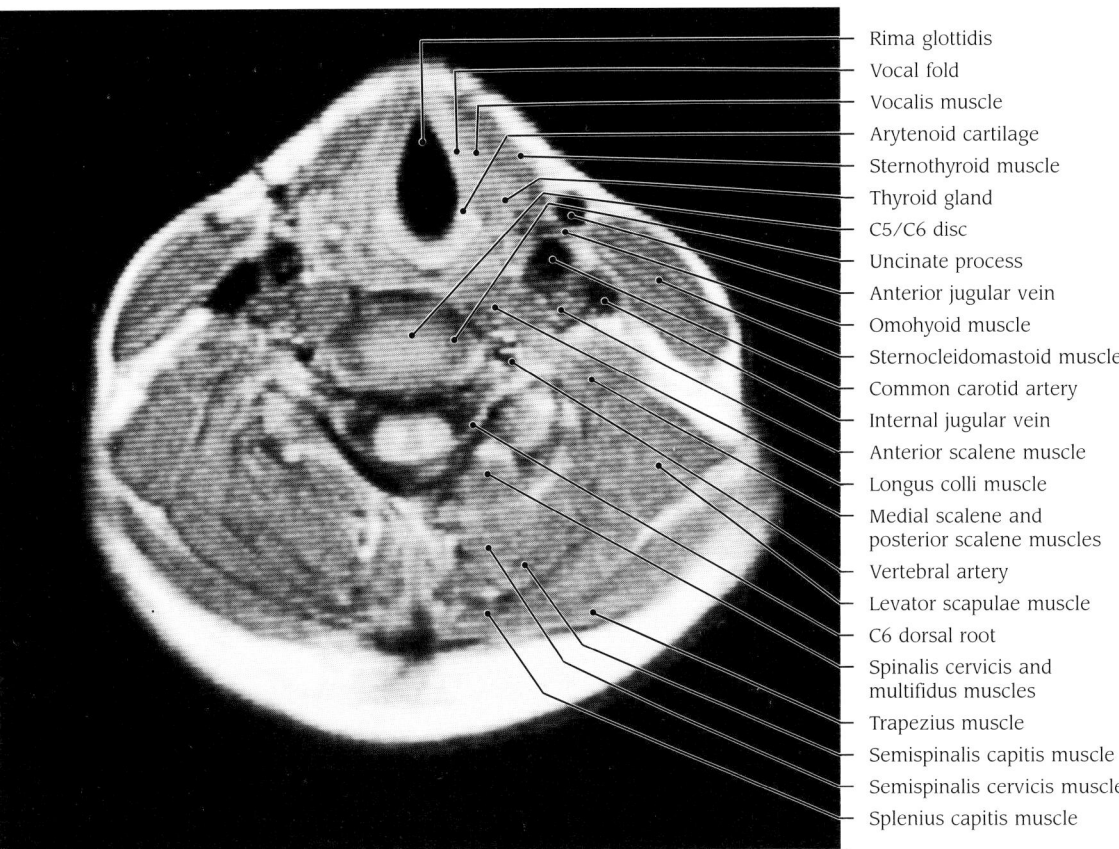

FIG. 7.30. TR = 500 msec, TE = 28 msec.

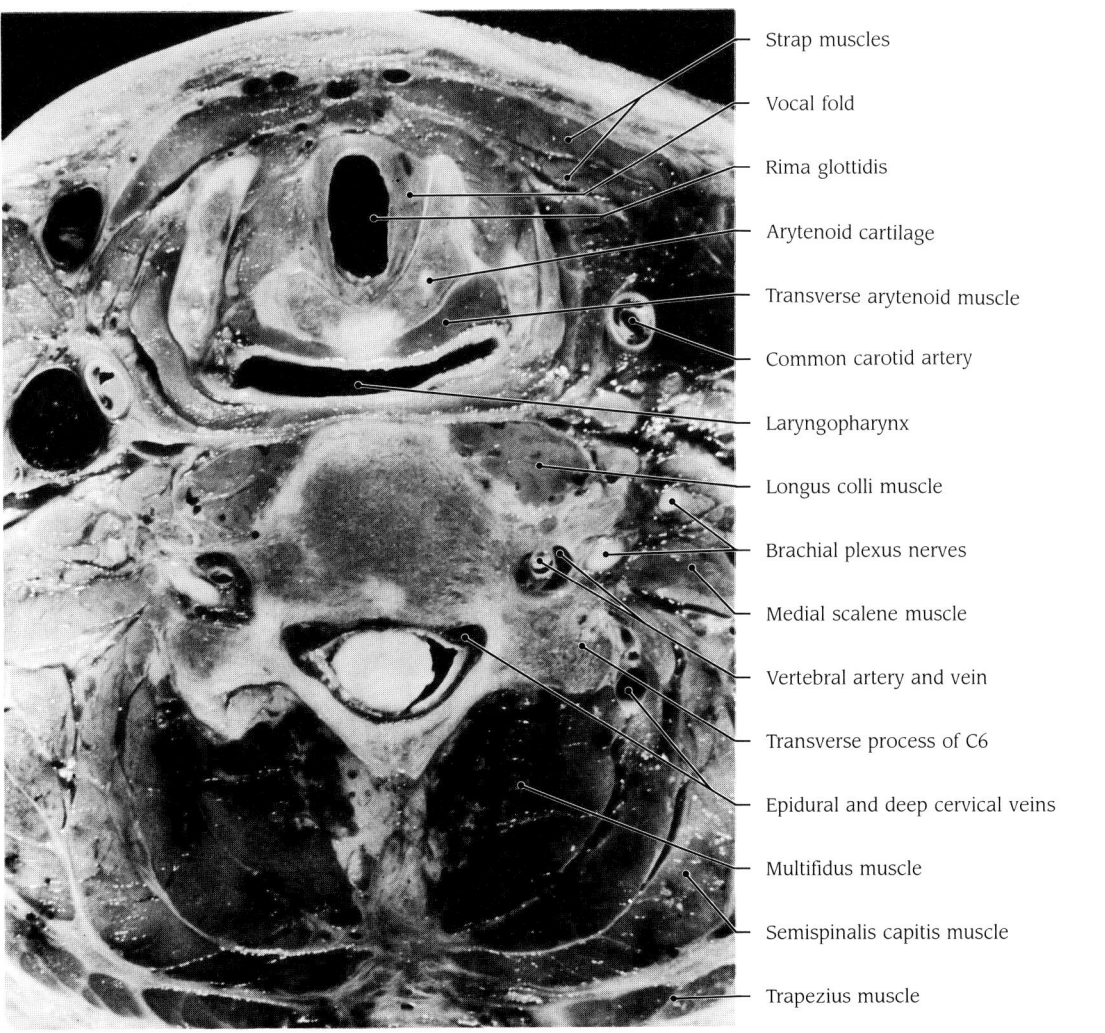

FIG. 7.31.

179

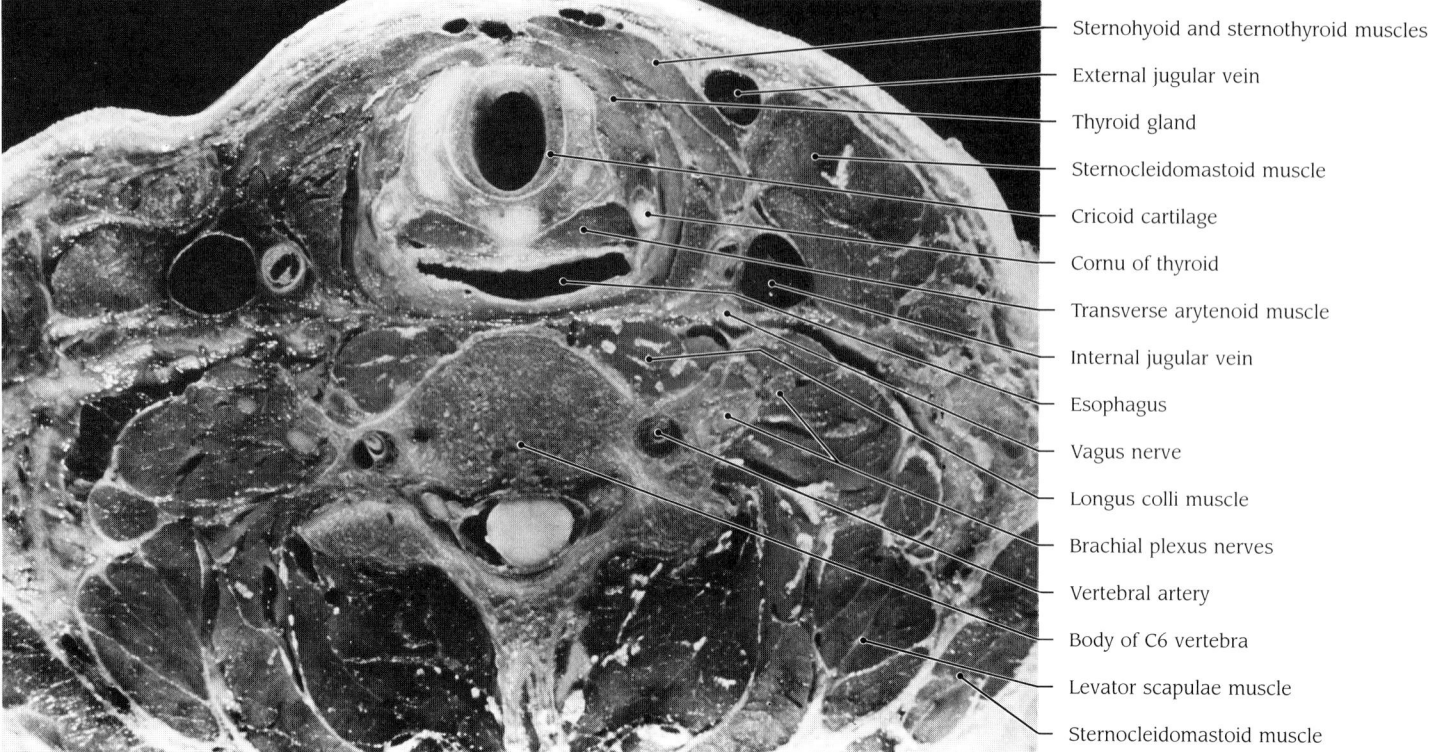

FIG. 7.32.

- Although smaller, the cricoid cartilage is thicker and stronger than the thyroid cartilage. It forms the inferior portion of the anterior and lateral walls and most of the posterior wall of the larynx.

- The lamina of the cricoid cartilage is broad and deep; its vertical dimension is from 2 to 3 cm. The arch of the cricoid is anteriorly narrow, and its vertical dimension measures from 5 to 7 mm. The arch, however, widens posteriorly as it approaches the lamina.

- The superior border of the cricoid cartilage attaches anteriorly to the conus elasticus and laterally to the cricothyroid ligament and the cricoarytenoid ligaments. Posteriorly, the cricoid cartilage articulates with the base of the arytenoid cartilage. The inferior border of the cricoid cartilage is connected to the trachea by the cricotracheal ligament.

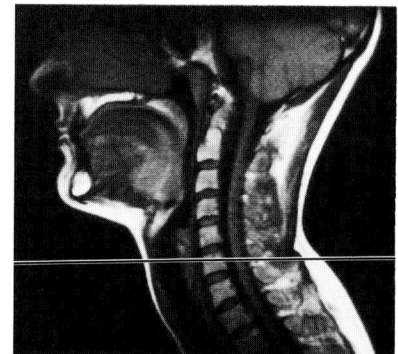

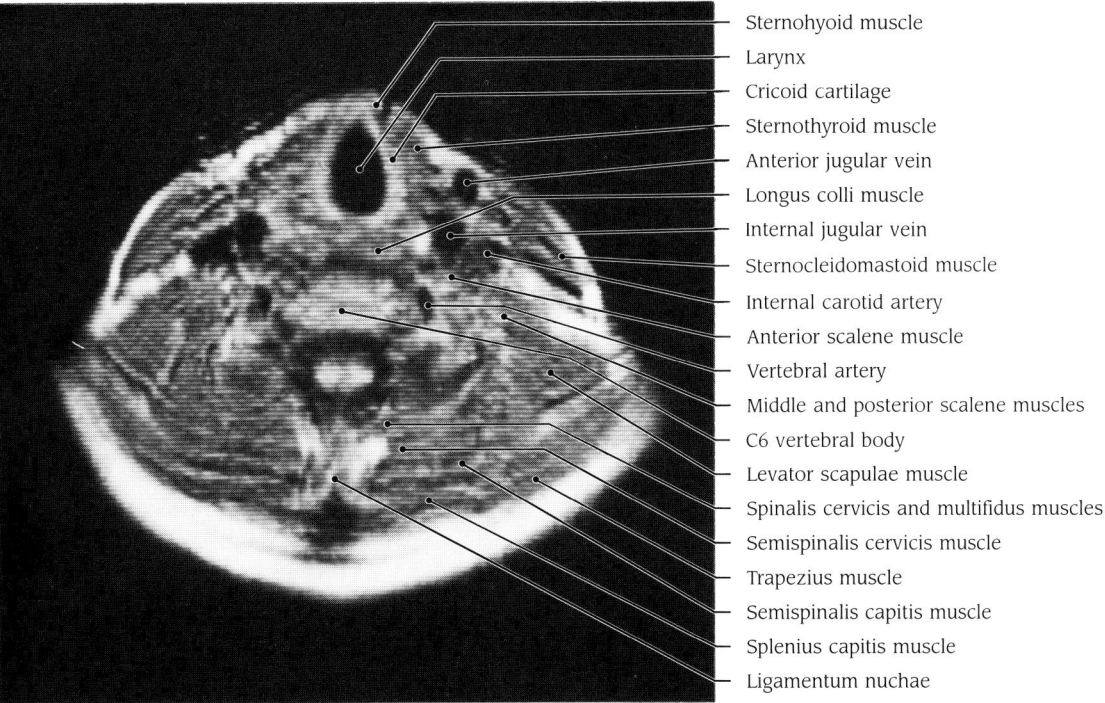

FIG. 7.33. TR = 500 msec, TE = 28 msec.

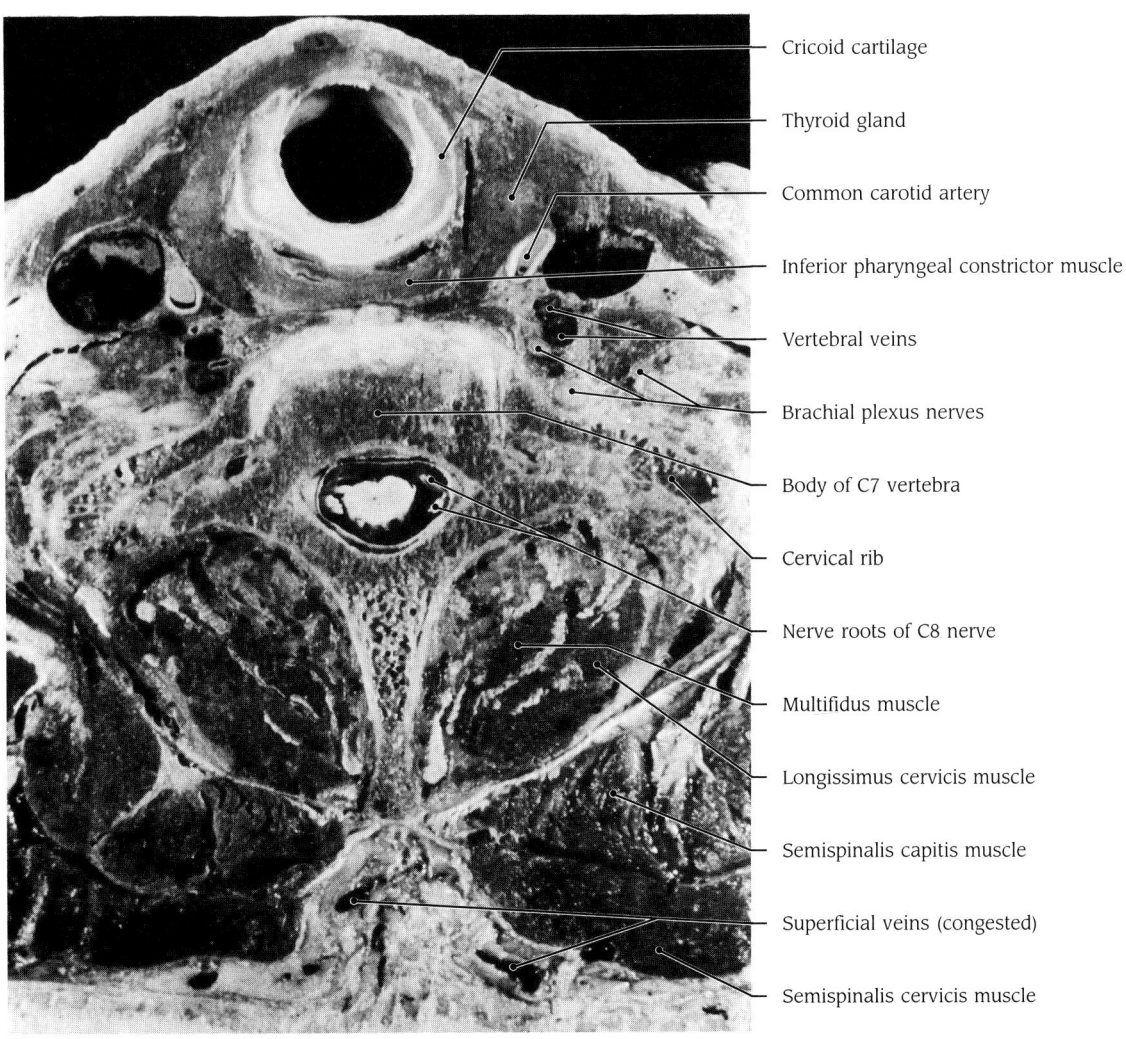

FIG. 7.34.

8
Neck and Cervical Spine, Coronal Plane

Anatomic Level	Figures
Larynx	8.1–8.10
Pharynx, carotid arteries, internal jugular veins	8.8–8.11
Spinal column, vertebral artery	8.11–8.21
Posterior musculature	8.18–8.26

A series of cadaveric coronal sections that extend through the cervical spine and neck is shown. These sections are matched with coronal magnetic resonance images of a volunteer. The magnetic resonance images were obtained with a 500 msec TR to highlight anatomic structures. Magnified anatomic sections are shown at several section planes to enhance detail.

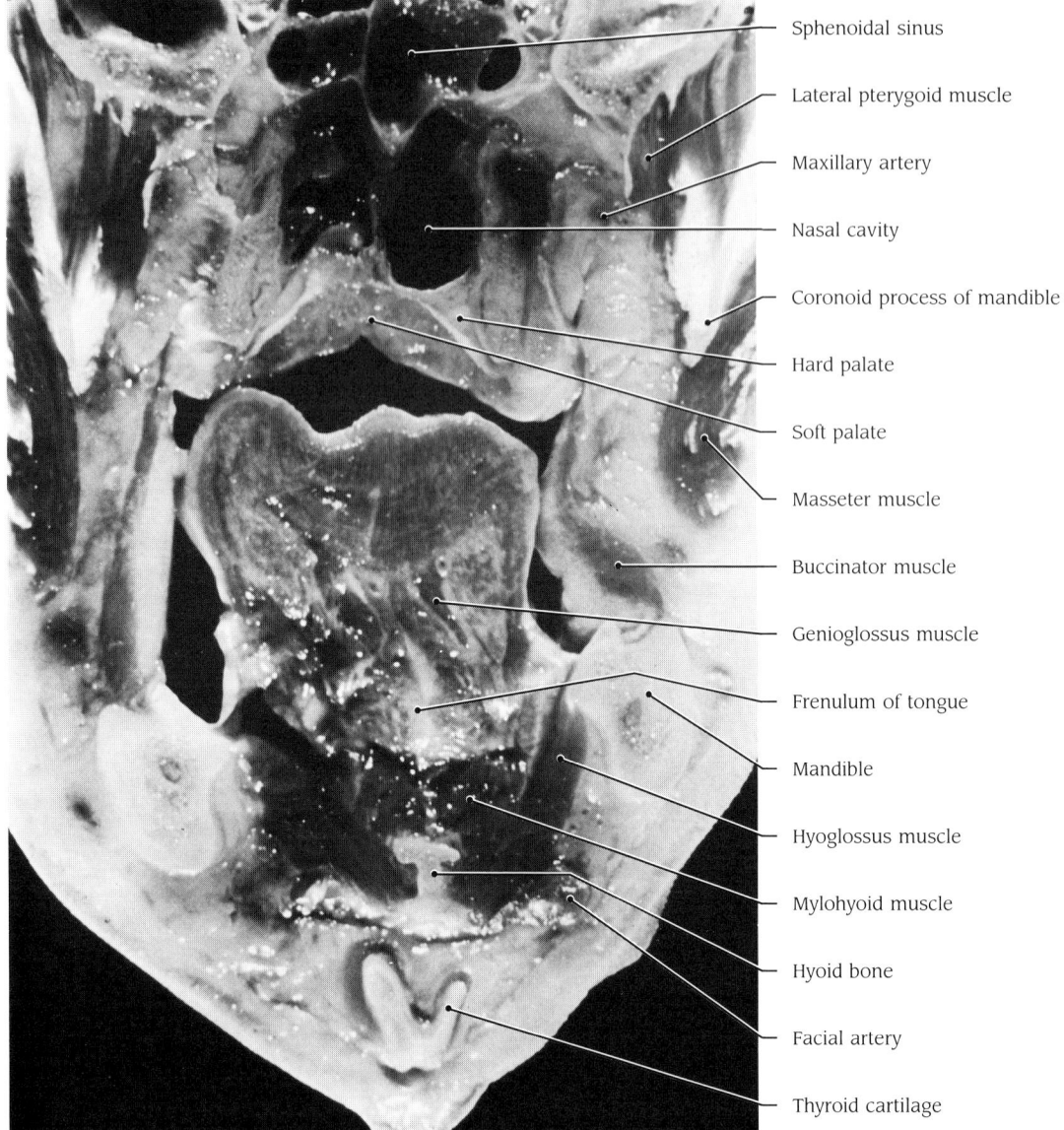

FIG. 8.1.

- The sphenoidal rostrum is a triangular spine that projects from the inferior surface of the sphenoid bone in the median plane. The rostrum is located in a fissure between the anterior portions of the alae of the vomer.

- The movement of the soft palate is vital in deglutition, in speech, and in blowing, acts that necessitate variable degrees of closure of the pharyngeal isthmus. The pharyngeal isthmus is closed when the levator veli palatini muscles pull the soft palate superiorly and posteriorly in the direction of the posterior pharyngeal wall. At the same time, a ridge is formed on the posterior pharyngeal wall by the fibers of the palatopharyngeal sphincter. This ridge meets the nasal surface of the soft palate, thereby closing the isthmus. The isthmus is maximally closed when blowing out through the mouth so that air cannot escape through the nose. Closure of the pharyngeal isthmus during deglutition prevents the passage of food into the nasopharynx. During speech, the closure is greatest for the generation of the explosive consonants, such as *b* or *p*.

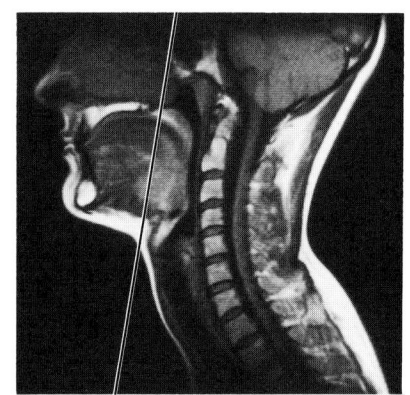

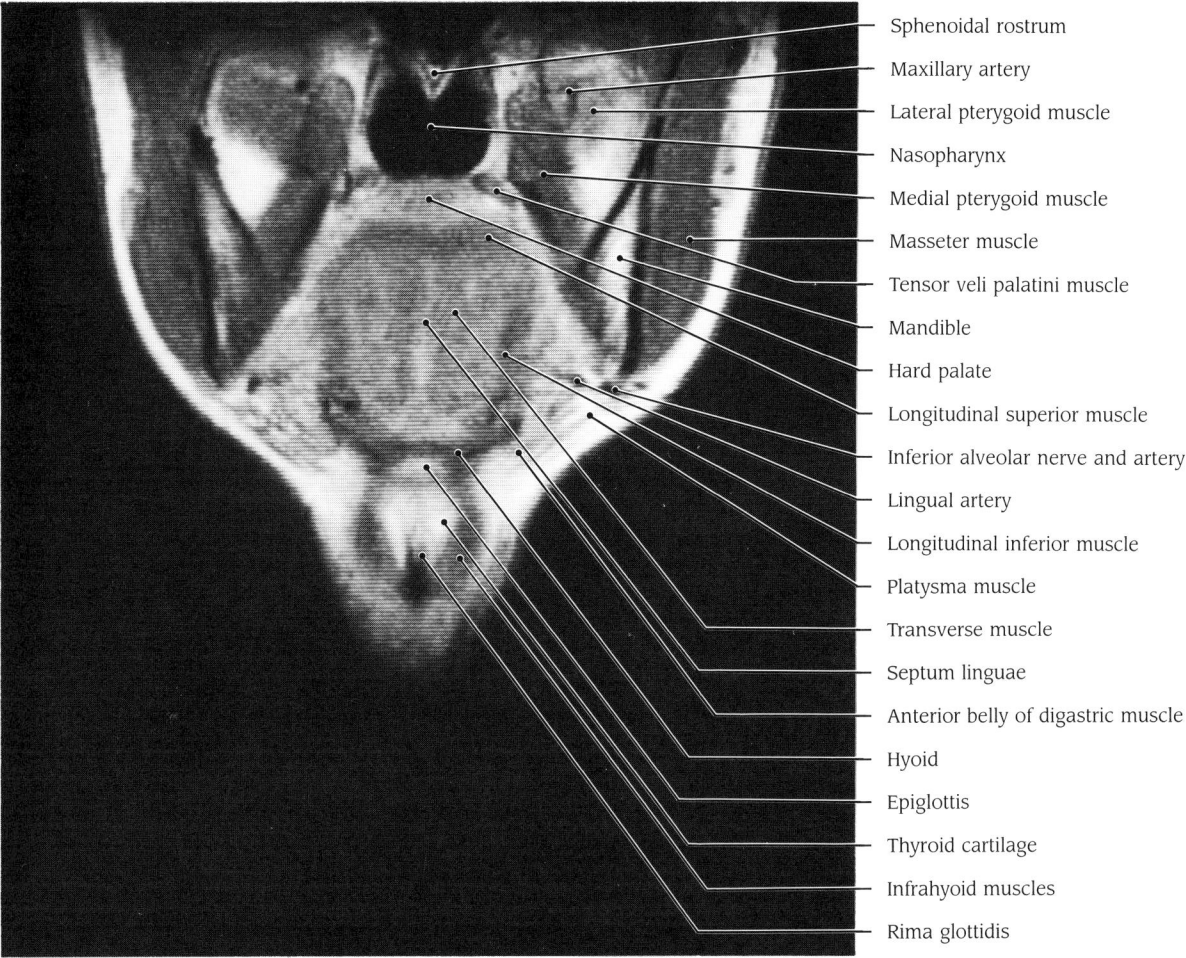

FIG. 8.2. TR = 500 msec, TE = 28 msec.

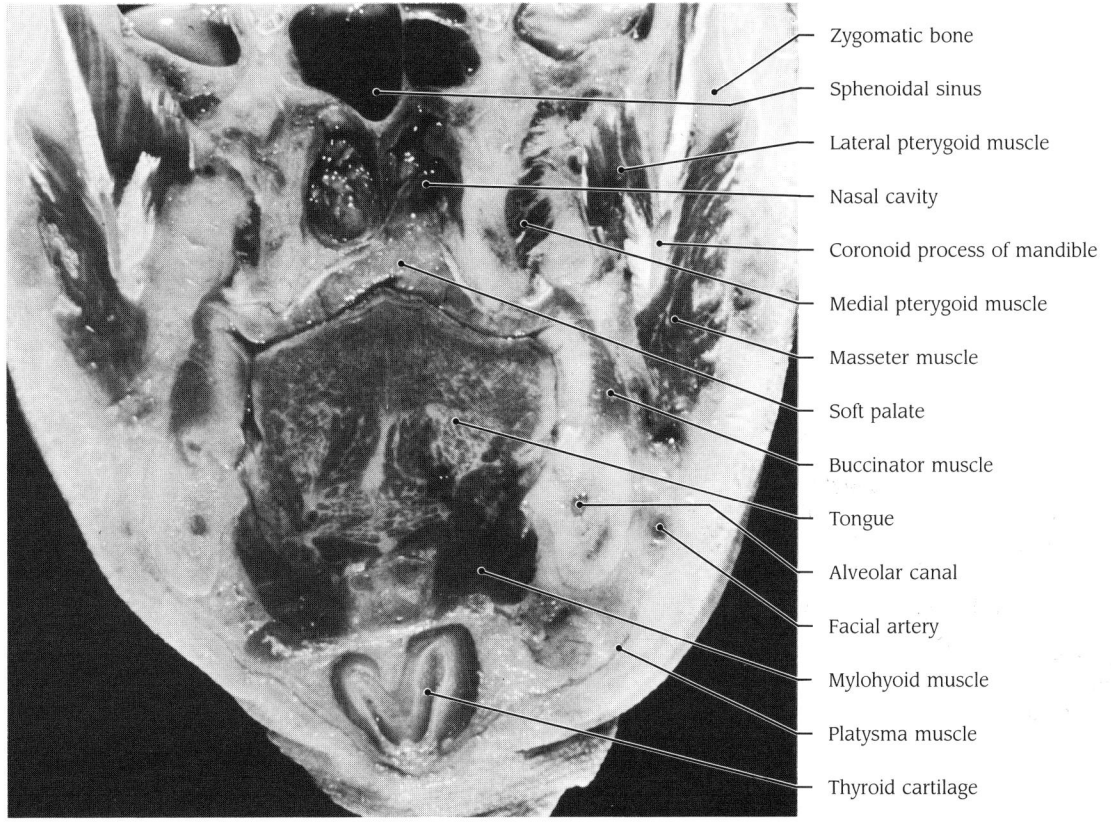

FIG. 8.3.

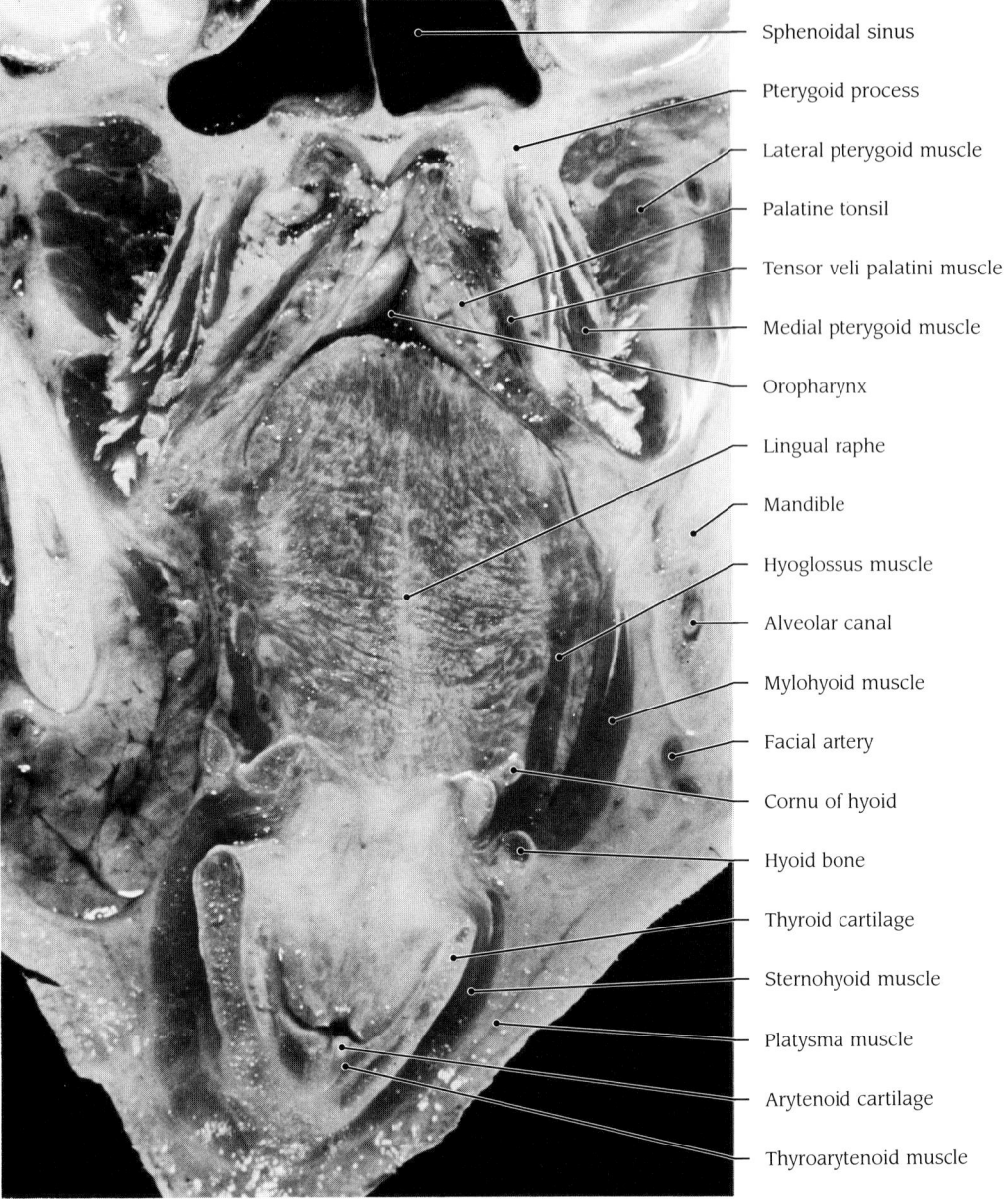

FIG. 8.4.

- The palatine musculature includes a levator and a tensor of the soft palate, the muscle of the uvula, and the muscles underlying the palatoglossal and palatopharyngeal folds, which extend into the palate.

- The levator veli palatini muscle arises from the petrous portion of the temporal bone, the fascia from the tympanic part of the temporal bone, and the auditory tube, and it inserts into the palatine aponeurosis. This muscle elevates the soft palate.

- The epiglottis moves superiorly and anteriorly during deglutition and is squeezed between the base of the tongue and the remainder of the larynx. The bolus of food moves over the posterior surface of the epiglottis and over the closed inlet of the larynx. In man, the epiglottis is not necessary for deglutition, respiration, or phonation.

- The nasopharynx communicates anteriorly with the nasal cavity via the posterior apertures of the nose (choanae). The nasopharynx and oropharynx communicate through an opening called the pharyngeal isthmus. The lateral aspect of the nasopharynx communicates with the pharyngeal opening of the auditory (eustachian) tube.

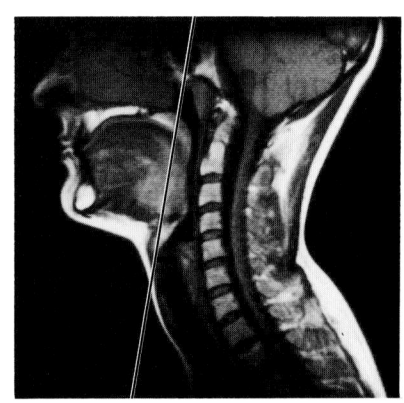

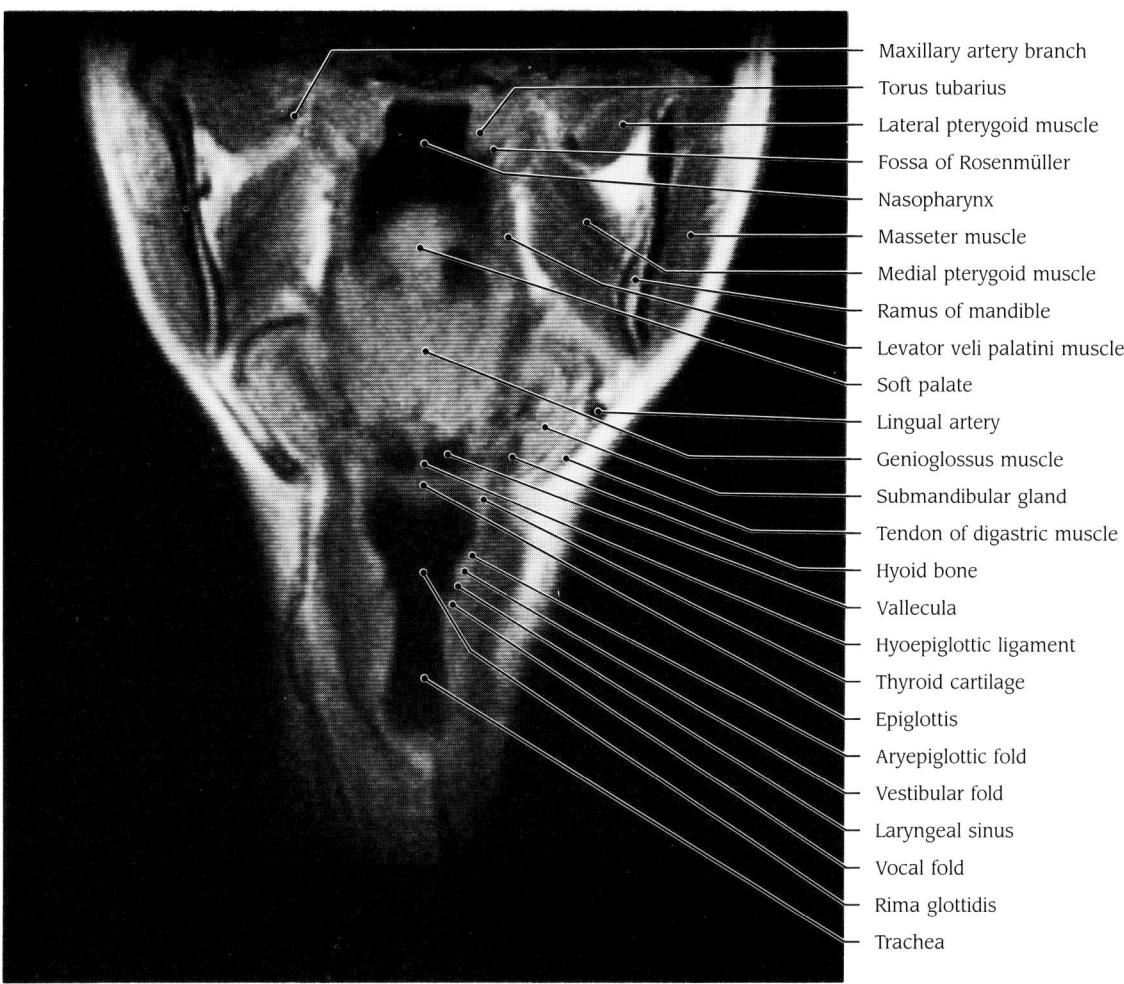

FIG. 8.5. TR = 500 msec, TE = 28 msec.

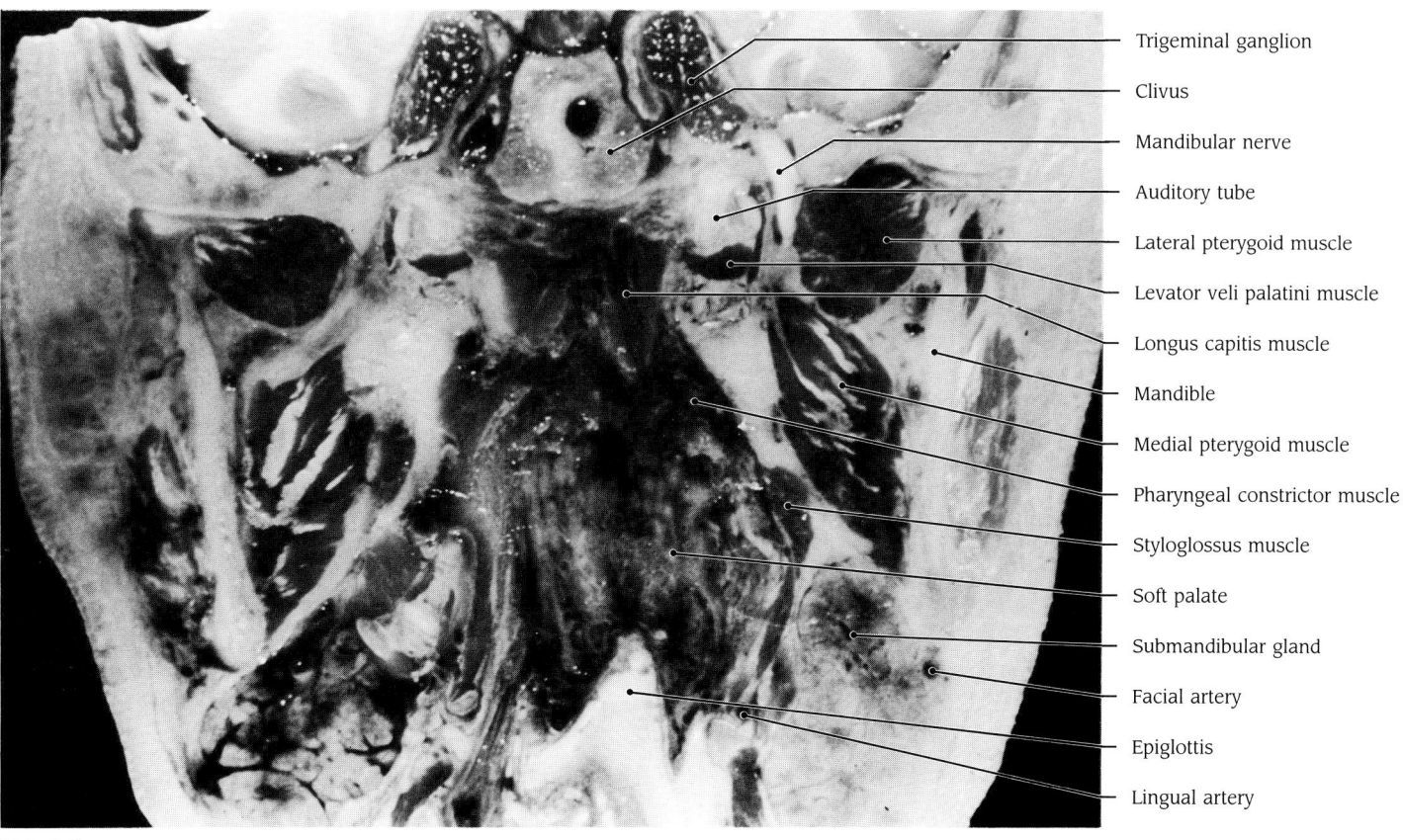

FIG. 8.6.

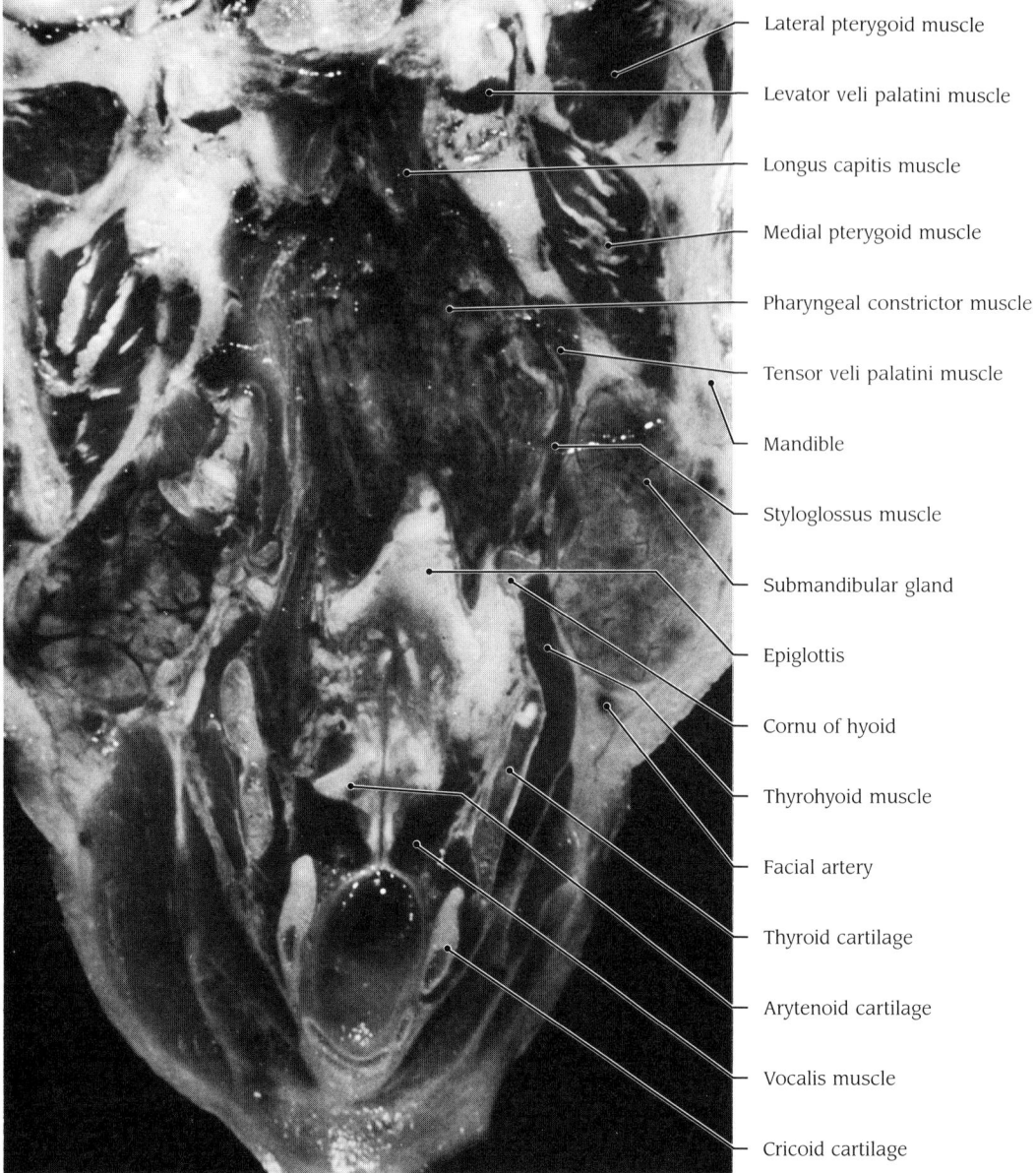

FIG. 8.7.

- The pyriform fossa is a small recess that lies on each side of the laryngeal orifice and is medially bounded by the aryepiglottic fold and laterally bounded by the thyroid cartilage and the thyrohyoid membrane.

- The arytenoid cartilages lie on the lateral part of the superior border of the lamina of the cricoid cartilage in the posterior larynx. These paired structures are pyramidal.

- The aryepiglottic folds connect the sides of the epiglottis to the arytenoid cartilages. The thyroepiglottic ligament connects the epiglottis to the angle formed by the two lamina of the thyroid cartilage.

- The parotid gland is drained by the parotid duct (Stensen's duct), which crosses the masseter muscle, then turns medially, piercing both the adipose tissue of the cheek and the buccinator muscle, and terminates opposite the second upper molar tooth at a small papilla.

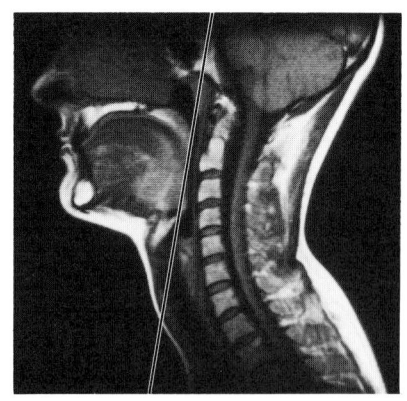

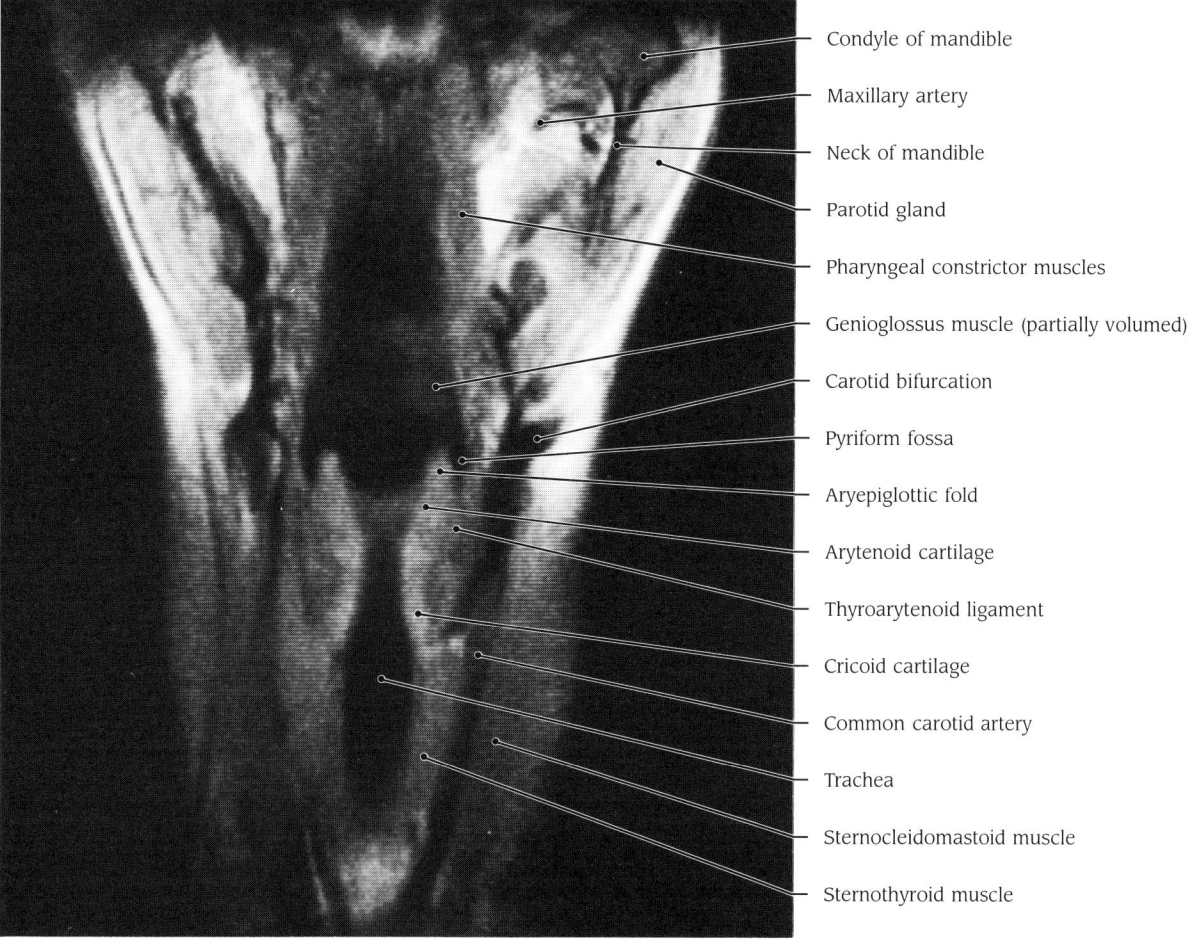

FIG. 8.8. TR = 500 msec, TE = 28 msec.

- Condyle of mandible
- Maxillary artery
- Neck of mandible
- Parotid gland
- Pharyngeal constrictor muscles
- Genioglossus muscle (partially volumed)
- Carotid bifurcation
- Pyriform fossa
- Aryepiglottic fold
- Arytenoid cartilage
- Thyroarytenoid ligament
- Cricoid cartilage
- Common carotid artery
- Trachea
- Sternocleidomastoid muscle
- Sternothyroid muscle

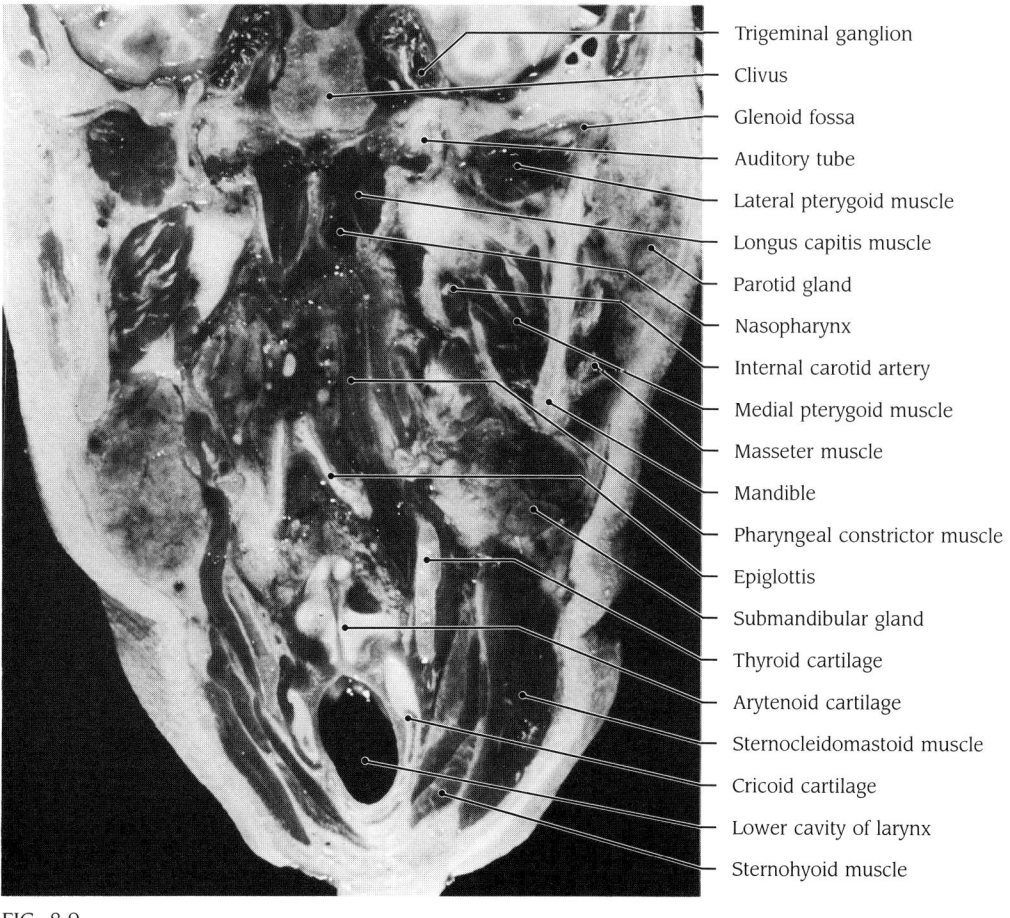

FIG. 8.9.

- Trigeminal ganglion
- Clivus
- Glenoid fossa
- Auditory tube
- Lateral pterygoid muscle
- Longus capitis muscle
- Parotid gland
- Nasopharynx
- Internal carotid artery
- Medial pterygoid muscle
- Masseter muscle
- Mandible
- Pharyngeal constrictor muscle
- Epiglottis
- Submandibular gland
- Thyroid cartilage
- Arytenoid cartilage
- Sternocleidomastoid muscle
- Cricoid cartilage
- Lower cavity of larynx
- Sternohyoid muscle

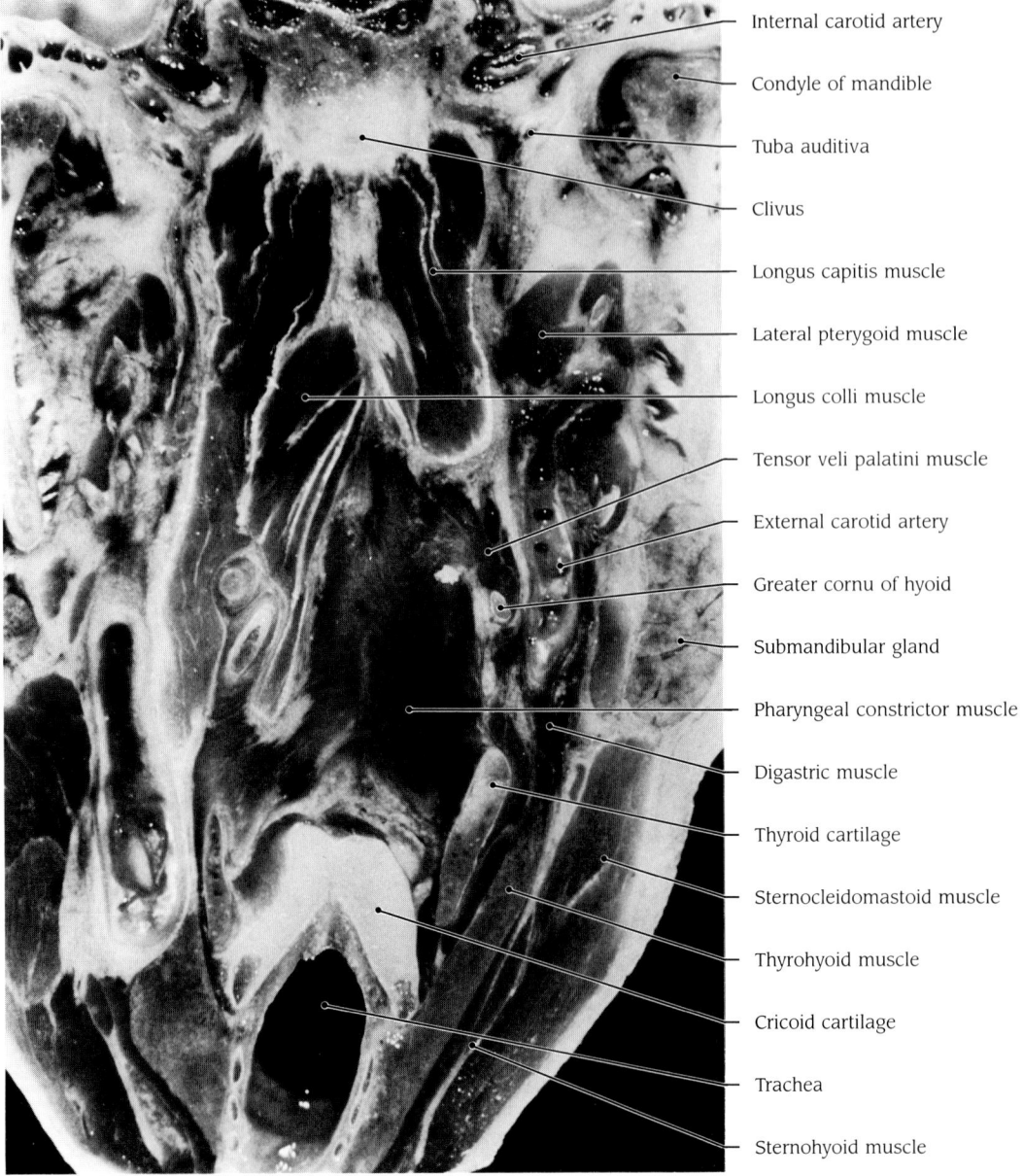

FIG. 8.10.

- The lateral masses of C1 are connected anteriorly by a short anterior arch and posteriorly by a longer posterior arch. The anterior tubercle of the anterior arch of the atlas serves as the point of attachment for the anterior longitudinal ligament and the superior oblique part of the longus colli muscle.
- The sternocleidomastoid muscle divides the neck into anterior and posterior triangles. The anterior triangle is delimited by the median line of the neck, the anterior margin of the sternocleidomastoid, the base of the mandible, and the sternum. The posterior triangle of the neck is bounded by the posterior border of the sternocleidomastoid muscle, the middle one third of the clavicle, and the anterior margin of the trapezius.
- The sinuous course of the internal carotid artery in the neck is contrasted with the almost linear course of the internal jugular vein as shown here.

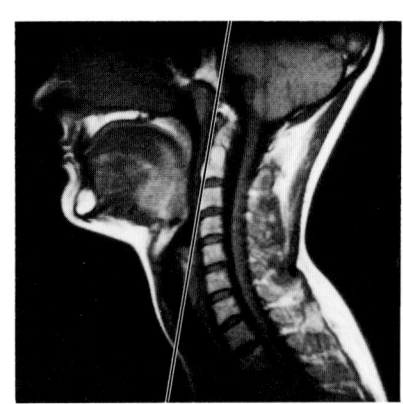

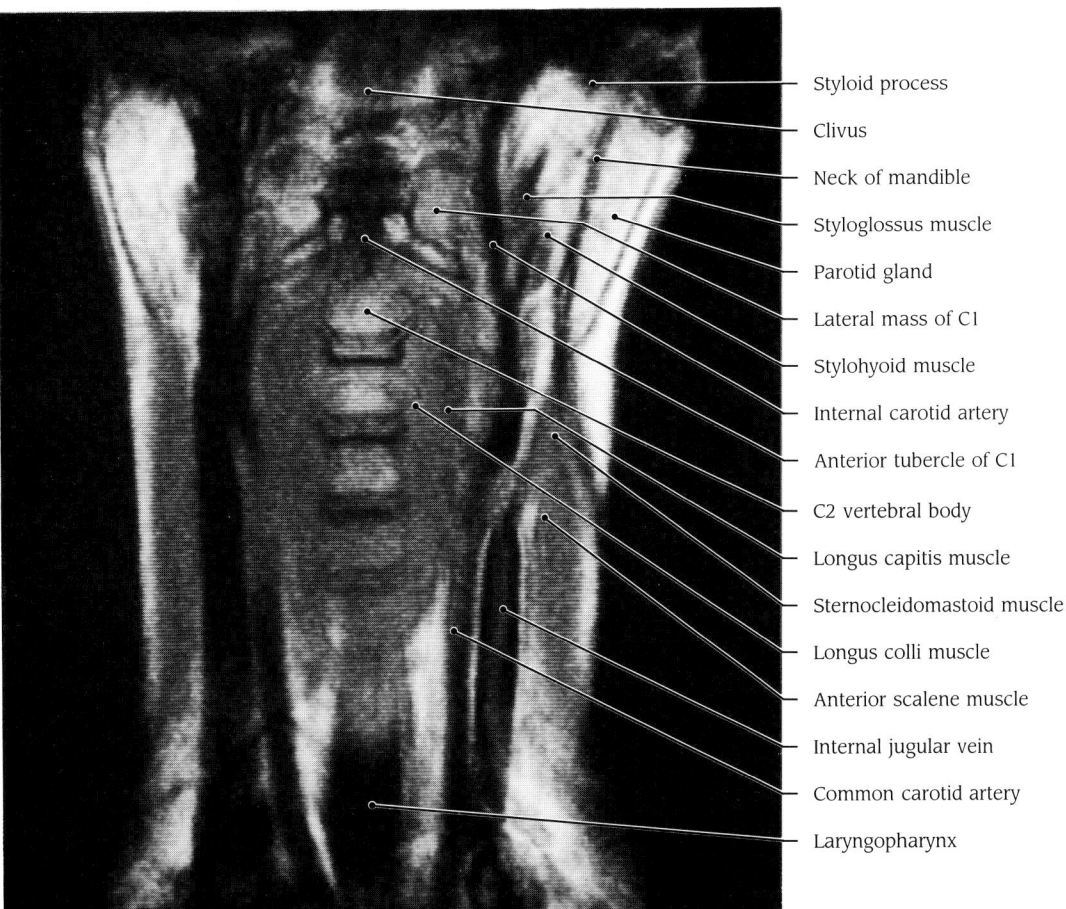

FIG. 8.11. TR = 500 msec, TE = 28 msec.

- Styloid process
- Clivus
- Neck of mandible
- Styloglossus muscle
- Parotid gland
- Lateral mass of C1
- Stylohyoid muscle
- Internal carotid artery
- Anterior tubercle of C1
- C2 vertebral body
- Longus capitis muscle
- Sternocleidomastoid muscle
- Longus colli muscle
- Anterior scalene muscle
- Internal jugular vein
- Common carotid artery
- Laryngopharynx

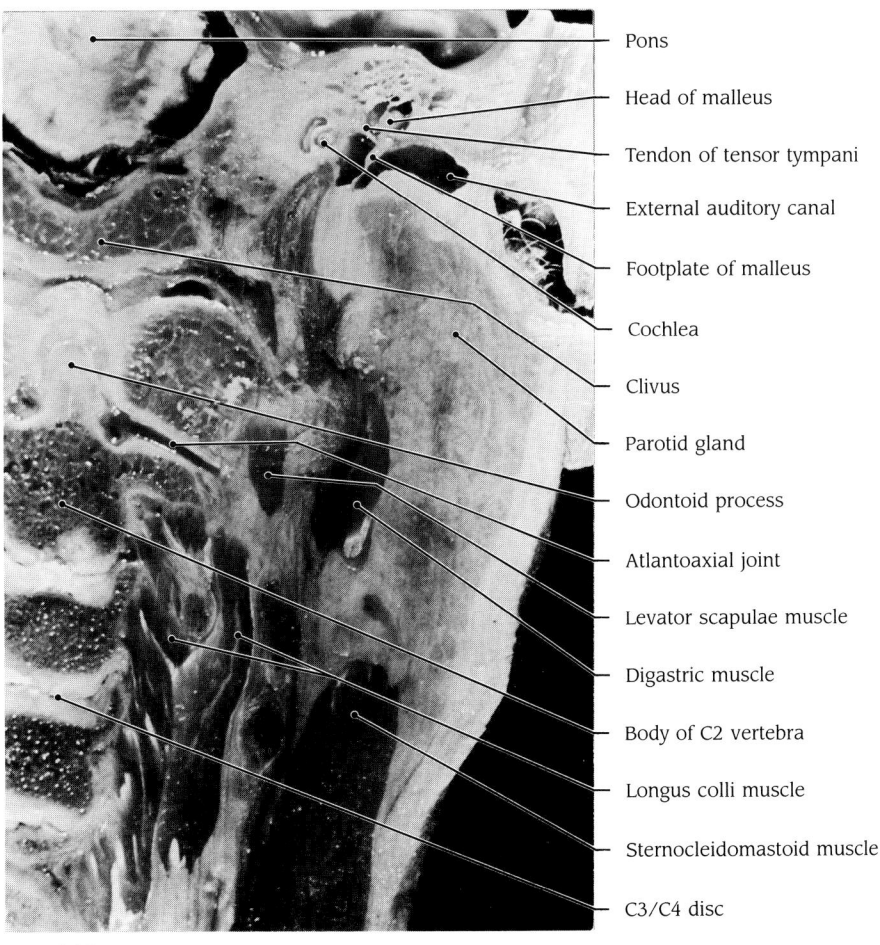

FIG. 8.12.

- Pons
- Head of malleus
- Tendon of tensor tympani
- External auditory canal
- Footplate of malleus
- Cochlea
- Clivus
- Parotid gland
- Odontoid process
- Atlantoaxial joint
- Levator scapulae muscle
- Digastric muscle
- Body of C2 vertebra
- Longus colli muscle
- Sternocleidomastoid muscle
- C3/C4 disc

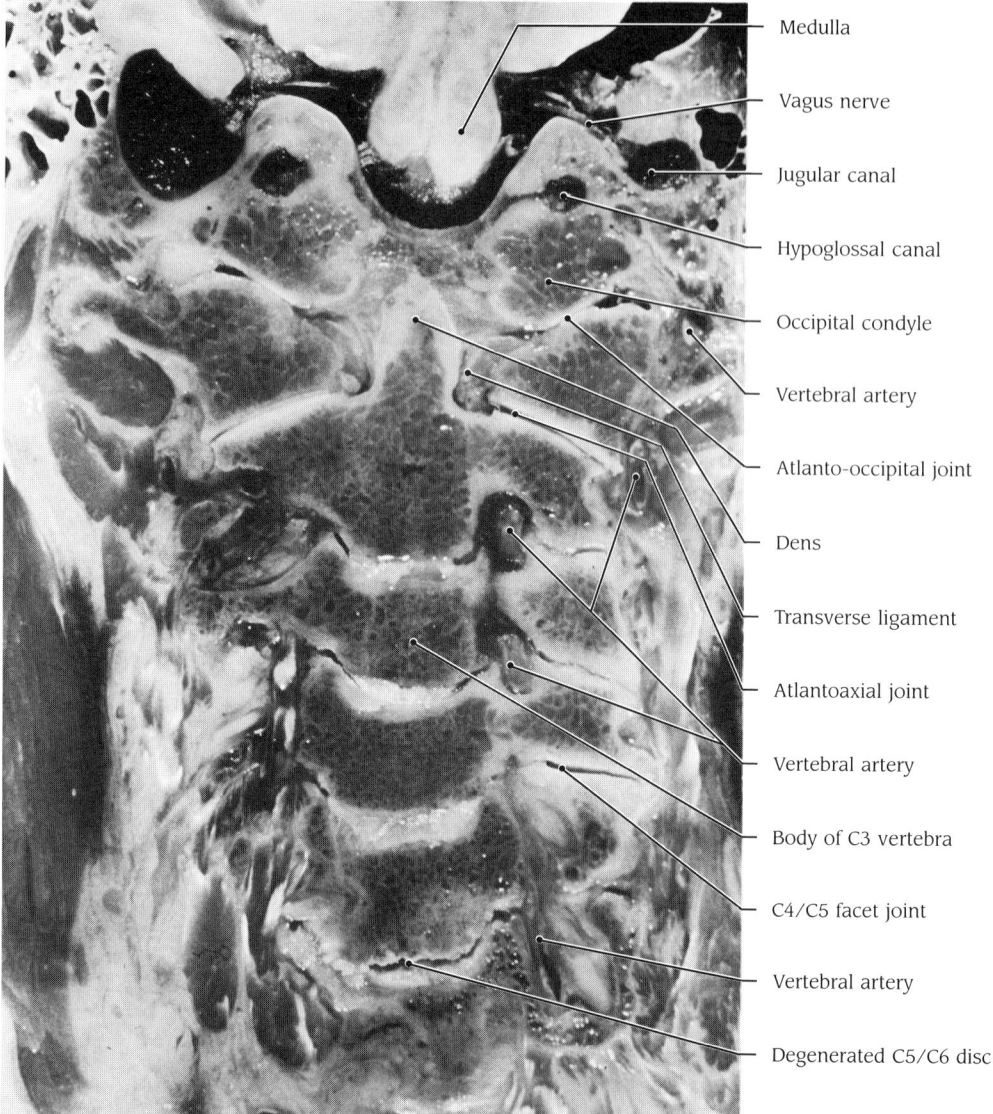

FIG. 8.13.

- The vertebral artery may be divided into four parts. The first segment extends from its origin to its point of entrance into the foramen of the transverse process of a cervical vertebra, usually the sixth. The second segment ascends through the foramina of the first six cervical vertebrae in a vertical course as far as the transverse process of the axis, through which it runs upward and laterally to the transverse foramen of the atlas. The lateral course of the artery is caused by the unusually long transverse process of C1. The third segment extends from the transverse foramen of the atlas, posteromedially behind the lateral mass of the atlas, in a groove on the upper surface of the posterior arch of the atlas. The artery then enters the vertebral canal by turning cephalad and piercing the posterior atlanto-occipital membrane. The fourth segment (not seen here) pierces the dura at the level of the rootlets of the C1 nerve, then ascends in front of the hypoglossal nerve, and terminates at the junction with the opposite vertebral artery to form the basilar artery.

- The lateral masses of C1 are interposed between the atlanto-occipital articulation and the atlantoaxial articulation. In this plane, the orientation of the atlantoaxial joint is approximately 30° from superomedial to inferolateral; in contrast, the atlanto-occipital joint is approximately 40° from inferomedial to superolateral.

- The superior surface of the lateral mass of C1 is concave for articulation with the occipital condyle. The inferior surface of each lateral mass is flat or minimally concave for articulation with the superior articular facet of the axis. The articular cartilage covering the cortical bone of the inferior surface is biconvex.

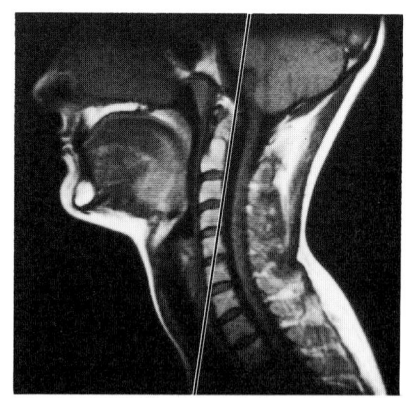

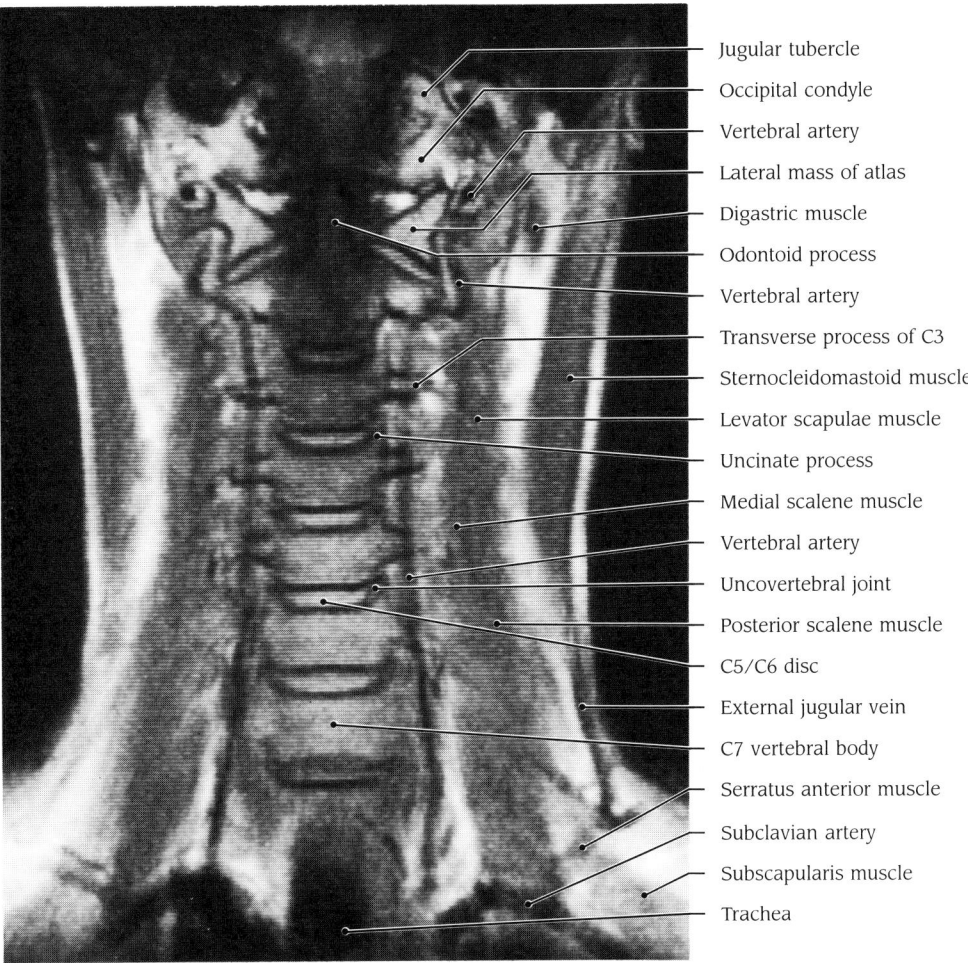

FIG. 8.14. TR = 500 msec, TE = 28 msec.

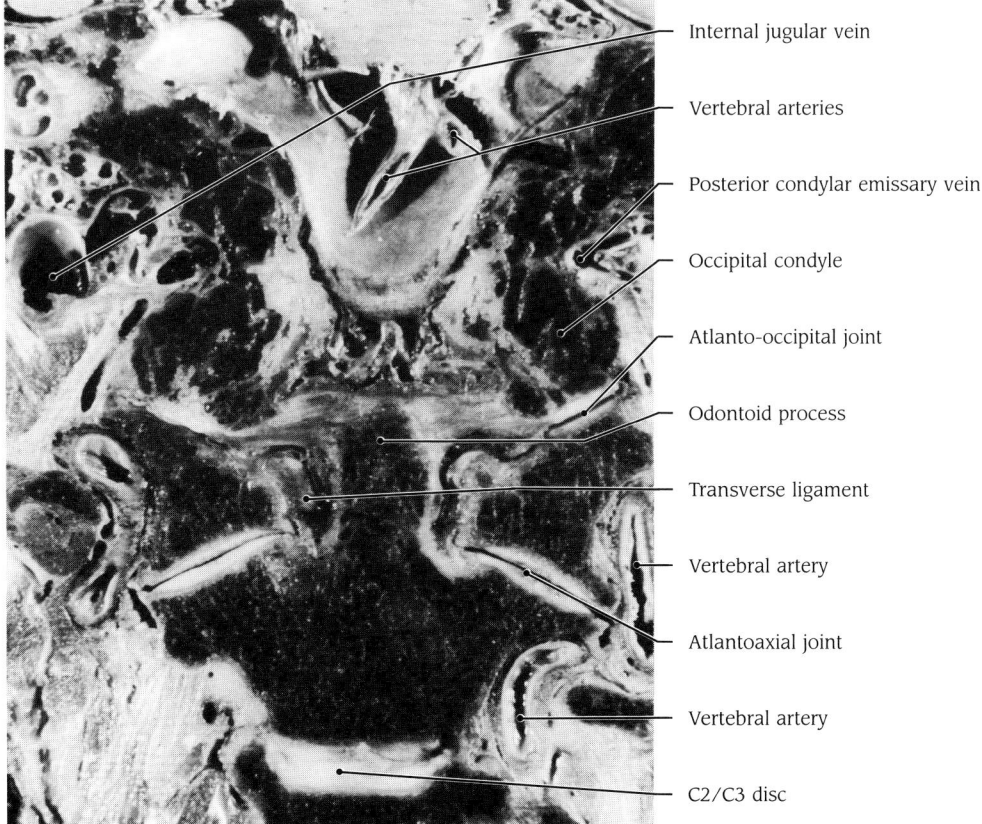

FIG. 8.15. From de Groot, J.: Correlative Neuroanatomy of Computed Tomography and Magnetic Resonance Imaging. Philadelphia, Lea & Febiger, 1984.

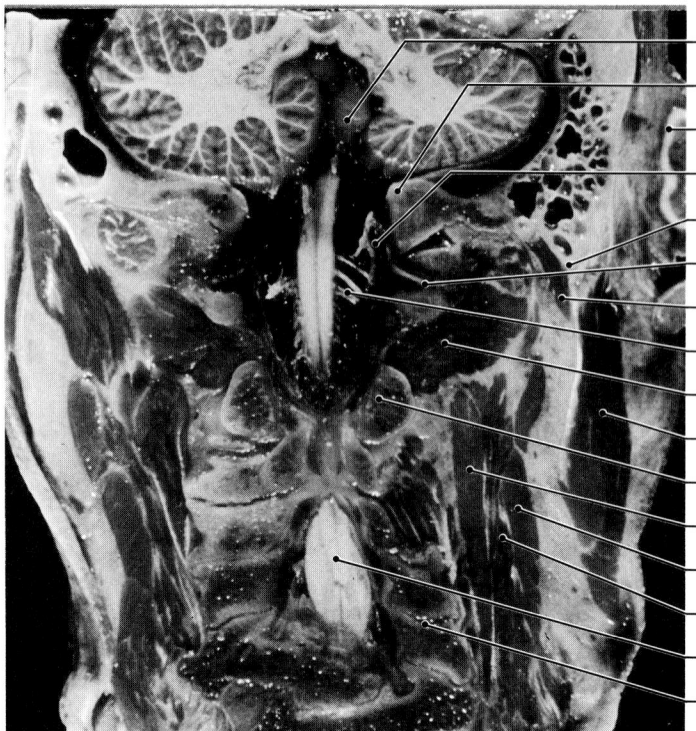
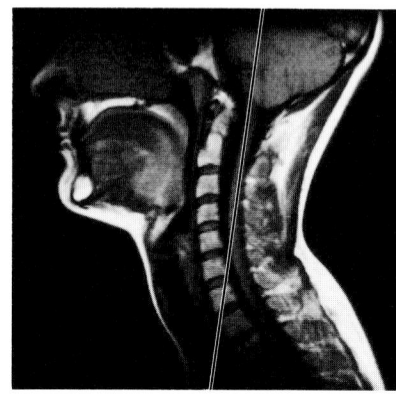

FIG. 8.16.

- The term "obex" is used frequently in the radiologic literature to define the inferior angle of the floor of the fourth ventricle, an opening that is continuous with the central canal or its remnant. The obex (Latin: barrier) is actually the thin triangular lamina formed by the convergence of taeniae of the fourth ventricle over the inferior angle of the ventricle.
- The gray matter of the cervical spinal cord consists of paired anterior or ventral gray columns and posterior or dorsal gray columns and of a connecting transverse gray commissure around the remnant of the central canal. The lateral gray column does not appear in the cervical cord. In the lower cervical levels, the ventral gray column is large and divided into four cell groups. The dorsal gray column is divided into several laminae of which the substantia gelatinosa and the nucleus proprius are prominent.
- During the development of the neuraxis, the central canal extends throughout the spinal cord and into the caudal medulla. This canal contains cerebrospinal fluid and is lined by ependyma. In adults, this central cavity becomes virtually obliterated except in the cervical cord. Enlargement of the central canal is termed hydromyelia, whereas a cleft separate from the central canal lined by glial cells is termed syringomyelia.

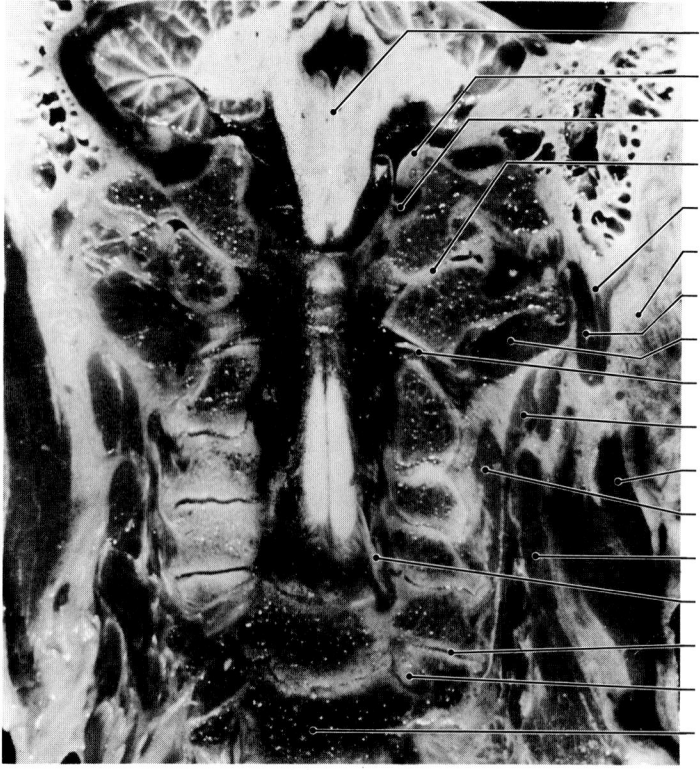

FIG. 8.17.

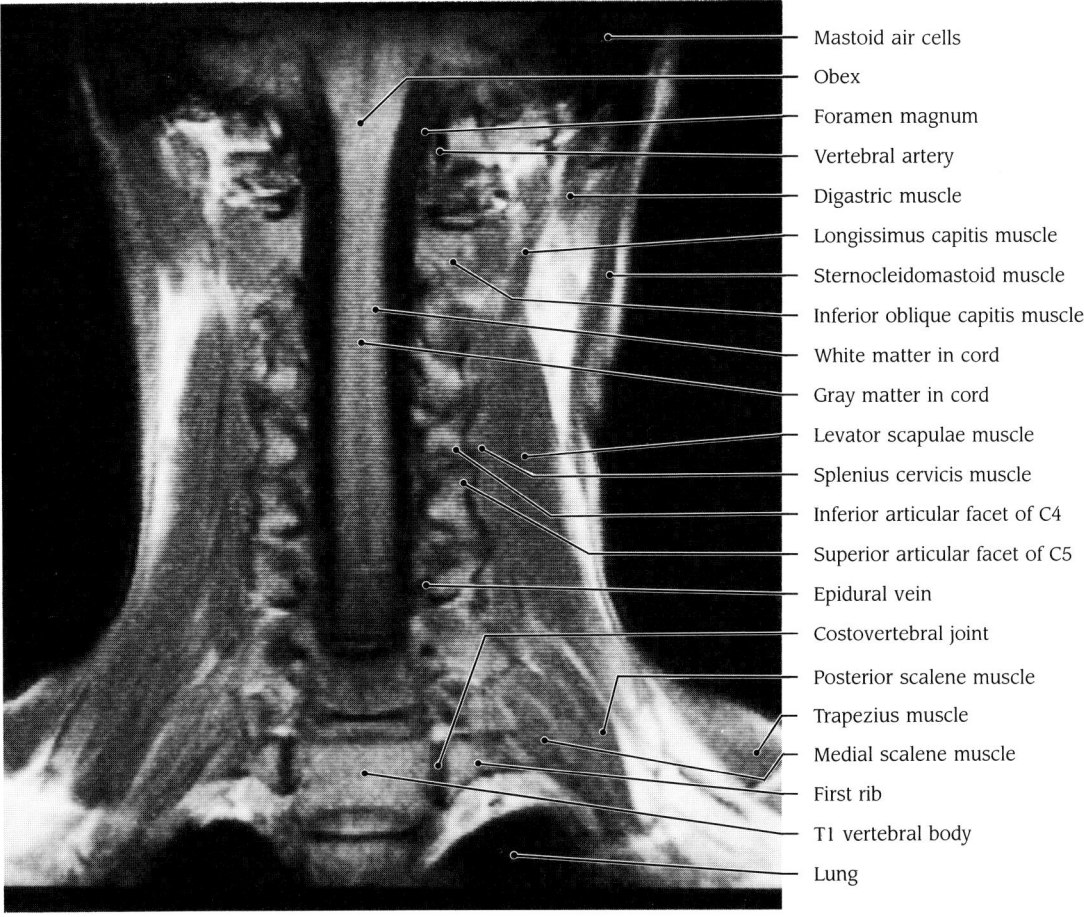

FIG. 8.18. TR = 500 msec, TE = 28 msec.

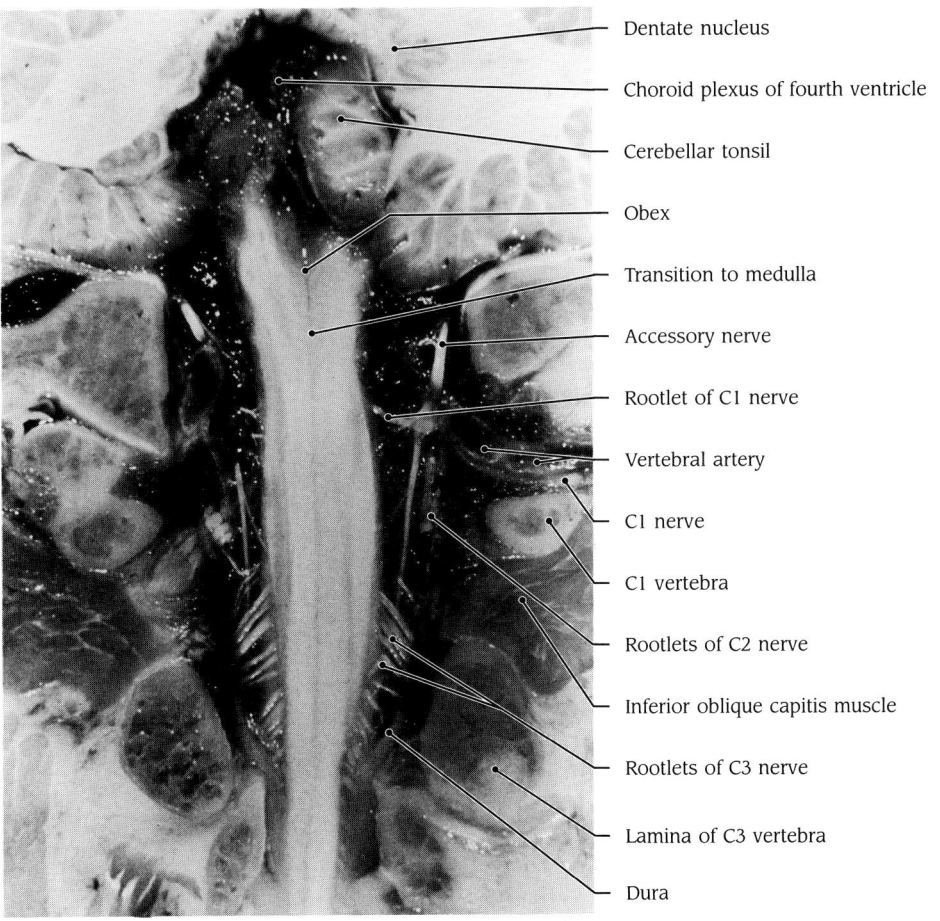

FIG. 8.19.

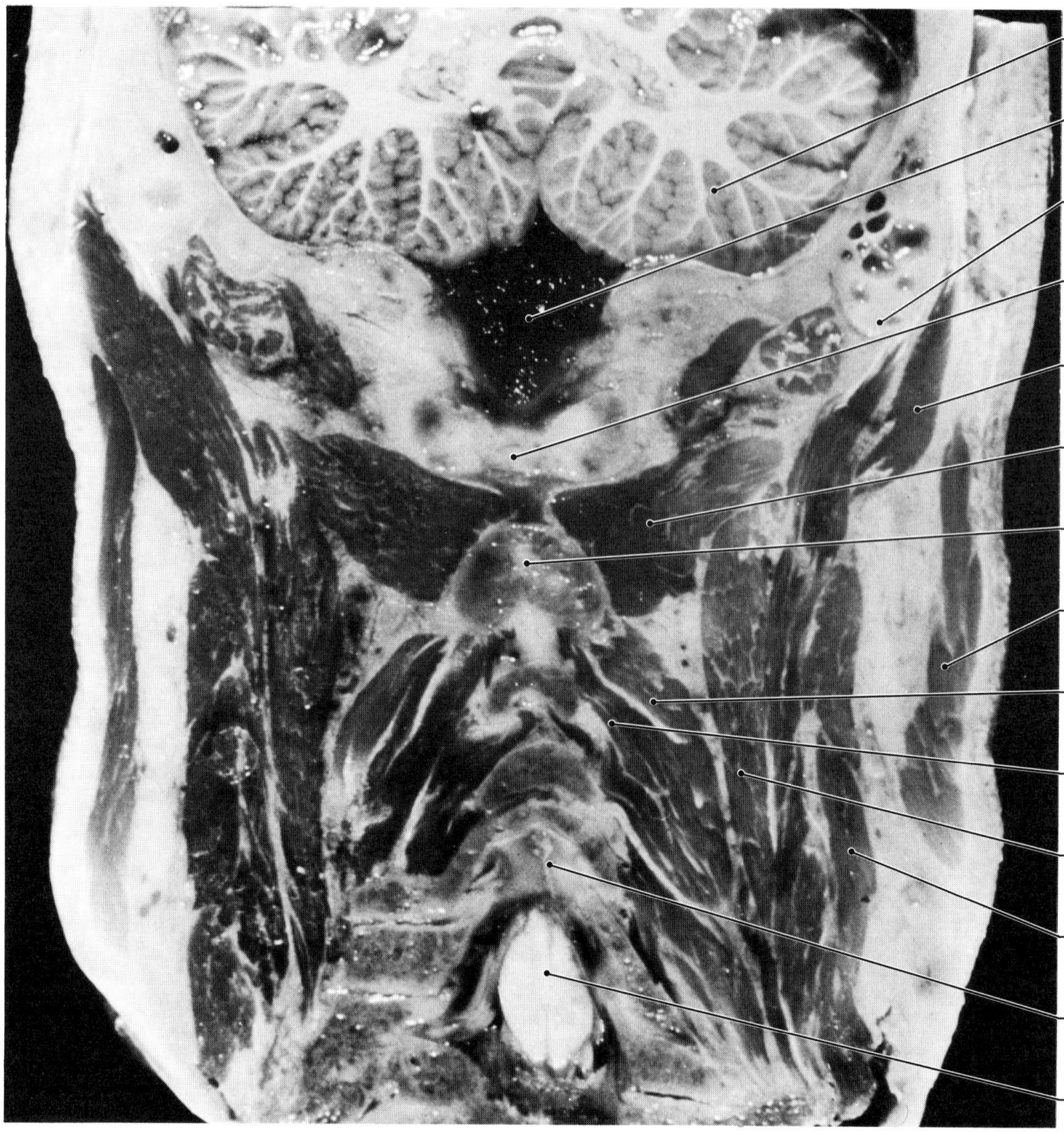

FIG. 8.20.

- Lateral cerebellum
- Cisterna magna
- Mastoid process
- Posterior arch of C1
- Splenius capitis muscle
- Inferior oblique capitis muscle
- Spinous process of C2
- Sternocleidomastoid muscle
- Multifidus muscle
- Rotator muscle
- Longissimus cervicis muscle
- Splenius cervicis muscle
- C5 vertebra
- Spinal cord

- The posterior arch of the atlas comprises about two fifths of the ring of C1. A wide groove is present on its upper surface behind each lateral mass, which contains the vertebral artery and the small first cervical spinal nerve.
- The lateral vertebral muscles include the anterior, middle, and posterior scalene muscles, which attach to the cervical transverse processes and extend to the first two ribs. The middle and posterior scalene muscles (seen here) bend the cervical part of the vertebral column to the same side. Additionally, as accessory respiratory muscles, the middle scalene muscle assists in elevating the first rib, whereas the posterior scalene muscle assists in elevating the second rib.

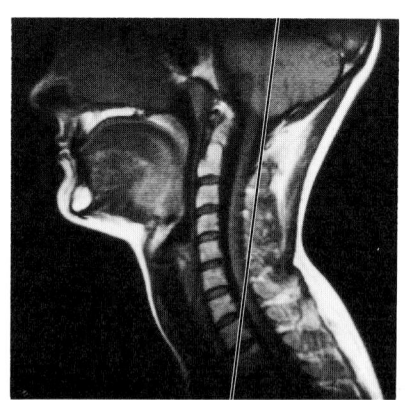

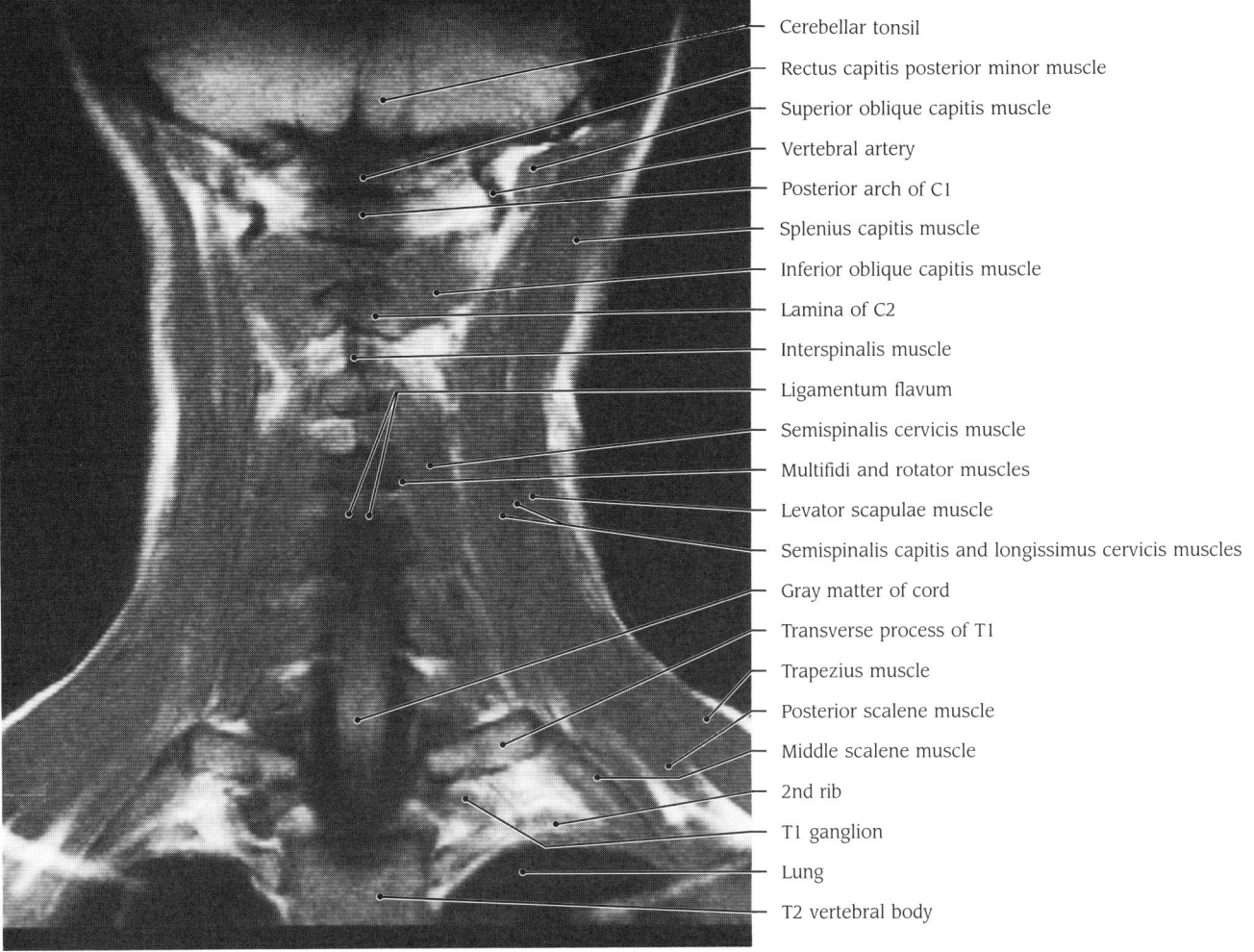

FIG. 8.21. TR = 500 msec, TE = 28 msec.

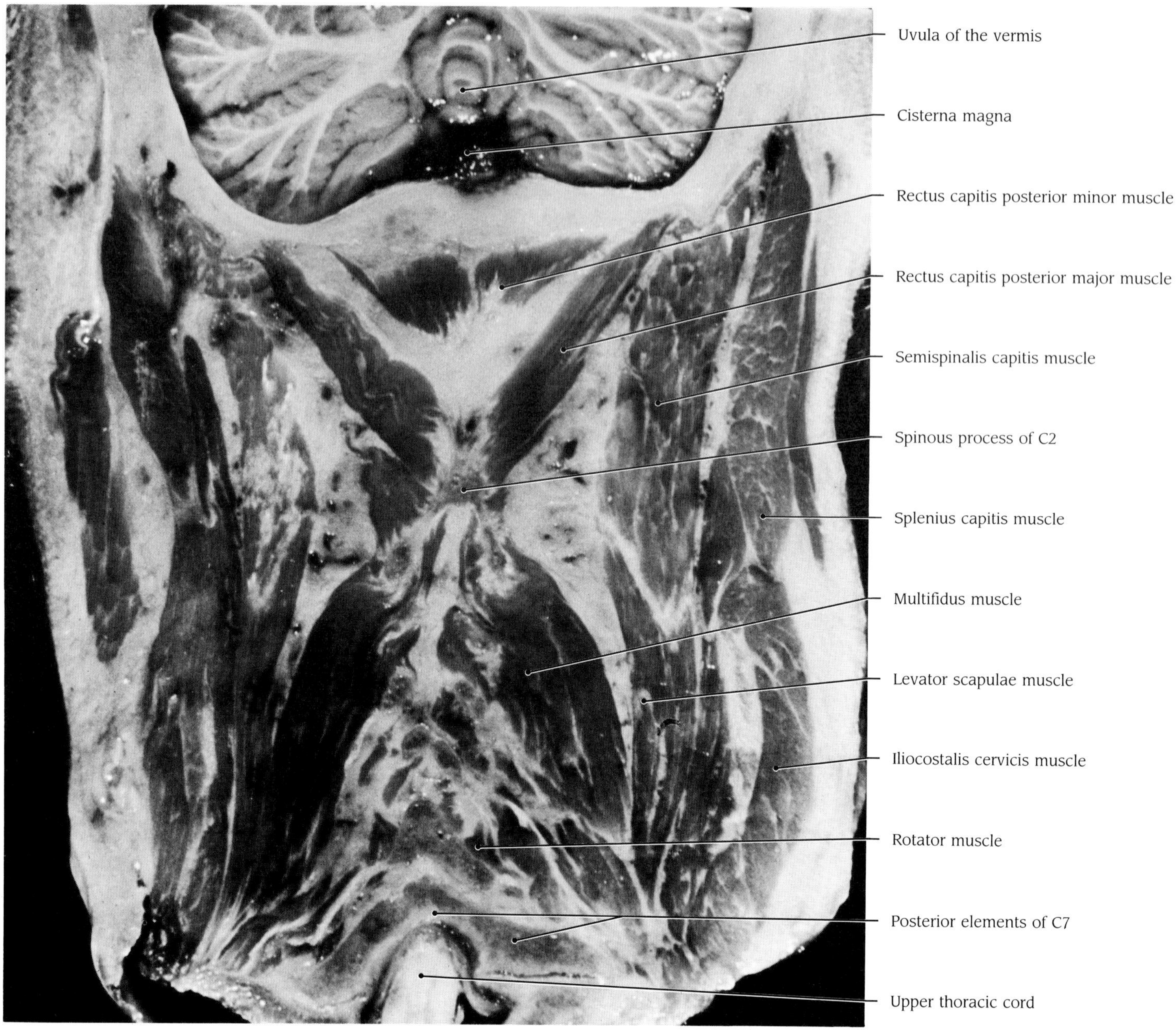

FIG. 8.22.

- Uvula of the vermis
- Cisterna magna
- Rectus capitis posterior minor muscle
- Rectus capitis posterior major muscle
- Semispinalis capitis muscle
- Spinous process of C2
- Splenius capitis muscle
- Multifidus muscle
- Levator scapulae muscle
- Iliocostalis cervicis muscle
- Rotator muscle
- Posterior elements of C7
- Upper thoracic cord

- The suboccipital muscles, which include the rectus capitis posterior major and minor and the obliquus capitis superior and inferior, function as extensors of the head and rotators of the head and atlas on the axis. The major attachments of these muscles are from the base of the occiput to the posterior arch of C1 (atlas) and C2 (axis) and their spinous processes and transverse processes.
- An irregular network of prominent cervical veins traverses the spaces between the suboccipital muscles. These veins and their continuation, the deep cervical veins, are particularly obvious when the patient is in the supine position for an extended period.

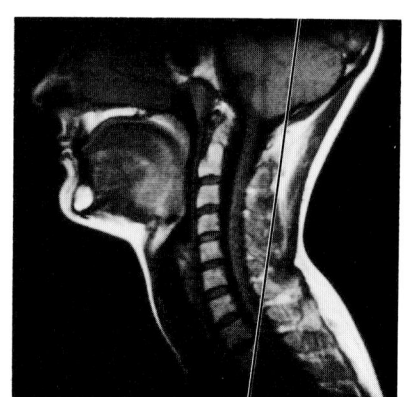

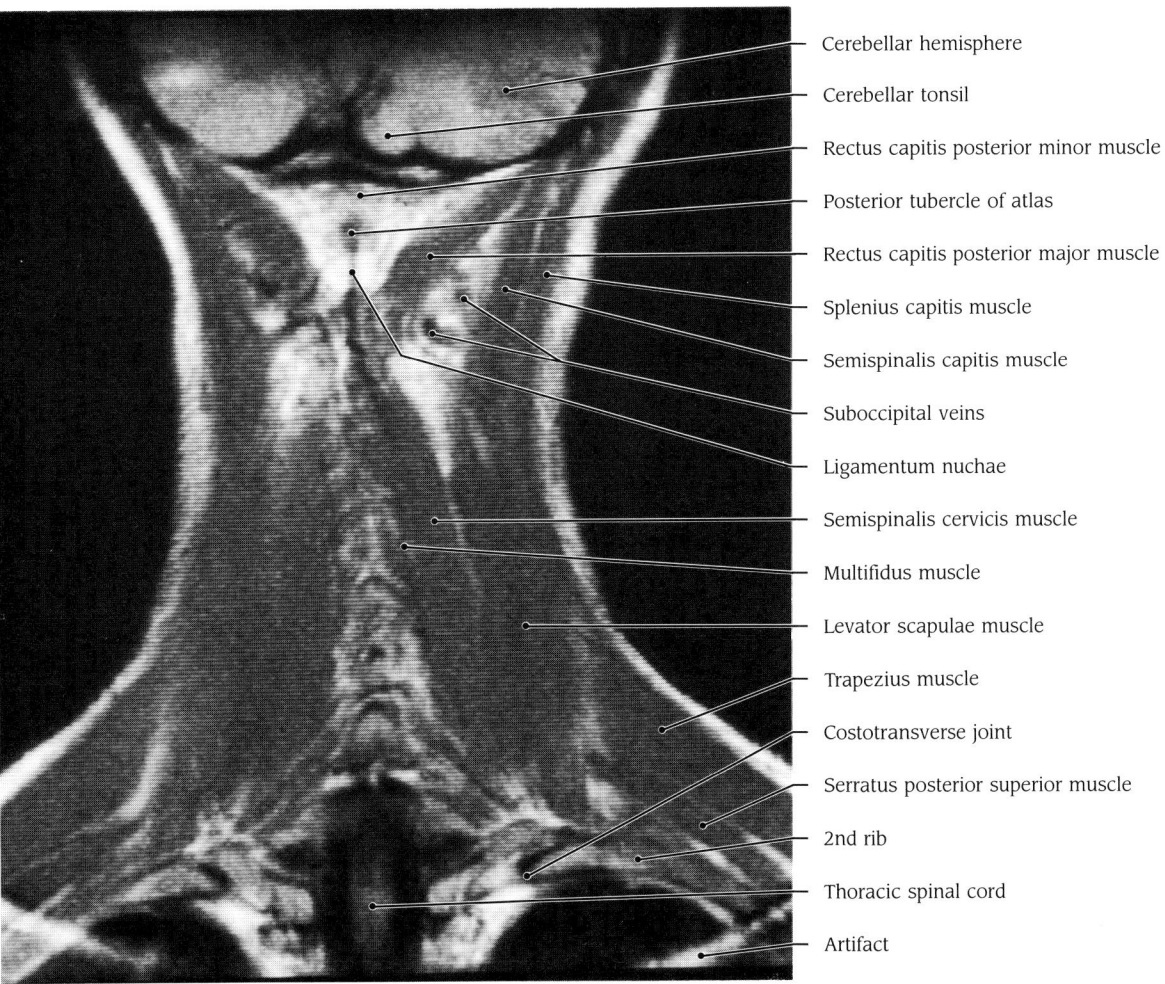

FIG. 8.23. TR = 500 msec, TE = 28 msec.

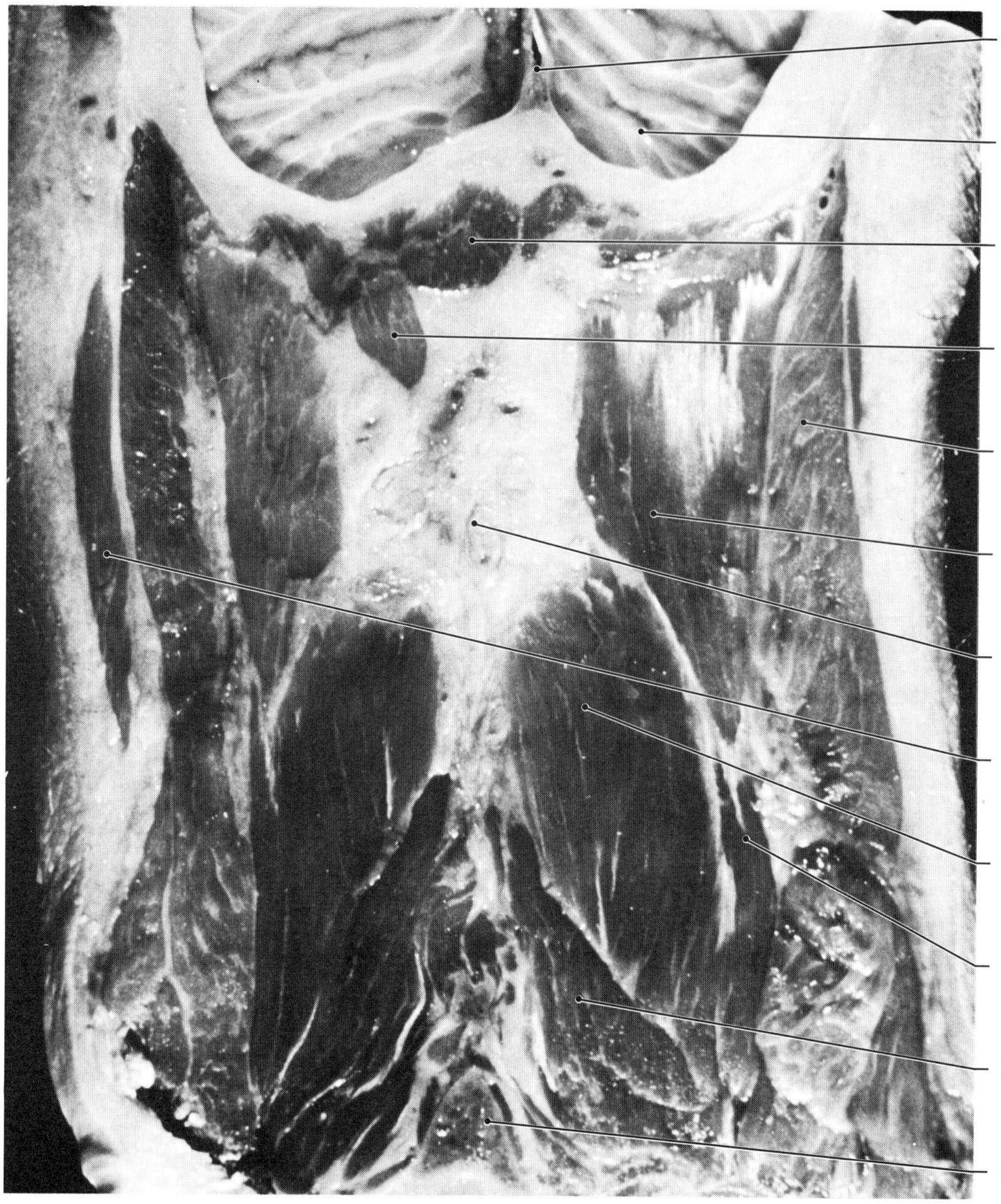

FIG. 8.24.

- Falx cerebelli
- Cerebellar hemisphere
- Rectus capitis posterior minor muscle
- Rectus capitis posterior major muscle
- Splenius capitis muscle
- Semispinalis capitis muscle
- Ligamentum nuchae
- Sternocleidomastoid muscle
- Semispinalis cervicis muscle
- Levator scapulae muscle
- Multifidus muscle
- Spinous process of C7

- The superficial muscles of the neck, which include the trapezius, splenius capitis, semispinalis capitis, and semispinalis cervicis, as well as the multifidus, lie in concentric layers between the superficial fascia and the vertebrae. These symmetrically paired groups of muscles attach to the midline ligamentum nuchae. In coronal sections, therefore, the more superficial muscle layers are seen lateral to the deeper muscle layers.

- The ligamentum nuchae is a fibroelastic membrane, or intermuscular septum, that extends from the external occipital protuberance and external occipital crest to the spine of the seventh cervical vertebra. It is homologous with the supraspinous and interspinous ligaments seen at lower levels.

- The ligamentum nuchae is favored as a surgical plane of dissection because it is relatively bloodless.

- The spinous process of the seventh cervical vertebra is seen readily, even in the coronal plane, because of its prominence. The spinous process of the first thoracic vertebra, however, is normally more prominent.

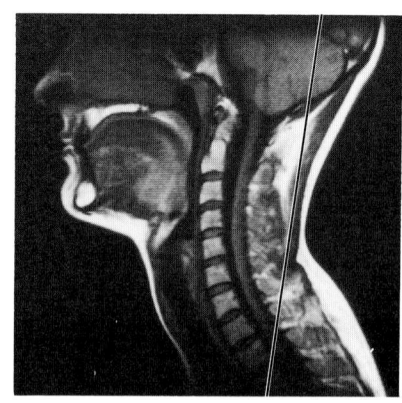

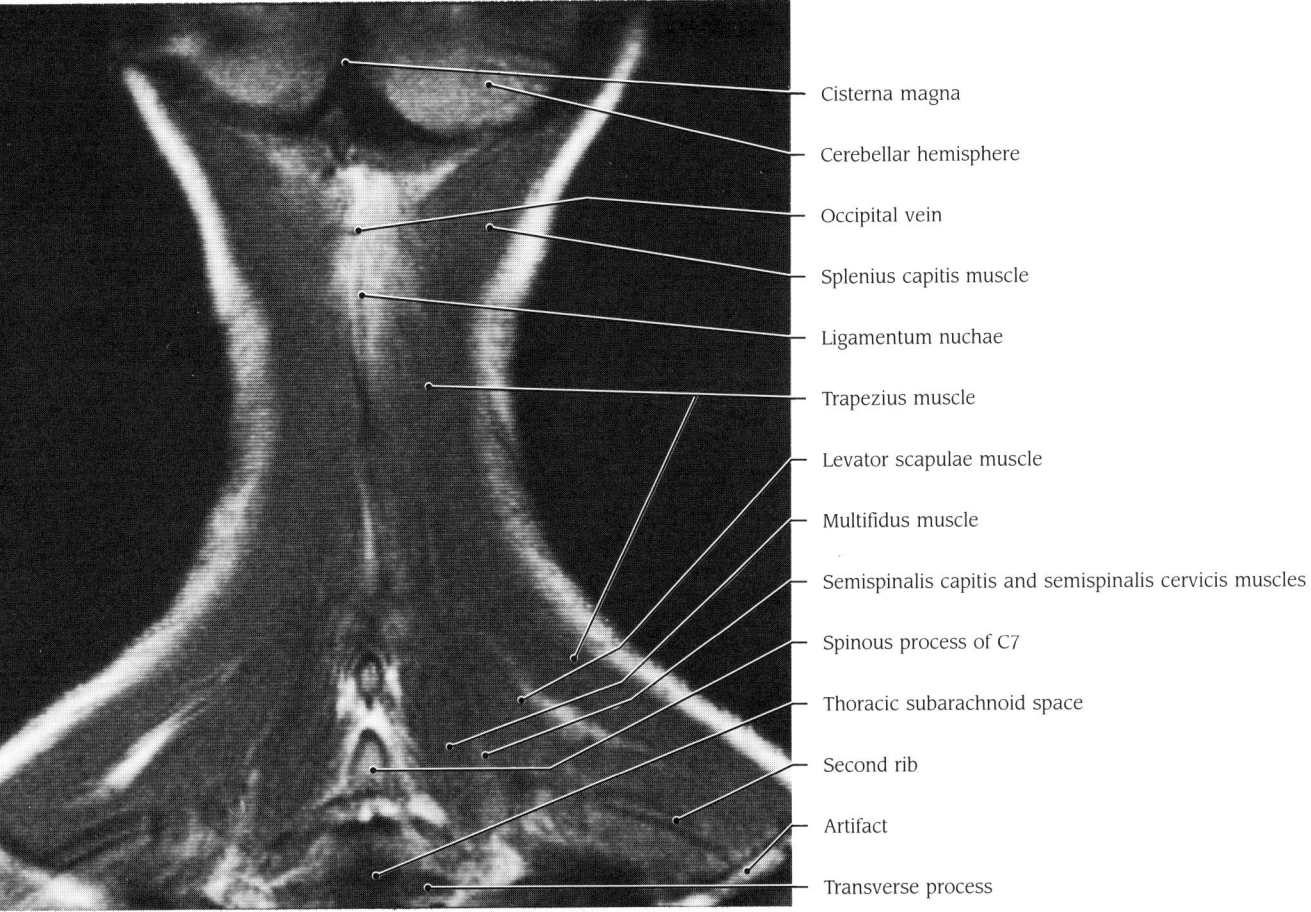

FIG. 8.25. TR = 500 msec, TE = 28 msec.

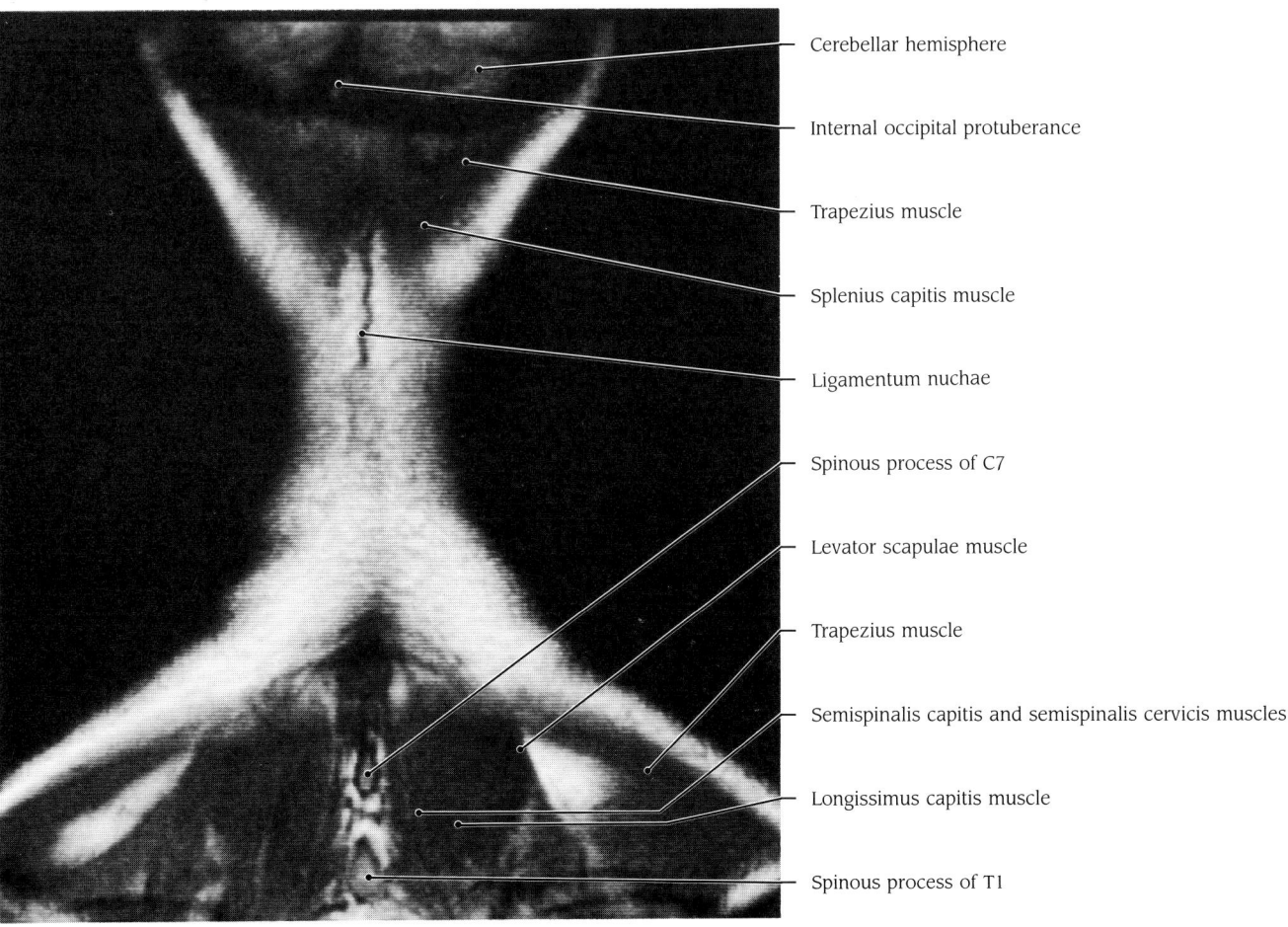

FIG. 8.26. TR = 500 msec, TE = 28 msec.

9

Neck and Cervical Spine, Sagittal Plane

Anatomic Level	Figures
Spinal cord, larynx	9.1–9.21
Lateral neck musculature	9.22–9.26

A series of cadaveric sagittal sections that extend through the cervical spine and neck is shown. These sections are matched with sagittal magnetic resonance images of a volunteer. The magnetic resonance images encompass the entire neck at 4-mm increments. Because of the symmetry of the neck, the right and left sides have been interleaved for purposes of display and are ordered from midline to most lateral. The magnetic resonance images were obtained with a short TR to highlight anatomic structures. Magnified anatomic sections are shown at several section planes to enhance detail.

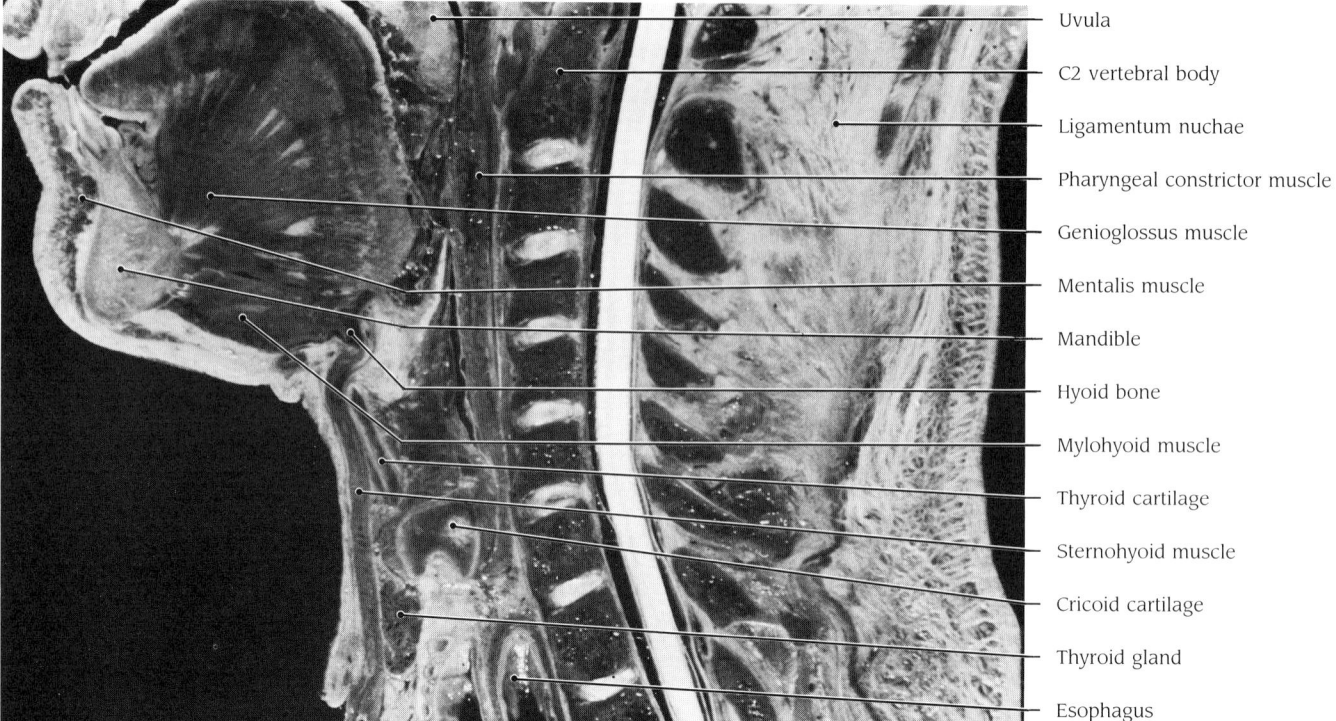

FIG. 9.1.

- The larynx extends from the root of the tongue to the trachea. The skeletal framework of the larynx is formed of cartilages, which include the epiglottis, thyroid, and cricoid, and the paired arytenoid, corniculate, and cuneiform. These cartilages are connected by ligaments and membranes, which are moved by muscles.

- The epiglottis is a thin projection of elastic fibrocartilage that extends obliquely posterior to the tongue and body of the hyoid bone, anterior to the opening of the larynx. The stalk of the epiglottis is attached to the thyroid cartilage just inferior to the thyroid notch by the thyroepiglottic ligament. The lateral margins of the epiglottis attach to the arytenoid cartilages by the aryepiglottic folds. The mucous membrane covering the anterior surface of the epiglottis is reflected on to the tongue and on to the lateral walls of the pharynx, thereby forming a median glossoepiglottic fold and two lateral glossoepiglottic folds. The valleculae are the depressions on each side of the median glossoepiglottic fold. The hyoepiglottic ligament connects the inferior aspect of the epiglottis to the hyoid bone.

- The corniculate cartilages are two small cone-shaped pieces of elastic fibrocartilage located in the posterior portions of the aryepiglottic folds. These cartilages articulate with the superior aspects of the arytenoid cartilages, to which they are sometimes fused.

- The cuneiform cartilages are two small club-shaped pieces of elastic fibrocartilage located in the aryepiglottic folds just anterior to the corniculate cartilages.

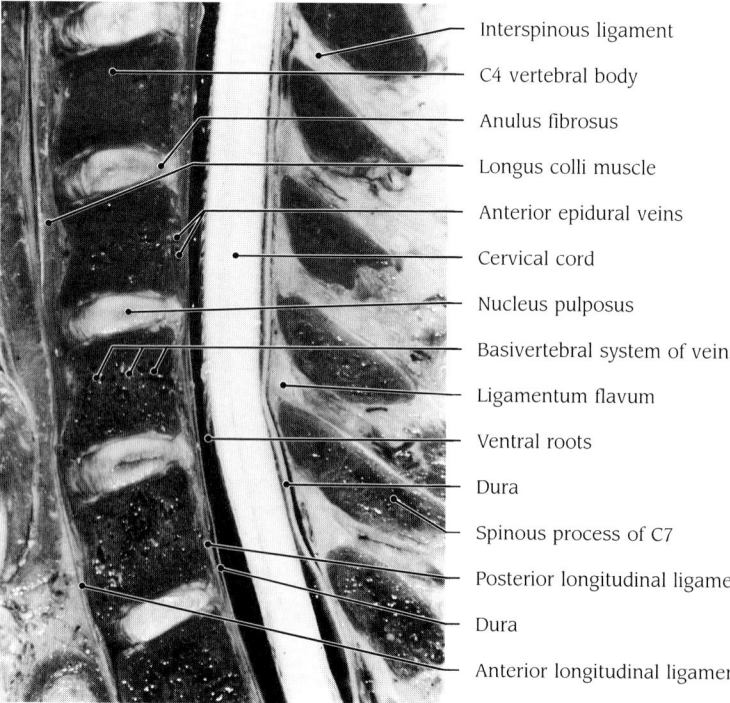

FIG. 9.2.

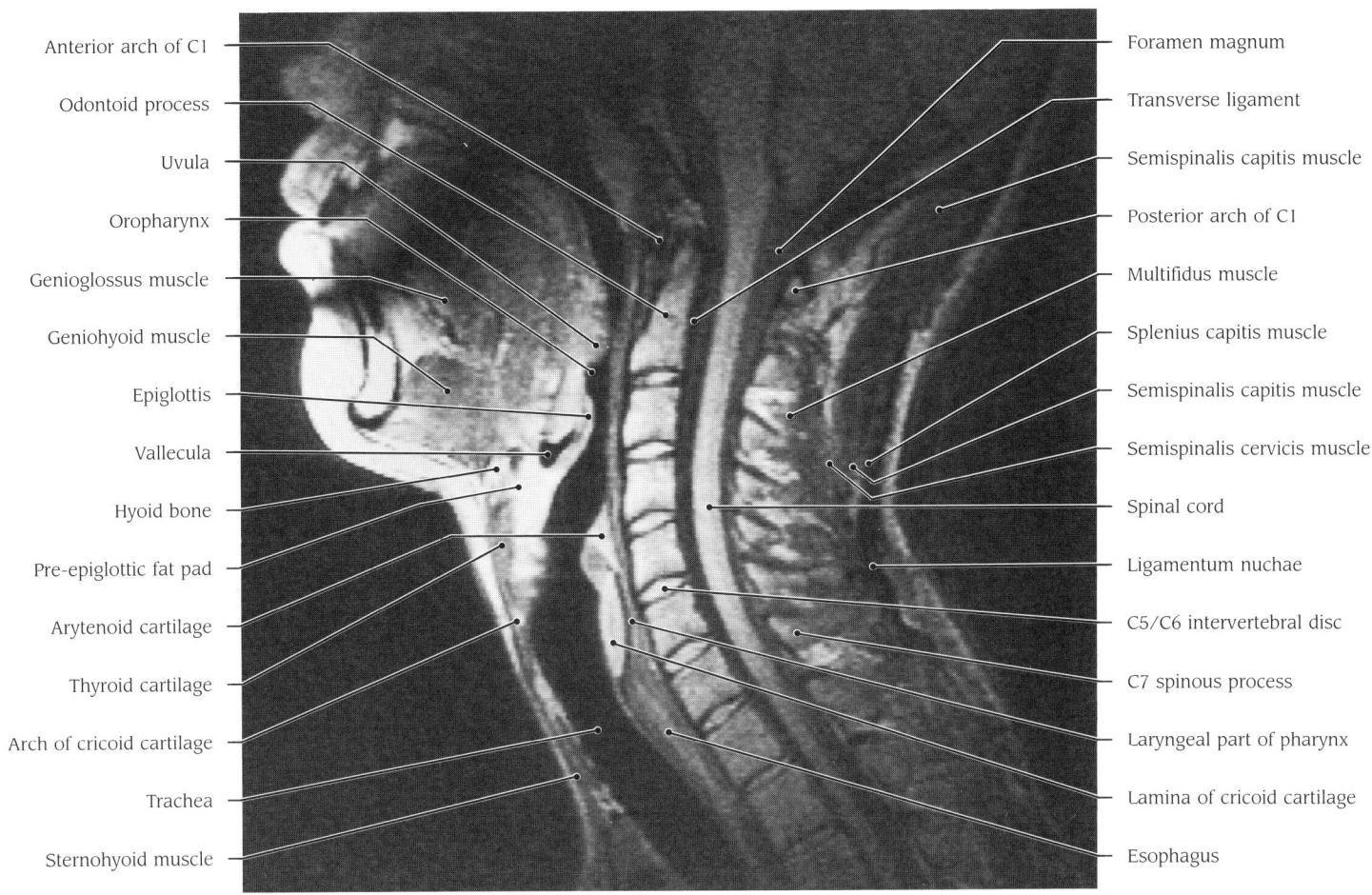

FIG. 9.3. TR = 739 msec, TE = 39 msec.

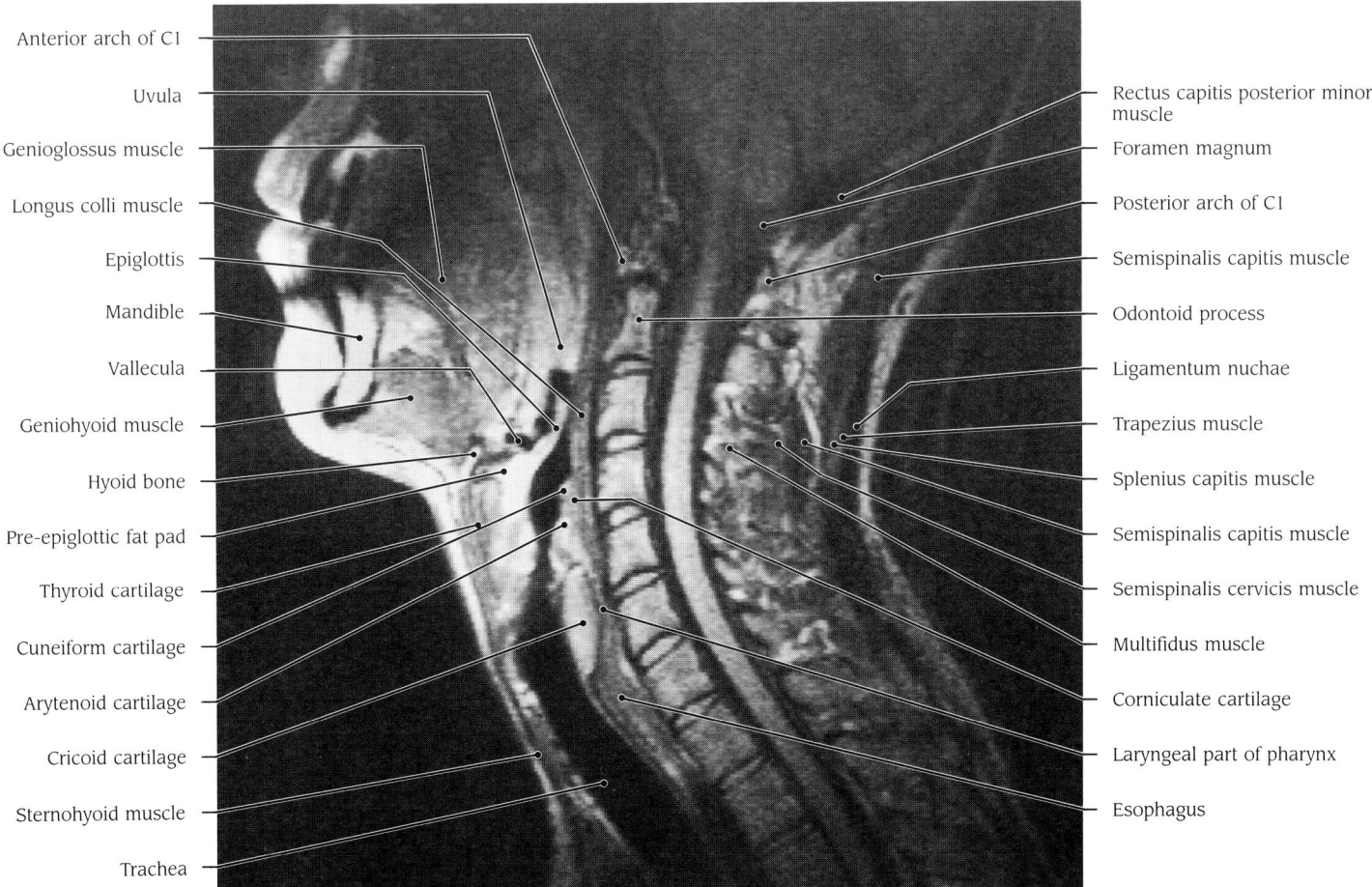

FIG. 9.4. TR = 739 msec, TE = 39 msec.

205

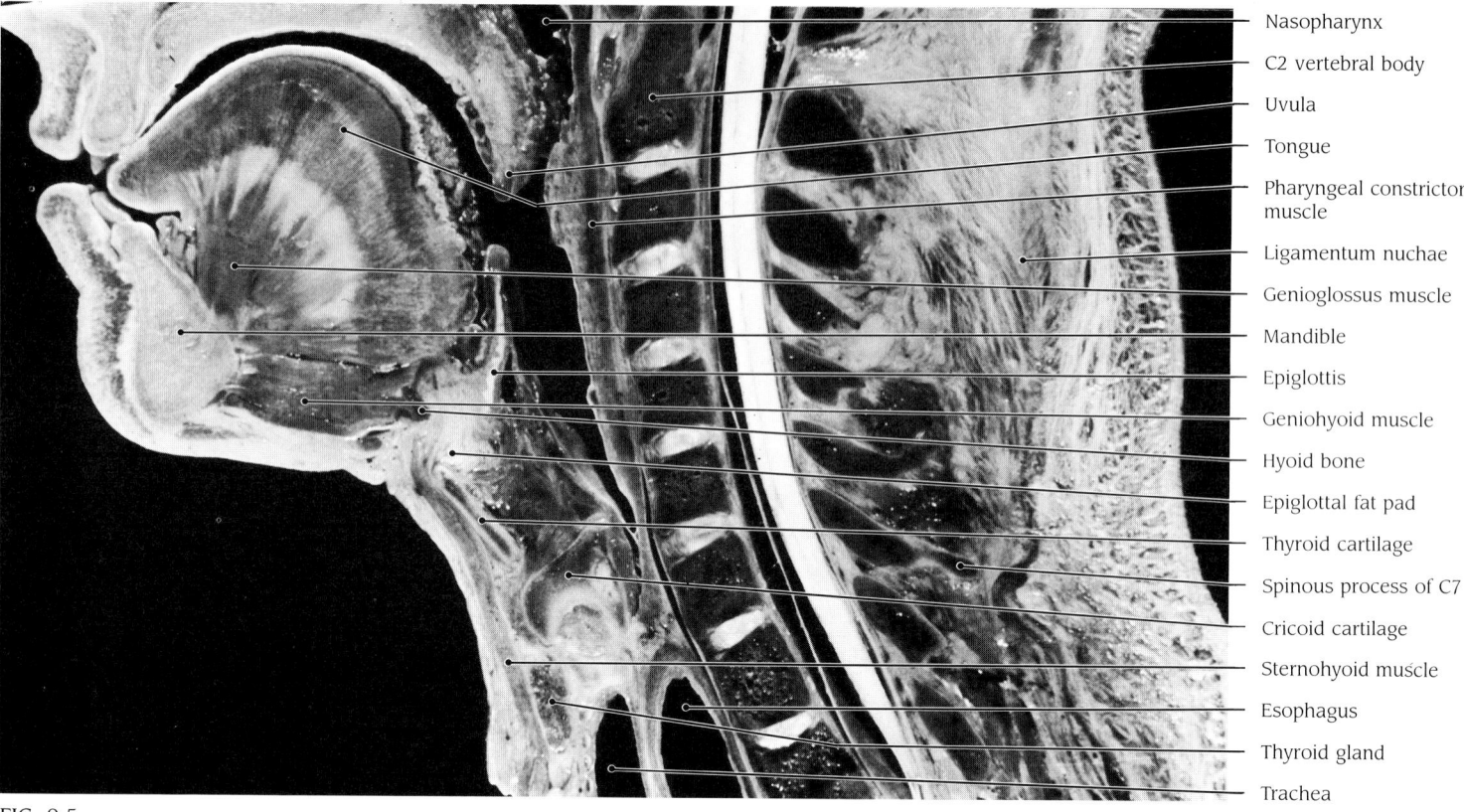

FIG. 9.5.

- The larynx is divided into three parts by the vestibular and vocal folds. The superior portion, or vestibule, of the larynx extends from the laryngeal inlet to the vestibular folds. The middle portion includes the area from the fissure between the vestibular folds, the rima vestibuli, to the fissure between the vocal folds, the rima glottidis. The inferior portion of the laryngeal cavity extends from the rima glottidis to the inferior border of the cricoid cartilage.

- The vestibular folds are two thick folds of mucous membrane, each of which envelops the vestibular ligament, a band of fibrous tissue. The vestibular folds attach to the thyroid cartilage anteriorly, just inferior to the point of attachment of the epiglottis, and to the arytenoid cartilage posteriorly, just above the vocal process.

- The vocal folds are two folds of mucous membrane, each of which encloses the vocal ligament. The vocal folds extend from the angle of the thyroid cartilage to the vocal processes of the arytenoid cartilages.

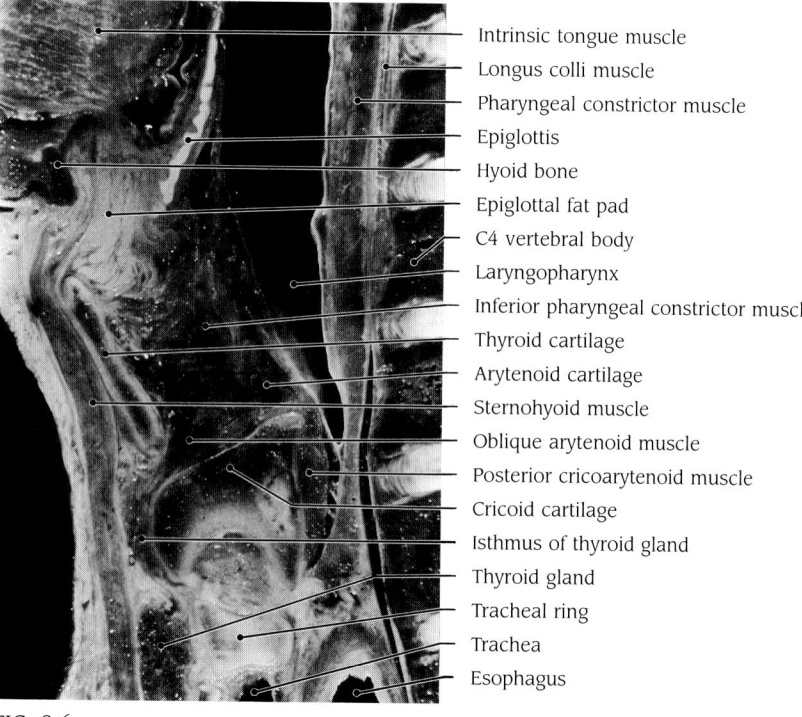

FIG. 9.6.

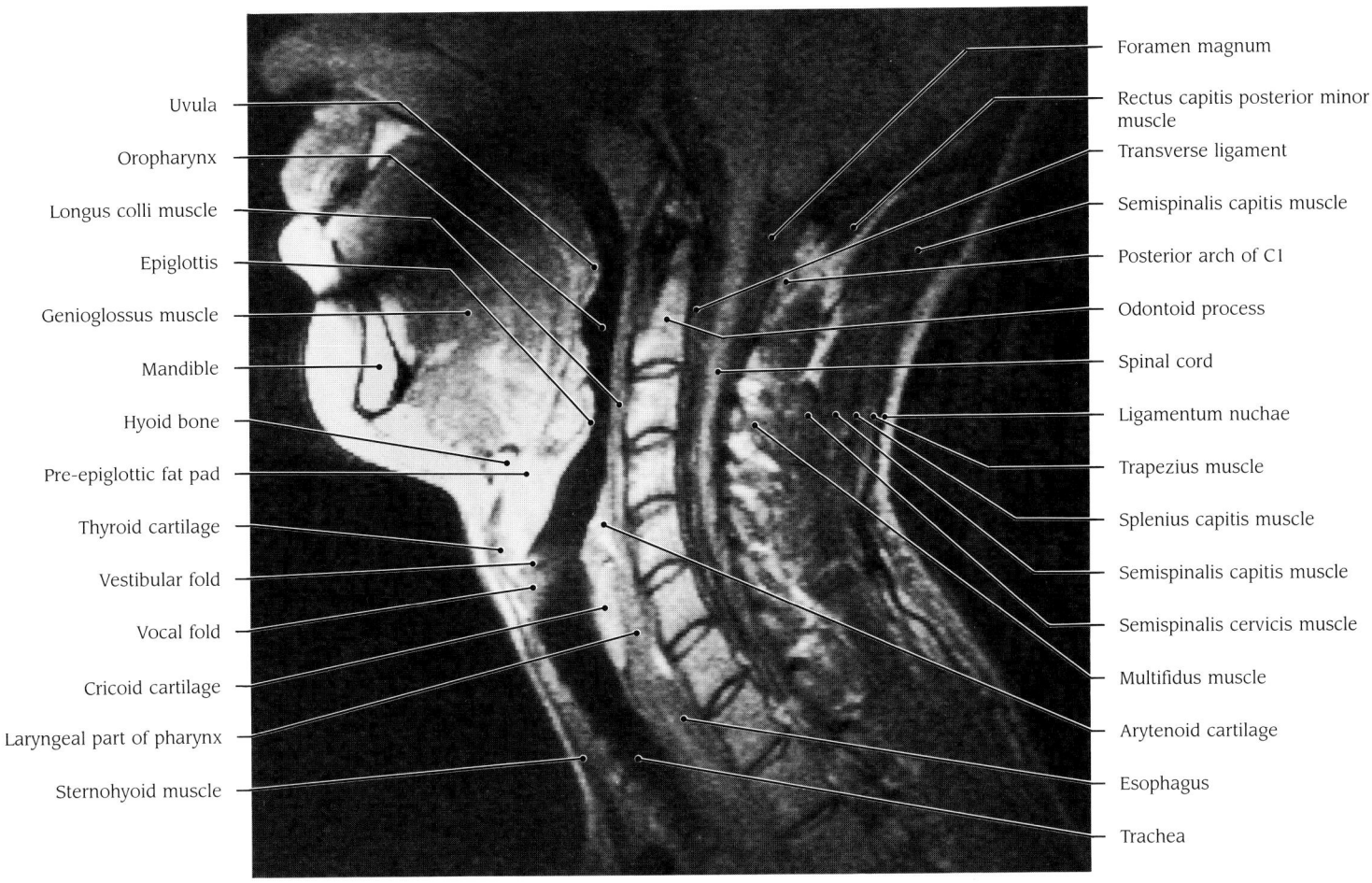

FIG. 9.7. TR = 739 msec, TE = 39 msec.

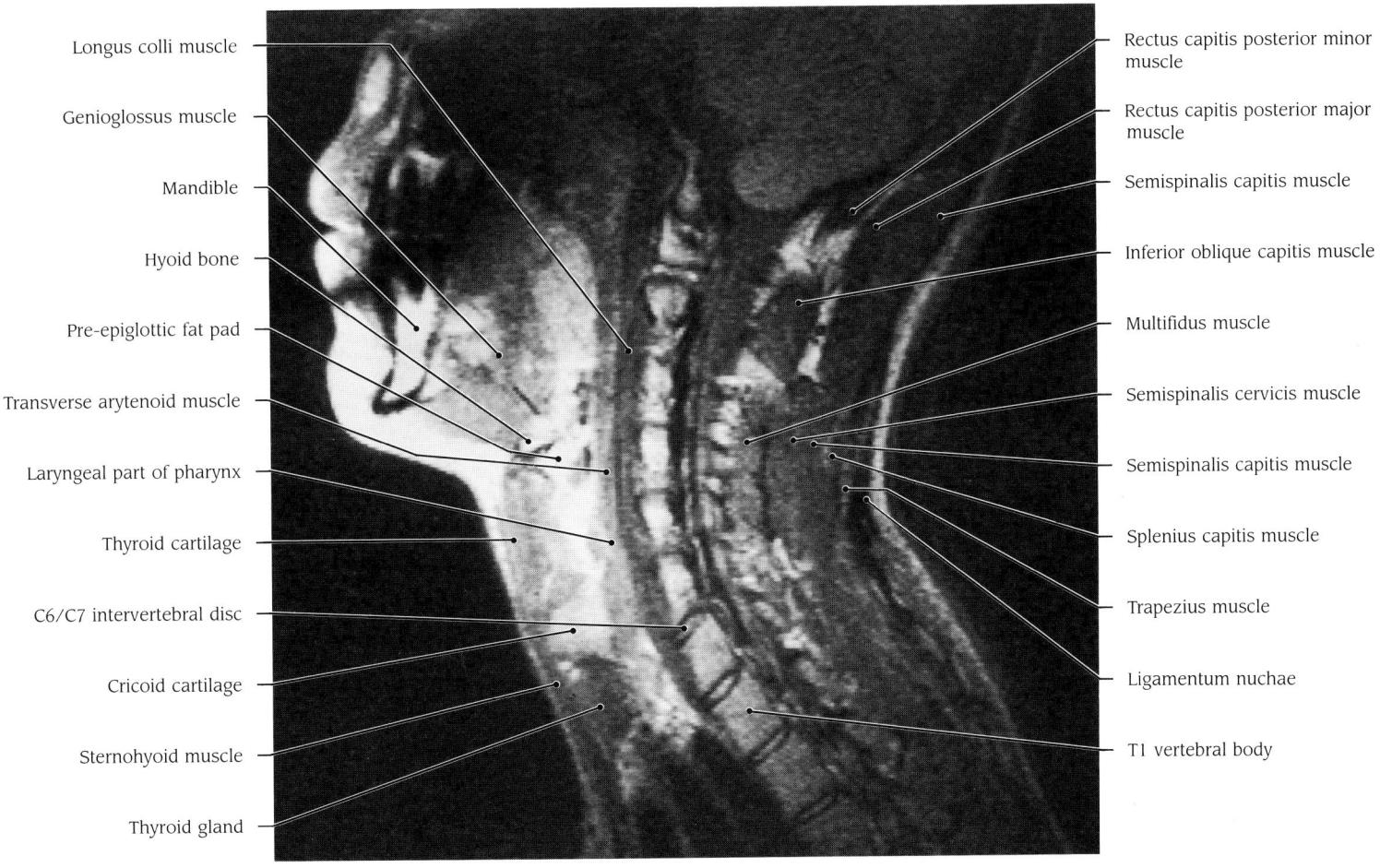

FIG. 9.8. TR = 739 msec, TE = 39 msec.

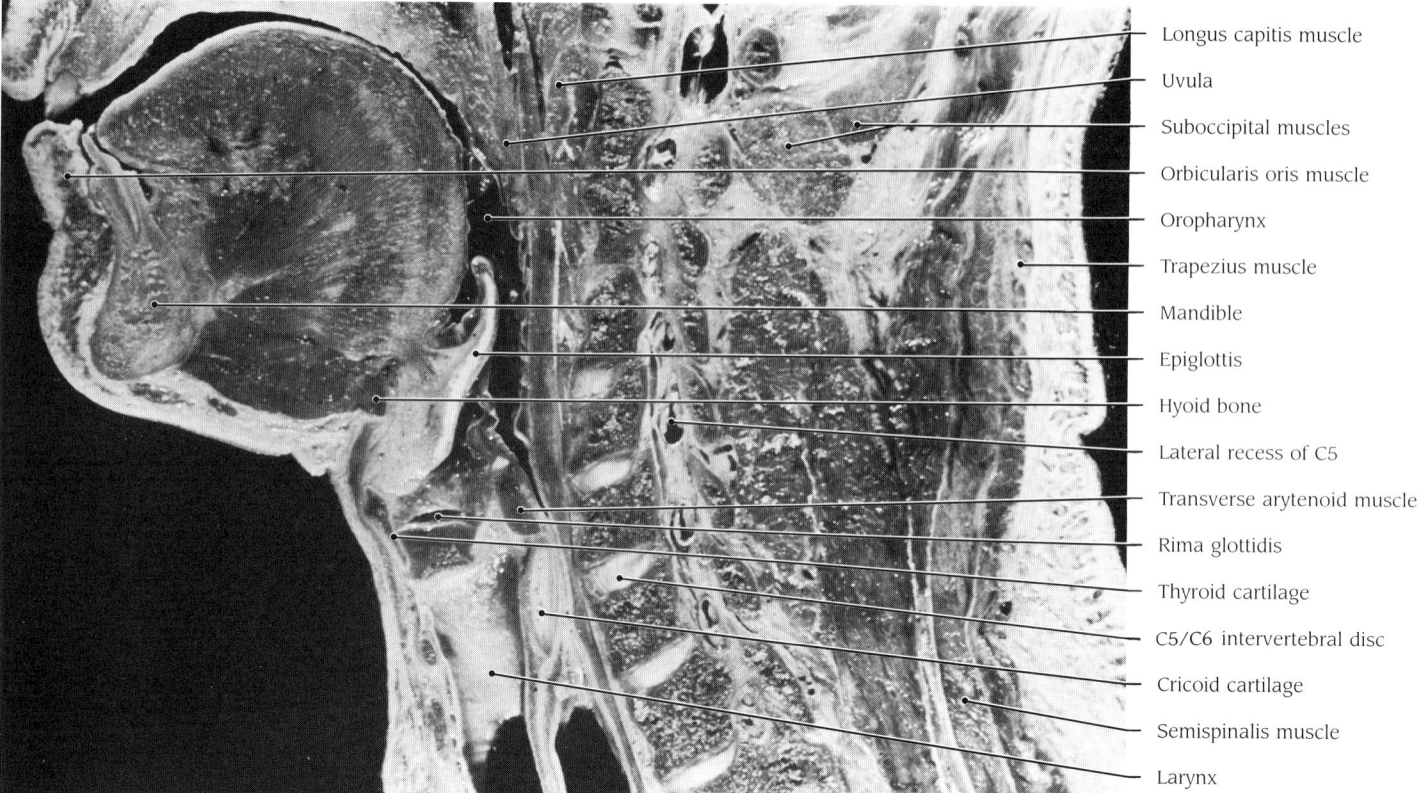

FIG. 9.9.

- The transverse arytenoid muscle, one of the intrinsic muscles of the larynx, attaches to the posterior aspect of the muscular process and to the lateral edge of each arytenoid cartilage. This muscle approximates the arytenoids and closes the opening of the glottis. The other intrinsic muscles, which, unlike the transverse arytenoid muscle, are all paired, are the cricothyroid, posterior cricoarytenoid, lateral cricoarytenoid, oblique arytenoid, aryepiglotticus, thyroarytenoid, vocalis, and thyroepiglotticus.

- These intrinsic muscles may be divided into three groups, according to their actions: (1) the muscles that alter the laryngeal inlet, the aryepiglottici and the thyroepiglottici; (2) the muscles that modify the vocal ligaments, the cricothyroids, the posterior cricoarytenoids, the vocales, and the thyroarytenoids; and (3) the muscles that change the glottis, the oblique and transverse arytenoids and the posterior and lateral cricoarytenoids.

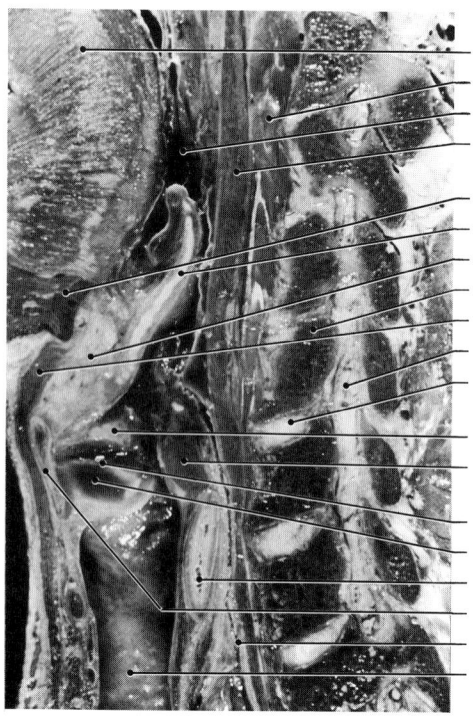

FIG. 9.10.

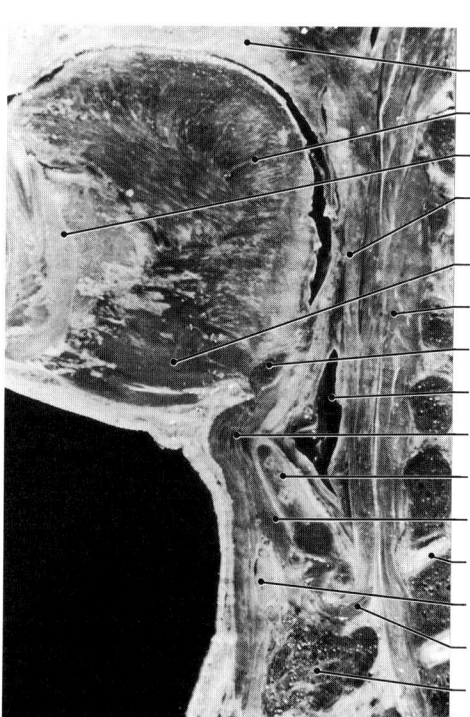

FIG. 9.11.

208

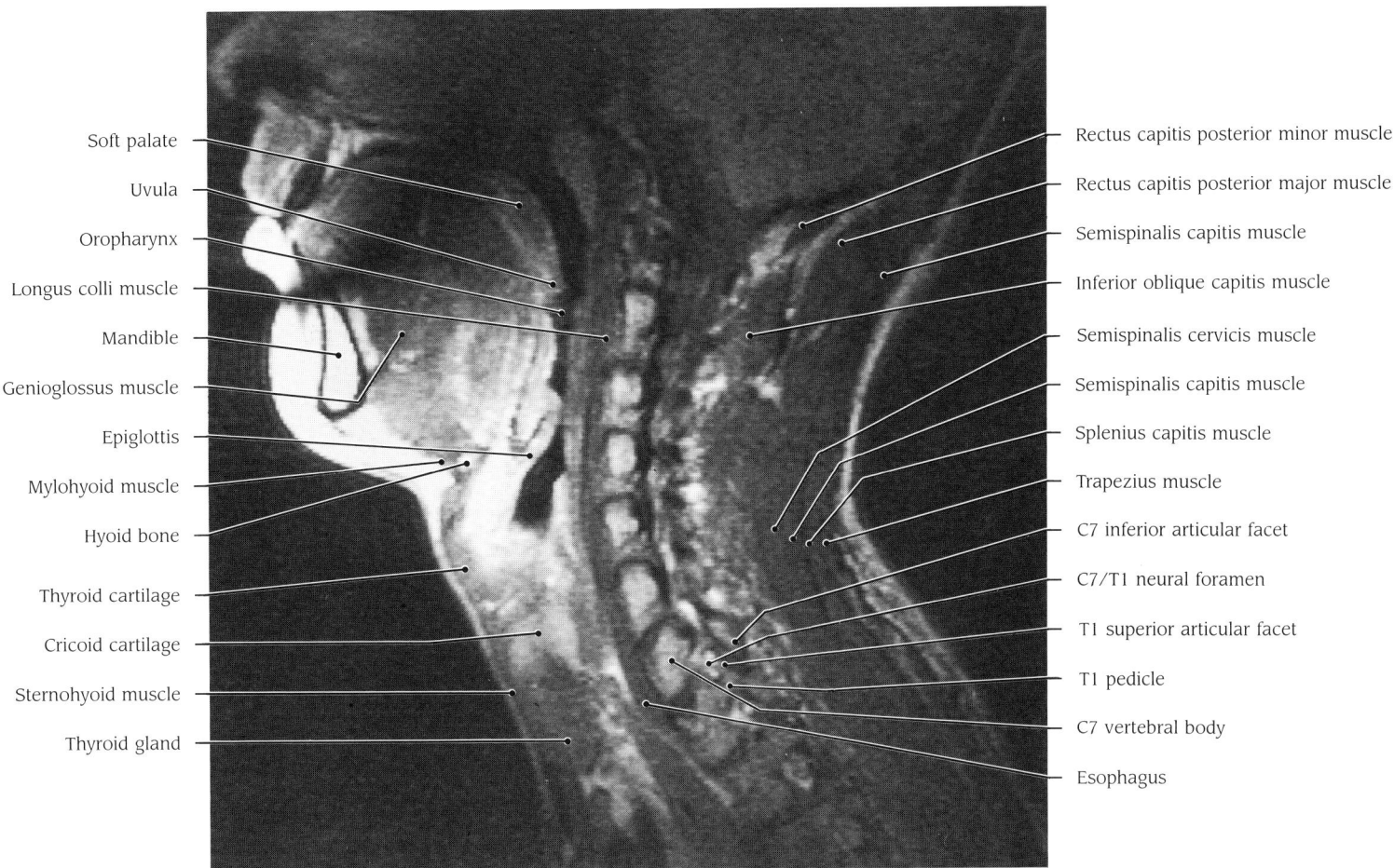

FIG. 9.12. TR = 739 msec, TE = 39 msec.

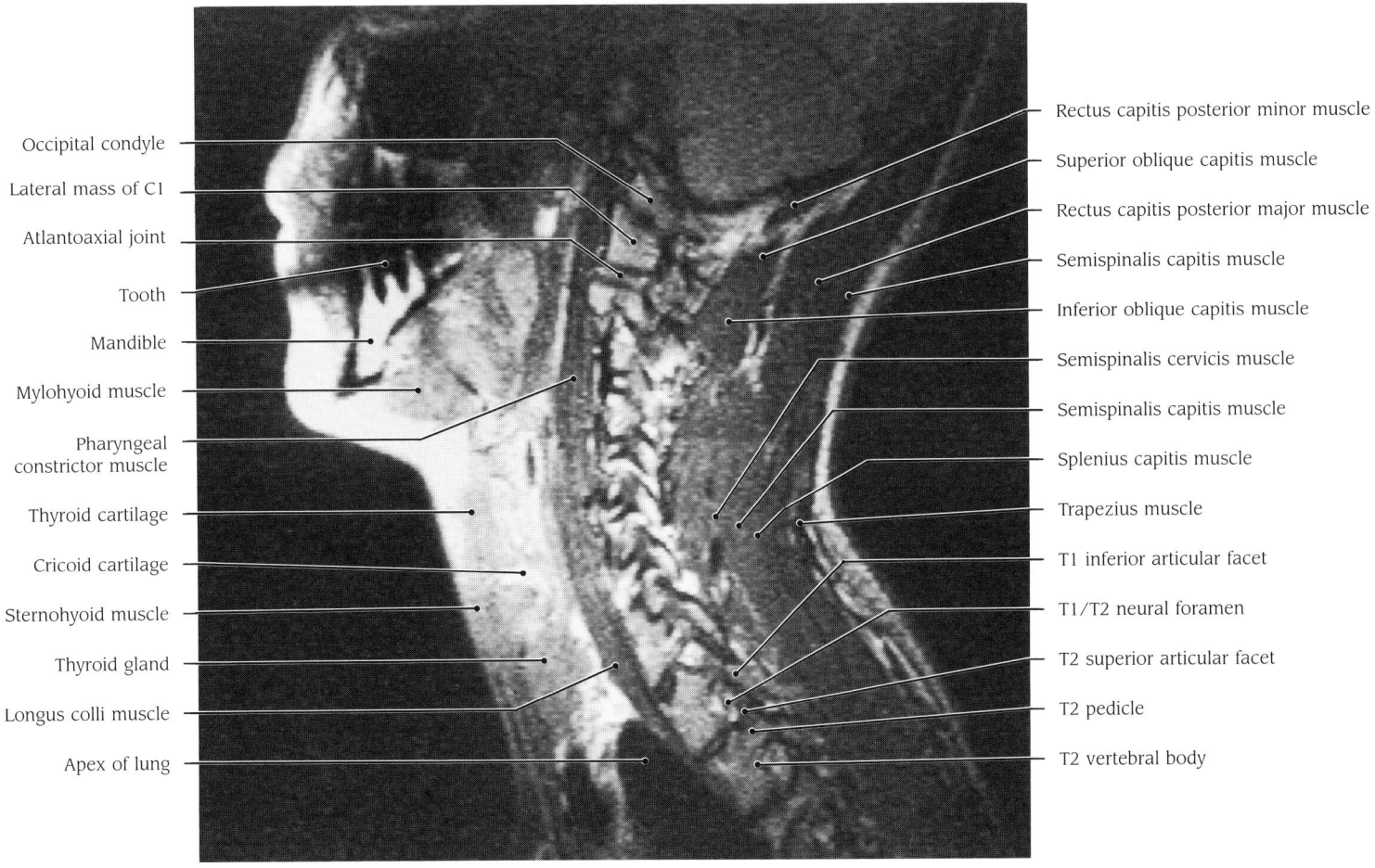

FIG. 9.13. TR = 739 msec, TE = 39 msec.

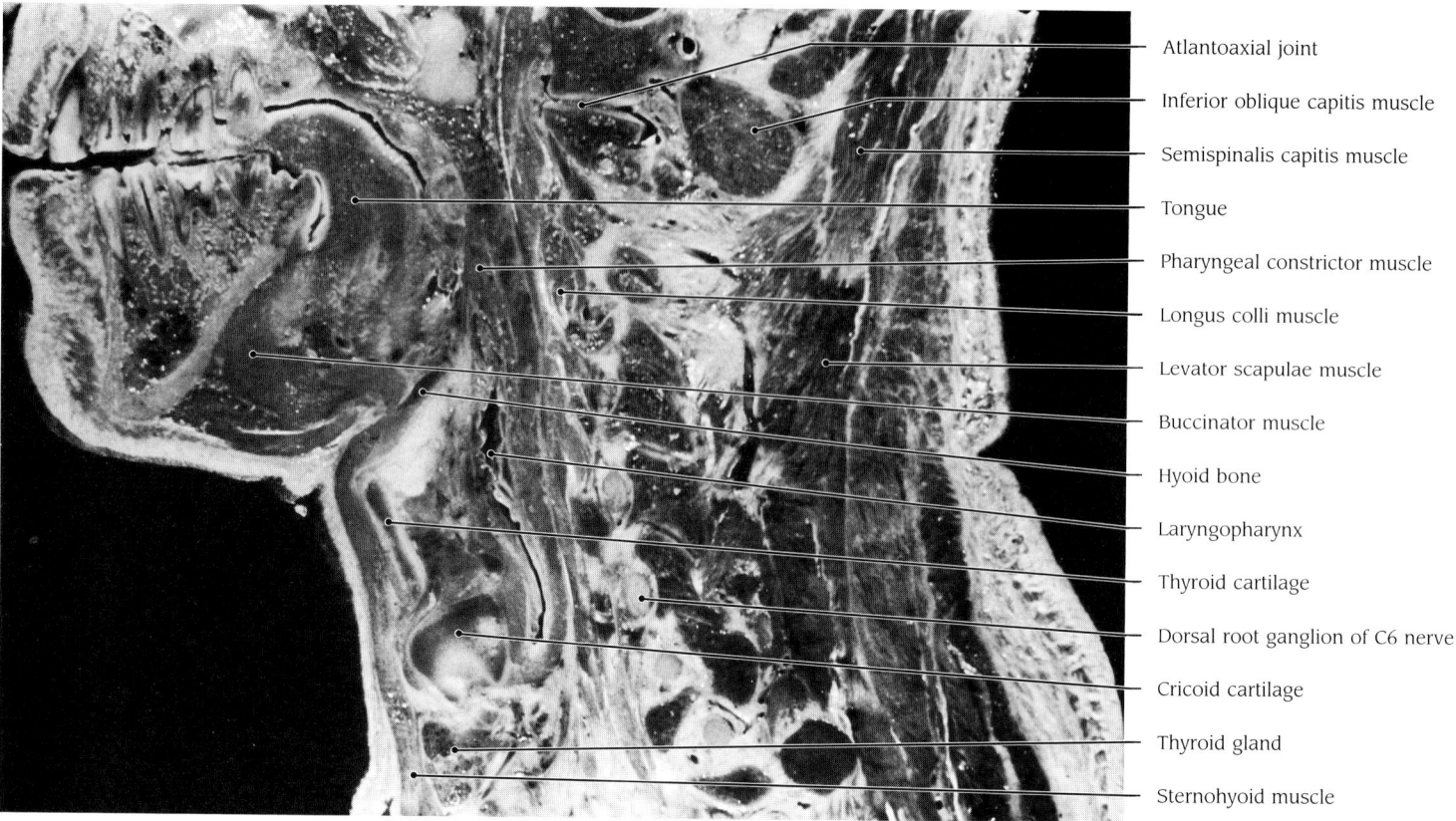

FIG. 9.14.

- The cricoid, thyroid, and the majority of the arytenoid cartilages are composed of hyaline cartilage and become ossified with aging. The thyroid cartilage ossifies first, beginning at approximately 25 years, and the cricoid and arytenoid begin later. These cartilages may be entirely bone by age 65. The apices of the arytenoids, the epiglottis, and the corniculate and cuneiform cartilages are elastic fibrocartilage and usually do not calcify.

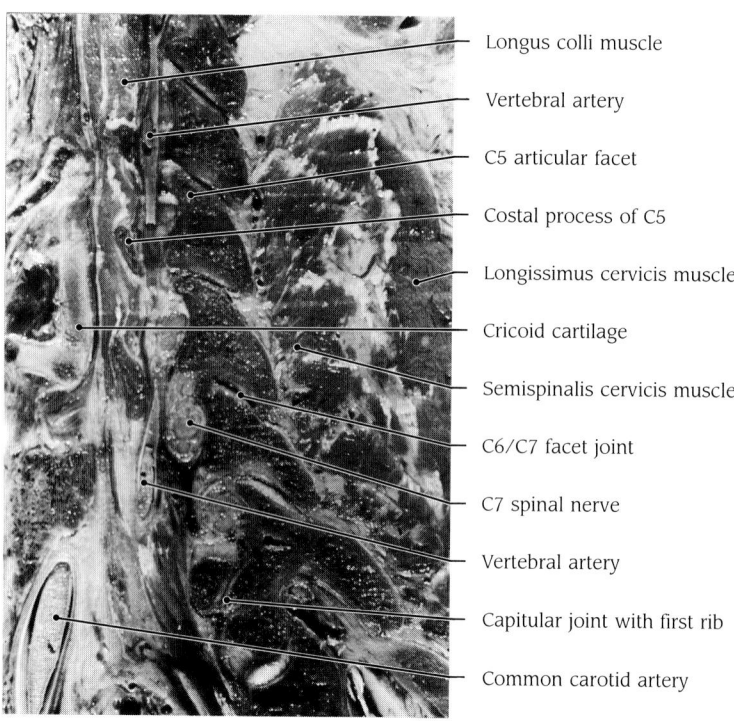

FIG. 9.15.

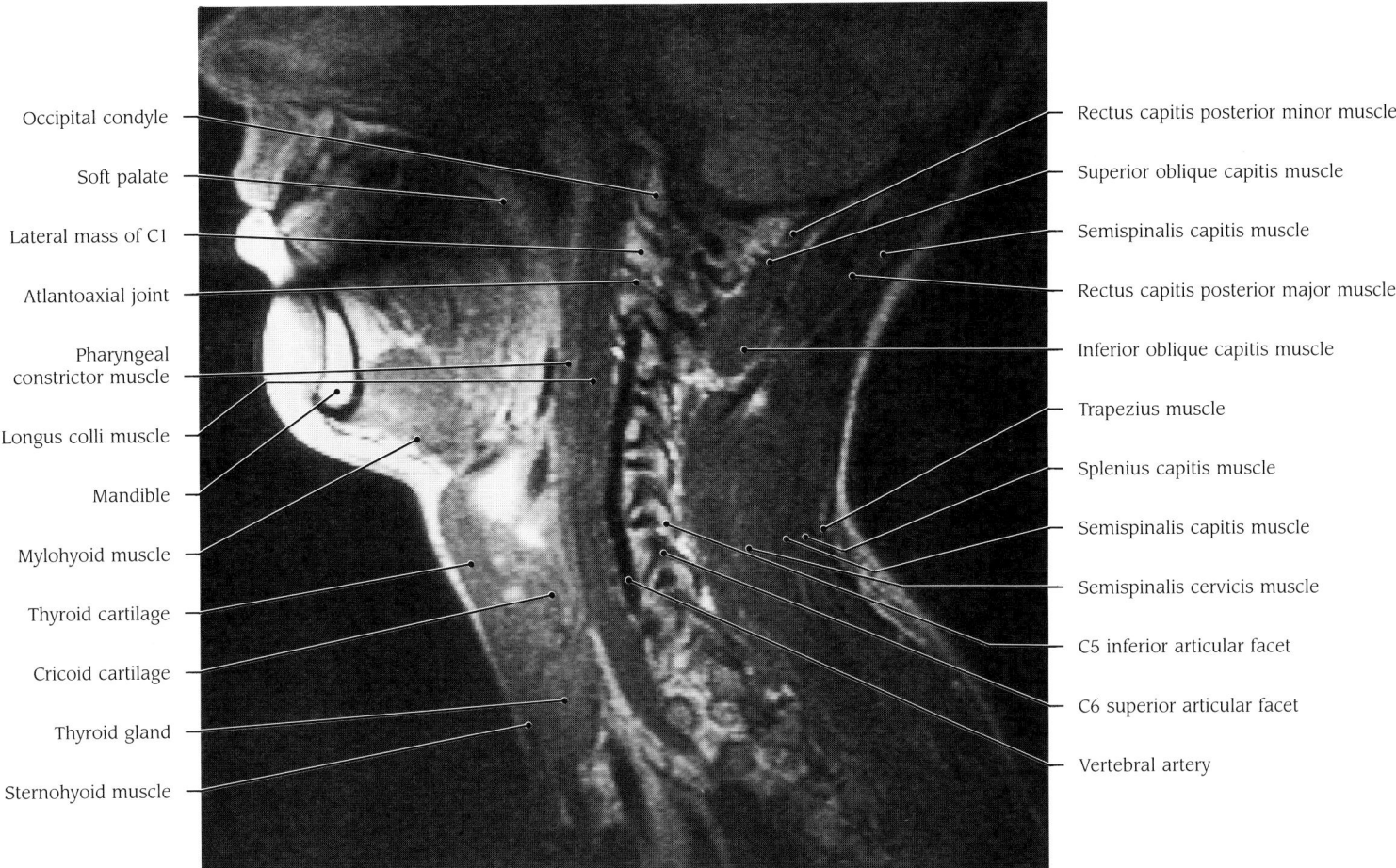

FIG. 9.16. TR = 739 msec, TE = 39 msec.

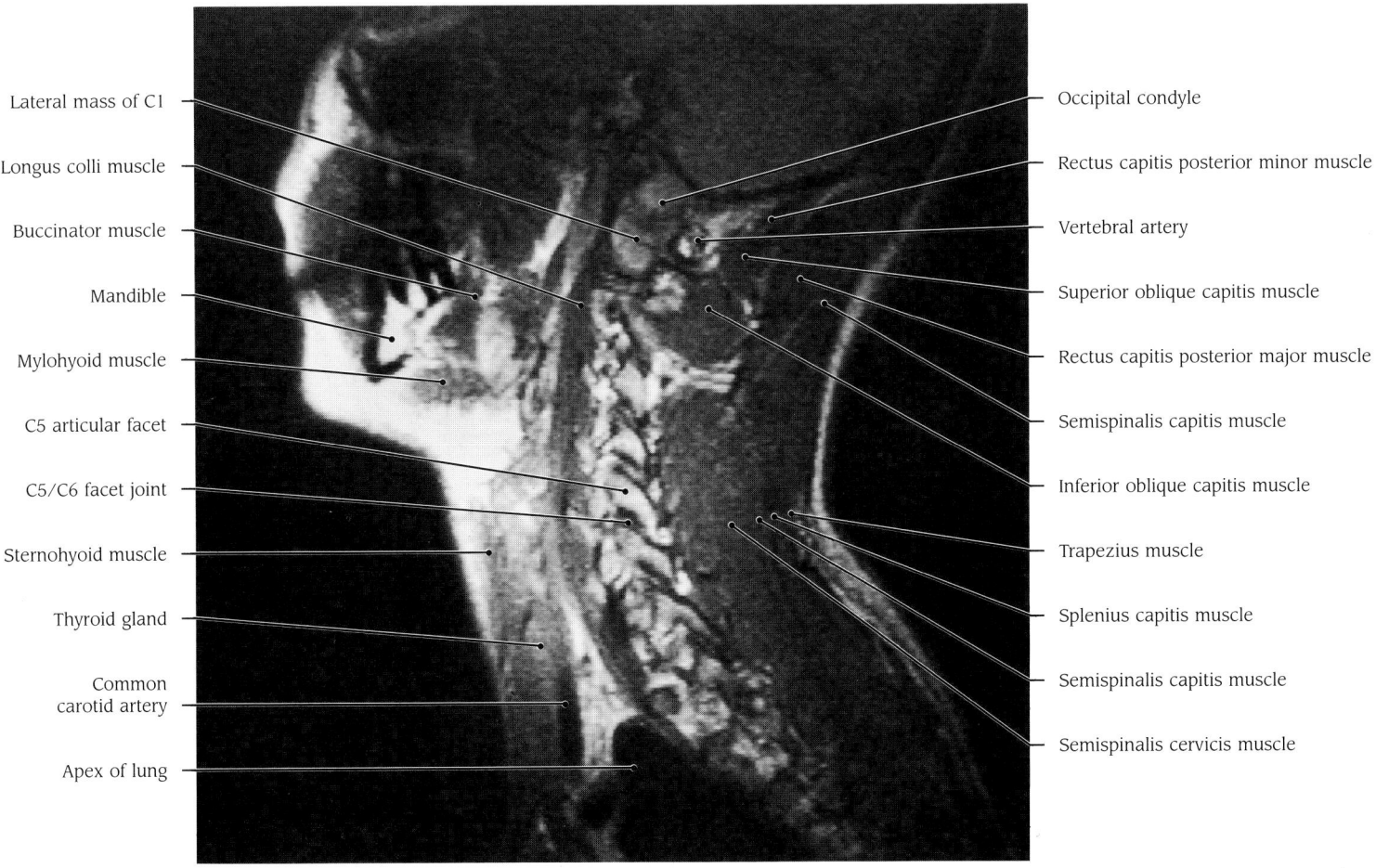

FIG. 9.17. TR = 739 msec, TE = 39 msec.

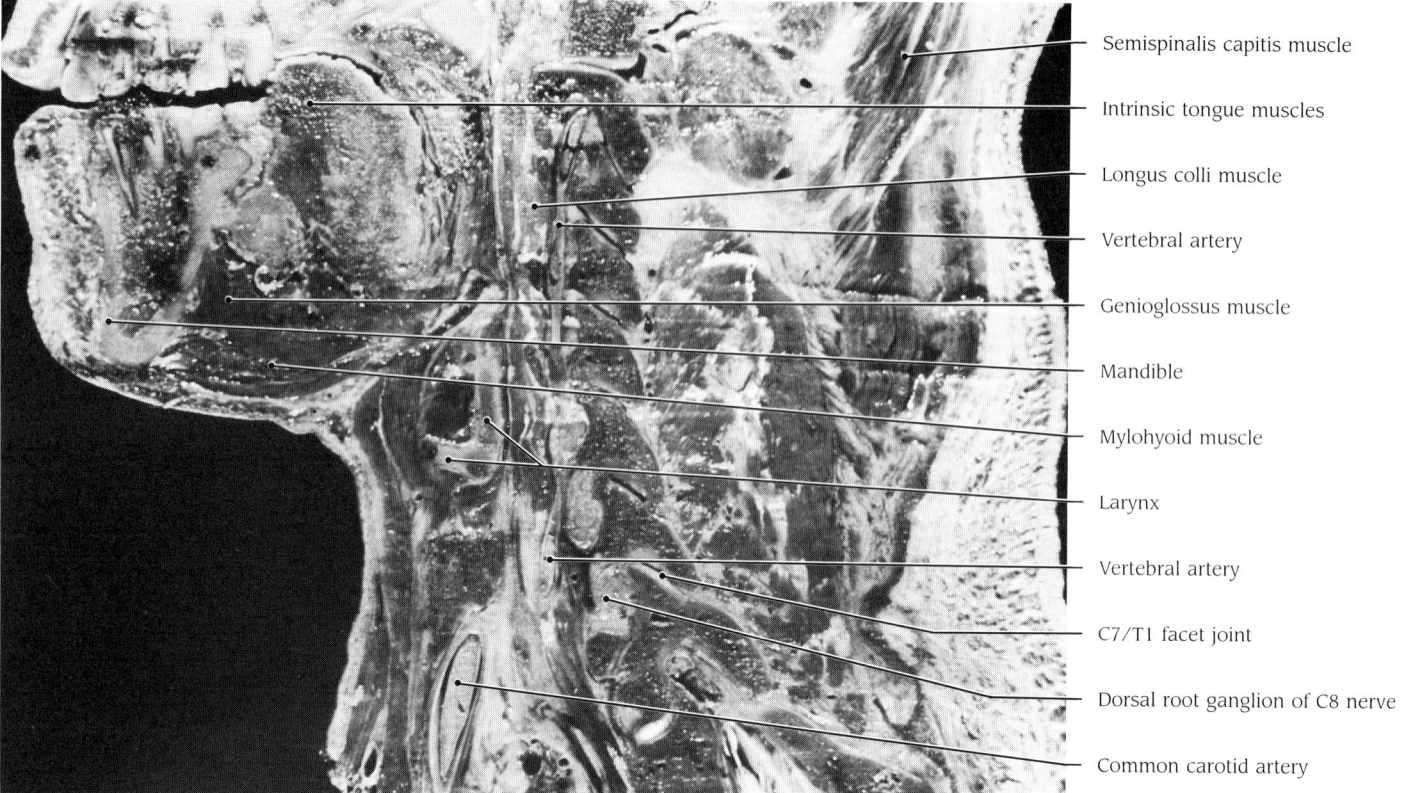

FIG. 9.18.

- The submandibular gland is an irregularly shaped salivary gland approximately the size of a walnut. It is divided into superficial and deep parts. The superficial portion is in the digastric triangle, and extends ventrally to the anterior belly of the digastric muscle and posteriorly to the stylomandibular ligament. The deep portion extends anteriorly to the sublingual gland between the mylohyoid muscle laterally and the hyoglossus and styloglossus muscles medially.

- The submandibular duct originates from many branches in the superficial region of the gland and emerges from the deep surface of the gland near the posterior edge of the mylohyoid muscle. It then traverses the deep portion of the gland and continues between the mylohyoid and the hyoglossus muscles. This duct runs between the sublingual gland and the genioglossus muscle and opens in the floor of the mouth at the side of the frenulum of the tongue.

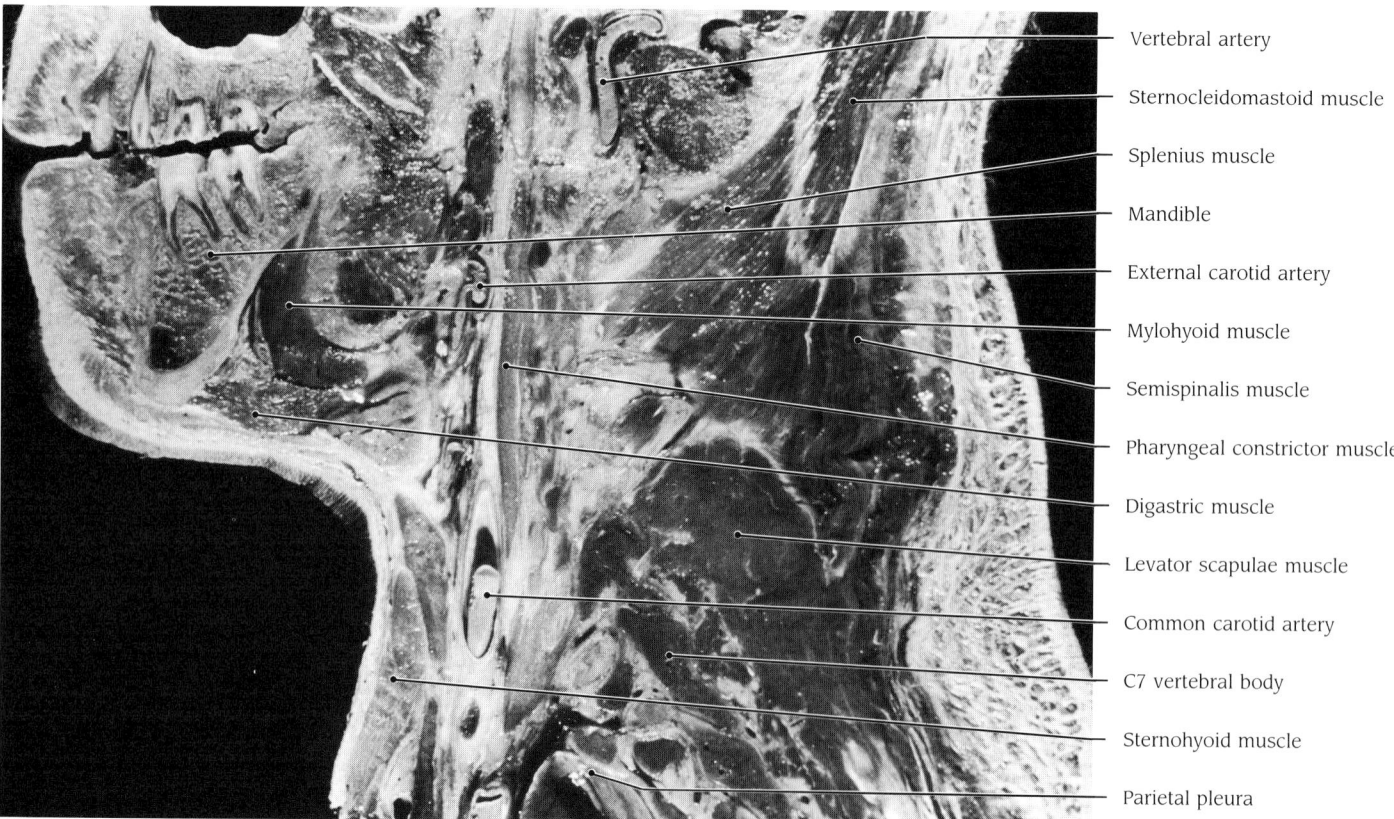

FIG. 9.19.

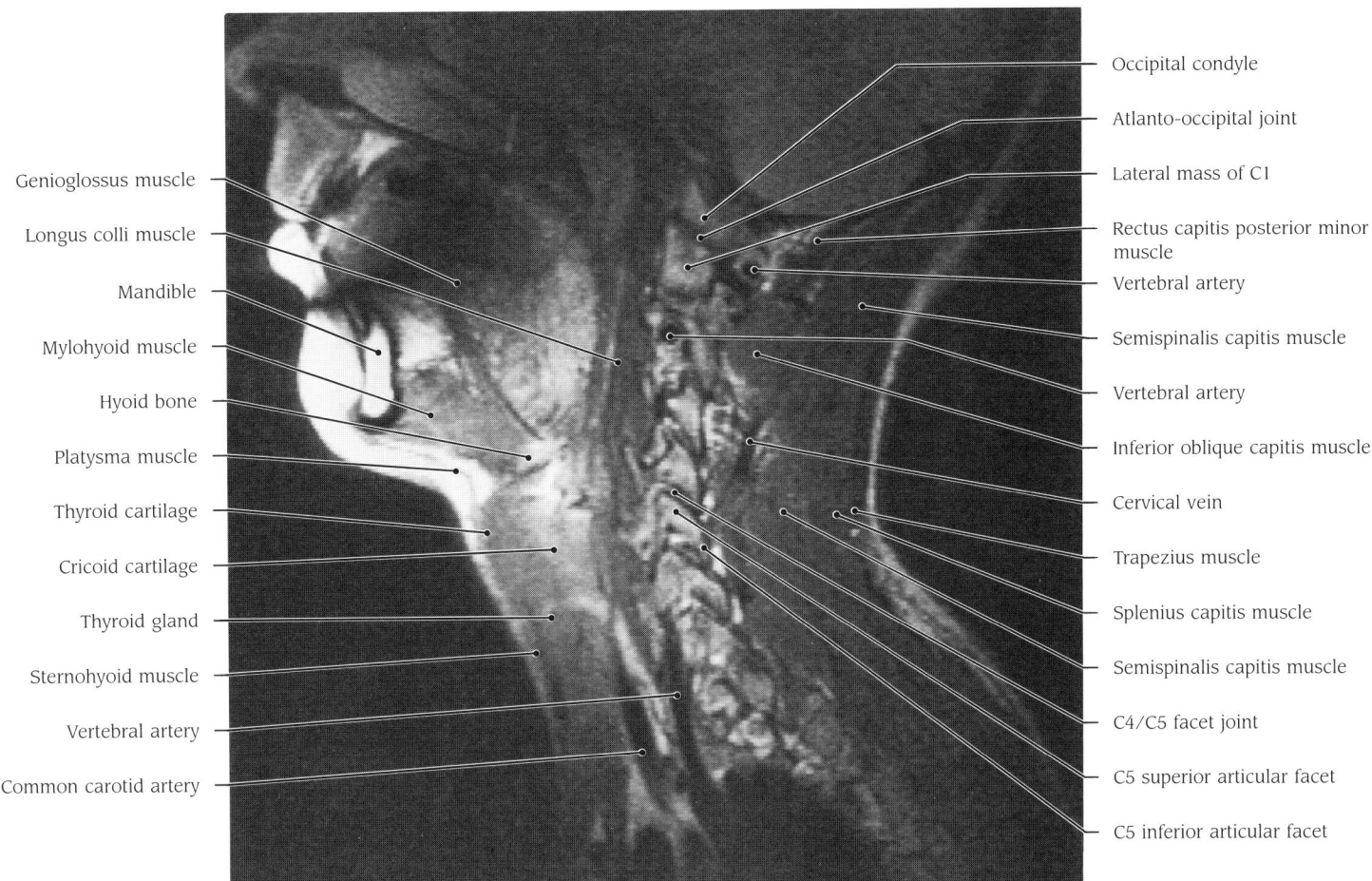

FIG. 9.20. TR = 739 msec, TE = 39 msec.

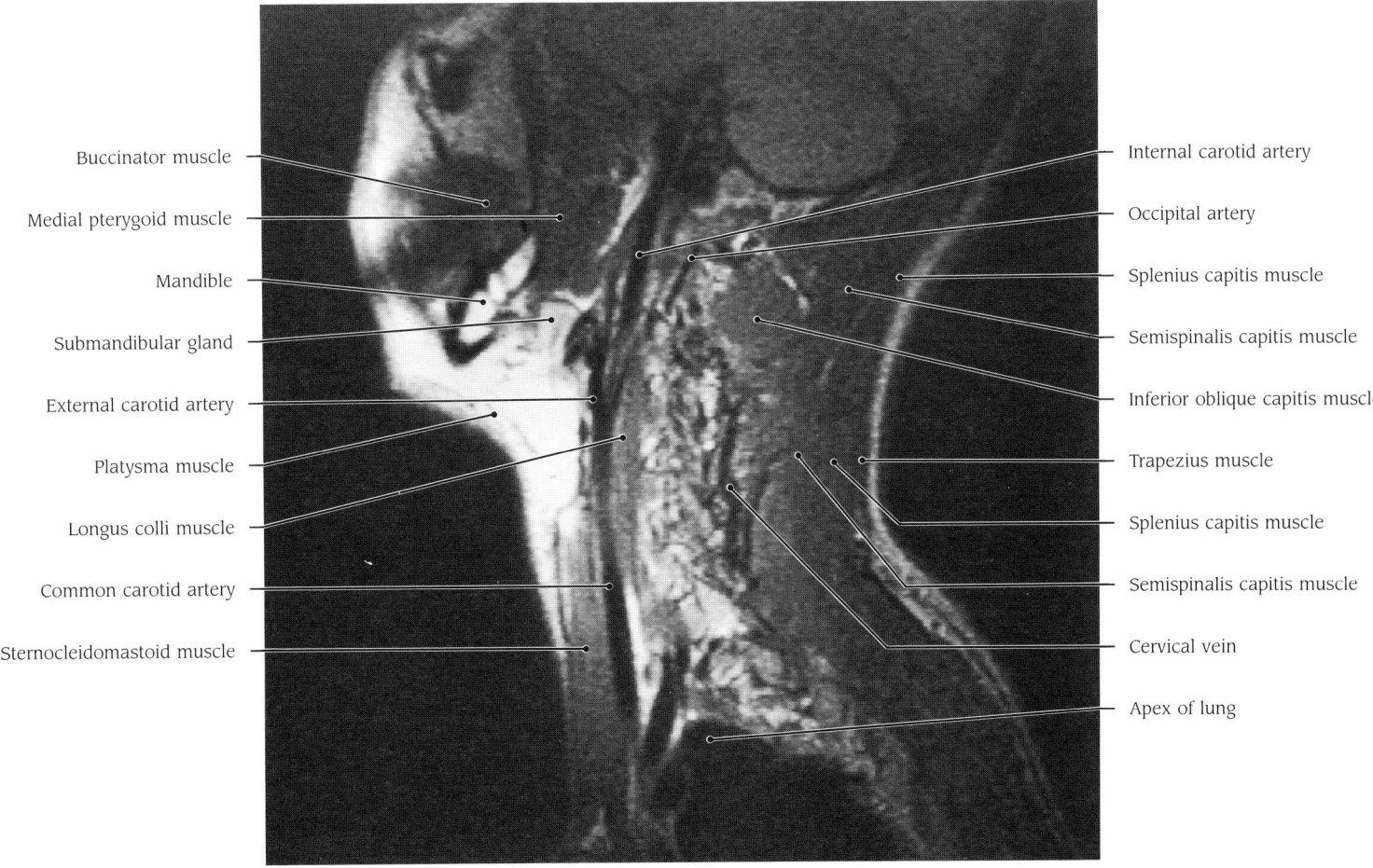

FIG. 9.21. TR = 739 msec, TE = 39 msec.

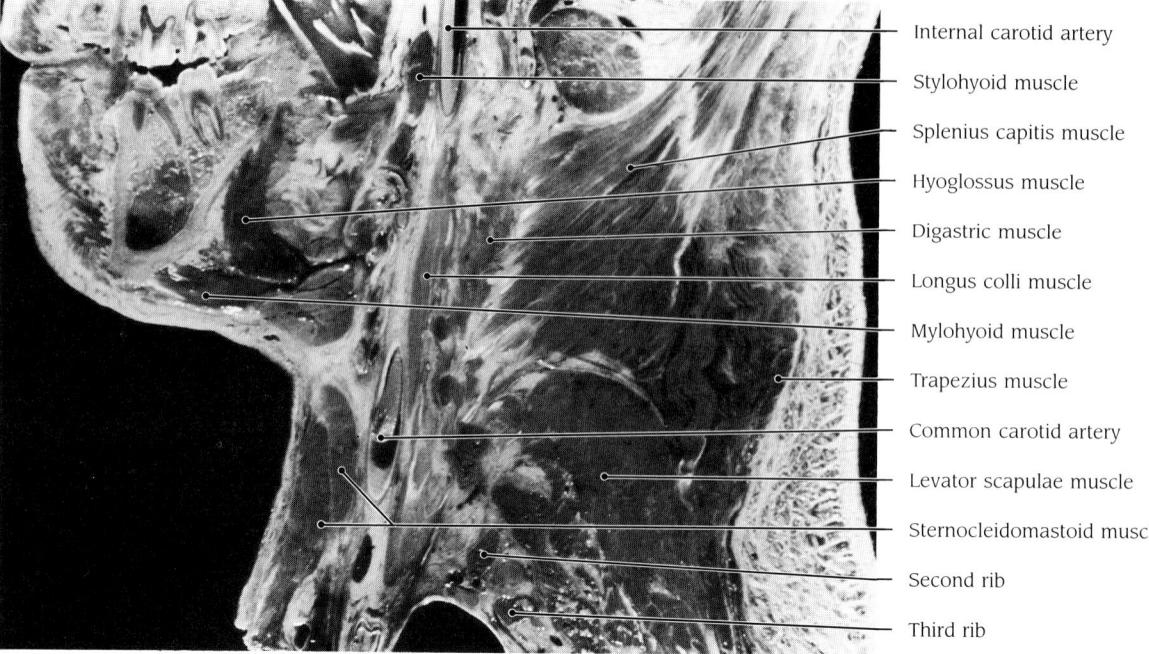

FIG. 9.22.

- The sternocleidomastoid muscle passes obliquely across the neck to divide the neck into two triangles, the anterior and posterior triangles. The anterior triangle is bounded anteriorly by the anterior median line of the neck, superiorly by the base of the mandible and a line from the angle of the mandible to the mastoid process, posteriorly by the anterior aspect of the sternocleidomastoid muscle, and inferiorly by the sternum. The posterior triangle is bounded anteriorly by the posterior aspect of the sternocleidomastoid muscle, inferiorly by the middle one third of the clavicle, posteriorly by the anterior margin of the trapezius muscle, and superiorly by the occipital bone between the sternocleidomastoid and the trapezius muscles.

- The anterior triangle may be subdivided into the muscular, carotid, digastric, and submental triangles. The muscular triangle is defined posteroinferiorly by the anterior margin of the sternocleidomastoid muscle, posterosuperiorly by the superior belly of the omohyoid muscle, and anteriorly by the anterior median line of the neck from the hyoid bone to the sternum. The carotid triangle is delimited posteriorly by the sternocleidomastoid muscle, anteroinferiorly by the superior belly of the omohyoid muscle, and superiorly by the stylohyoid muscle and the posterior belly of the digastric muscle. The digastric triangle is bounded superiorly by the base of the mandible and a line drawn from the angle of the mandible to the mastoid process, posteroinferiorly by the posterior belly of the digastric and the stylohyoid muscles, and anteroinferiorly by the anterior belly of the digastric muscle. The submental triangle is delimited laterally on each side by the anterior belly of the digastric muscle, superiorly by the mandible, and inferiorly by the hyoid bone and mylohyoid muscle.

- The posterior triangle may be subdivided into the occipital and supraclavicular triangles. The occipital triangle is bordered anteriorly by the sternocleidomastoid muscle, posteriorly by the trapezius muscle, and inferiorly by the inferior belly of the omohyoid muscle. The supraclavicular triangle is defined superiorly by the inferior belly of the omohyoid muscle, inferiorly by the clavicle, and anteriorly by the sternocleidomastoid muscle.

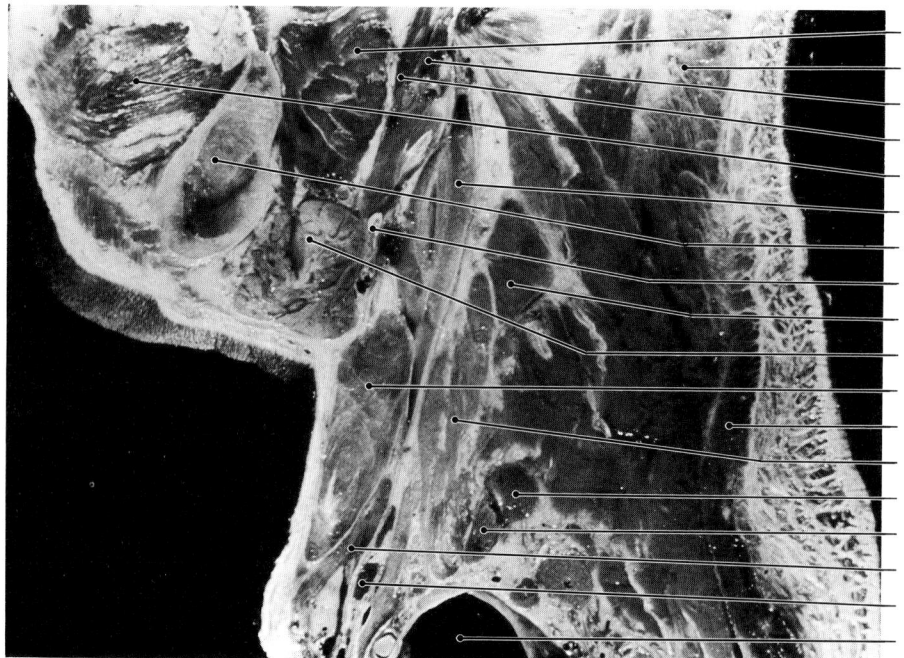

FIG. 9.23.

10

Thoracic Spine

Anatomic Level	Figures
Thoracic spine, axial series	10.1–10.22
Thoracic spine, coronal series	10.23–10.57
Thoracic spine, sagittal series	10.58–10.89

Sections from the thoracic spine of cadavers are shown in the axial, coronal, and sagittal planes. These sections are matched with corresponding magnetic resonance images of a normal volunteer. Additional anatomic sections and detailed views of the bony skeleton are included for clarification at some levels. The effect of the pulsatile motion of cerebrospinal fluid, which produces low signal intensity artifacts, is evident, particularly in the axial and sagittal planes.

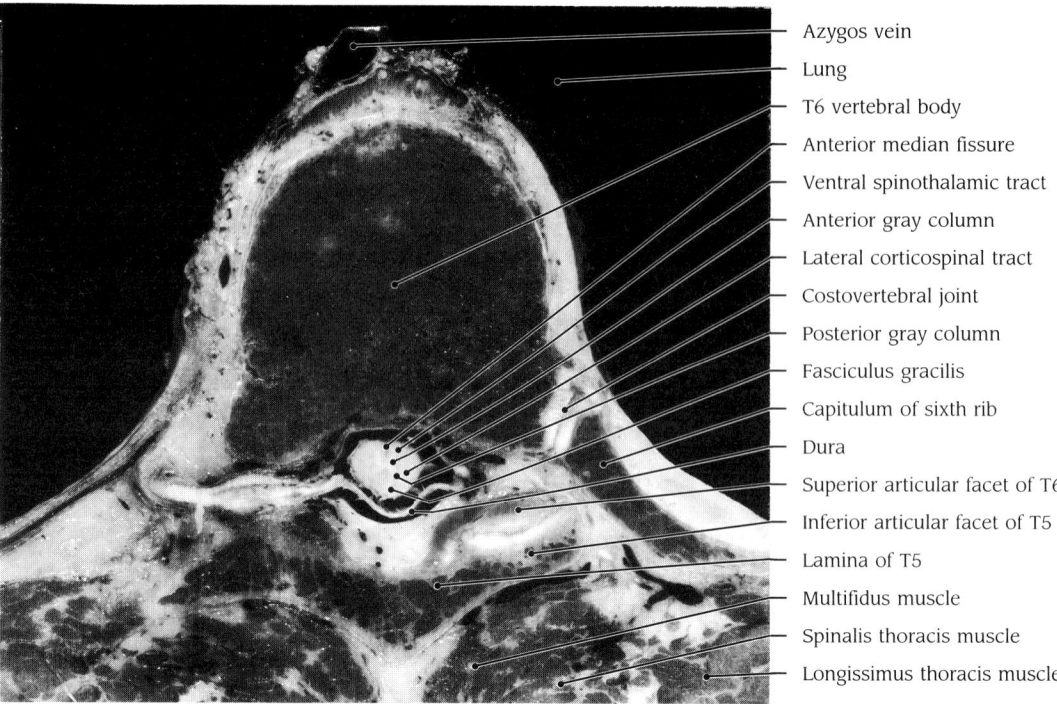

FIG. 10.1.

- The origin of the azygos vein is variable, although developmentally this vein should originate from the posterior aspect of the inferior vena cava at or inferior to the renal veins. At the T12 level, the lumbar azygos vein is joined by a prominent vessel formed by the right ascending lumbar and right subcostal veins. This common trunk may form the azygos vein if the lumbar azygos vein is absent. The azygos vein ascends in the posterior mediastinum to the level of the fourth thoracic vertebra, where it arches anteriorly, superior to the root of the right lung, and ends in the superior vena cava.

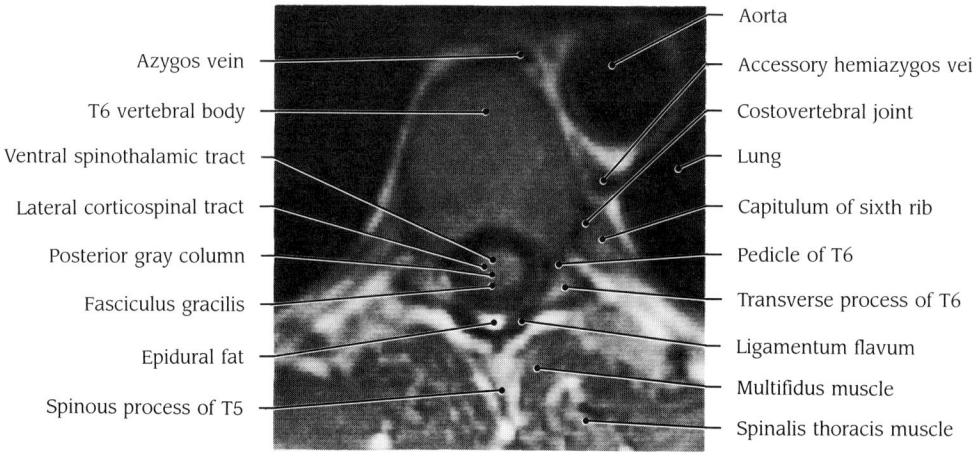

FIG. 10.2. TR = 537 msec, TE = 37 msec.

FIG. 10.3. TR = 5000 msec, TE = 64 msec.

218

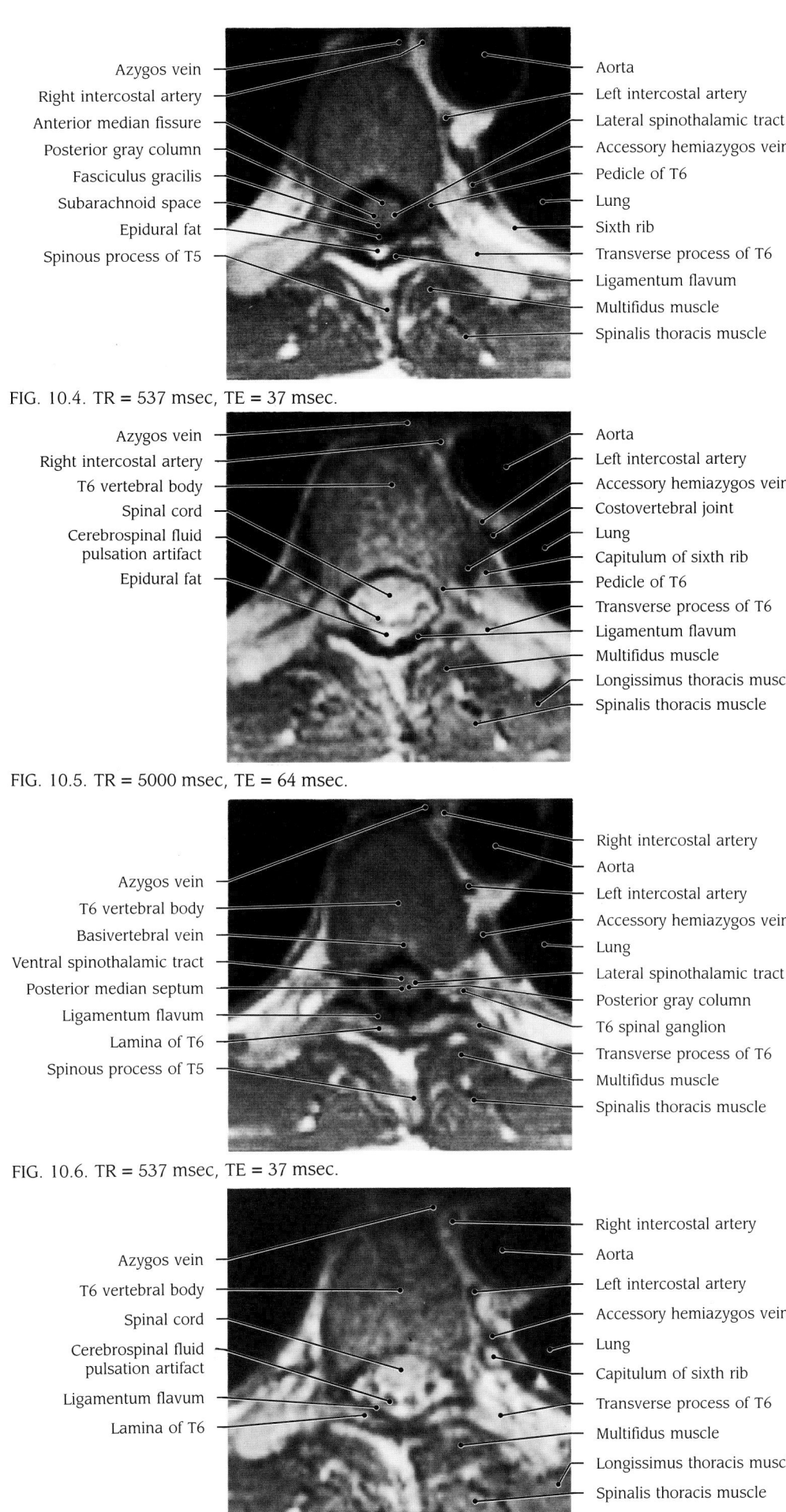

FIG. 10.4. TR = 537 msec, TE = 37 msec.

FIG. 10.5. TR = 5000 msec, TE = 64 msec.

FIG. 10.6. TR = 537 msec, TE = 37 msec.

FIG. 10.7. TR = 5000 msec, TE = 64 msec.

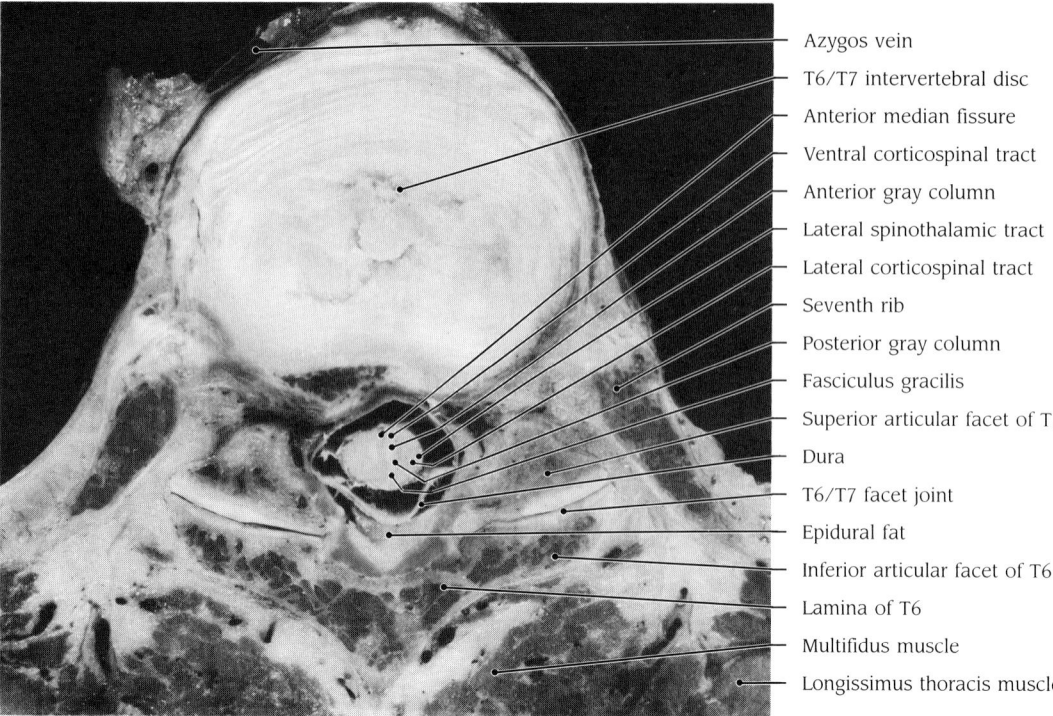

FIG. 10.8.

- The hemiazygos vein originates on the left, similar to the azygos vein on the right, from the union of the left lumbar azygos vein, the left ascending lumbar vein, and the left subcostal vein. It ascends along the anterior aspect of the vertebral column to the level of the eighth thoracic vertebra, where it crosses posterior to the aorta, esophagus, and thoracic duct to end in the azygos vein.

- The accessory hemiazygos vein is on the left side of the thoracic vertebrae, above the hemiazygos vein. After crossing the body of the seventh thoracic vertebra, the accessory hemiazygos vein joins the azygos vein. The accessory hemiazygos vein may join the hemiazygos vein to form a common trunk, which communicates with the azygos vein.

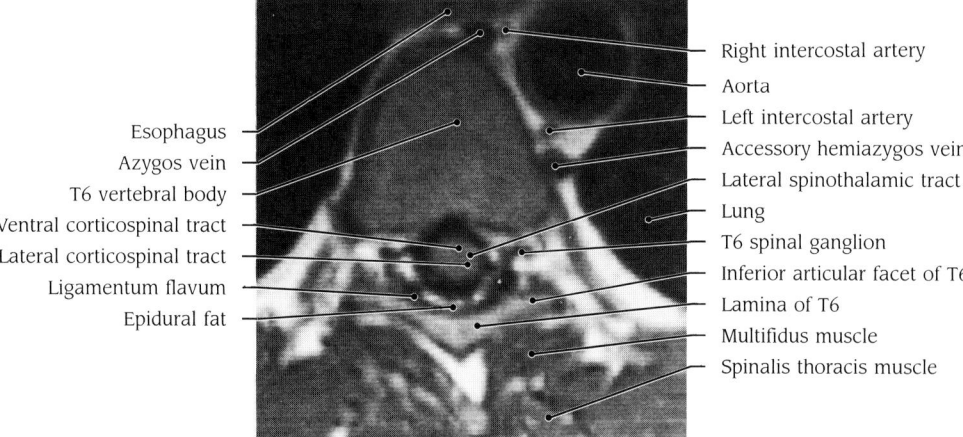

FIG. 10.9. TR = 537 msec, TE = 37 msec.

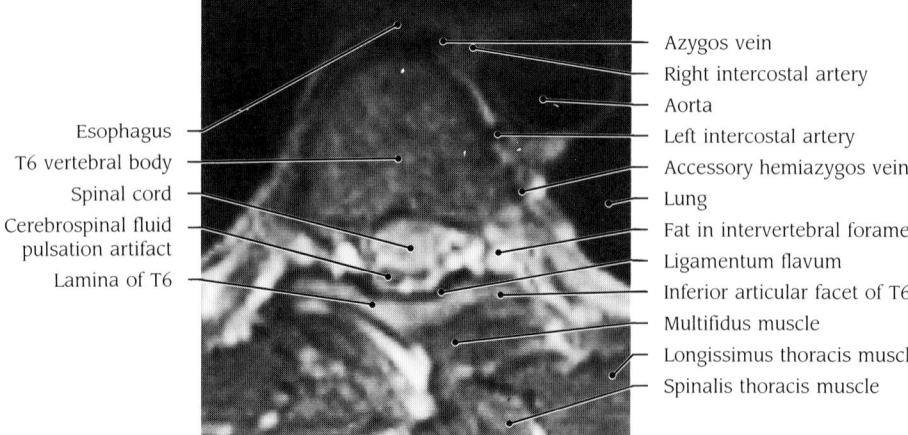

FIG. 10.10. TR = 5000 msec, TE = 64 msec.

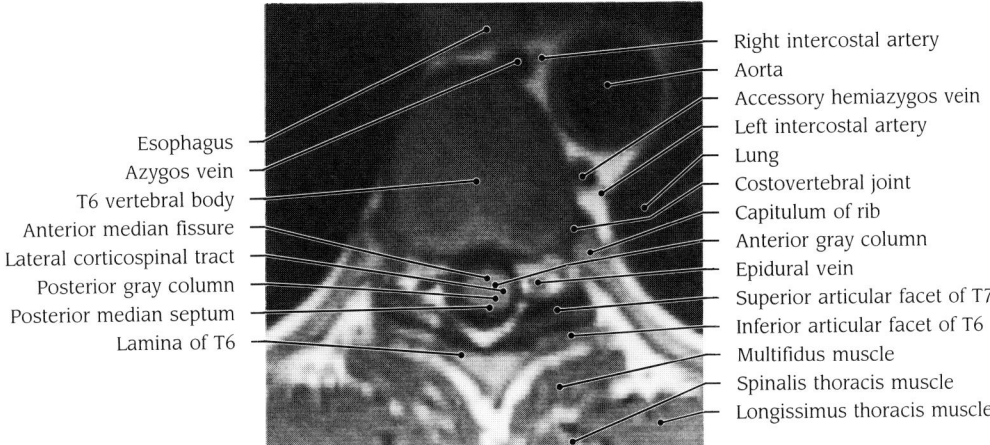

FIG. 10.11. TR = 537 msec, TE = 37 msec.

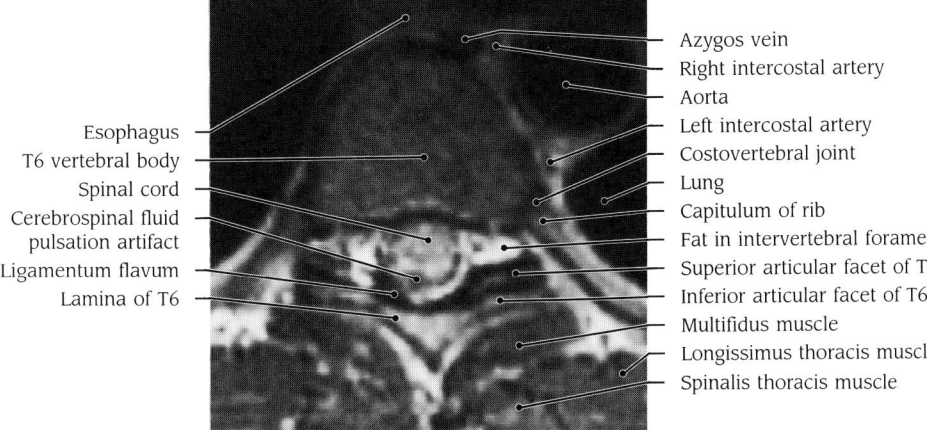

FIG. 10.12. TR = 5000 msec, TE = 64 msec.

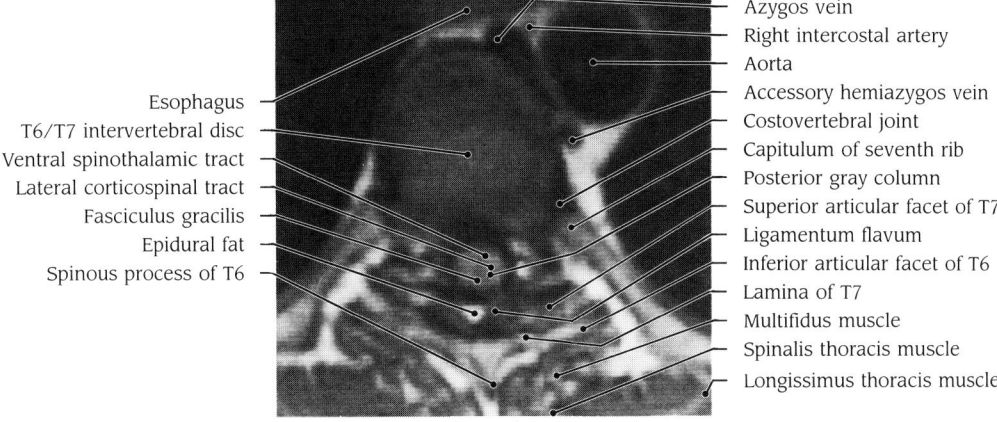

FIG. 10.13. TR = 537 msec, TE = 37 msec.

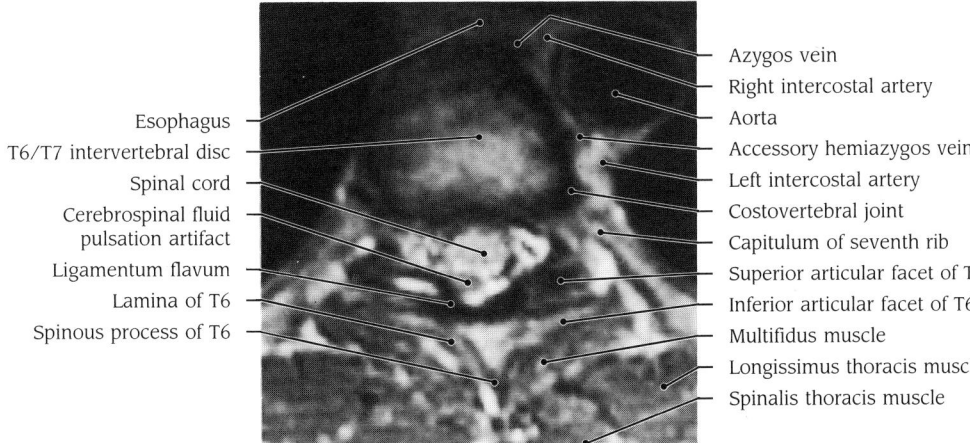

FIG. 10.14. TR = 5000 msec, TE = 64 msec.

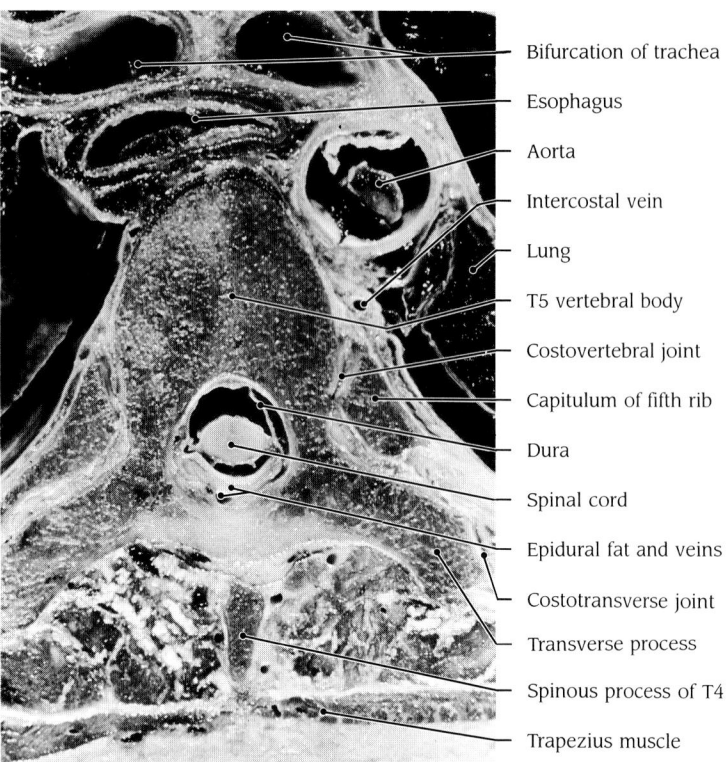

FIG. 10.15.

- The anterior median fissure and posterior median sulcus and septum divide the spinal cord almost completely into symmetric right and left halves, which are joined in the midline by a commissural band of tissue. The anterior median fissure extends approximately 3 mm into the ventral surface of the spinal cord to the anterior white commissure. The posterior median sulcus is not as deep as the anterior median fissure; however, a posterior median septum of neuroglia extends into the cord almost to the central canal.

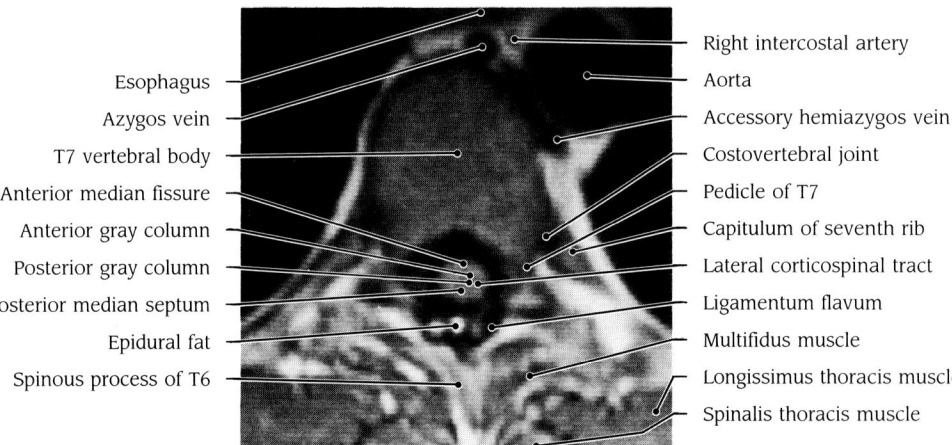

FIG. 10.16. TR = 537 msec, TE = 37 msec.

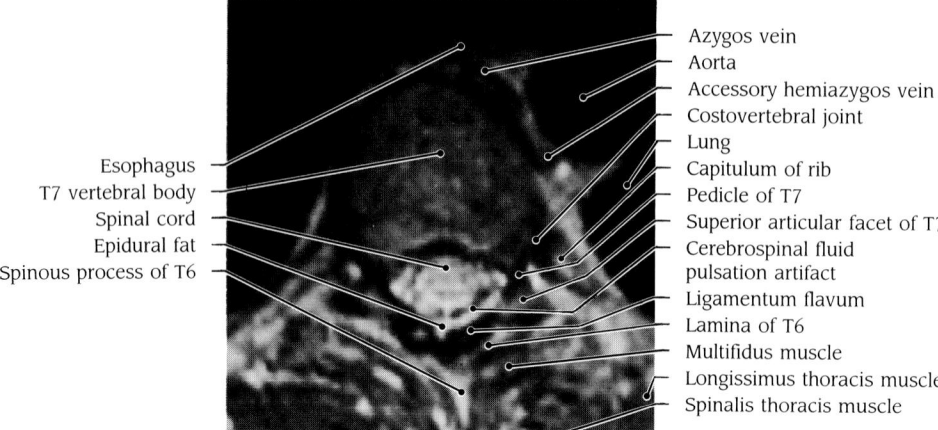

FIG. 10.17. TR = 5000 msec, TE = 64 msec.

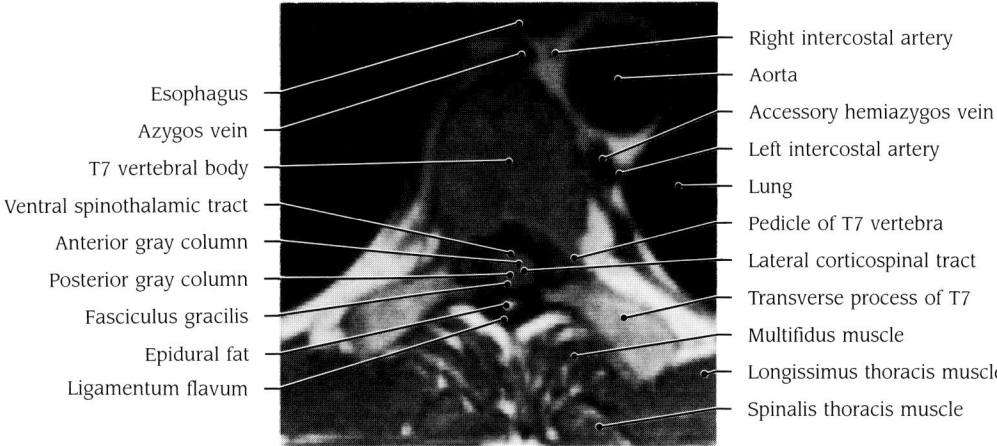

FIG. 10.18. TR = 537 msec, TE = 37 msec.

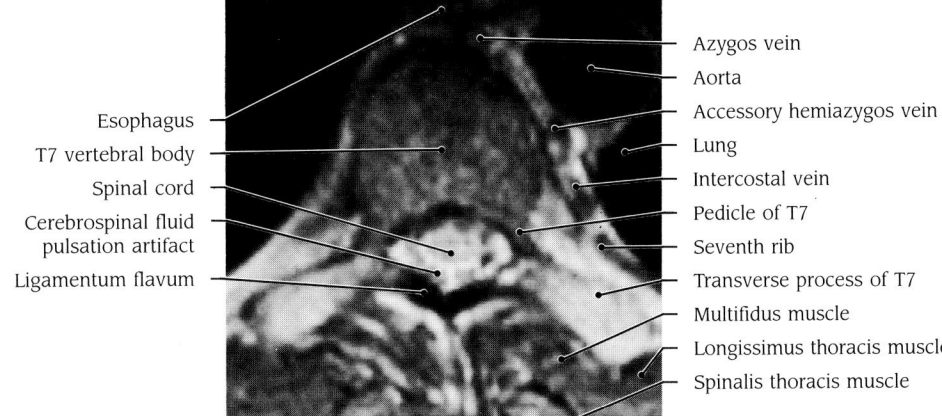

FIG. 10.19. TR = 5000 msec, TE = 64 msec.

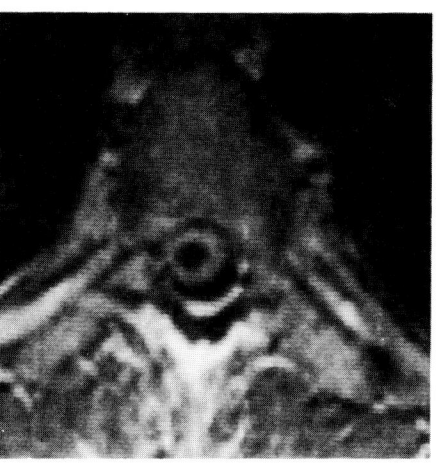

FIG. 10.20. TR = 539 msec, TE = 39 msec. A low signal intensity syrinx is present within the thoracic spinal cord.

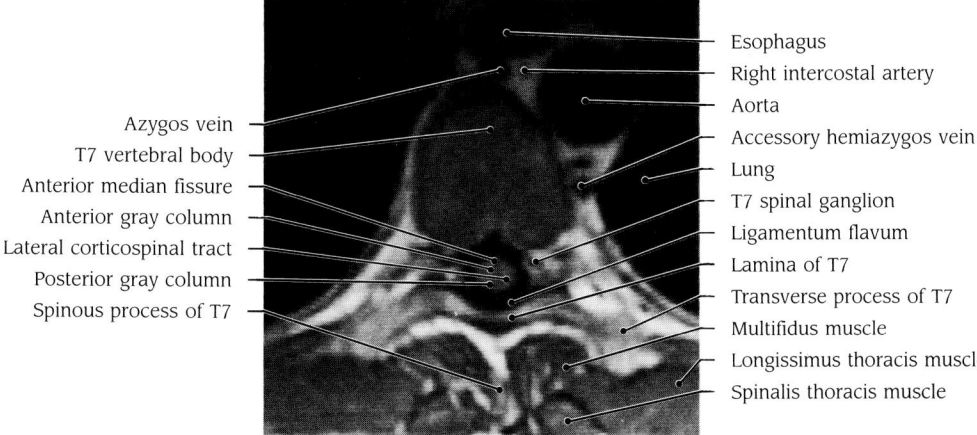

FIG. 10.21. TR = 537 msec, TE = 37 msec.

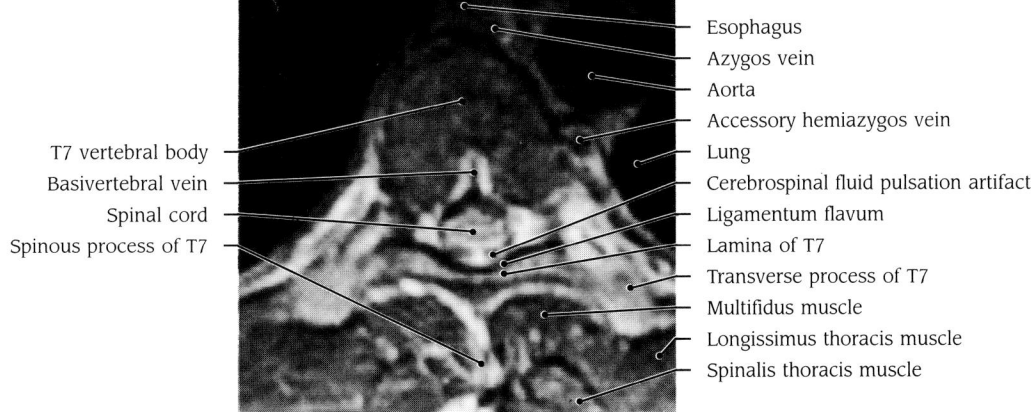

FIG. 10.22. TR = 5000 msec, TE = 64 msec.

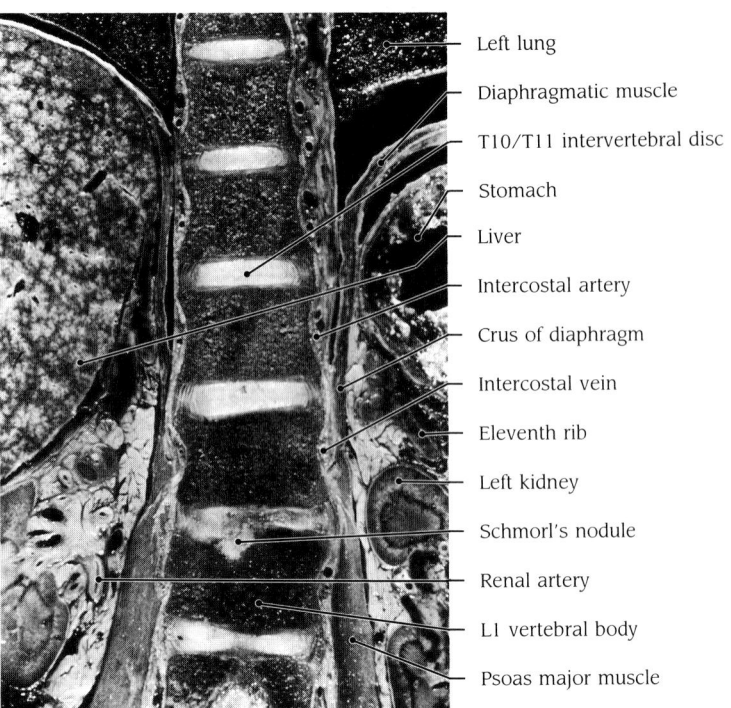

FIG. 10.23.

- The thoracic vertebrae gradually increase in size from superior to inferior, as seen in the cervical and lumbar areas, because of the increasing weight that must be supported. The thoracic vertebral foramen, or canal, is relatively small and circular. This configuration results because the pedicles are relatively parallel, rather than diverging as in the cervical spine, and the lamina are short, thick, and broad.

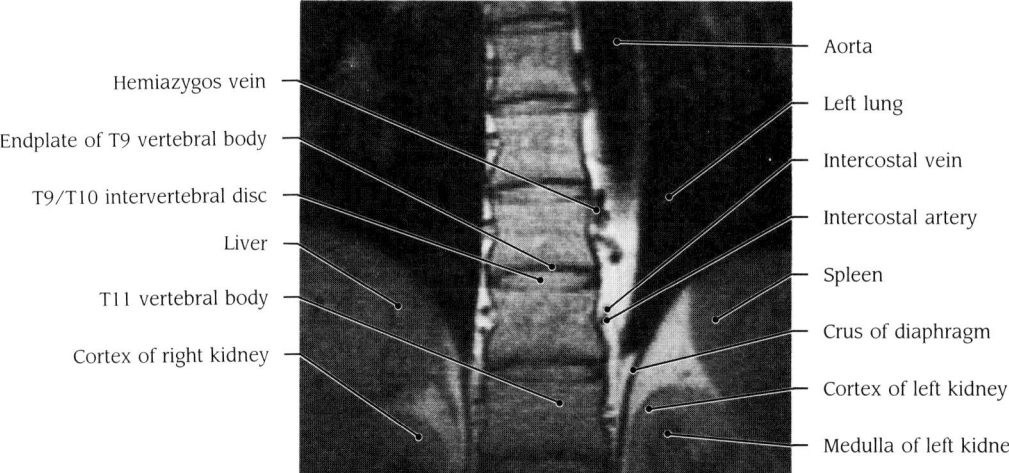

FIG. 10.24. TR = 737 msec, TE = 37 msec.

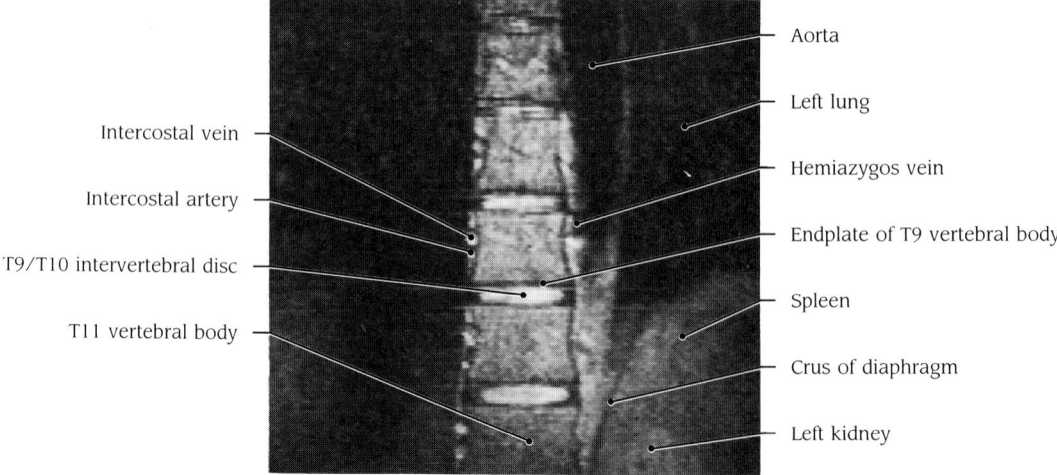

FIG. 10.25. TR = 5000 msec, TE = 64 msec.

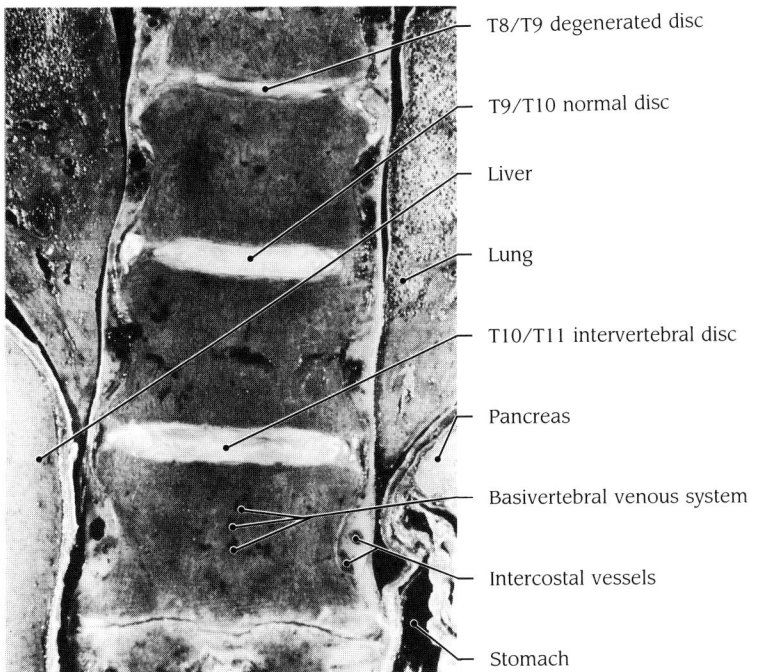

FIG. 10.26.

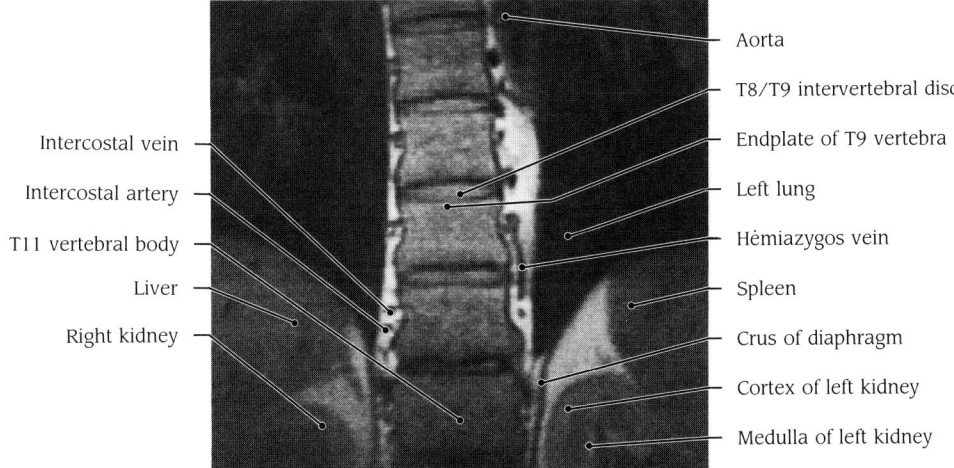

FIG. 10.27. TR = 737 msec, TE = 37 msec.

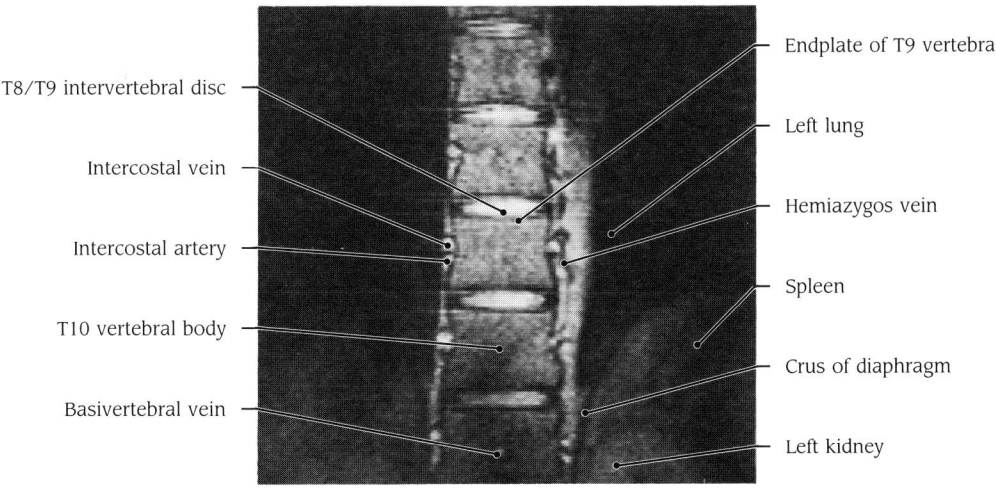

FIG. 10.28. TR = 5000 msec, TE = 64 msec.

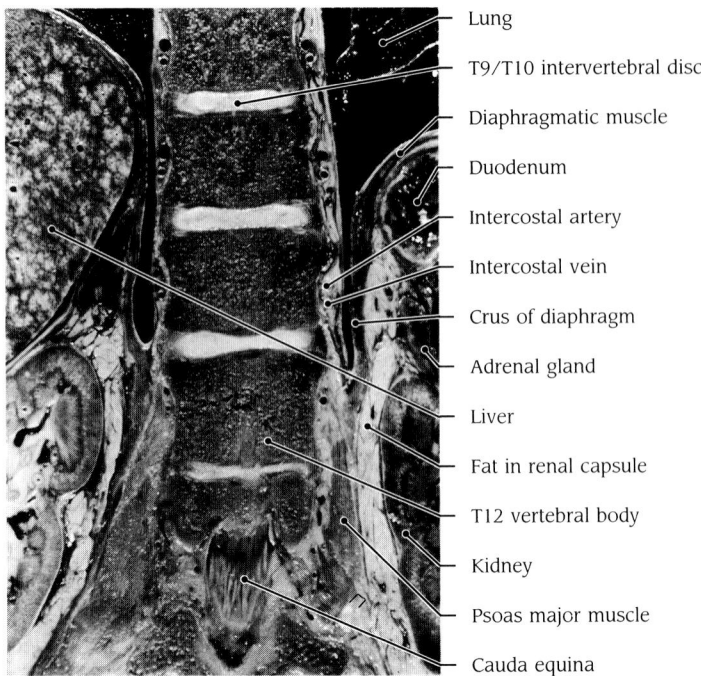

FIG. 10.29.

- The posterior longitudinal ligament is continuous with the membrana tectoria superiorly and extends from the body of the axis inferiorly to the sacrum. This ligament attaches to the intervertebral discs and to the vertebral bodies, and is separated by the basivertebral veins and the veins that drain into the anterior internal vertebral plexus. The posterior longitudinal ligament is broad and almost uniform in width in the cervical and upper thoracic regions; however, in the lower thoracic and lumbar spine, it is narrow over the vertebral bodies and wide over the discs. The posterior longitudinal ligament is composed of superficial fibers that extend between three or four vertebrae and deep fibers that extend between adjacent vertebrae.

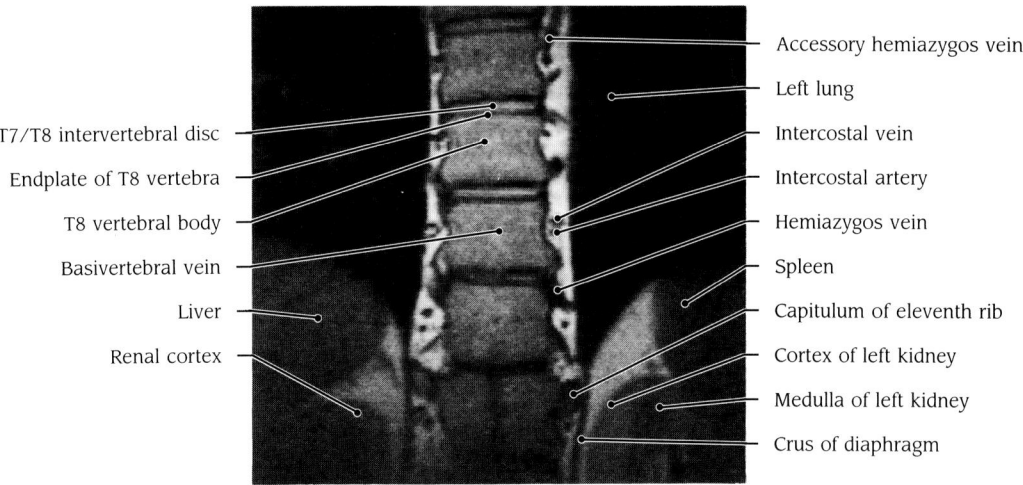

FIG. 10.30. TR = 737 msec, TE = 37 msec.

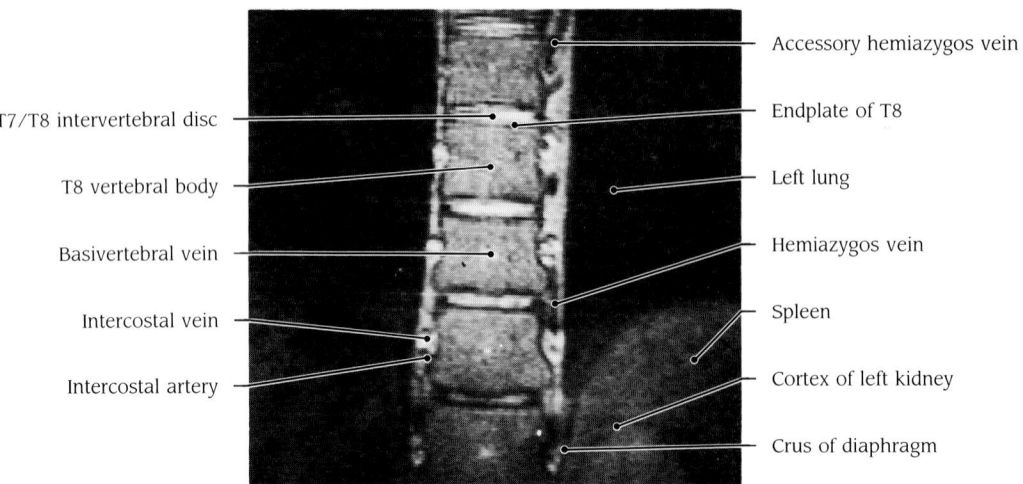

FIG. 10.31. TR = 5000 msec, TE = 64 msec.

226

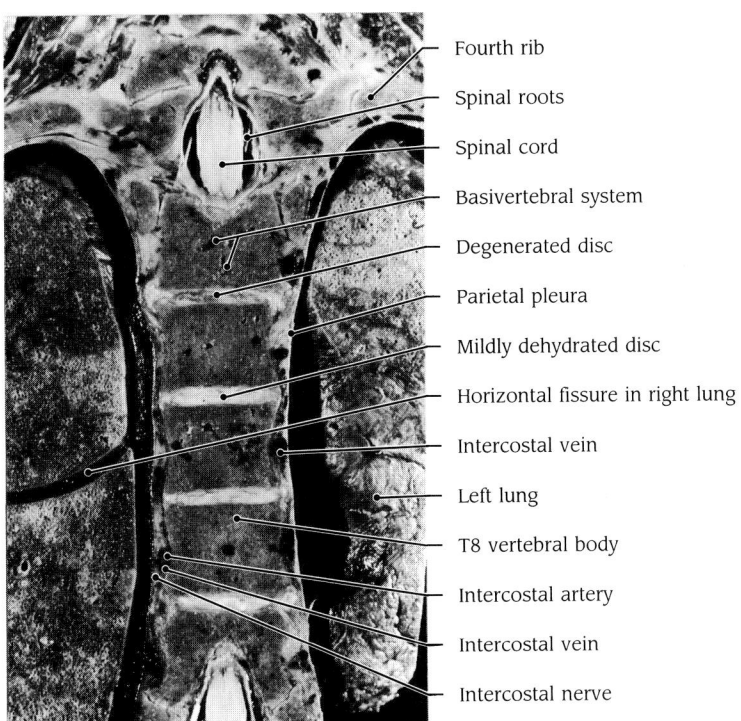

FIG. 10.32.

- Fourth rib
- Spinal roots
- Spinal cord
- Basivertebral system
- Degenerated disc
- Parietal pleura
- Mildly dehydrated disc
- Horizontal fissure in right lung
- Intercostal vein
- Left lung
- T8 vertebral body
- Intercostal artery
- Intercostal vein
- Intercostal nerve

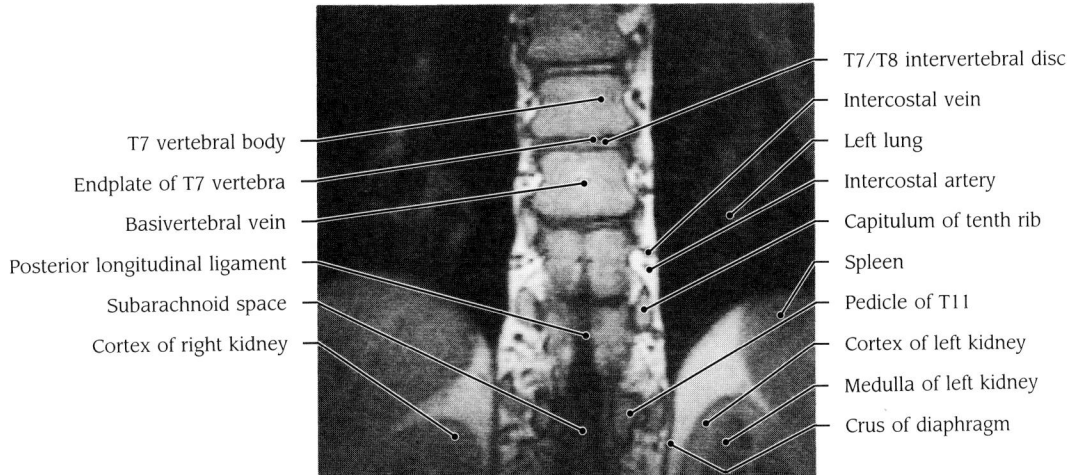

FIG. 10.33. TR = 737 msec, TE = 37 msec.

- T7 vertebral body
- Endplate of T7 vertebra
- Basivertebral vein
- Posterior longitudinal ligament
- Subarachnoid space
- Cortex of right kidney
- T7/T8 intervertebral disc
- Intercostal vein
- Left lung
- Intercostal artery
- Capitulum of tenth rib
- Spleen
- Pedicle of T11
- Cortex of left kidney
- Medulla of left kidney
- Crus of diaphragm

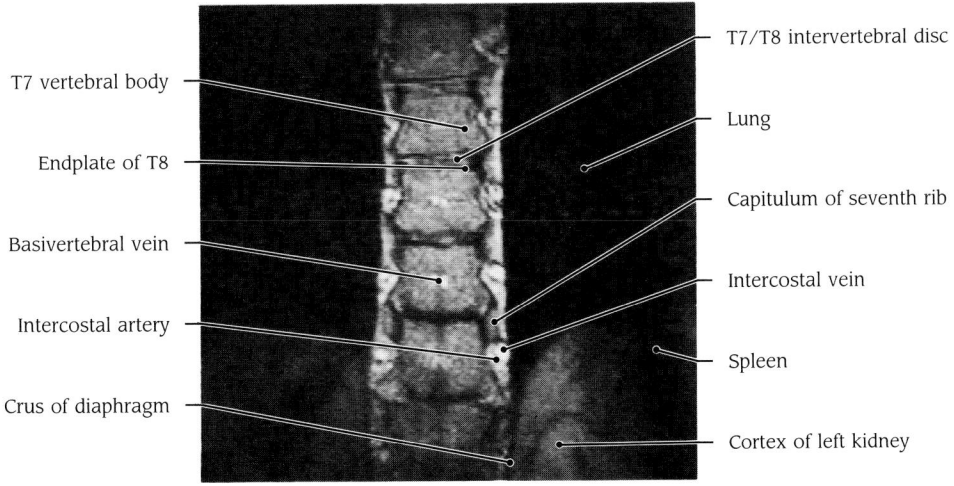

FIG. 10.34. TR = 5000 msec, TE = 64 msec.

- T7 vertebral body
- Endplate of T8
- Basivertebral vein
- Intercostal artery
- Crus of diaphragm
- T7/T8 intervertebral disc
- Lung
- Capitulum of seventh rib
- Intercostal vein
- Spleen
- Cortex of left kidney

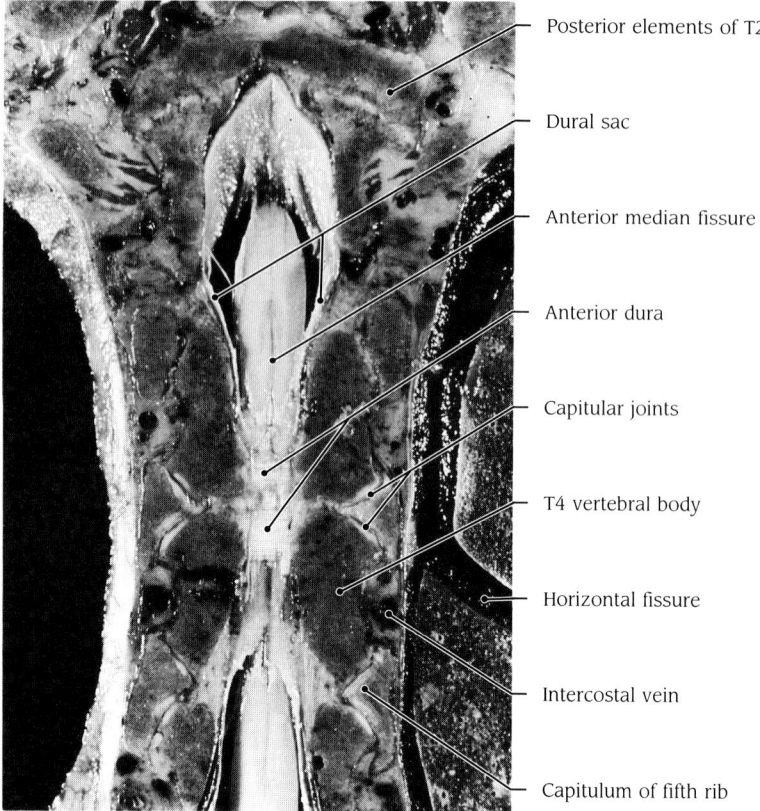

FIG. 10.35.

- Posterior elements of T2
- Dural sac
- Anterior median fissure
- Anterior dura
- Capitular joints
- T4 vertebral body
- Horizontal fissure
- Intercostal vein
- Capitulum of fifth rib

- There are two articulations of the ribs and the vertebral column. One connects the heads of the ribs with the vertebral bodies, and one is between the necks and tubercles of the ribs and the transverse processes.

- The articulations of the capitulae, or heads, of the ribs (shown here) are with facets on the margins of the vertebrae and with the intervertebral discs. The first, tenth, eleventh, and twelfth ribs each articulate with one vertebra. In the other joints, an intra-articular ligament separates the joint into two portions. The articulations at the first, tenth, eleventh, and twelfth ribs have capsular and radiate ligaments, whereas the other levels also have an intra-articular ligament.

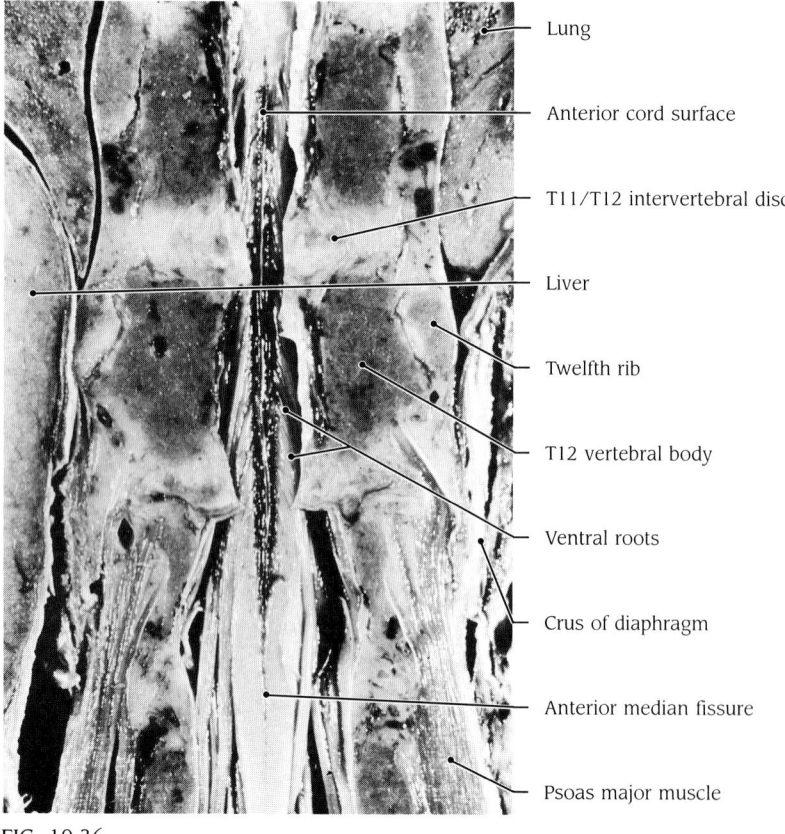

FIG. 10.36.

- Lung
- Anterior cord surface
- T11/T12 intervertebral disc
- Liver
- Twelfth rib
- T12 vertebral body
- Ventral roots
- Crus of diaphragm
- Anterior median fissure
- Psoas major muscle

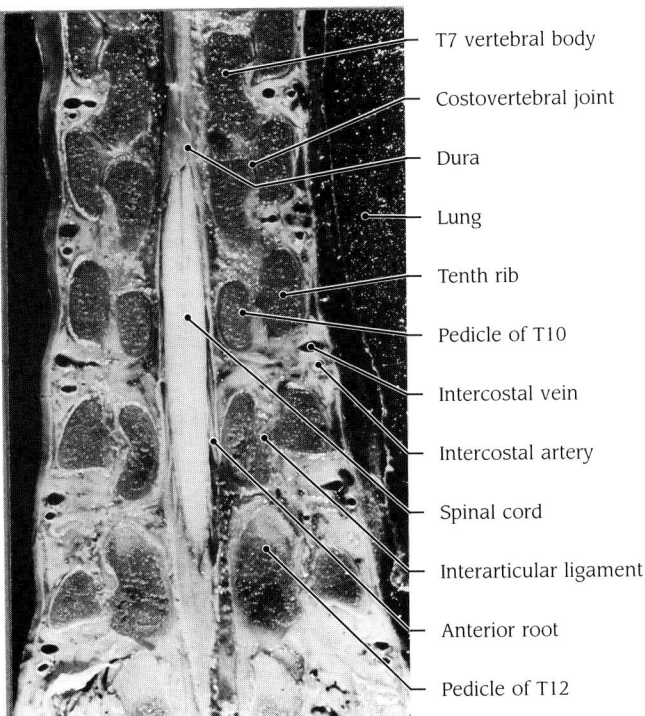

FIG. 10.37.

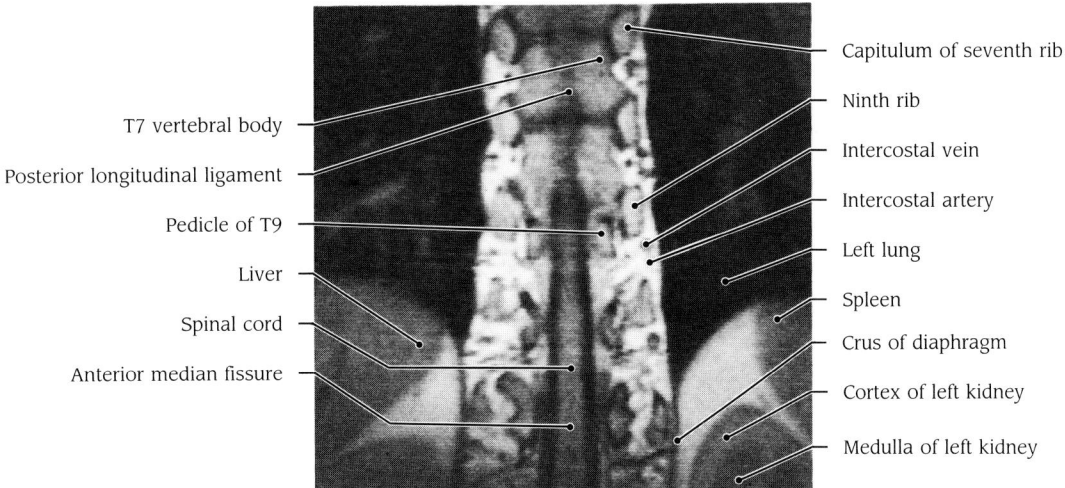

FIG. 10.38. TR = 737 msec, TE = 37 msec.

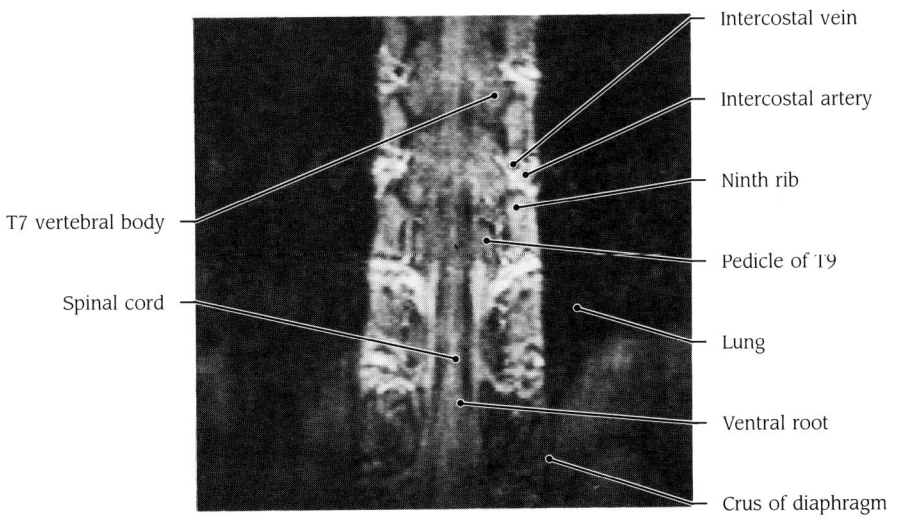

FIG. 10.39. TR = 5000 msec, TE = 64 msec.

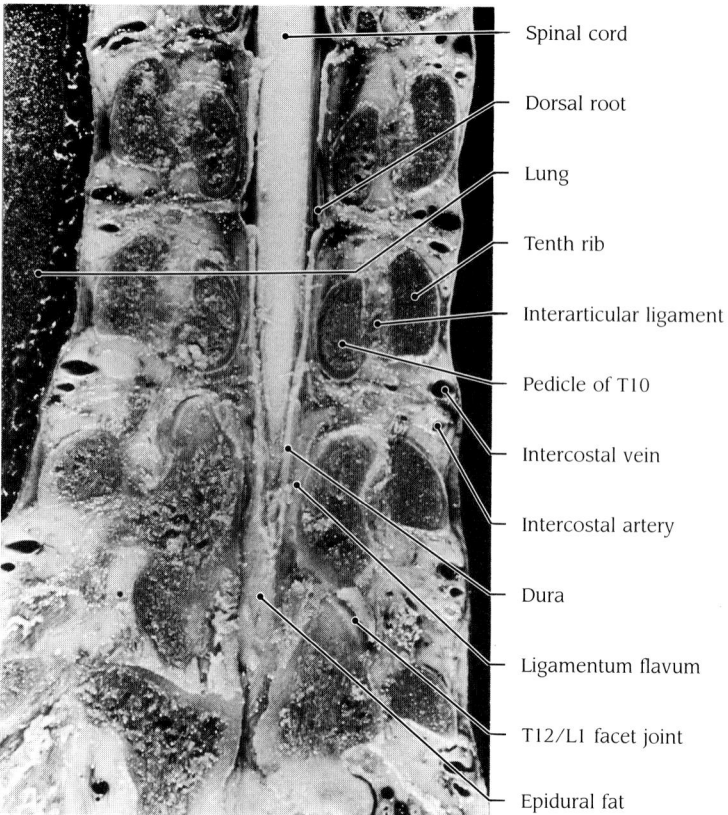

FIG. 10.40.

- Usually, nine pairs of posterior intercostal arteries arise from the thoracic aorta and are distributed to the nine lower intercostal spaces. The superior intercostal artery supplies the first and second spaces. The subcostal arteries are the last pair of branches from the thoracic aorta. They follow the same course as do the posterior intercostal arteries, but are named subcostal because they are located below the twelfth rib and are not intercostal. Each intercostal artery is accompanied by an intercostal vein and a nerve. The intercostal vein is superior to and the nerve is inferior to the intercostal artery, except in the upper intercostal spaces, where the nerve is at first superior to the artery.

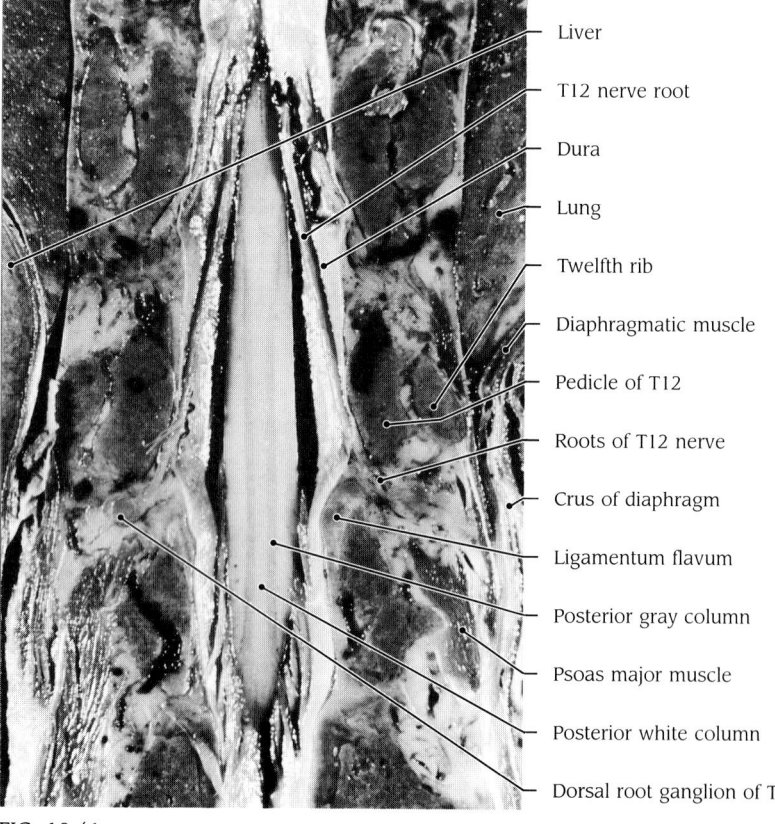

FIG. 10.41.

230

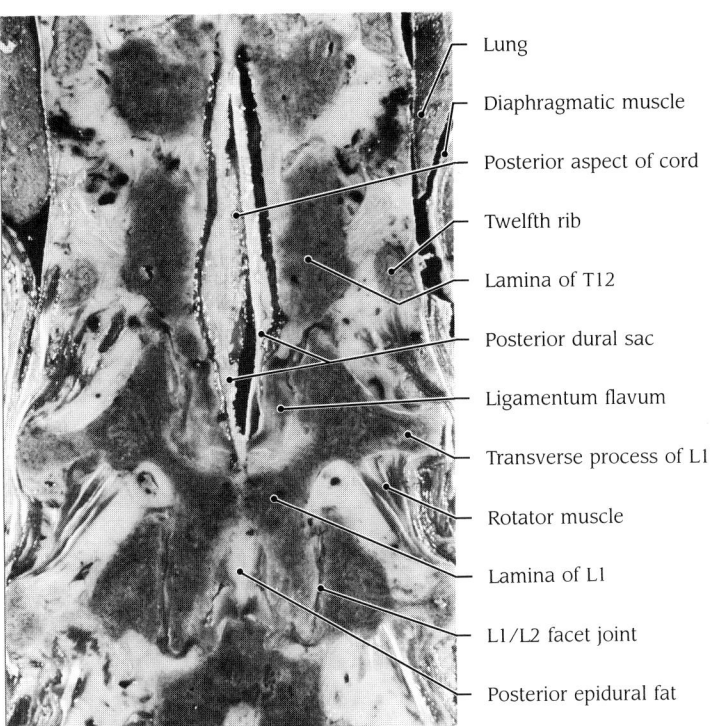

FIG. 10.42.

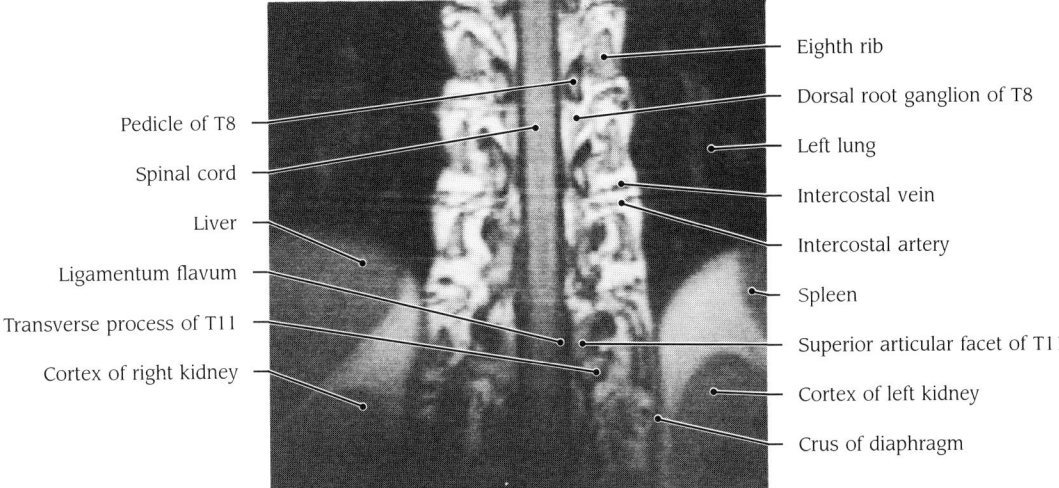

FIG. 10.43. TR = 737 msec, TE = 37 msec.

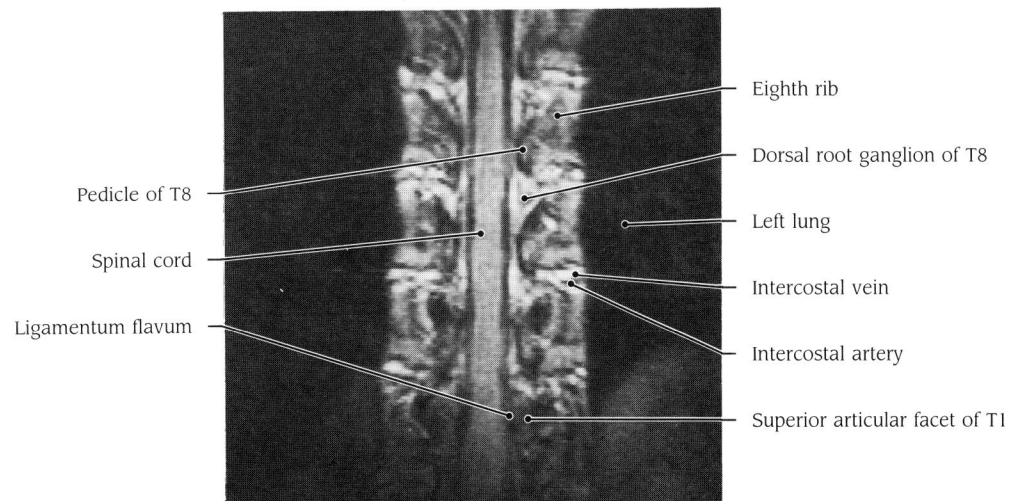

FIG. 10.44. TR = 5000 msec, TE = 64 msec.

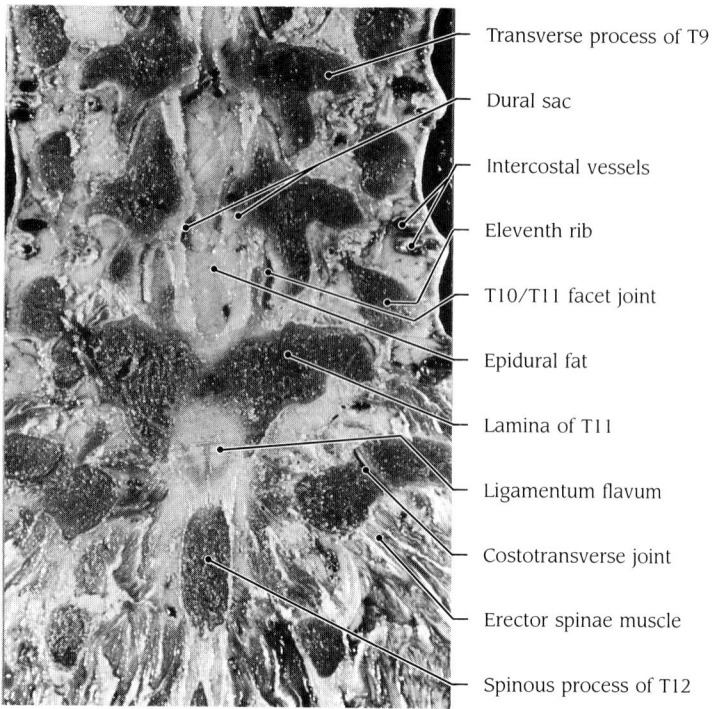

FIG. 10.45.

- The tubercle of each rib articulates with a facet on the transverse process of its corresponding vertebra at every level except eleven and twelve. The ligaments of the costotransverse joints include the costotransverse, superior and lateral costotransverse, and the fibrous capsule. These ligaments limit the movement of the costotransverse joints to minimal gliding, similar to the movement at the articulation with the head of each rib.

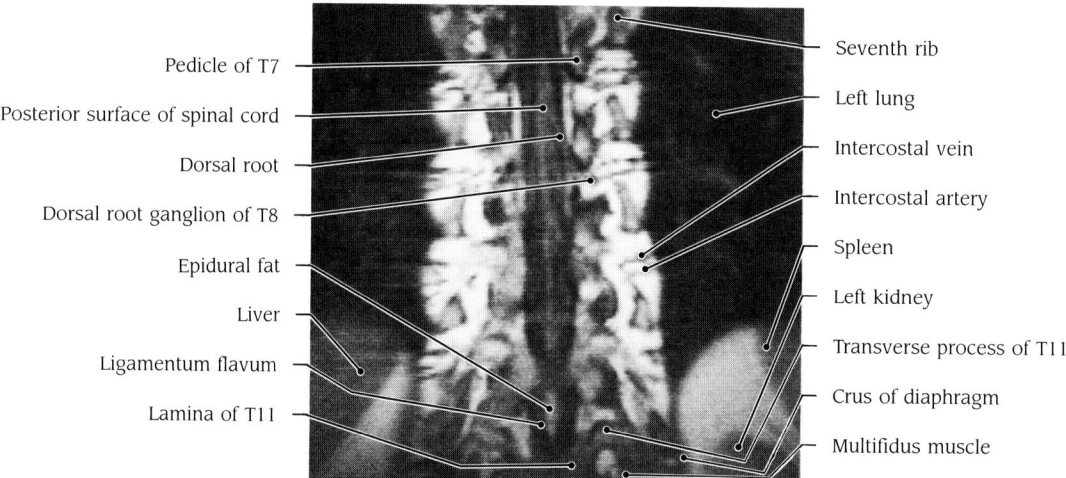

FIG. 10.46. TR = 737 msec, TE = 37 msec.

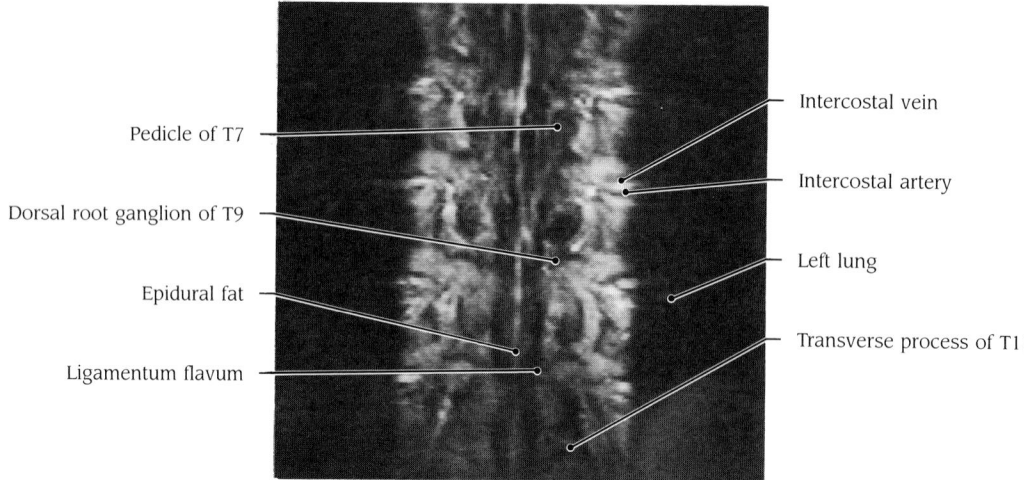

FIG. 10.47. TR = 5000 msec, TE = 64 msec.

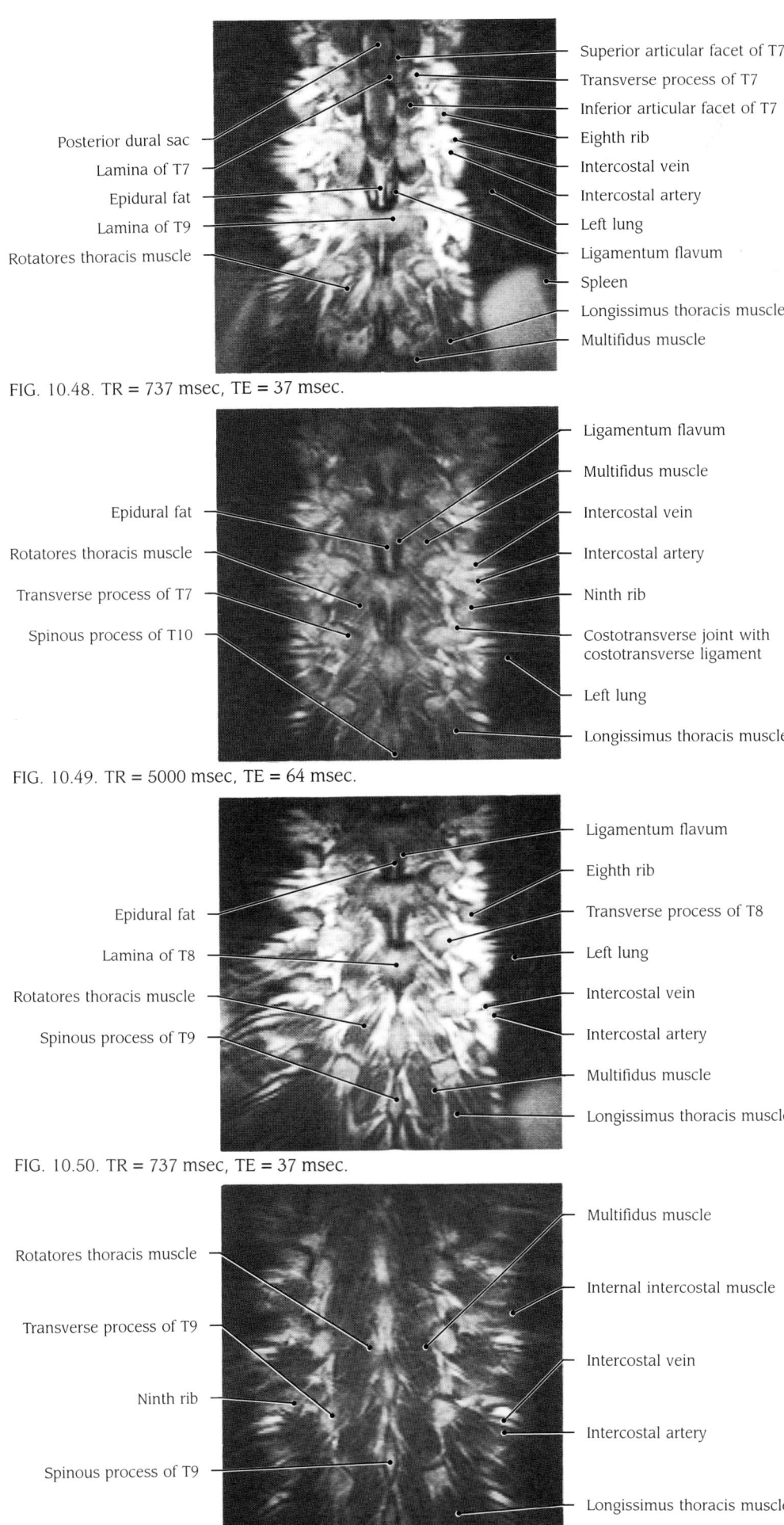

FIG. 10.48. TR = 737 msec, TE = 37 msec.

FIG. 10.49. TR = 5000 msec, TE = 64 msec.

FIG. 10.50. TR = 737 msec, TE = 37 msec.

FIG. 10.51. TR = 5000 msec, TE = 64 msec.

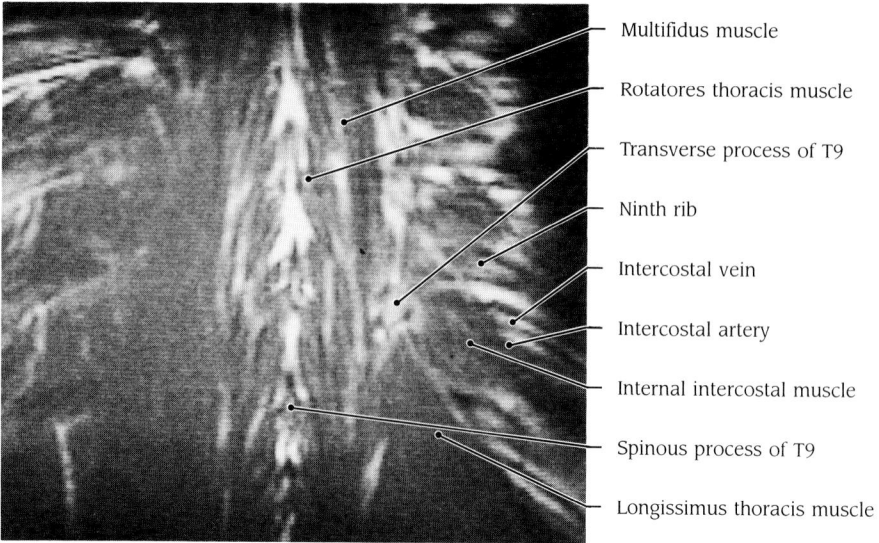

FIG. 10.52. TR = 737 msec, TE = 37 msec.

- The tendinous portions of the back muscles produce linear low signal intensity structures extending from superior to inferior. The long tendons of the semispinalis thoracis muscles are prominent in these sections.

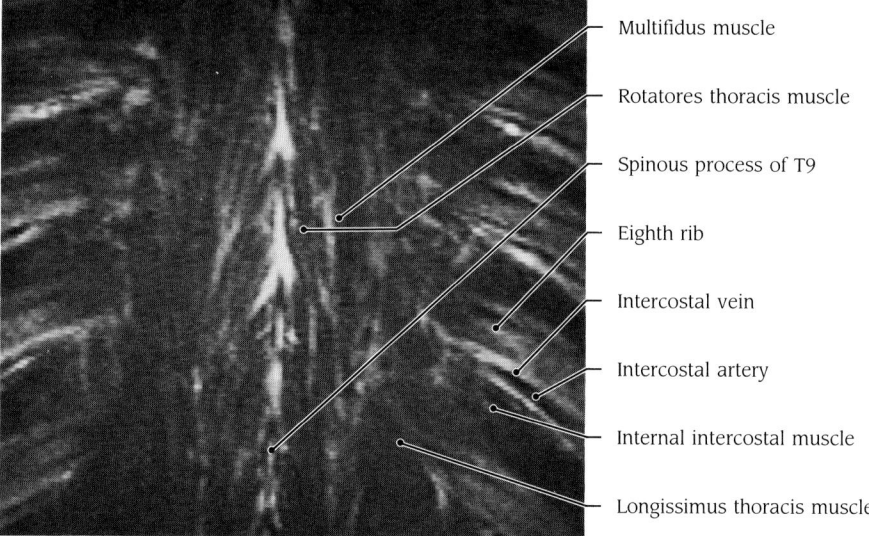

FIG. 10.53. TR = 5000 msec, TE = 64 msec.

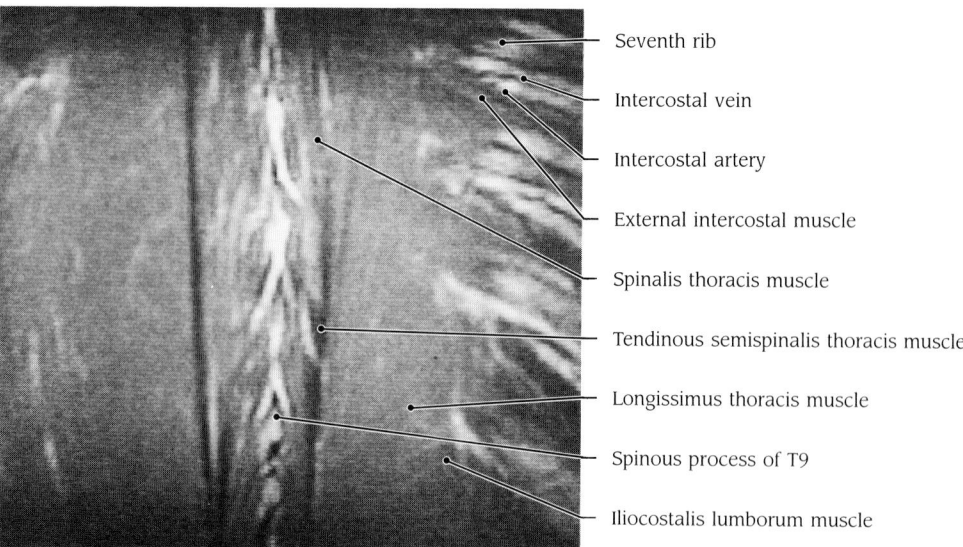

FIG. 10.54. TR = 737 msec, TE = 37 msec.

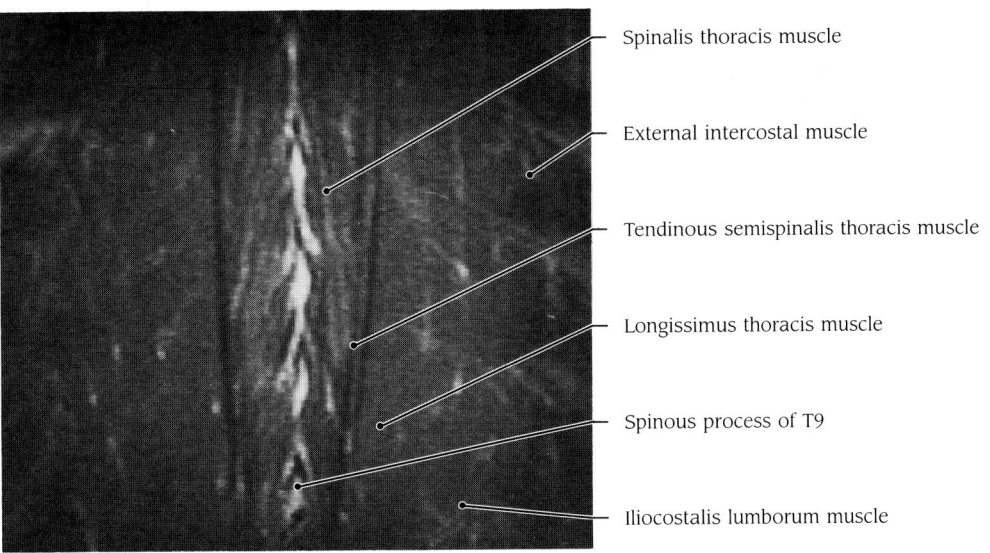

FIG. 10.55. TR = 5000 msec, TE = 64 msec.

- Spinalis thoracis muscle
- External intercostal muscle
- Tendinous semispinalis thoracis muscle
- Longissimus thoracis muscle
- Spinous process of T9
- Iliocostalis lumborum muscle

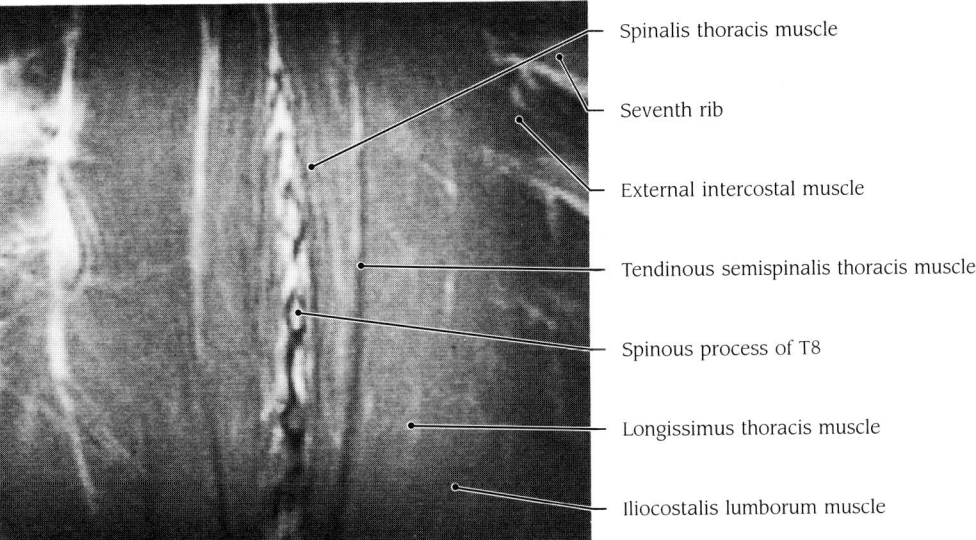

FIG. 10.56. TR = 737 msec, TE = 37 msec.

- Spinalis thoracis muscle
- Seventh rib
- External intercostal muscle
- Tendinous semispinalis thoracis muscle
- Spinous process of T8
- Longissimus thoracis muscle
- Iliocostalis lumborum muscle

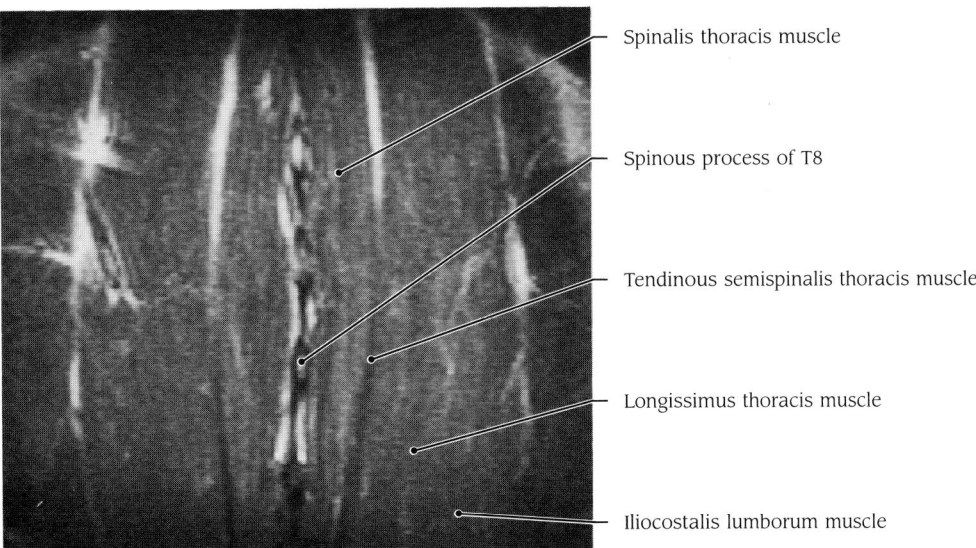

FIG. 10.57. TR = 5000 msec, TE = 64 msec.

- Spinalis thoracis muscle
- Spinous process of T8
- Tendinous semispinalis thoracis muscle
- Longissimus thoracis muscle
- Iliocostalis lumborum muscle

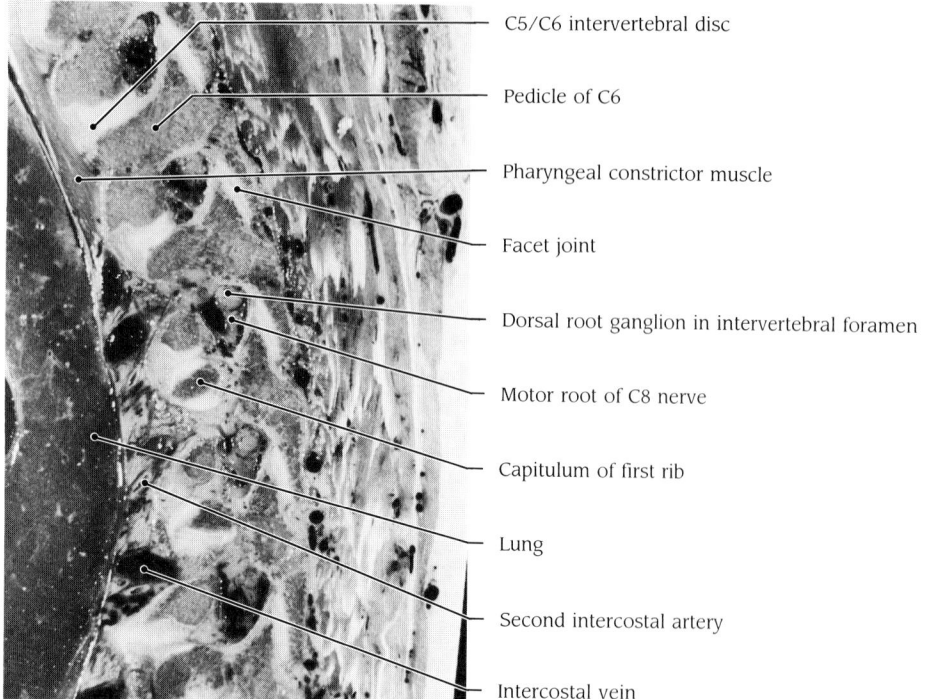

FIG. 10.58.

- Eleven pairs of posterior intercostal veins run with the posterior intercostal arteries. On both the right and the left sides, the first posterior intercostal vein drains into the corresponding brachiocephalic or vertebral vein. On the right side, the second, the third, and usually the fourth posterior intercostal veins join to form the right superior intercostal vein, which opens into the azygos vein. The posterior intercostal veins inferior to the fourth posterior intercostal vein on the right side open directly into the azygos vein. On the left side, the second, third, and occasionally the fourth posterior intercostal veins unite to form the left superior intercostal vein, which opens into the left brachiocephalic vein. The left fourth or fifth through the eighth posterior intercostal veins open into the accessory hemiazygos vein, and the ninth through the eleventh posterior intercostal veins open into the hemiazygos vein.

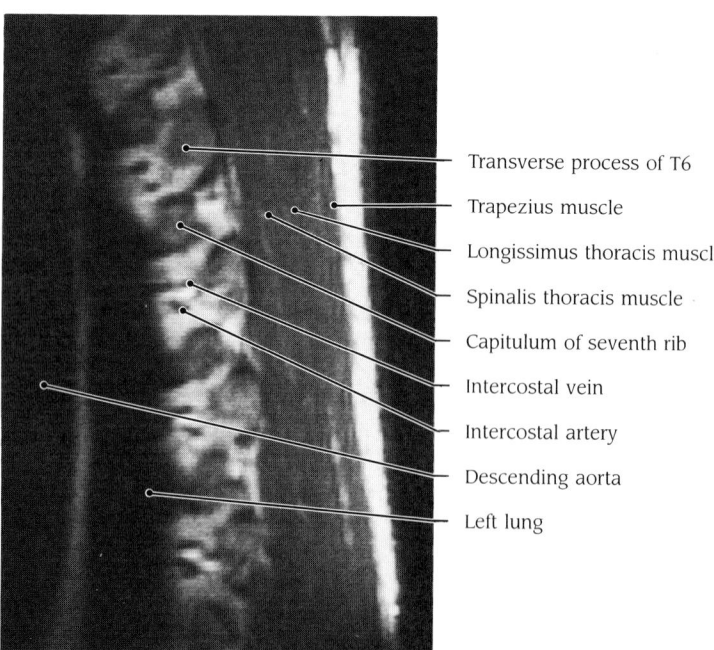

FIG. 10.59. TR = 637 msec, TE = 39 msec.

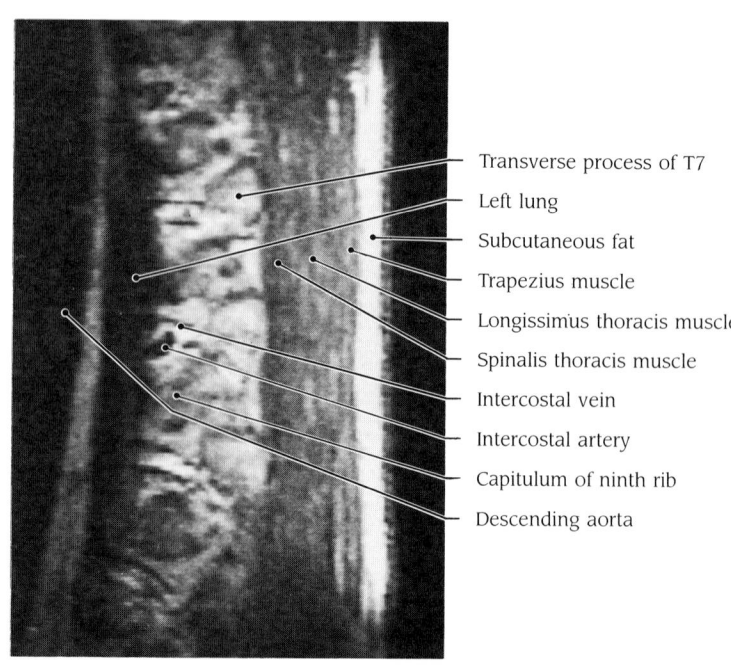

FIG. 10.60. TR = 5000 msec, TE = 60 msec.

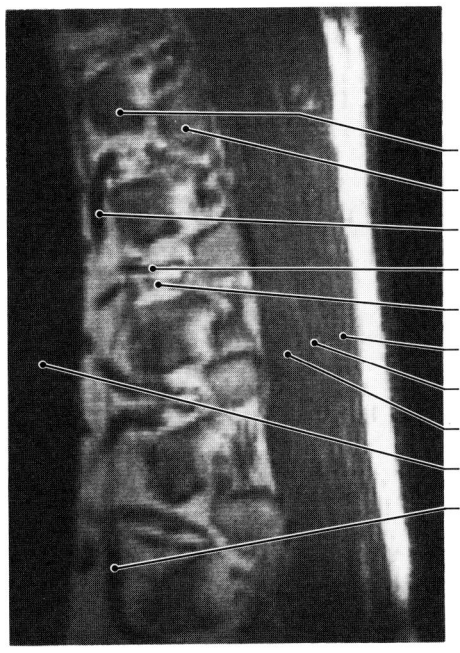

FIG. 10.61. TR = 637 msec, TE = 39 msec.

- Capitulum of sixth rib
- Transverse process of T6
- Accessory hemiazygos vein
- Intercostal vein
- Intercostal artery
- Trapezius muscle
- Longissimus thoracis muscle
- Spinalis thoracis muscle
- Descending aorta
- Hemiazygos vein

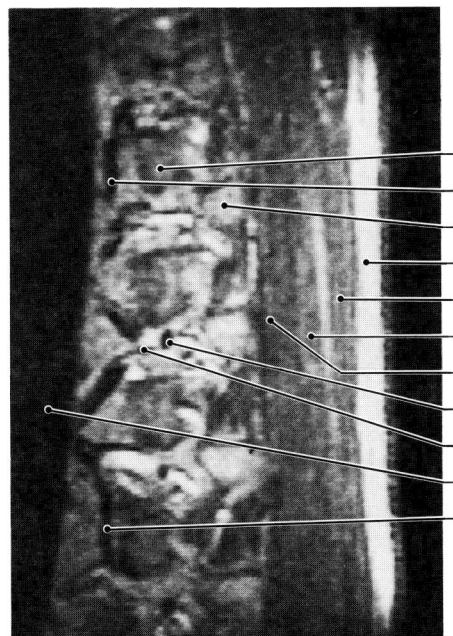

FIG. 10.62. TR = 5000 msec, TE = 60 msec.

- Capitulum of seventh rib
- Accessory hemiazygos vein
- Transverse process of T7
- Subcutaneous fat
- Trapezius muscle
- Longissimus thoracis muscle
- Spinalis thoracis muscle
- Intercostal vein
- Intercostal artery
- Descending aorta
- Hemiazygos vein

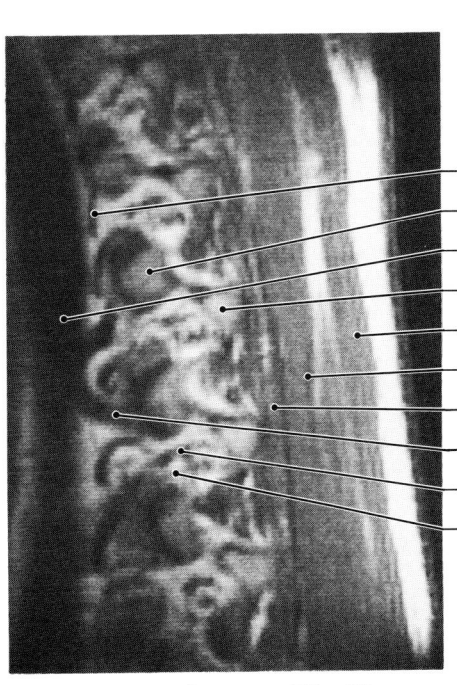

FIG. 10.63. TR = 637 msec, TE = 39 msec.

- Accessory hemiazygos vein
- Capitulum of seventh rib
- Descending aorta
- Transverse process of T7
- Trapezius muscle
- Spinalis thoracis muscle
- Multifidus muscle
- Hemiazygos vein
- Intercostal vein
- Intercostal artery

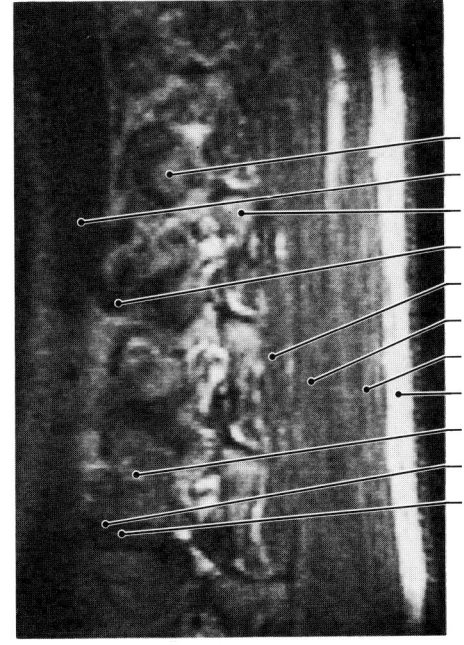

FIG. 10.64. TR = 5000 msec, TE = 60 msec.

- Capitulum of seventh rib
- Descending aorta
- Transverse process of T7
- Hemiazygos vein
- Multifidus muscle
- Spinalis thoracis muscle
- Trapezius muscle
- Subcutaneous fat
- T9 vertebral body
- Endplate of T9 vertebral body
- T9/T10 intervertebral disc

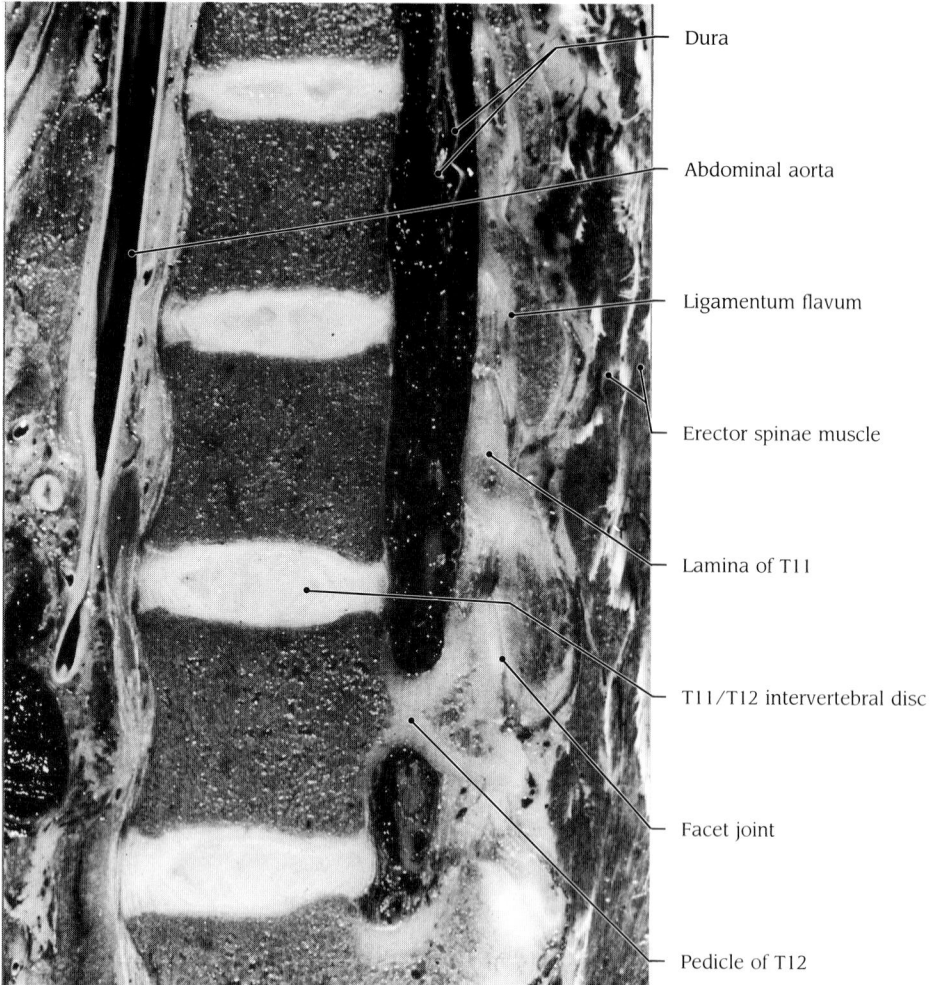

FIG. 10.65.

- The thoracic facets are oriented in a plane that is almost coronal. The superior articular processes are thin plates that project superiorly and face posteriorly and slightly laterally and superiorly. The inferior articular processes face anteriorly and slightly medially and superiorly. The change from the thoracic to the lumbar type of facet usually occurs at the eleventh thoracic vertebra, but it may occur one level higher or lower. The transitional vertebra is characterized by superior articular processes that are thoracic in type and by inferior articular processes that are slightly convex and face laterally and anteriorly, as in the lumbar area. The joints of the vertebral arches of the transitional vertebra usually interlock, thereby preventing all movement except flexion.

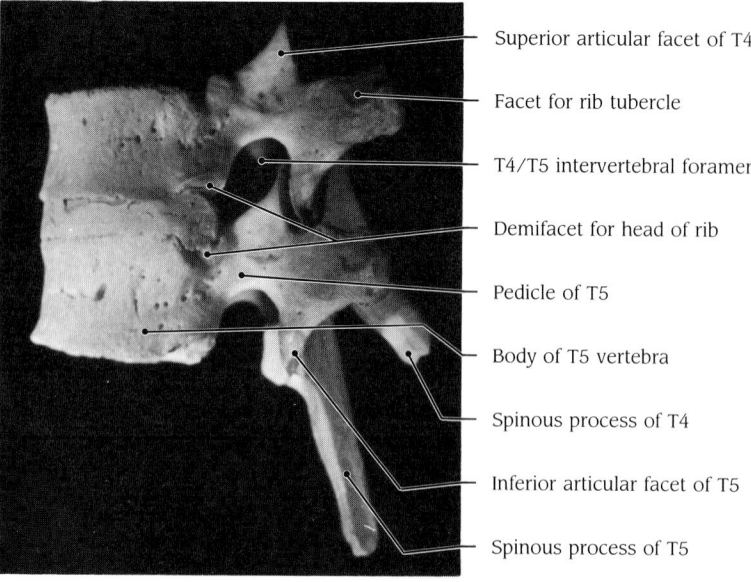

FIG. 10.66. (From de Groot, J.: Correlative Neuroanatomy of Computed Tomography and Magnetic Resonance Imaging. Philadelphia, Lea & Febiger, 1984.)

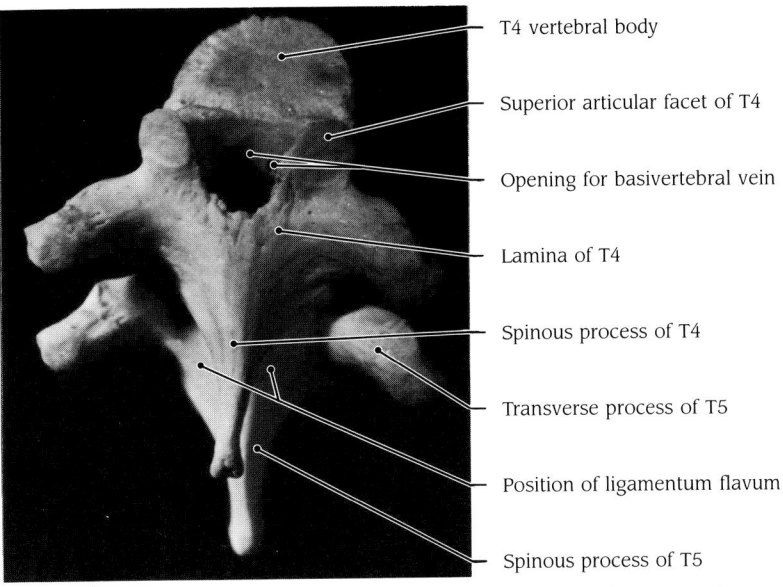

FIG. 10.67. (From de Groot, J.: Correlative Neuroanatomy of Computed Tomography and Magnetic Resonance Imaging. Philadelphia, Lea & Febiger, 1984.)

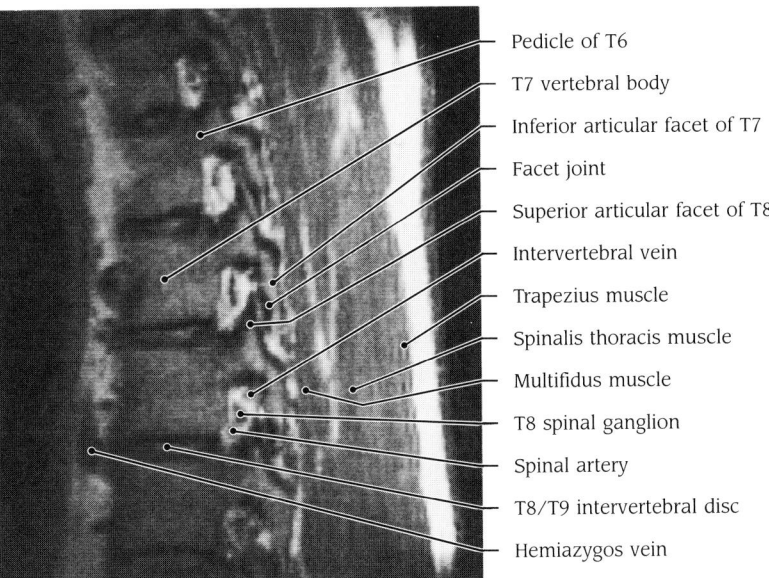

FIG. 10.68. TR = 637 msec, TE = 39 msec.

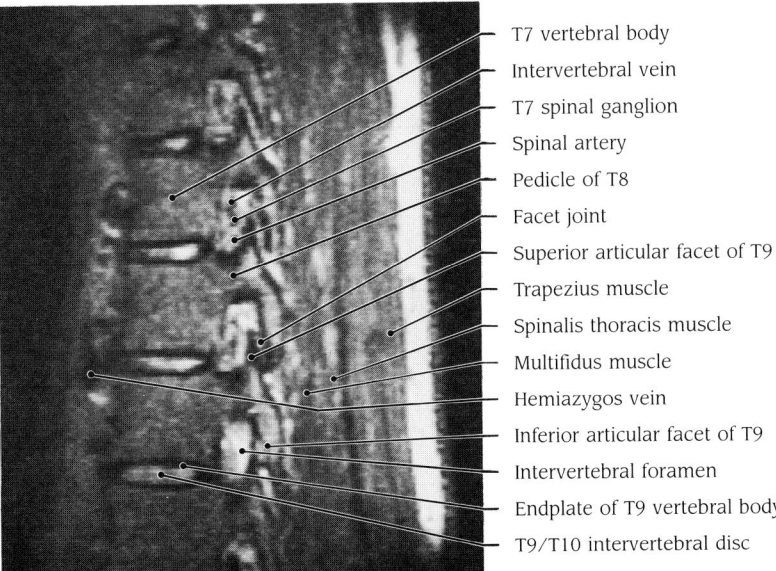

FIG. 10.69. TR = 5000 msec, TE = 60 msec.

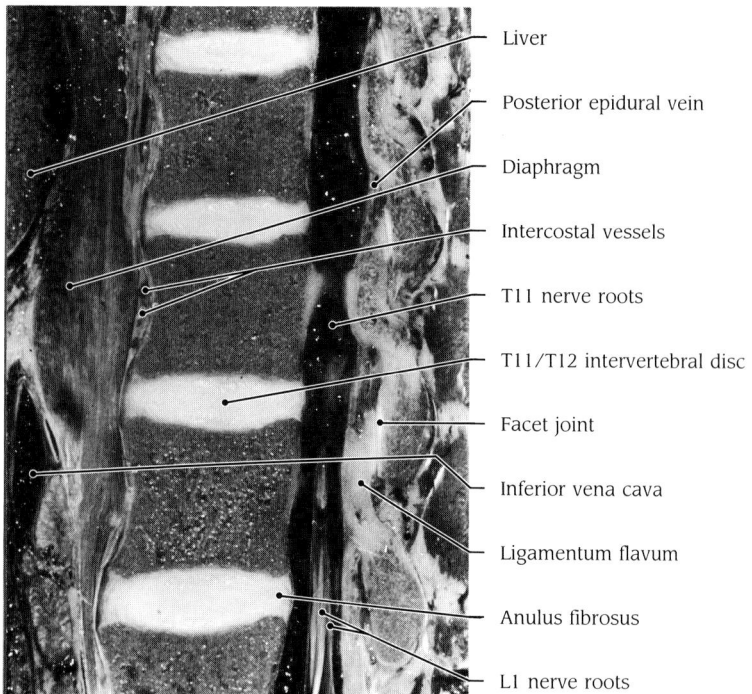

FIG. 10.70.

- The ligamenta flava are predominantly composed of elastic tissue and are attached to the inferior aspect of the lamina of one vertebral body and the posterior surface and superior margin of the lamina of the vertebral body below. The attachments of the ligamenta flava extend from the articular capsules to the fusion of the lamina. The right and left ligamenta flava are partially united; small openings remain for veins to communicate from the posterior internal to the posterior external venous plexuses. The ligaments progressively increase in thickness from the cervical to the lumbar levels. They function to slow the movement of flexion and assist in resuming an erect posture following flexion.

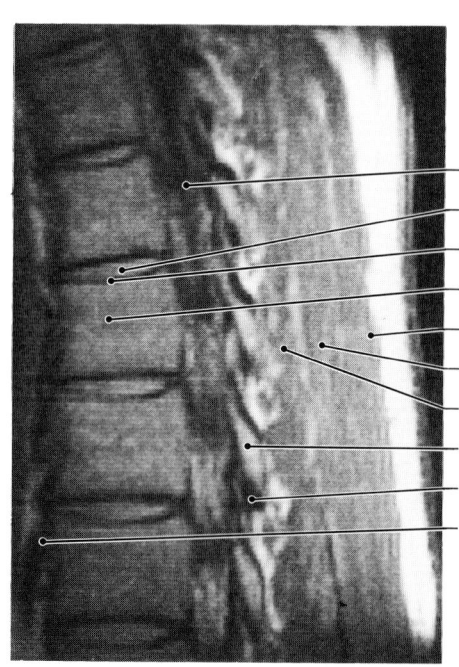

FIG. 10.71. TR = 637 msec, TE = 39 msec.

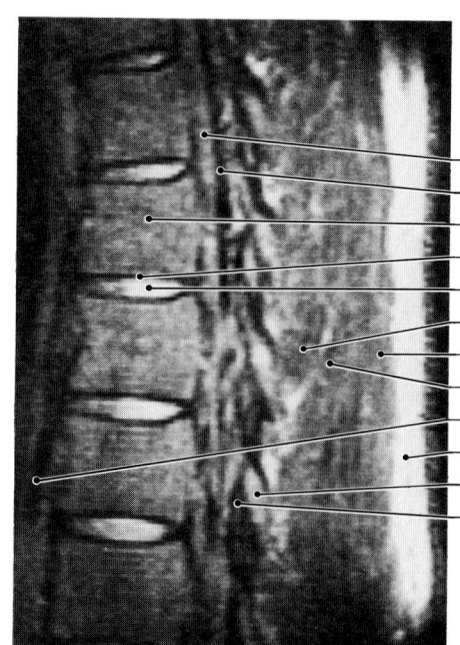

FIG. 10.72. TR = 5000 msec, TE = 60 msec.

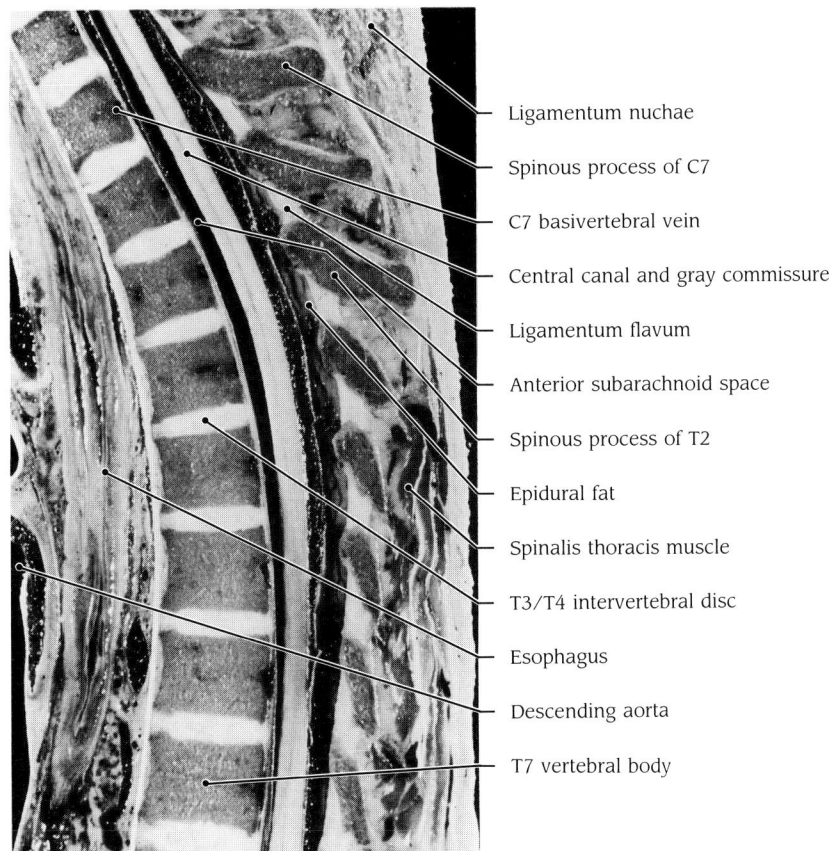

FIG. 10.73.

- Ligamentum nuchae
- Spinous process of C7
- C7 basivertebral vein
- Central canal and gray commissure
- Ligamentum flavum
- Anterior subarachnoid space
- Spinous process of T2
- Epidural fat
- Spinalis thoracis muscle
- T3/T4 intervertebral disc
- Esophagus
- Descending aorta
- T7 vertebral body

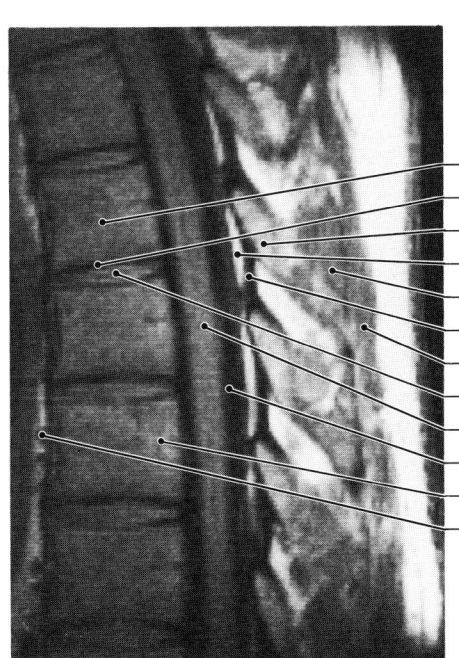

- T6 vertebral body
- Endplate of T6 vertebral body
- Spinous process of T6
- Epidural fat
- Multifidus muscle
- Ligamentum flavum
- Spinalis thoracis muscle
- T6/T7 intervertebral disc
- Spinal cord
- Subarachnoid space
- Basivertebral vein
- Intercostal artery

FIG. 10.74. TR = 637 msec, TE = 39 msec.

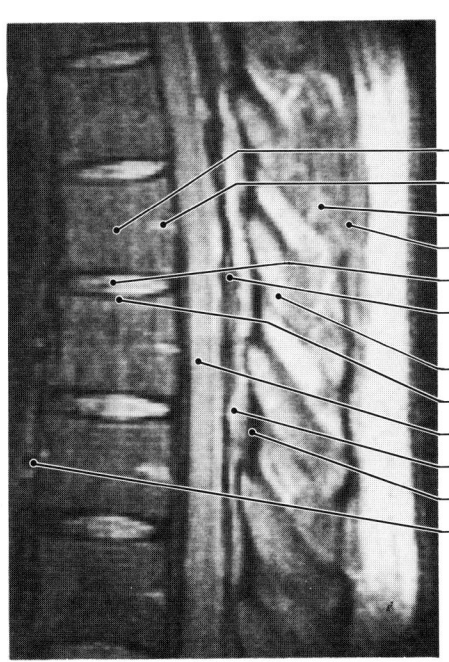

- T7 vertebral body
- Basivertebral vein
- Multifidus muscle
- Spinalis thoracis muscle
- T7/T8 intervertebral disc
- Cerebrospinal fluid pulsation artifact
- Spinous process of T7
- Endplate of T8 vertebral body
- Spinal cord
- Epidural fat
- Ligamentum flavum
- Intercostal artery

FIG. 10.75. TR = 5000 msec, TE = 60 msec.

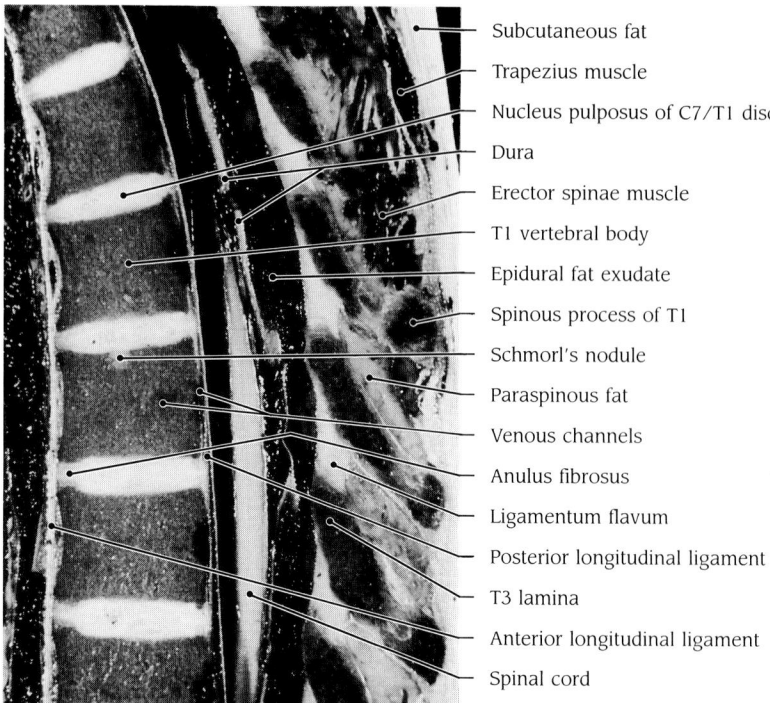

FIG. 10.76.

- The shape and direction of the articular facets determine the extent and type of vertebral movements. In the thoracic spine, particularly the superior portion, movements are limited to prevent respiratory problems. Extreme flexion is prevented by the minimal superior inclination of the superior articular processes, and extension is limited by the contact of the spinous processes with one another and the contact of the inferior articular processes with the lamina. Lateral flexion is checked in the upper thoracic region by the resistance of the ribs and sternum. Rotation is free in the thoracic spine and is accompanied by lateral displacement of the vertebral bodies at levels other than the midthoracic region. This displacement is secondary to the shift of the axis of rotation from within the vertebral bodies in the midthoracic spine to anterior to the vertebrae at other levels.

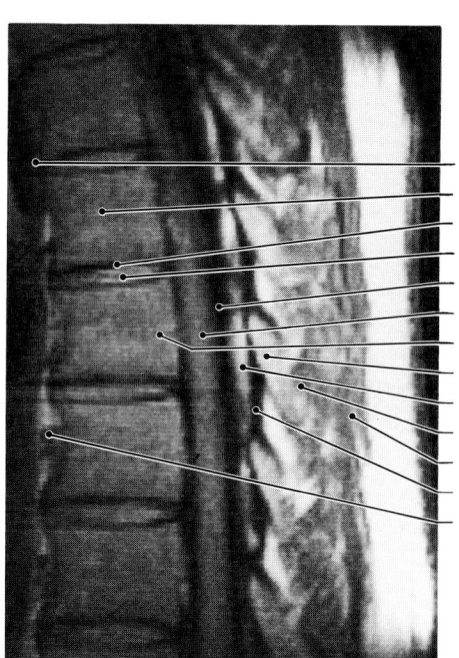

FIG. 10.77. TR = 637 msec, TE = 39 msec.

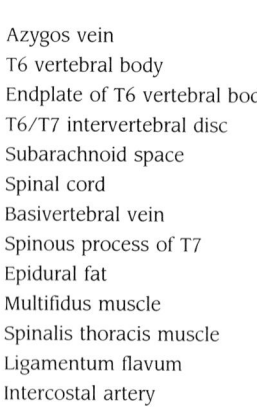

FIG. 10.78. TR = 5000 msec, TE = 60 msec.

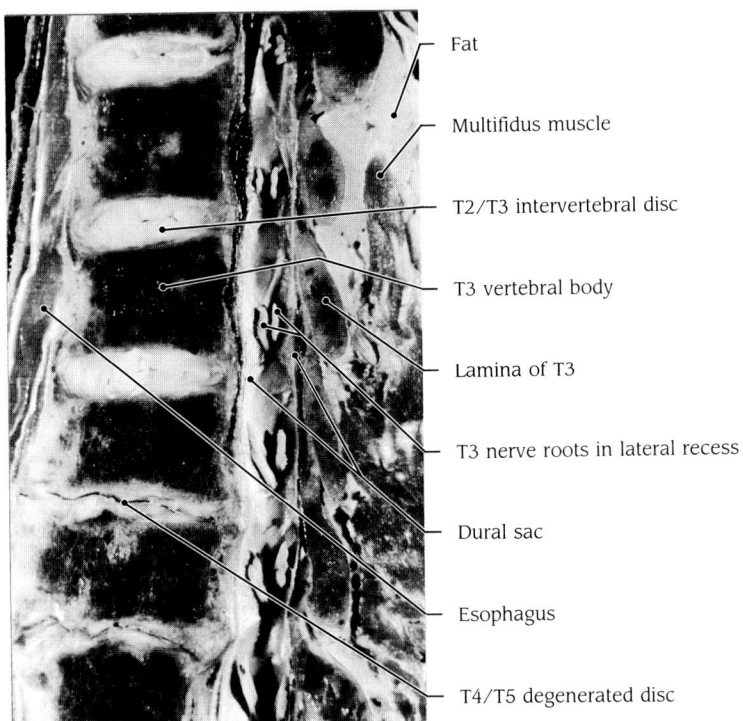

FIG. 10.79.

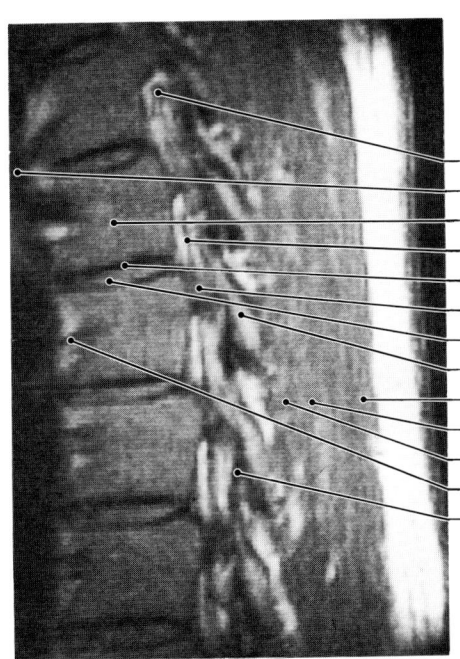

FIG. 10.80. TR = 637 msec, TE = 39 msec.

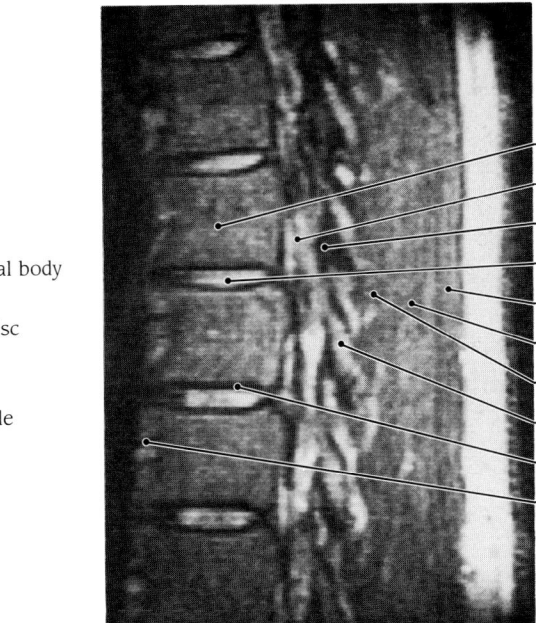

FIG. 10.81. TR = 5000 msec, TE = 60 msec.

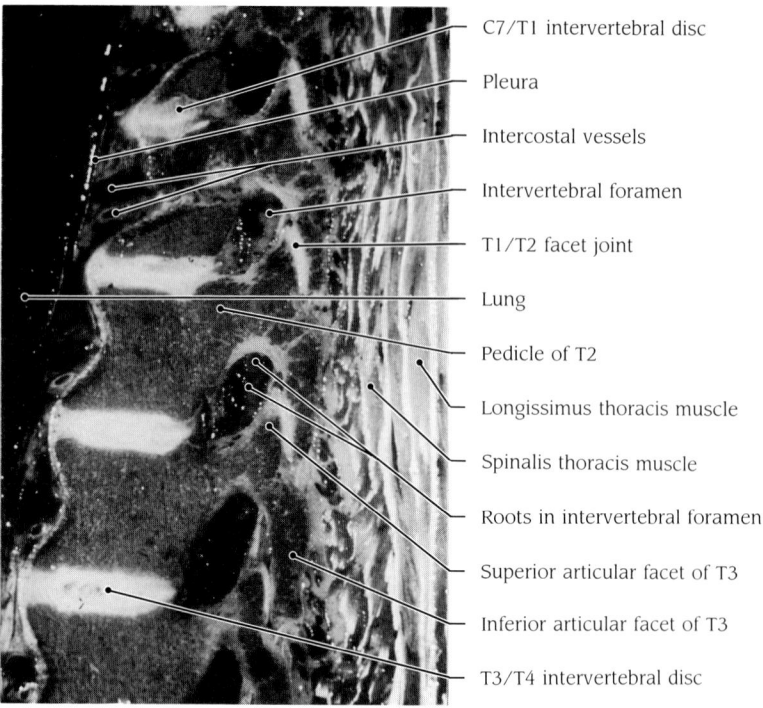

FIG. 10.82.

- The thoracic transverse processes are club-shaped projections that extend laterally and slightly posteriorly. The length of the transverse processes gradually decreases from superior to inferior. Near the ends of the transverse processes, facets are present for articulation with the tubercles of the ribs. The transverse processes serve as points of attachment for the intertransverse muscles and the deep muscles of the back.

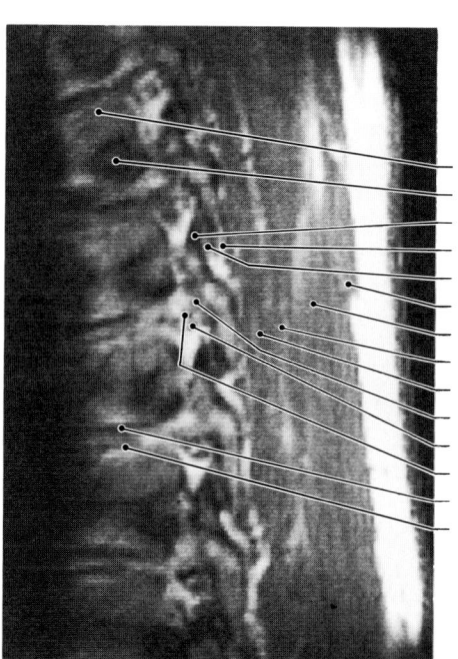

FIG. 10.83. TR = 637 msec, TE = 39 msec.

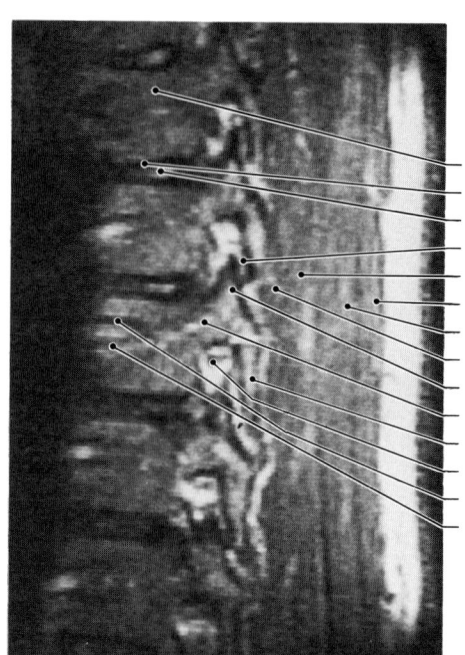

FIG. 10.84. TR = 5000 msec, TE = 60 msec.

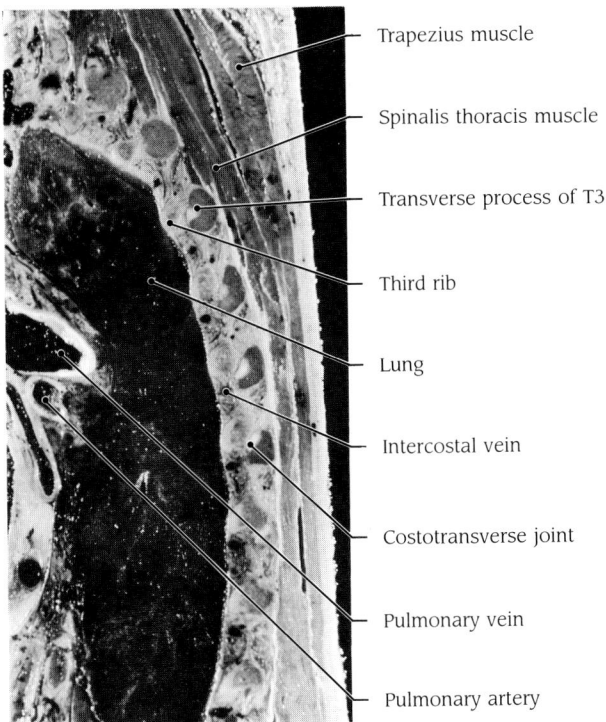

FIG. 10.85.

- Trapezius muscle
- Spinalis thoracis muscle
- Transverse process of T3
- Third rib
- Lung
- Intercostal vein
- Costotransverse joint
- Pulmonary vein
- Pulmonary artery

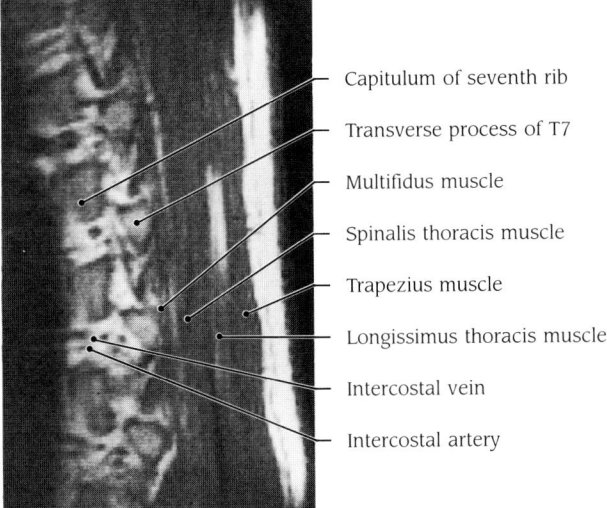

FIG. 10.86. TR = 637 msec, TE = 39 msec.

- Capitulum of seventh rib
- Transverse process of T7
- Multifidus muscle
- Spinalis thoracis muscle
- Trapezius muscle
- Longissimus thoracis muscle
- Intercostal vein
- Intercostal artery

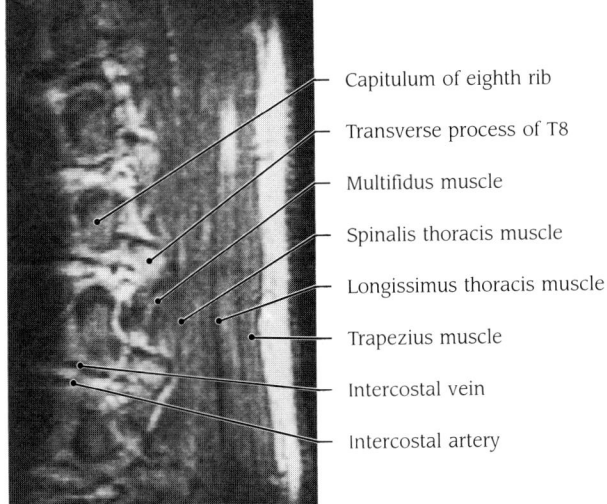

FIG. 10.87. TR = 5000 msec, TE = 60 msec.

- Capitulum of eighth rib
- Transverse process of T8
- Multifidus muscle
- Spinalis thoracis muscle
- Longissimus thoracis muscle
- Trapezius muscle
- Intercostal vein
- Intercostal artery

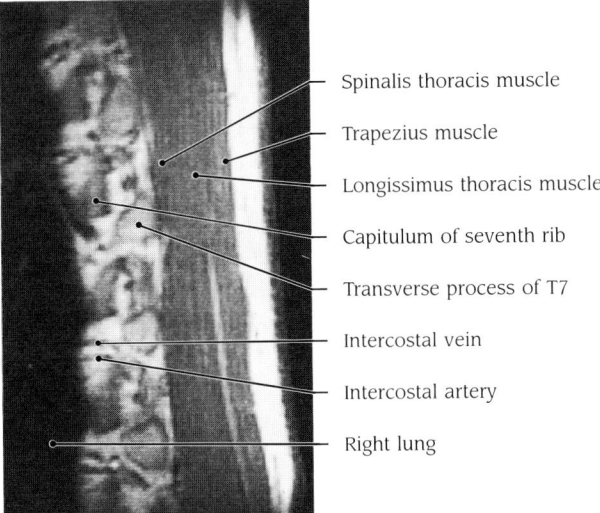

FIG. 10.88. TR = 637 msec, TE = 39 msec.

- Spinalis thoracis muscle
- Trapezius muscle
- Longissimus thoracis muscle
- Capitulum of seventh rib
- Transverse process of T7
- Intercostal vein
- Intercostal artery
- Right lung

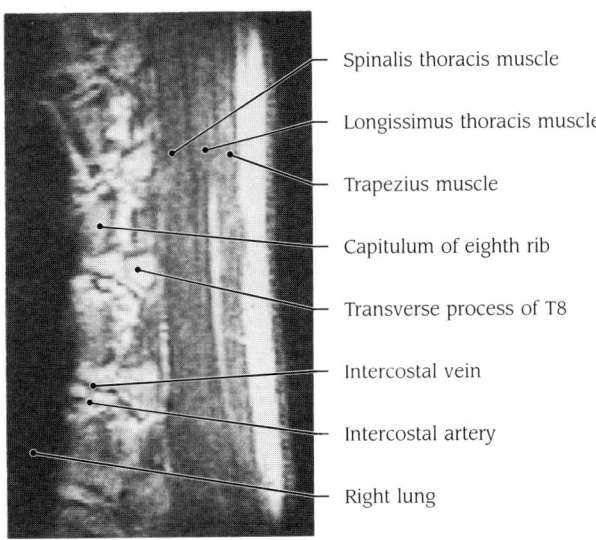

FIG. 10.89. TR = 5000 msec, TE = 60 msec.

- Spinalis thoracis muscle
- Longissimus thoracis muscle
- Trapezius muscle
- Capitulum of eighth rib
- Transverse process of T8
- Intercostal vein
- Intercostal artery
- Right lung

11

Lumbar Spine

Anatomic Level	Figures
Lumbar spine, axial series	11.1–11.27
Lumbar spine, coronal series	11.28–11.69
Lumbar spine, sagittal series	11.70–11.103

Sections from the lumbar spine of cadavers are shown in the axial, coronal, and sagittal planes. These sections are matched with corresponding magnetic resonance images of a normal volunteer. Additional anatomic sections and detailed views of the bony skeleton are included for clarification at some levels.

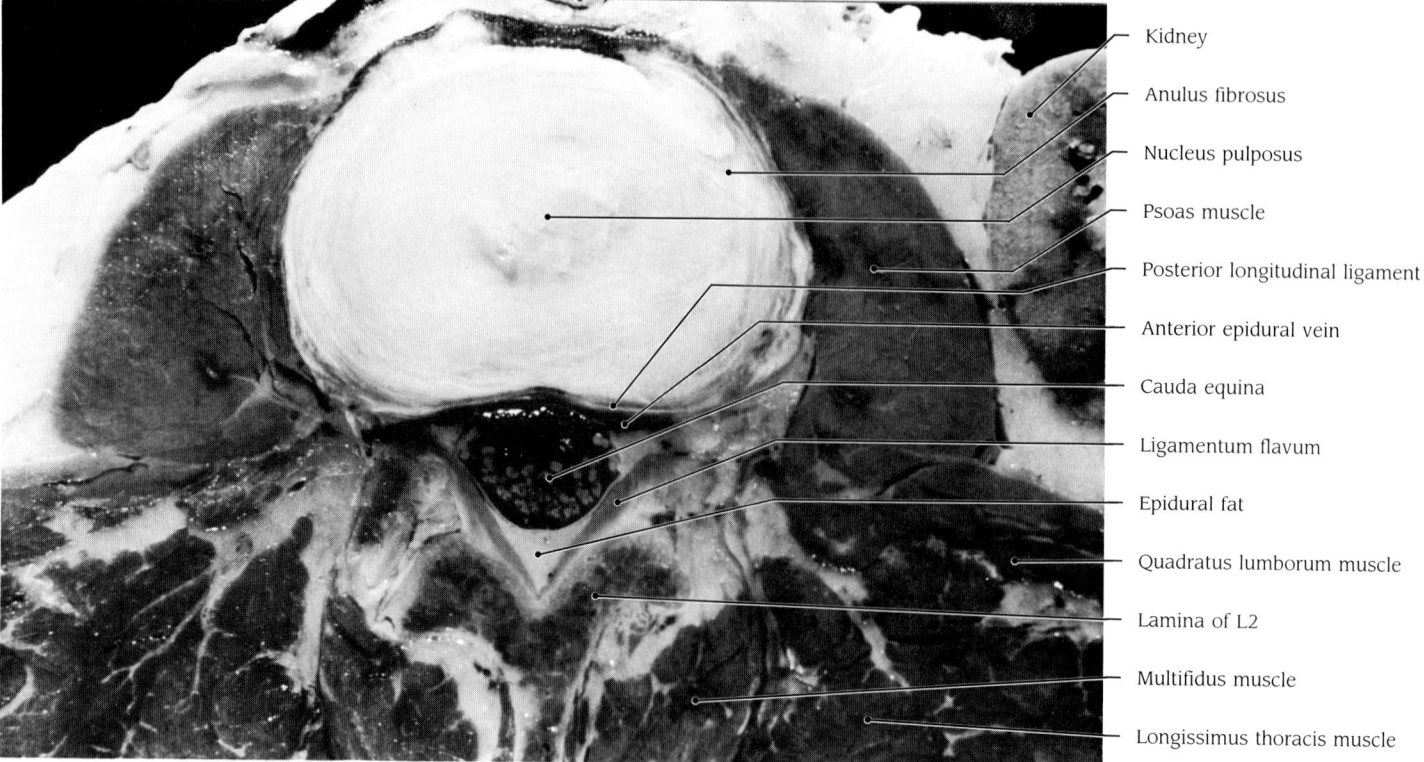

FIG. 11.1.

- The superior articular processes of the lumbar vertebrae have concave vertical articular facets that face medially and posteriorly. The inferior articular processes have convex vertical articular facets that face laterally and anteriorly. The inferior articular process of L5 faces anteriorly to articulate with the superior articular facet of the sacrum.

- The shape and direction of the articular facets influence the extent and variety of vertebral movements. In the lumbar spine, extension is free and wider in range than is flexion. In addition, a considerable degree of lateral flexion and a small amount of rotation are possible.

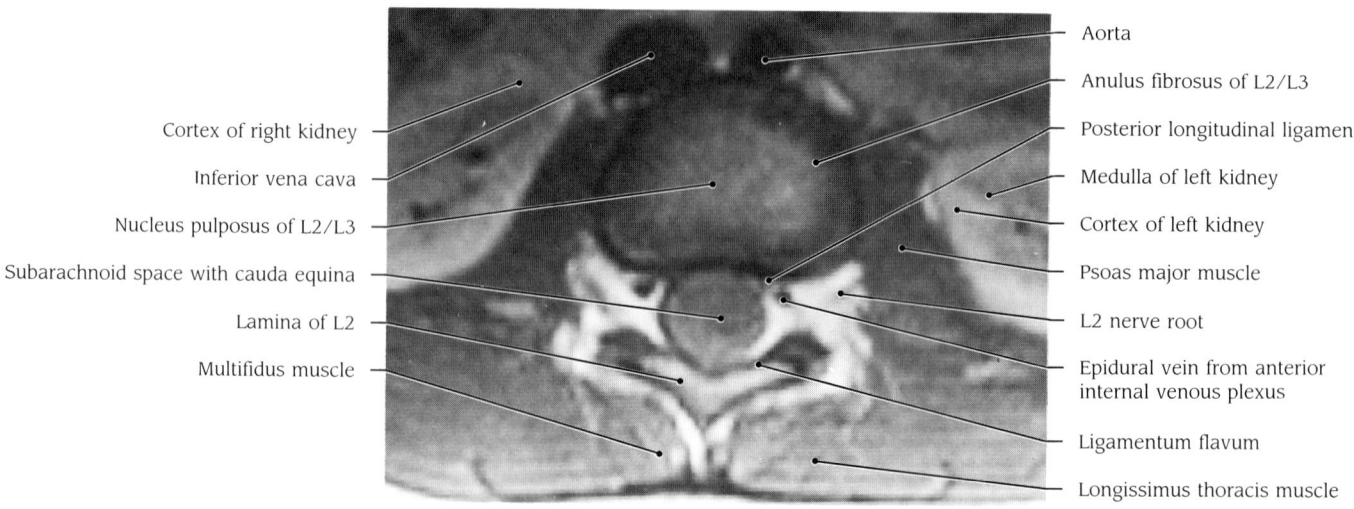

FIG. 11.2. TR = 1500 msec, TE = 40 msec.

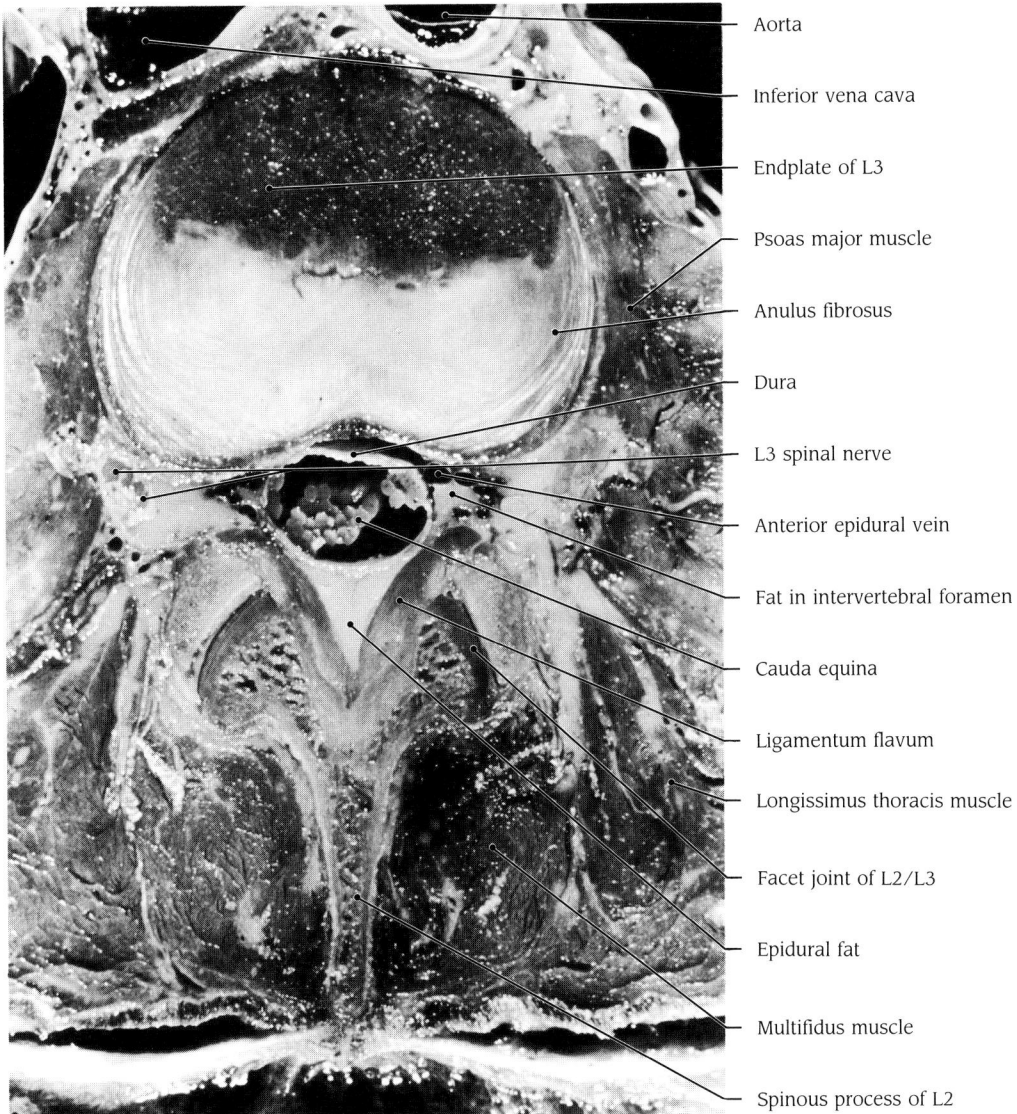

FIG. 11.3.

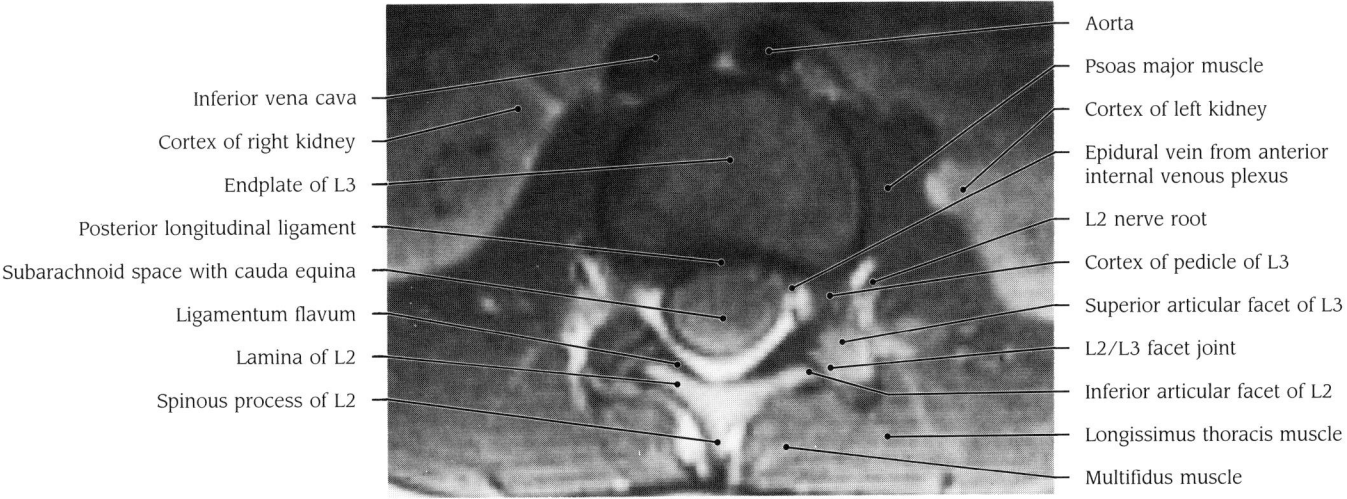

FIG. 11.4. TR = 1500 msec, TE = 40 msec.

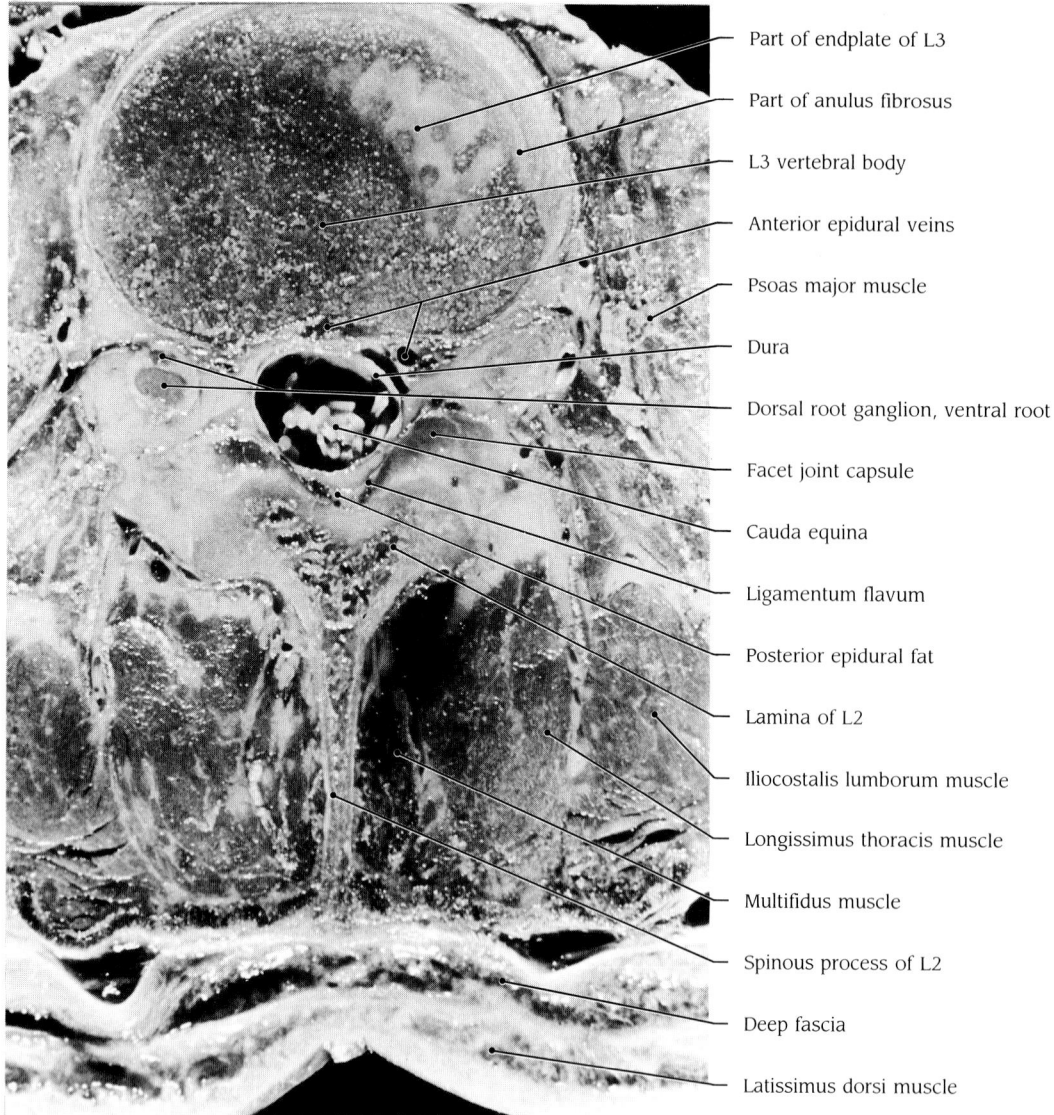

FIG. 11.5.

- The distinguishing features of the lumbar vertebrae are their larger size and the absence of costal facets. The vertebral foramen, or canal, is triangular and is larger than in the thoracic spine, but smaller than in the cervical spine. The laminae are broad, short, and strong, and are clearly separated from each other by a space filled with ligamentum flavum. The ligamenta flava function to permit separation of the laminae in flexion while simultaneously slowing the movement so that its limit is not reached abruptly.

- The intervertebral discs, which constitute approximately one fifth of the length of the vertebral column, excluding the first two vertebrae, vary in shape and thickness at different spinal levels. The lumbar intervertebral discs are thicker anteriorly than posteriorly, as in the cervical region. This change in thickness contributes to the anterior convexities at these levels.

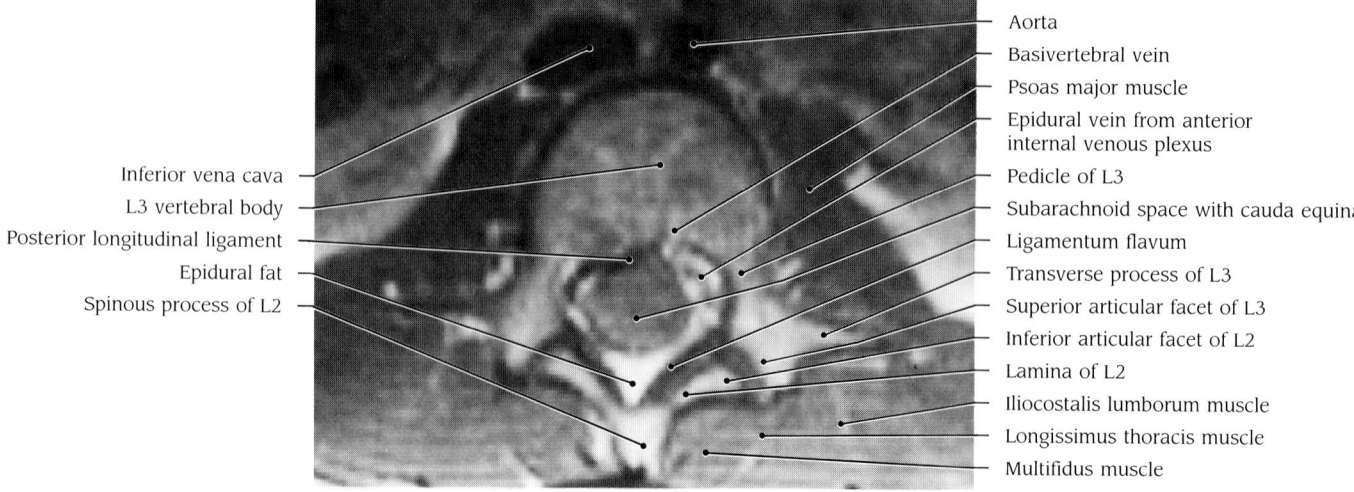

FIG. 11.6. TR = 1500 msec, TE = 40 msec.

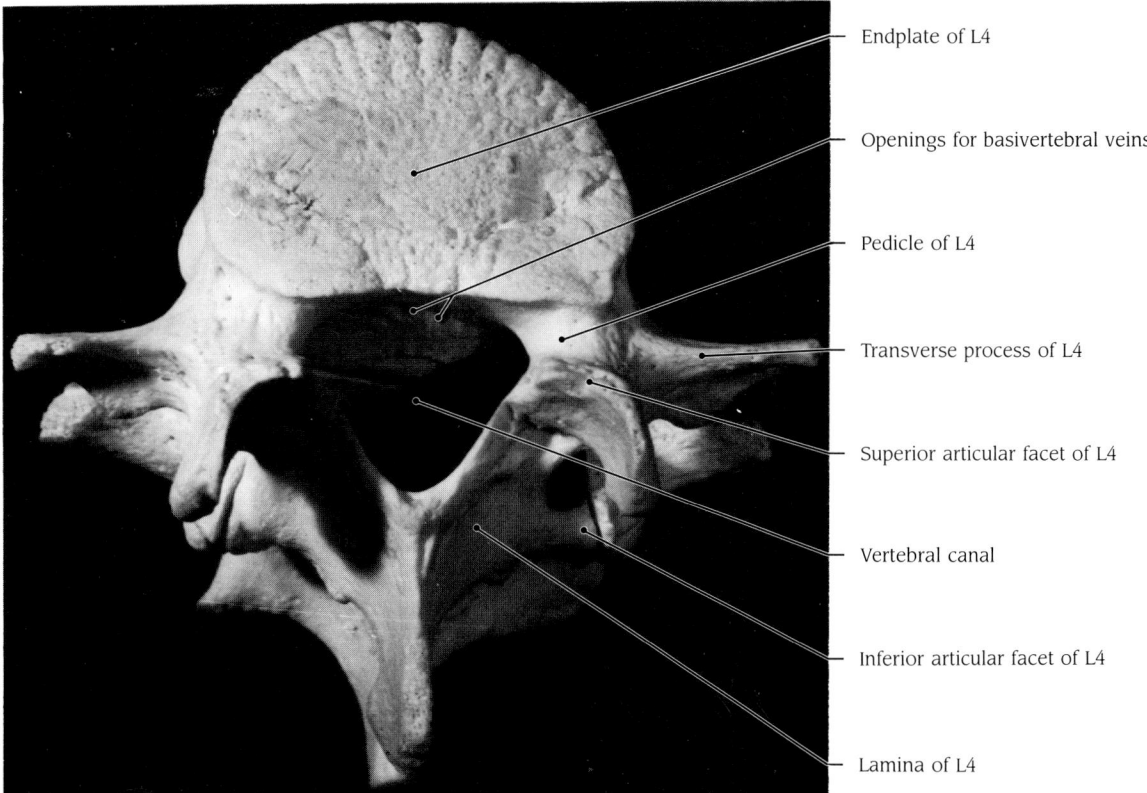

FIG. 11.7.

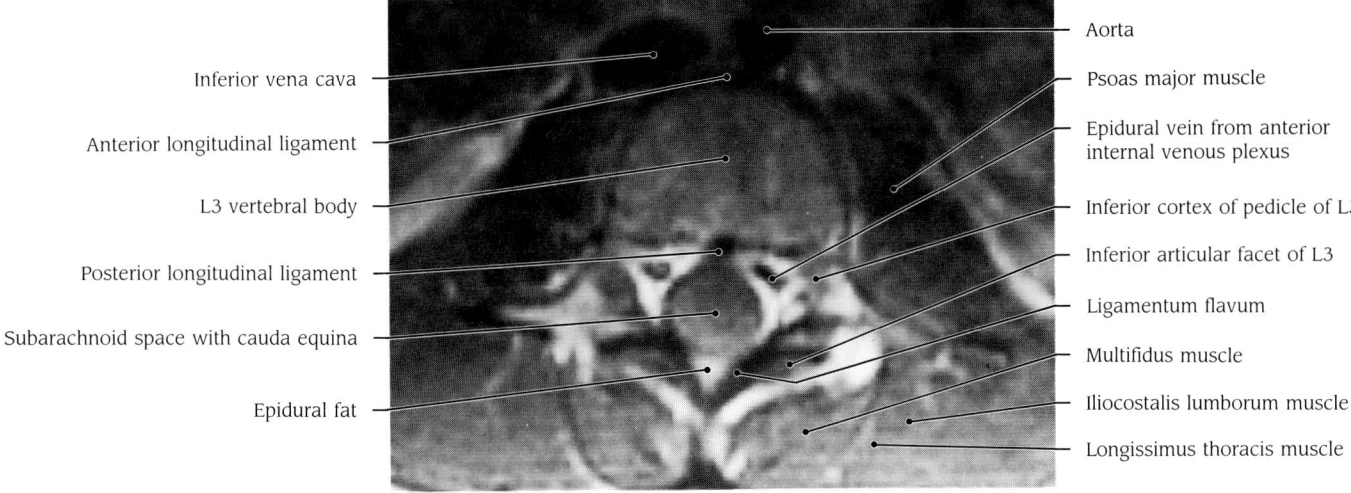

FIG. 11.8. TR = 1500 msec, TE = 40 msec.

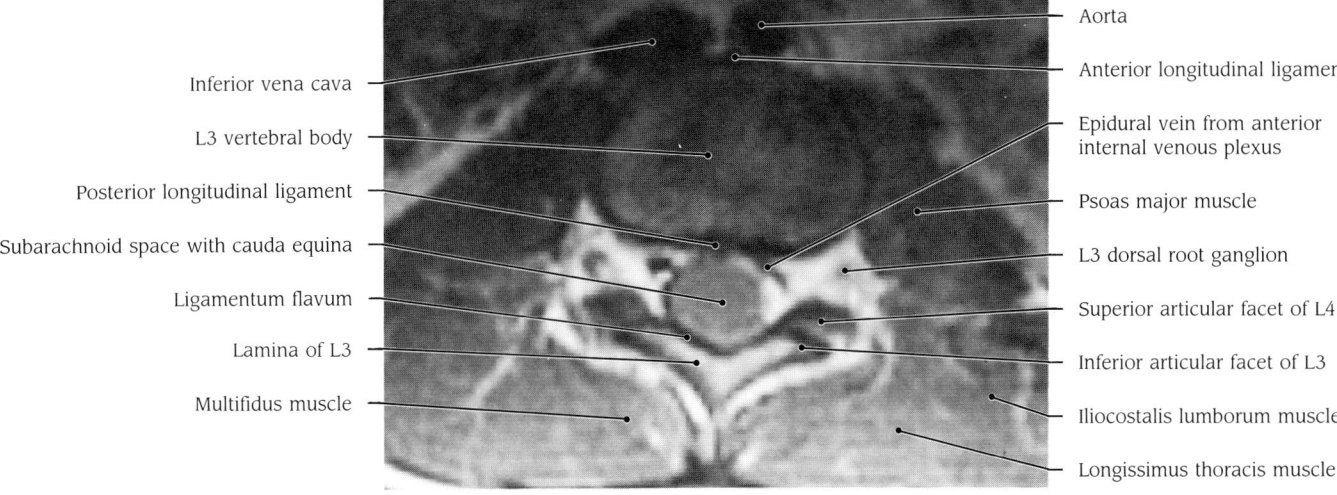

FIG. 11.9. TR = 1500 msec, TE = 40 msec.

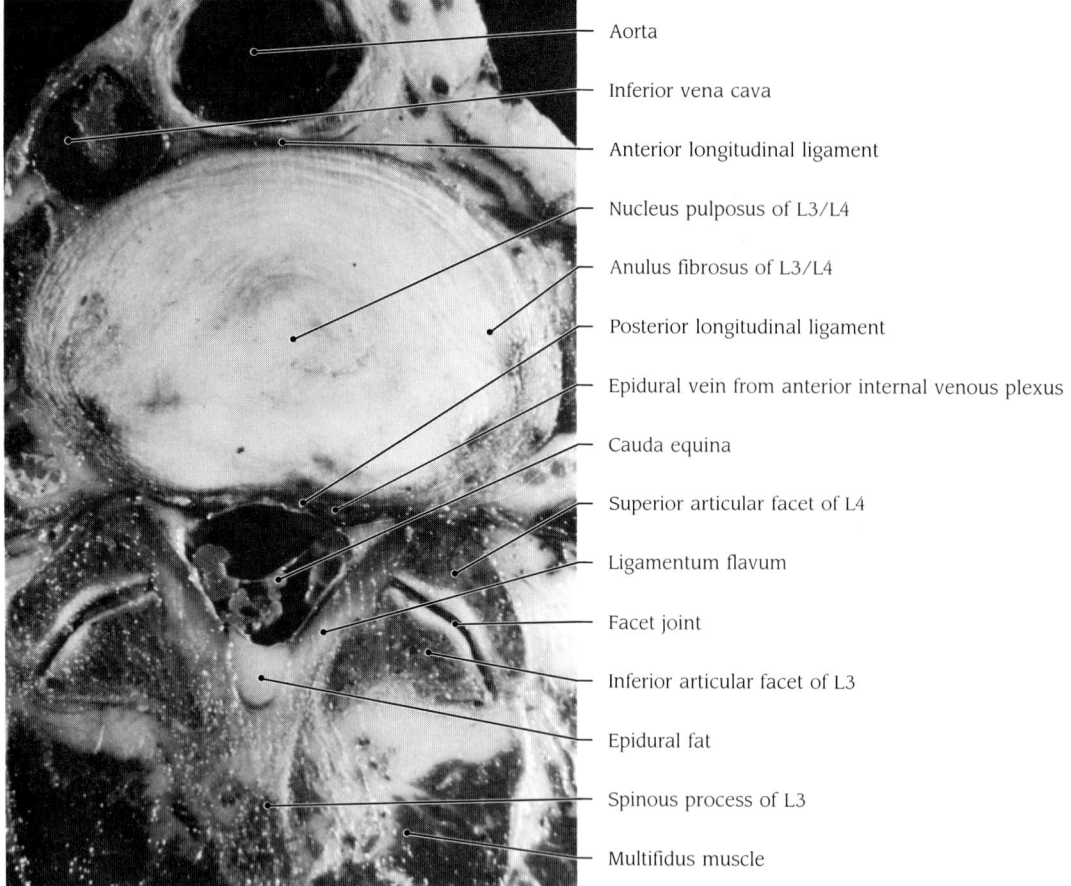

FIG. 11.10.

- The veins of the vertebral column form plexuses that are divided into internal or external groups; they anastomose freely with each other, are devoid of valves, and end in the intervertebral veins. The external vertebral venous plexus is composed of an anterior external plexus, which lies in front of the bodies of the vertebrae, and a posterior external plexus, which is located on the posterior surface of the laminae and around the spinous and transverse and articular processes. The internal vertebral venous plexus is divided into an anterior internal plexus, which lies on the posterior surfaces of the vertebral bodies and intervertebral discs, and a posterior internal plexus, which is anterior to the vertebral arch and ligamentum flavum.

- The basivertebral veins are large tortuous channels in the middle of the vertebral bodies that emerge from foramina on the posterior surfaces of the vertebral bodies and drain into the anterior internal venous plexus. Additionally, they drain into the anterior external plexus through openings on the front and sides of the vertebrae.

- The intervertebral veins drain veins from the spinal cord and the internal and external venous plexuses, accompany the spinal nerves through the intervertebral foramina, and end in the vertebral, posterior intercostal, lumbar, and lateral sacral veins.

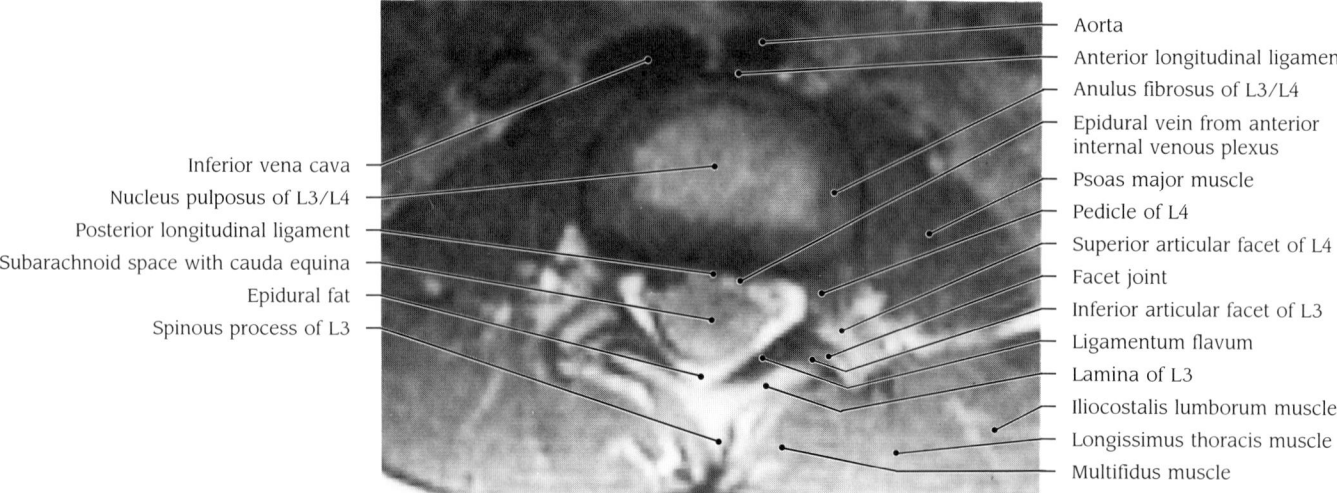

FIG. 11.11. TR = 1500 msec, TE = 40 msec.

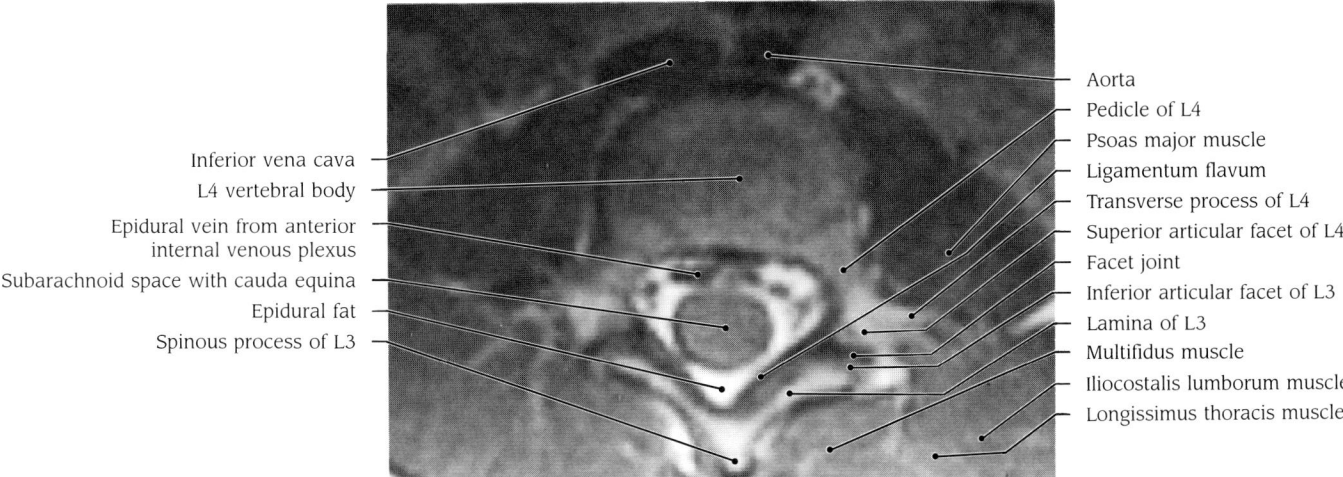

FIG. 11.12. TR = 1500 msec, TE = 40 msec.

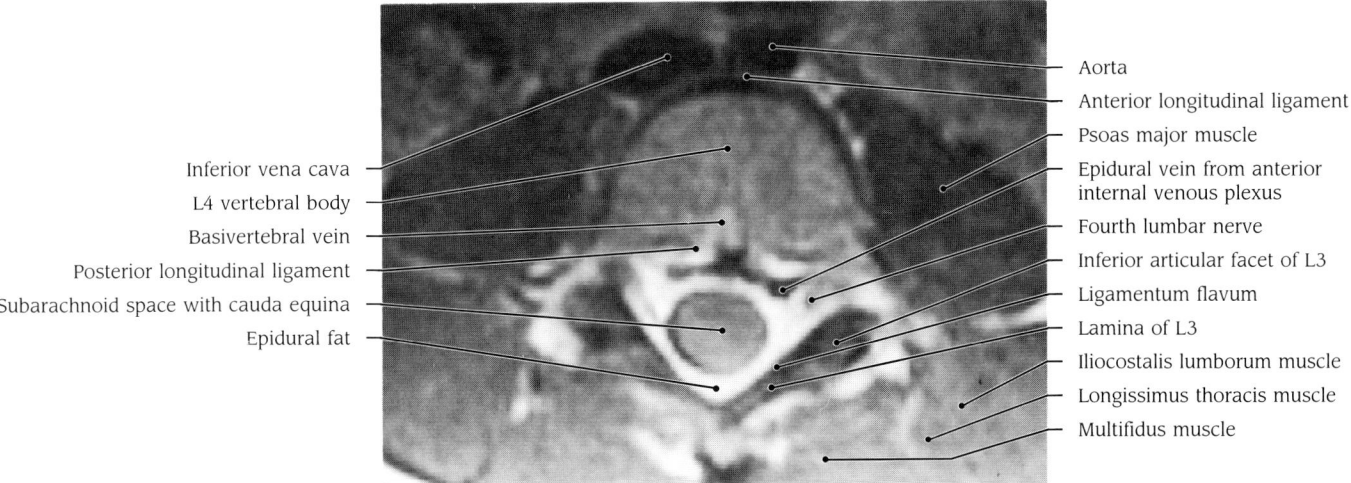

FIG. 11.13. TR = 1500 msec, TE = 40 msec.

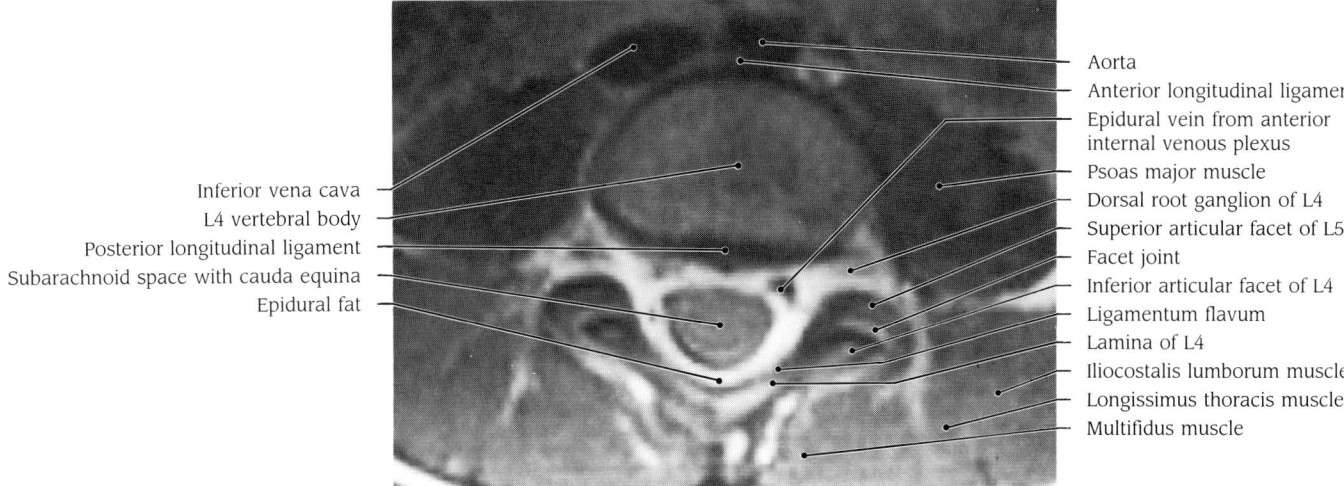

FIG. 11.14. TR = 1500 msec, TE = 40 msec.

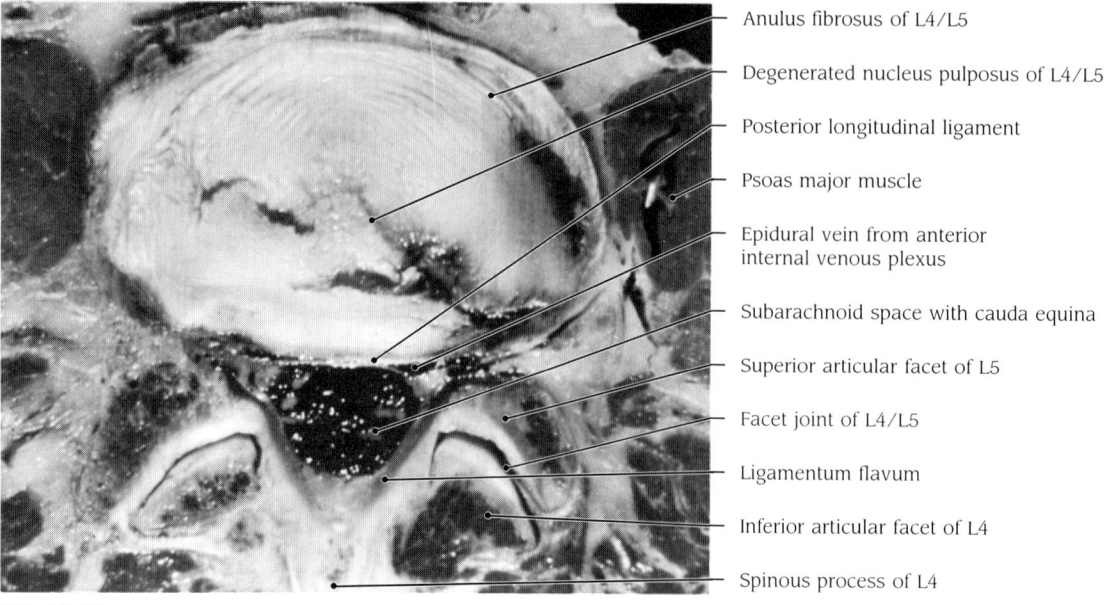

FIG. 11.15.

- Usually, four lumbar arteries on each side arise from the back of the aorta. A fifth pair of arteries may arise from the median sacral artery, but the lumbar branches of the iliolumbar arteries usually take their place. Each lumbar artery gives off a dorsal ramus, which goes posteriorly to the muscles and skin of the back. The posterior ramus has a spinal branch that enters the vertebral canal to supply its contents and adjacent vertebrae.

- The ganglia of the lower lumbar and sacral nerves are spindle-shaped structures that course inferiorly and outward.

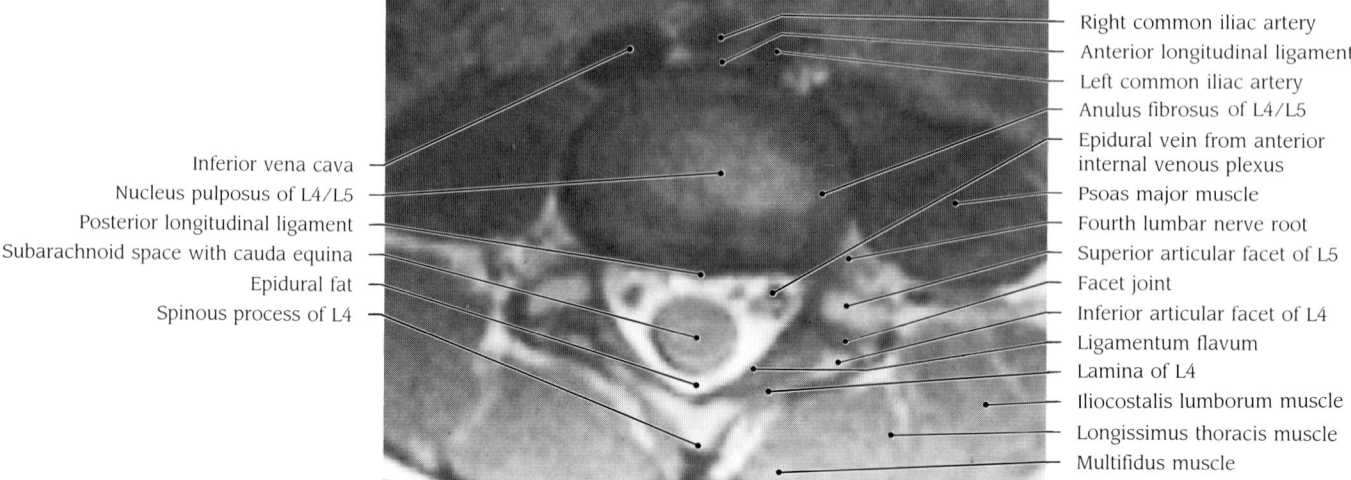

FIG. 11.16. TR = 1500 msec, TE = 40 msec.

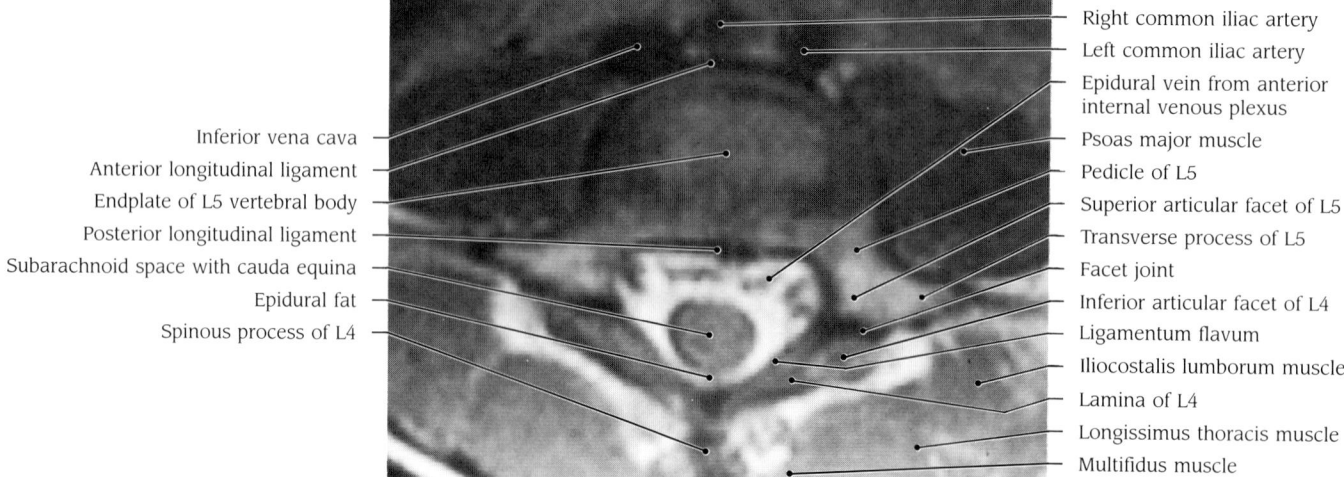

FIG. 11.17. TR = 1500 msec, TE = 40 msec.

254

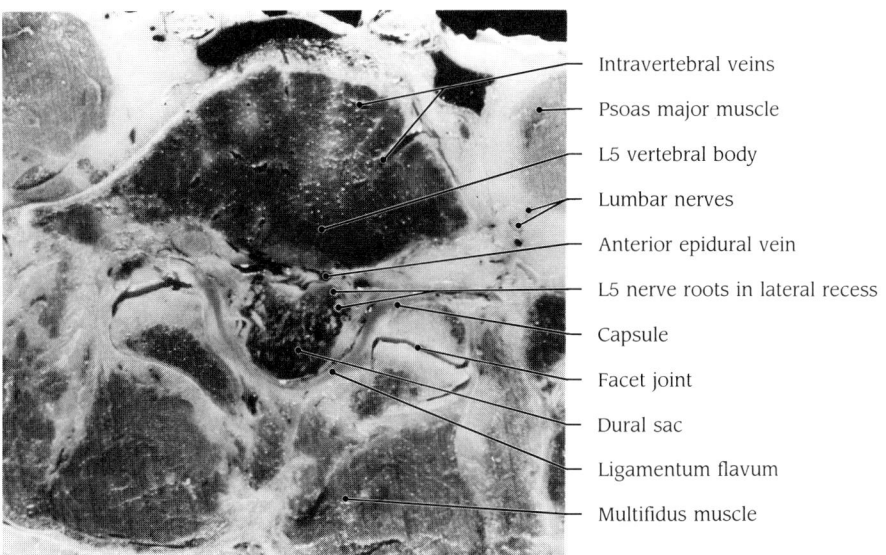

FIG. 11.18.

- Intravertebral veins
- Psoas major muscle
- L5 vertebral body
- Lumbar nerves
- Anterior epidural vein
- L5 nerve roots in lateral recess
- Capsule
- Facet joint
- Dural sac
- Ligamentum flavum
- Multifidus muscle

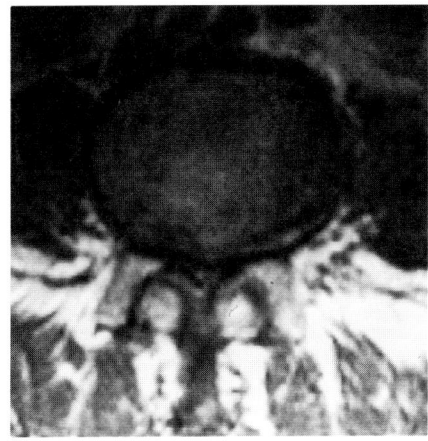

FIG. 11.19. TR = 739 msec, TE = 39 msec. Marked spinal stenosis present at the L4/L5 level is caused by congenitally short pedicles, facet joint hypertrophy, and a circumferential disc protrusion.

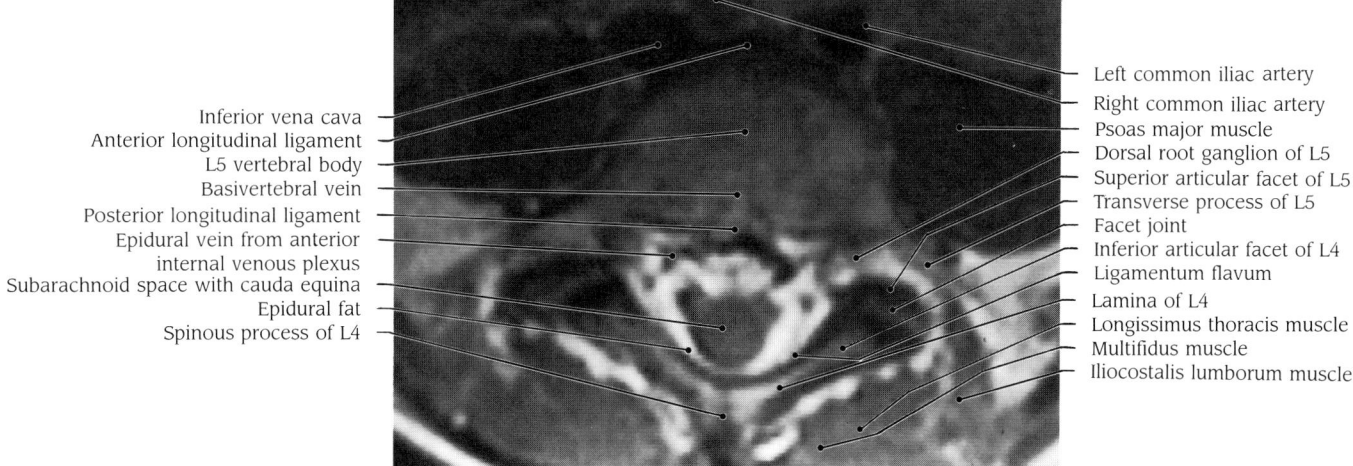

FIG. 11.20. TR = 1500 msec, TE = 40 msec.

- Inferior vena cava
- Anterior longitudinal ligament
- L5 vertebral body
- Basivertebral vein
- Posterior longitudinal ligament
- Epidural vein from anterior internal venous plexus
- Subarachnoid space with cauda equina
- Epidural fat
- Spinous process of L4
- Left common iliac artery
- Right common iliac artery
- Psoas major muscle
- Dorsal root ganglion of L5
- Superior articular facet of L5
- Transverse process of L5
- Facet joint
- Inferior articular facet of L4
- Ligamentum flavum
- Lamina of L4
- Longissimus thoracis muscle
- Multifidus muscle
- Iliocostalis lumborum muscle

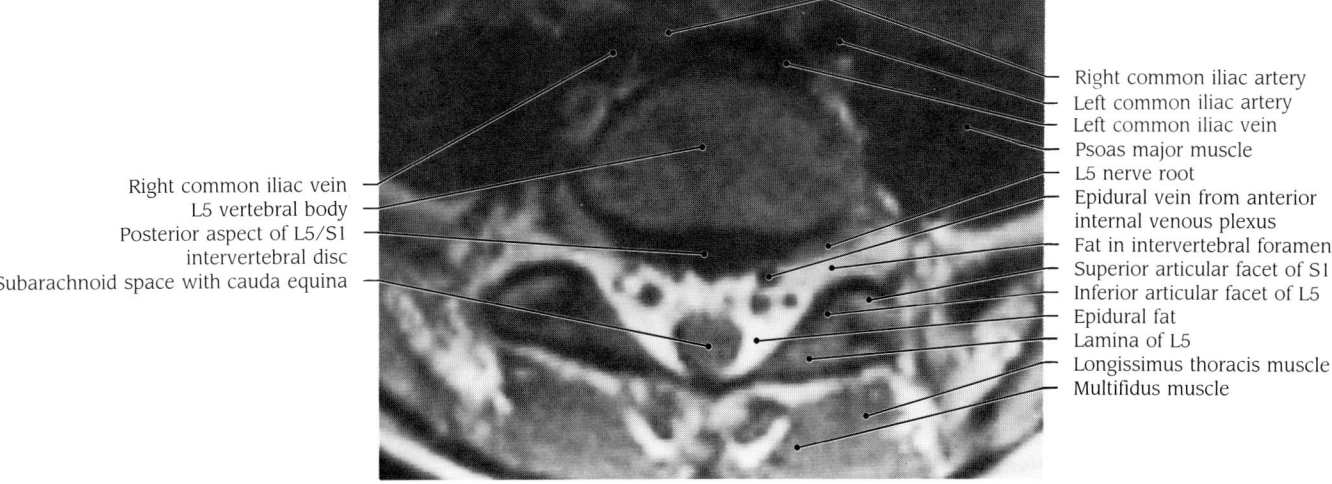

FIG. 11.21. TR = 1500 msec, TE = 40 msec.

- Right common iliac vein
- L5 vertebral body
- Posterior aspect of L5/S1 intervertebral disc
- Subarachnoid space with cauda equina
- Right common iliac artery
- Left common iliac artery
- Left common iliac vein
- Psoas major muscle
- L5 nerve root
- Epidural vein from anterior internal venous plexus
- Fat in intervertebral foramen
- Superior articular facet of S1
- Inferior articular facet of L5
- Epidural fat
- Lamina of L5
- Longissimus thoracis muscle
- Multifidus muscle

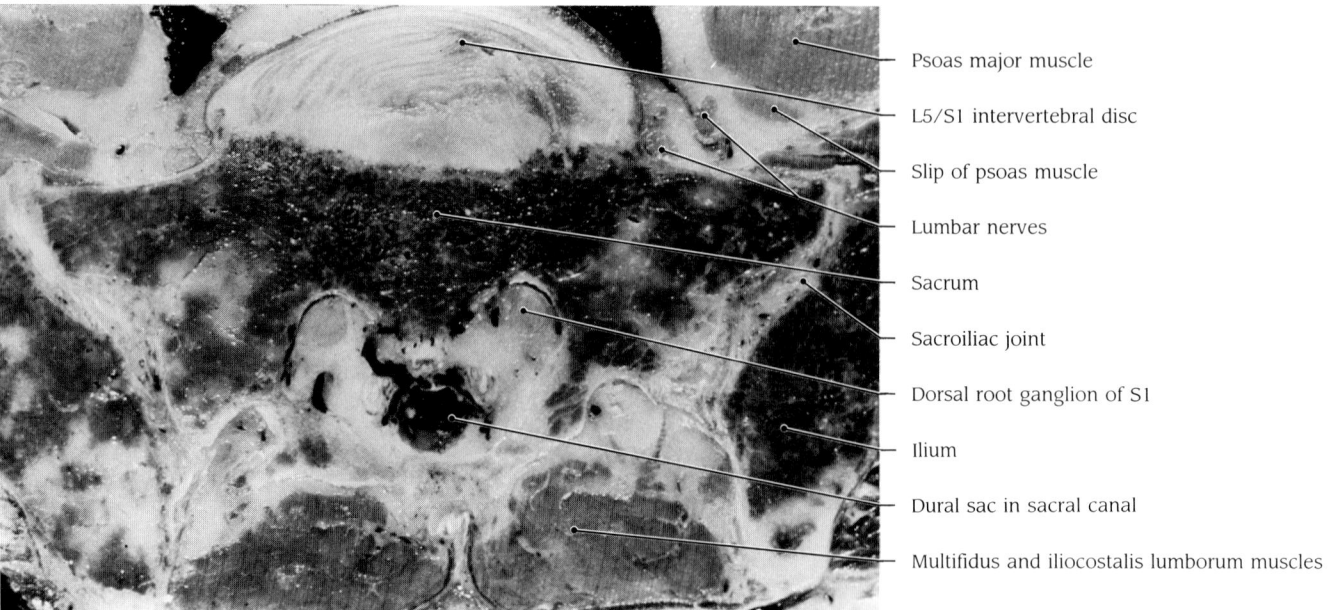

FIG. 11.22.

- The filum terminale externa, which is composed of connective tissue, courses within the sacral canal and extends from the lower end of the dural sac and attaches to the first coccygeal vertebra. The filum terminale interna, which courses within the subarachnoid space and extends from the tip of the conus to the distal aspect of the dural sac, is composed of pia and glial fibers and often is accompanied by a vein.

- The sacrum contains anterior and posterior foramina at each level that transmit the larger anterior ramus and the smaller posterior ramus, respectively. The sacral dorsal root ganglion is situated within the sacral canal, an extension of the vertebral canal.

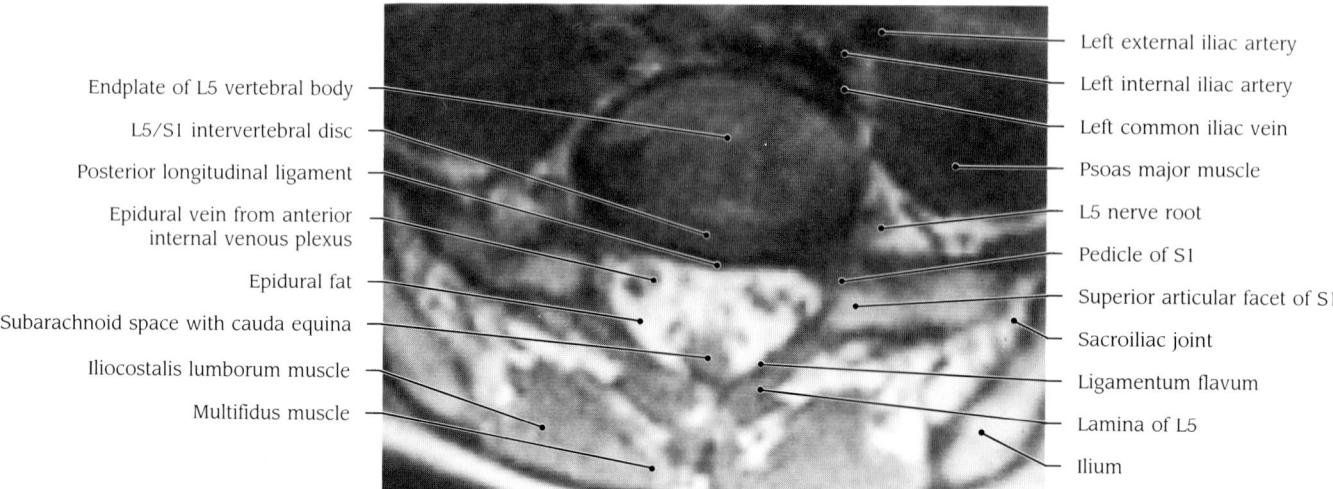

FIG. 11.23. TR = 1500 msec, TE = 40 msec.

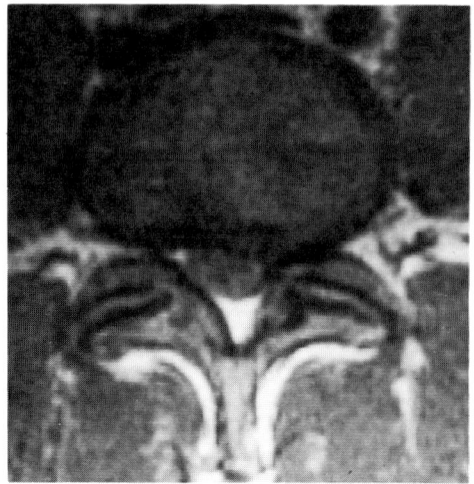

FIG. 11.24. TR = 739 msec, TE = 39 msec. Spinal stenosis and an intervertebral disc herniation on the left are present at L4/L5.

256

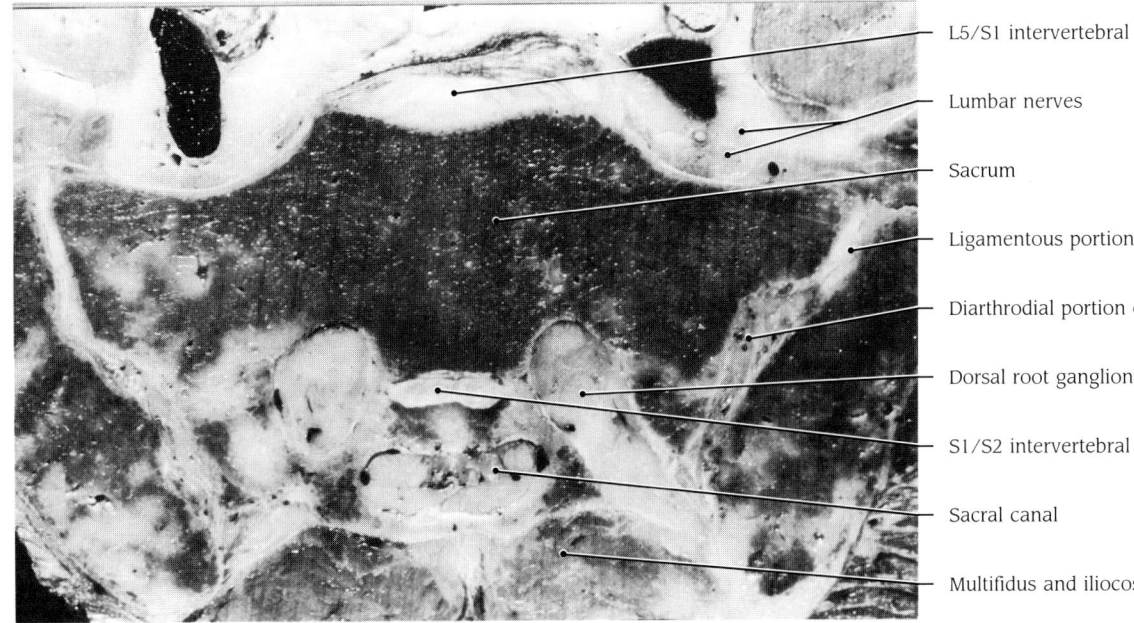

FIG. 11.25.

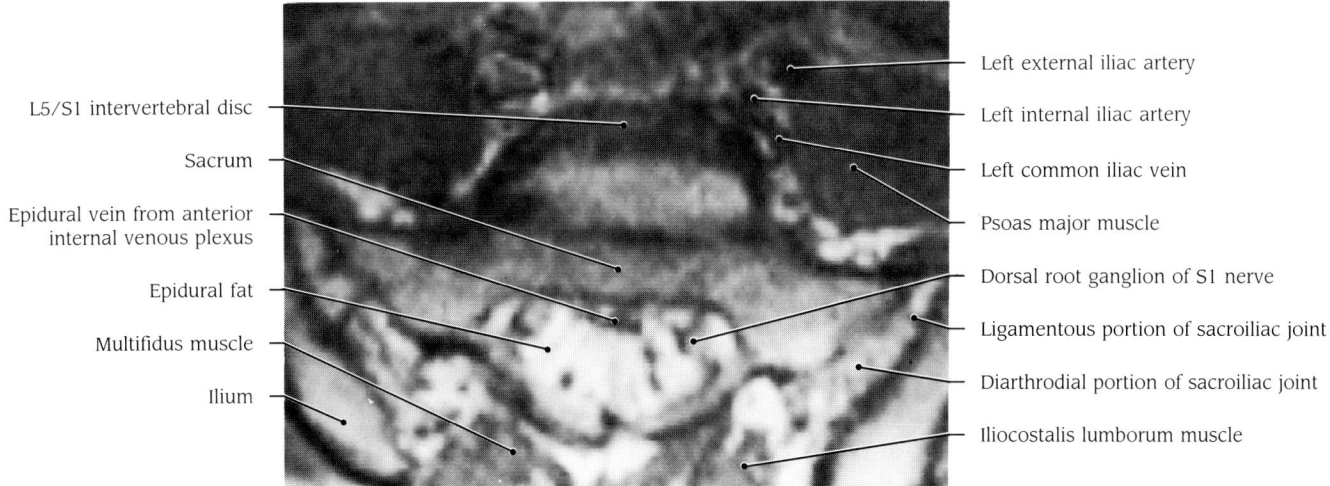

FIG. 11.26. TR = 1500 msec, TE = 40 msec.

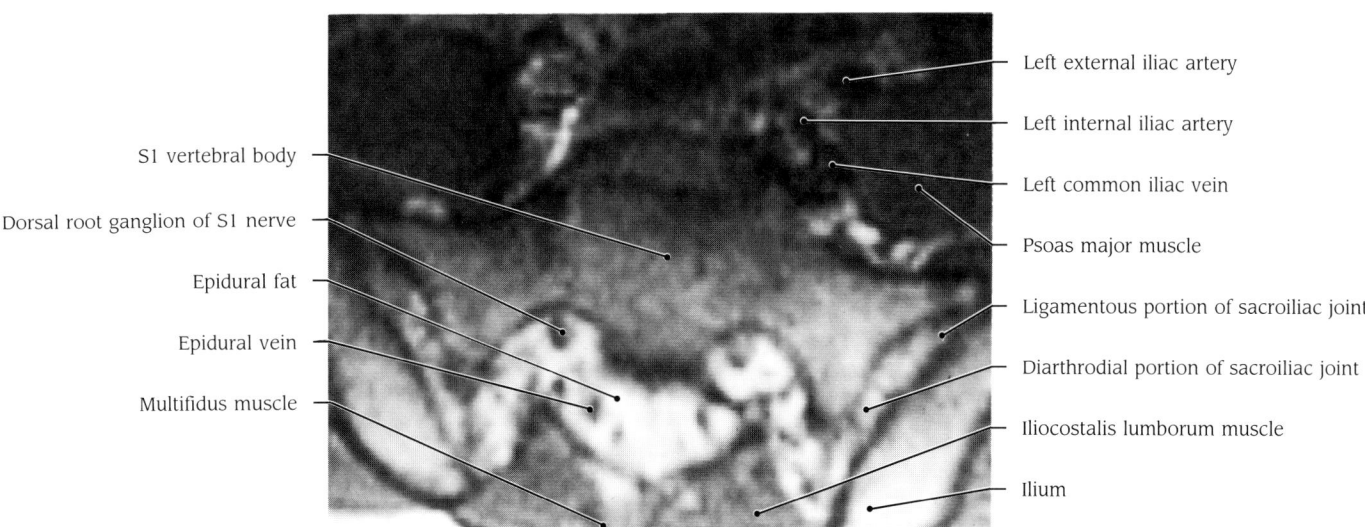

FIG. 11.27. TR = 1500 msec, TE = 40 msec.

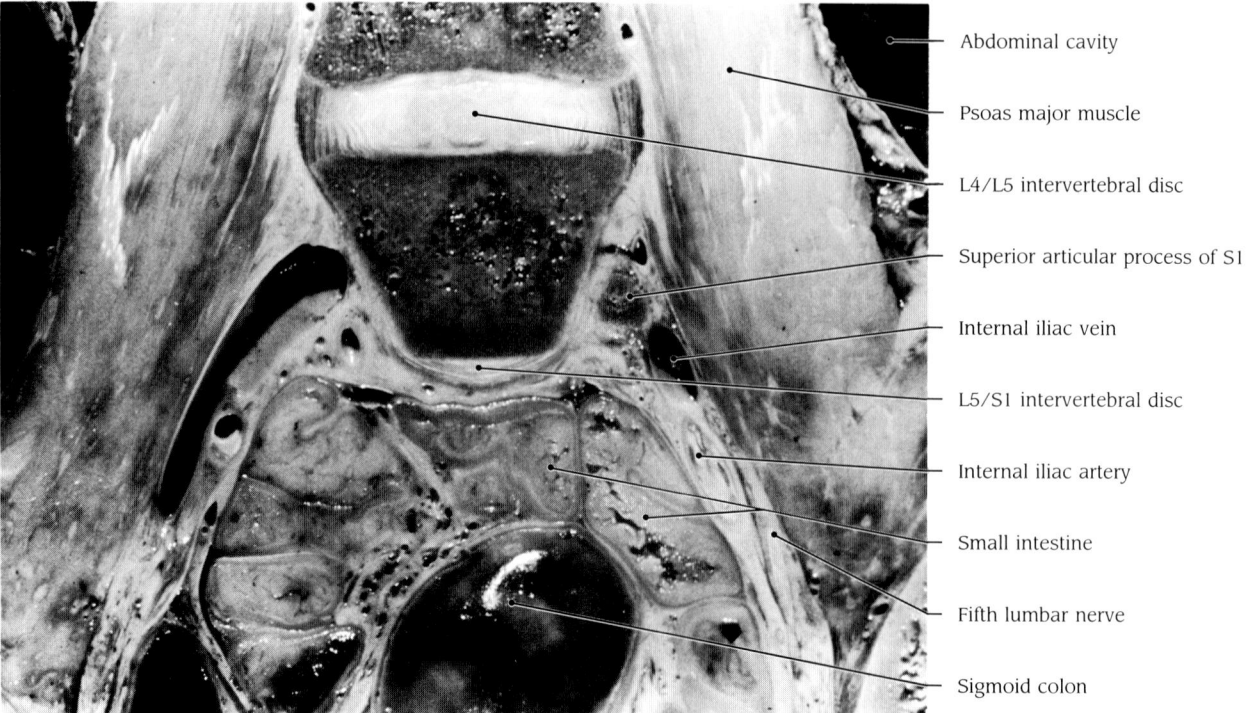

FIG. 11.28.

- The psoas major muscle arises from the bodies, the transverse processes, and the intervertebral discs of all the lumbar vertebrae, as well as of the twelfth thoracic vertebra. It descends along the pelvic brim and attaches to the lesser trochanter of the femur. The psoas major muscle functions with the iliacus muscle to flex the thigh, and when both the right and left pairs of muscles act in concert, they contract to bend the trunk and pelvis forward against resistance. When the neck of the femur is fractured, the psoas major muscle acts as a lateral rotator of the femur.

- The iliacus muscle is a large fan-shaped muscle that lies along the lower lateral side of the psoas major muscle. It arises from the iliac fossa, the inner lip of the iliac crest, the lateral part of the sacrum, and the sacroiliac and iliolumbar ligaments. Its fibers primarily insert into the lateral side of the tendon of the psoas major muscle; however, some of the fibers attach directly to the femur.

- Epidural abscesses in the lower thoracic and upper lumbar region may track into the thigh within the fascial sheath of the psoas major muscle.

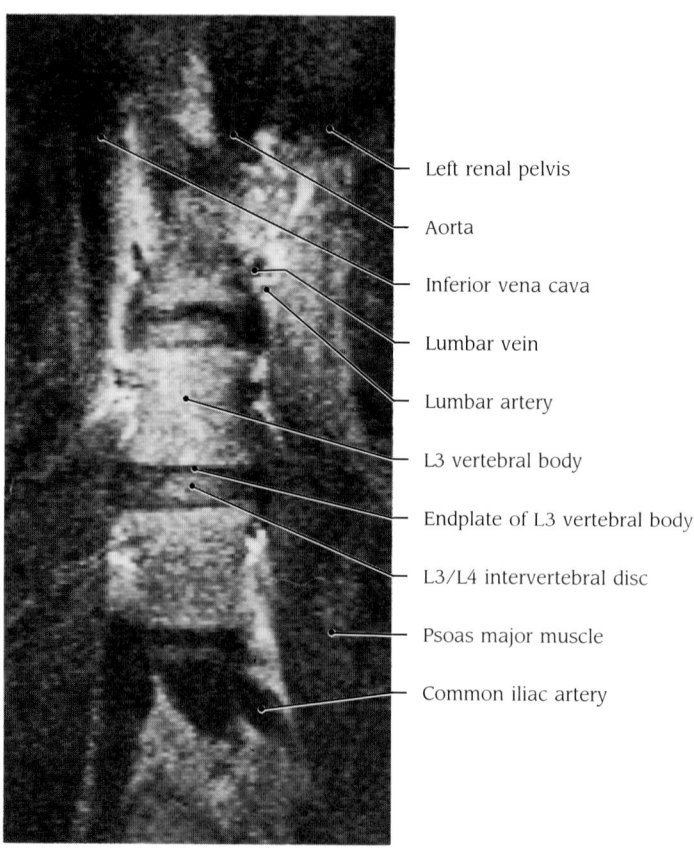

FIG. 11.29. TR = 837 msec, TE = 37 msec.

FIG. 11.30. TR = 5000 msec, TE = 64 msec.

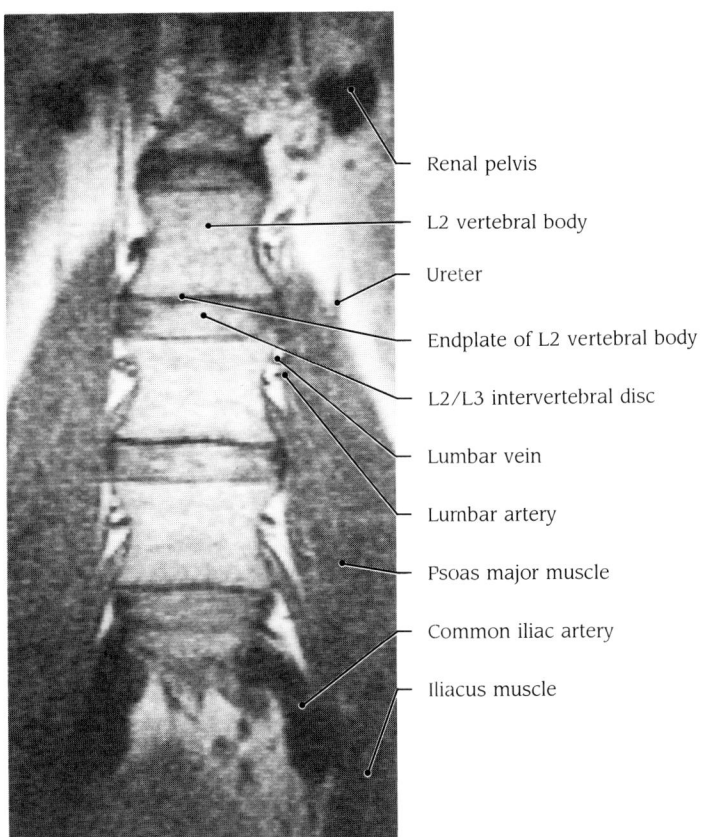

FIG. 11.31. TR = 837 msec, TE = 37 msec.

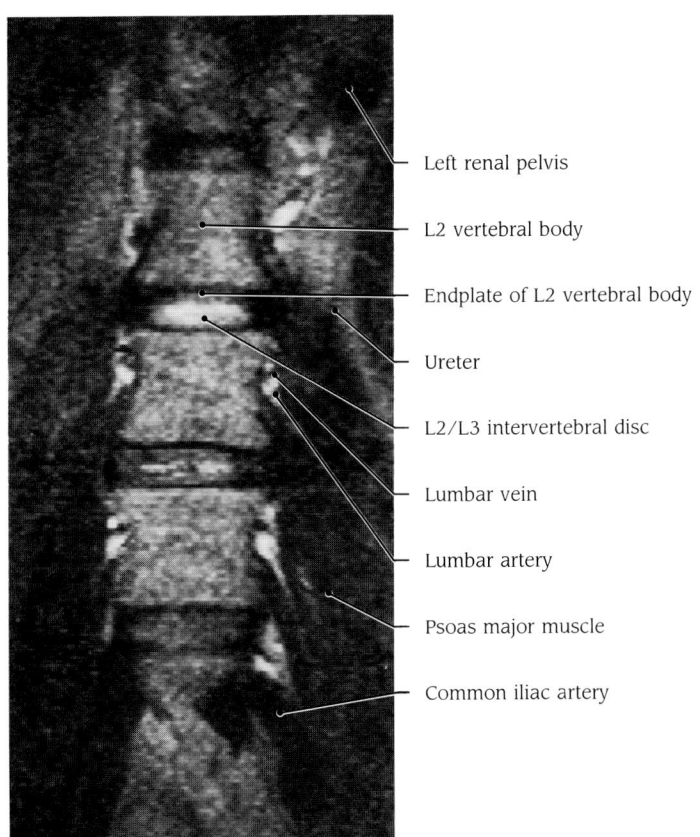

FIG. 11.32. TR = 5000 msec, TE = 64 msec.

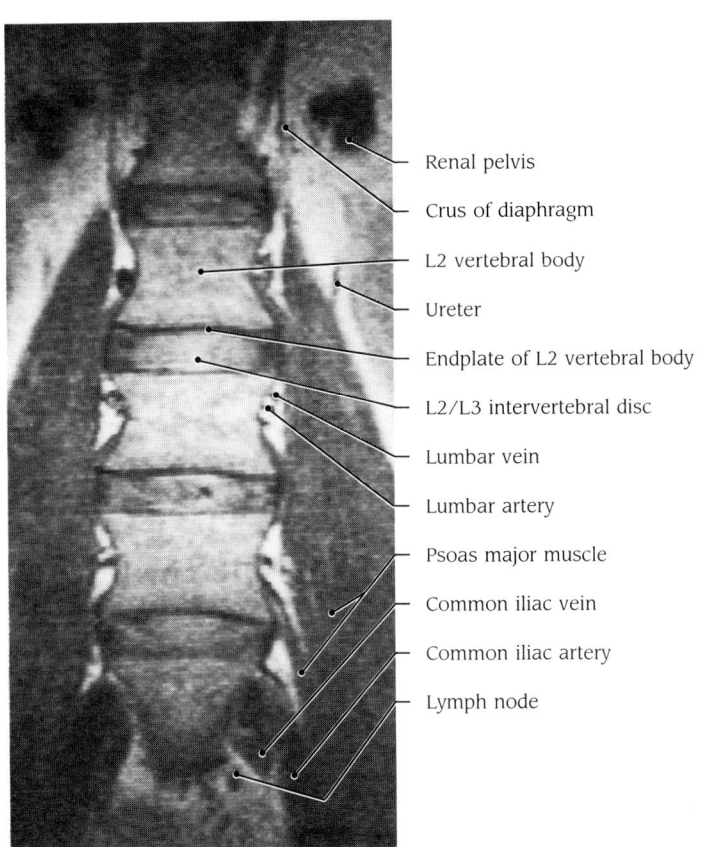

FIG. 11.33. TR = 837 msec, TE = 37 msec.

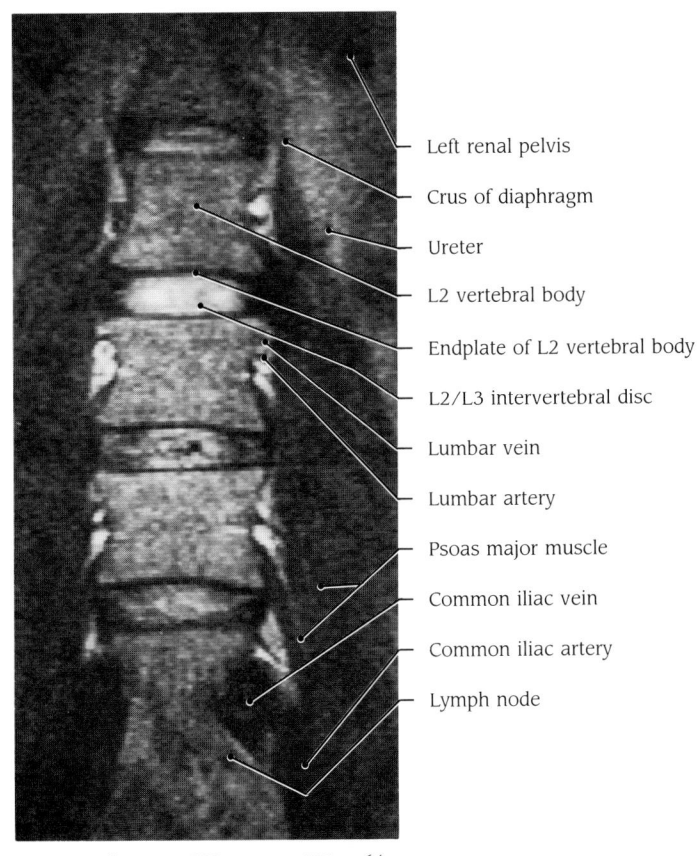

FIG. 11.34. TR = 5000 msec, TE = 64 msec.

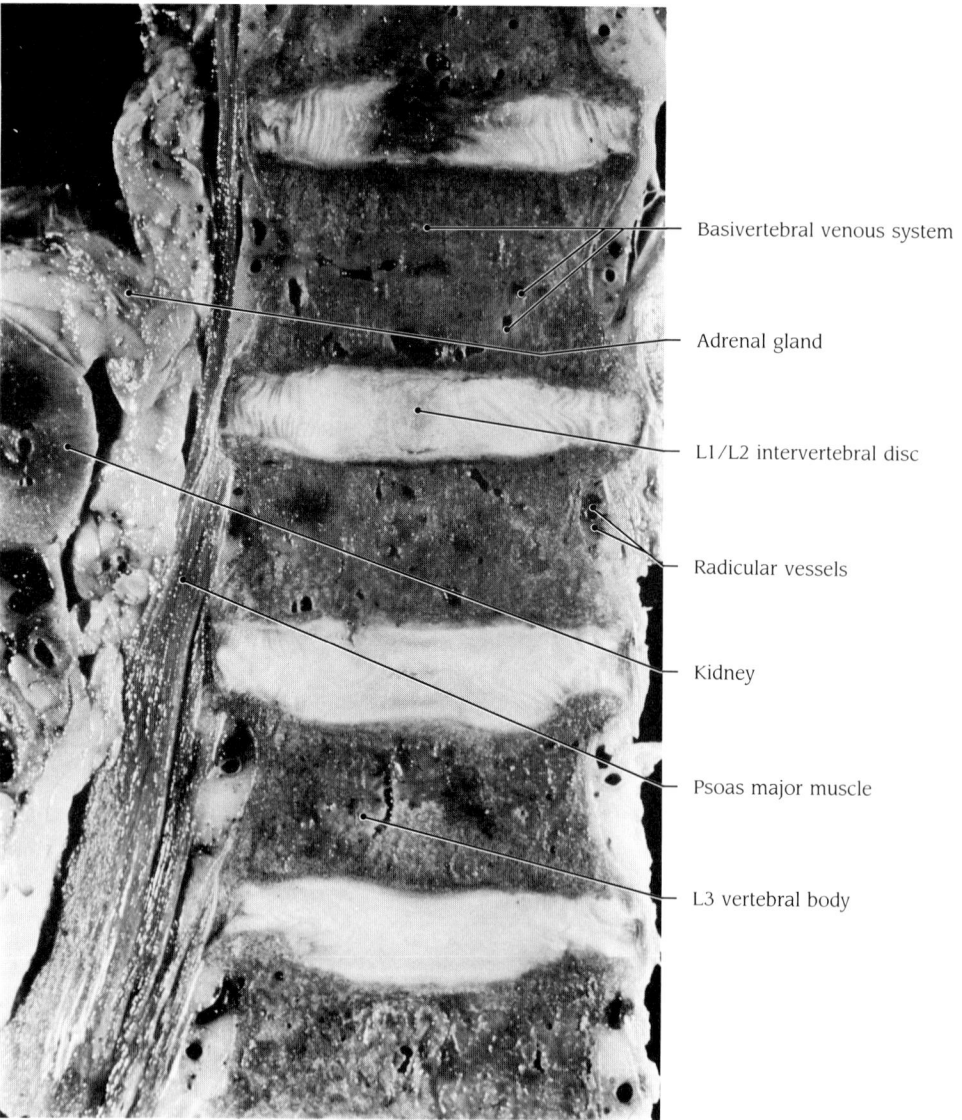

FIG. 11.35.

- The crura of the diaphragm are tendinous at their attachments and blend with the anterior longitudinal ligament of the vertebral column. The right crus arises from the anterolateral surfaces of the bodies and intervertebral discs of the upper three lumbar vertebrae, whereas the left crus arises from the corresponding parts of the upper two lumbar vertebrae. The crura meet in the median plane to form an arch across the anterior aspect of the aorta, called the median arcuate ligament.

- The lumbar arteries and veins and branches of the sympathetic trunk are medial to the psoas major muscle.

- The intervertebral discs are thicker anteriorly than posteriorly in both the cervical spine and the lumbar spine. This difference contributes to the anterior convexities of these levels. The greater thickness of the intervertebral discs in the lumbar area, as well as in the cervical area, is associated with wider individual range of motion when compared to the thoracic area.

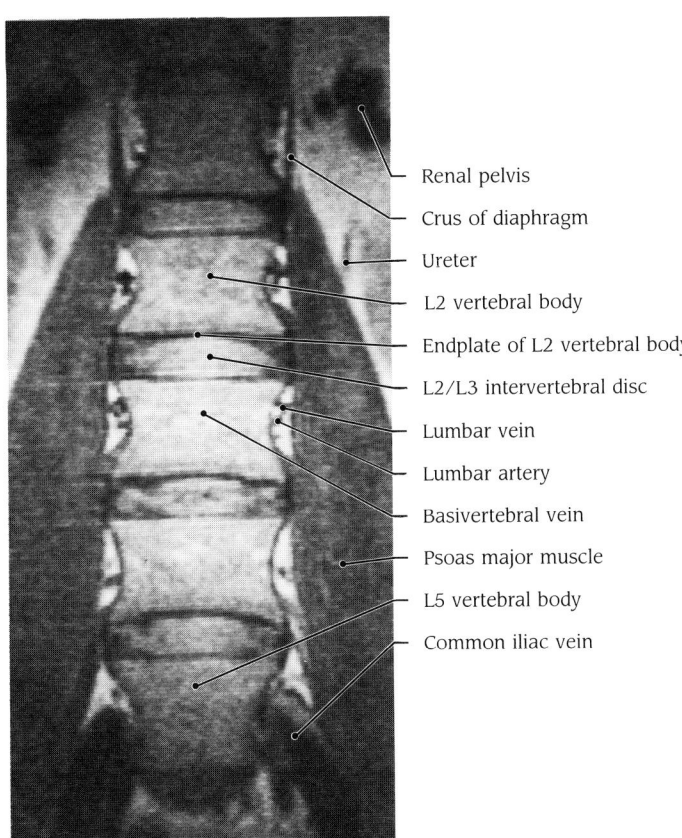

FIG. 11.36. TR = 837 msec, TE = 37 msec.

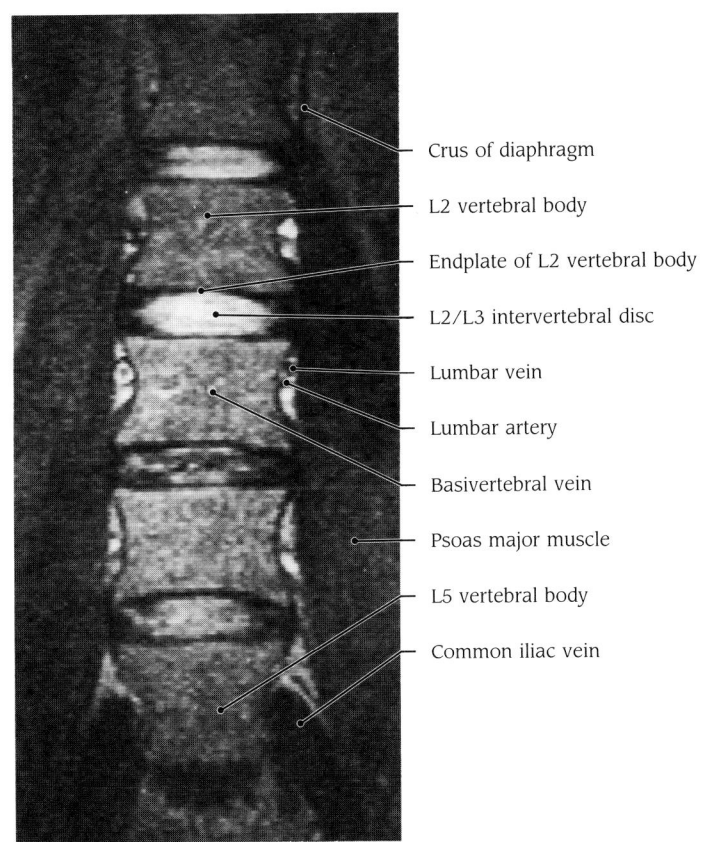

FIG. 11.37. TR = 5000 msec, TE = 64 msec.

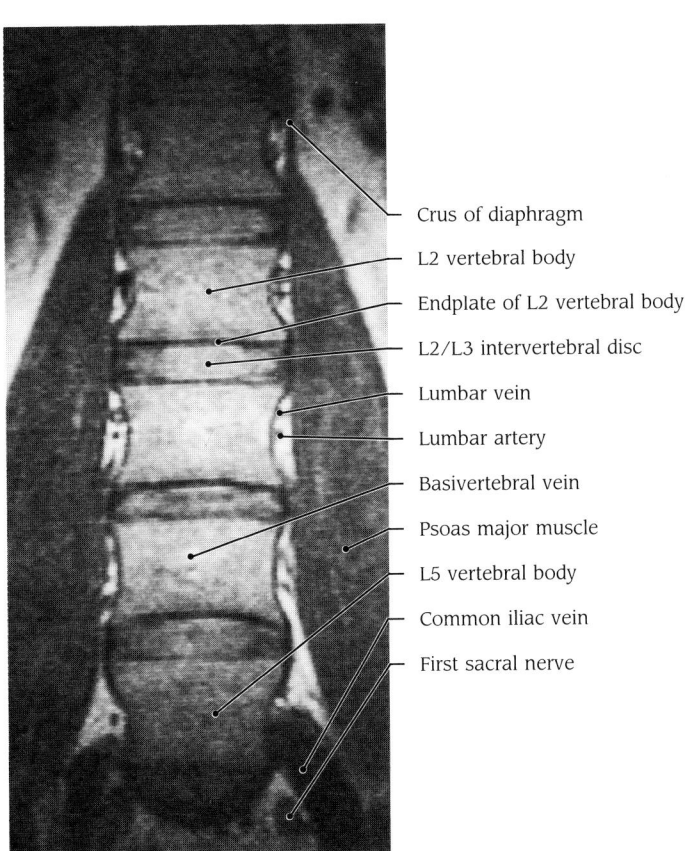

FIG. 11.38. TR = 837 msec, TE = 37 msec.

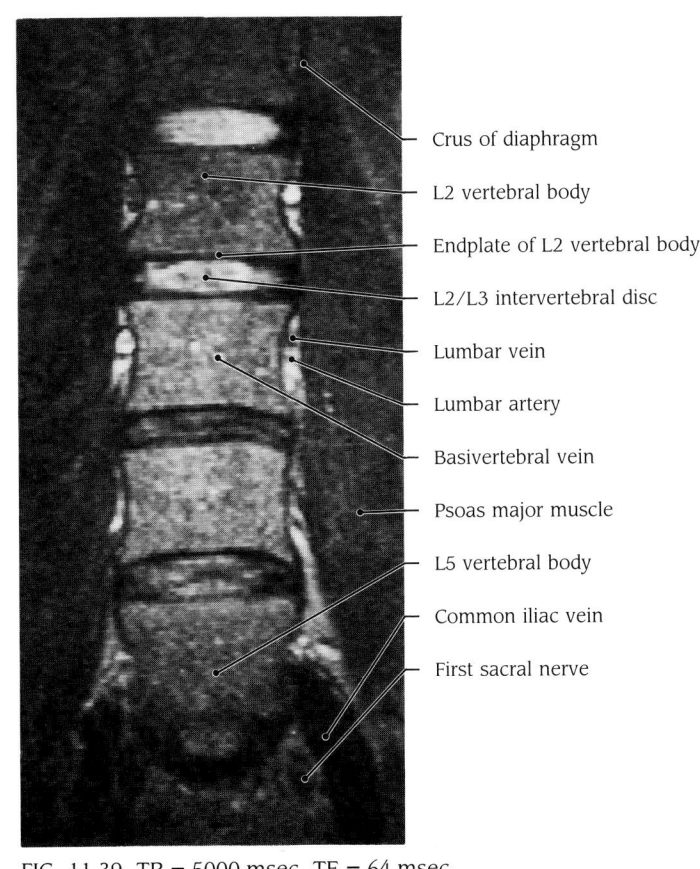

FIG. 11.39. TR = 5000 msec, TE = 64 msec.

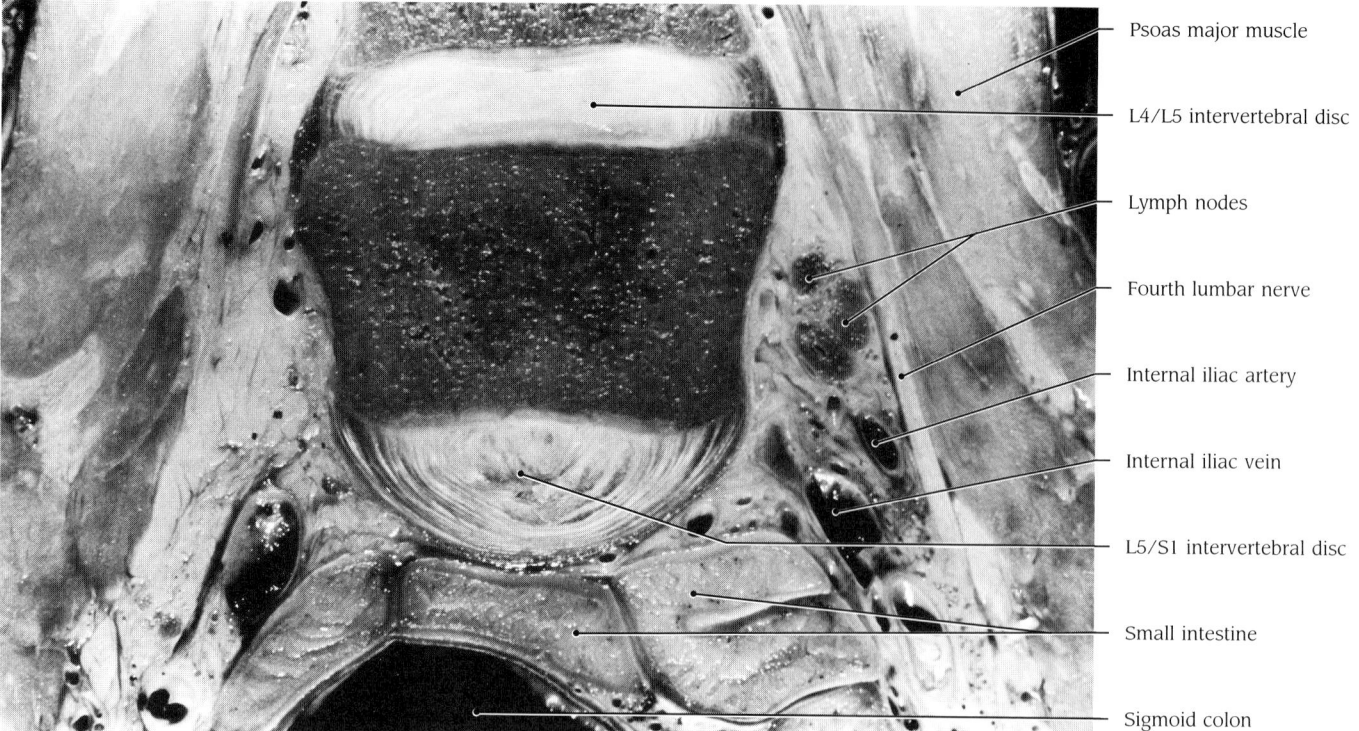

FIG. 11.40.

- In flexion, the anterior longitudinal ligament is relaxed and the anterior aspects of the intervertebral discs are compressed. The posterior longitudinal ligament, the ligamenta flava, the interspinous and supraspinous ligaments, and the extensor muscles of the back function to limit flexion. Extension is limited by the anterior longitudinal ligament and by the approximation of the spines. In the lumbar region, extension is free and wider in range than flexion.

- The lumbar plexus lies anterior to the transverse processes of the lumbar vertebrae, within the posterior portion of the psoas major muscle. It is formed by the ventral rami of the first three lumbar nerves, part of the fourth, and a branch from the twelfth thoracic nerve.

- The obturator nerve arises from the anterior branches of the ventral rami of the second, third, and fourth lumbar nerves.

- The femoral nerve, the largest branch of the lumbar plexus, arises from the posterior branches of the ventral rami of the second, third, and fourth lumbar nerves.

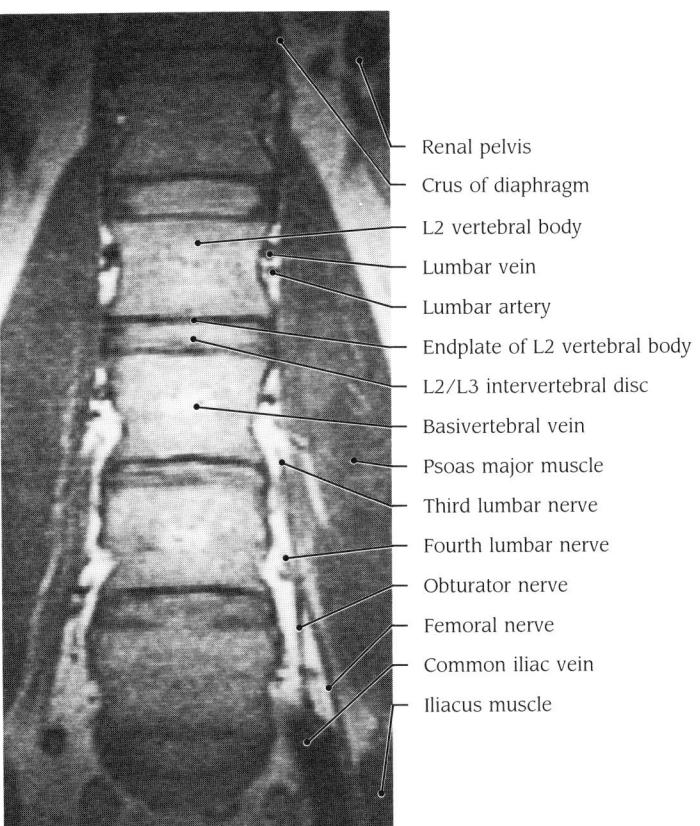

FIG. 11.41. TR = 837 msec, TE = 37 msec.

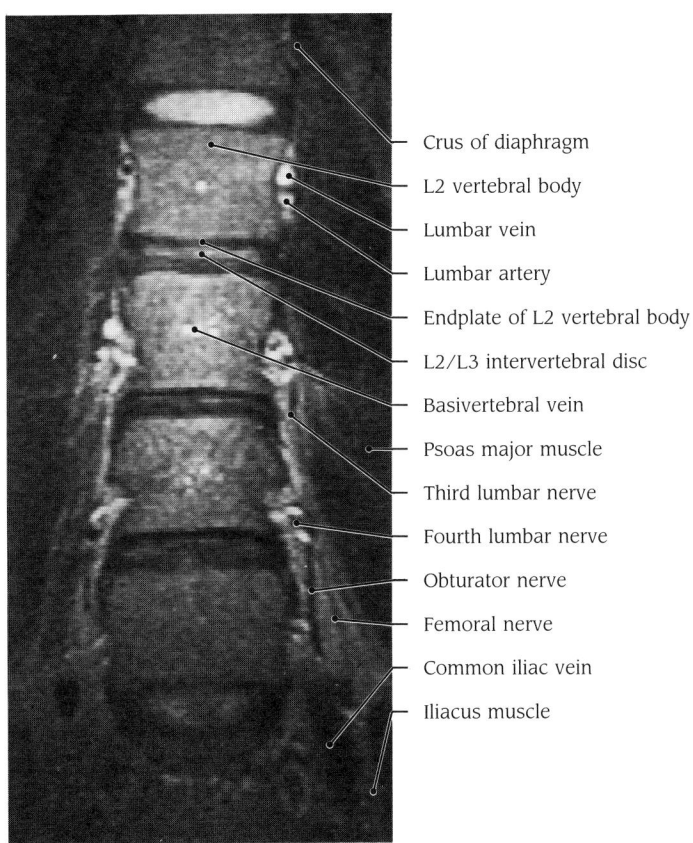

FIG. 11.42. TR = 5000 msec, TE = 64 msec.

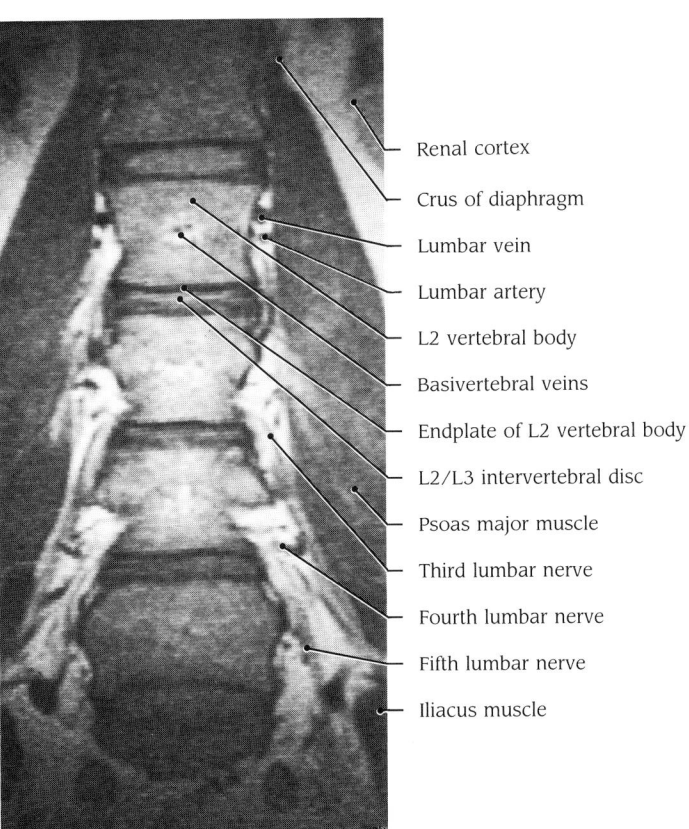

FIG. 11.43. TR = 837 msec, TE = 37 msec.

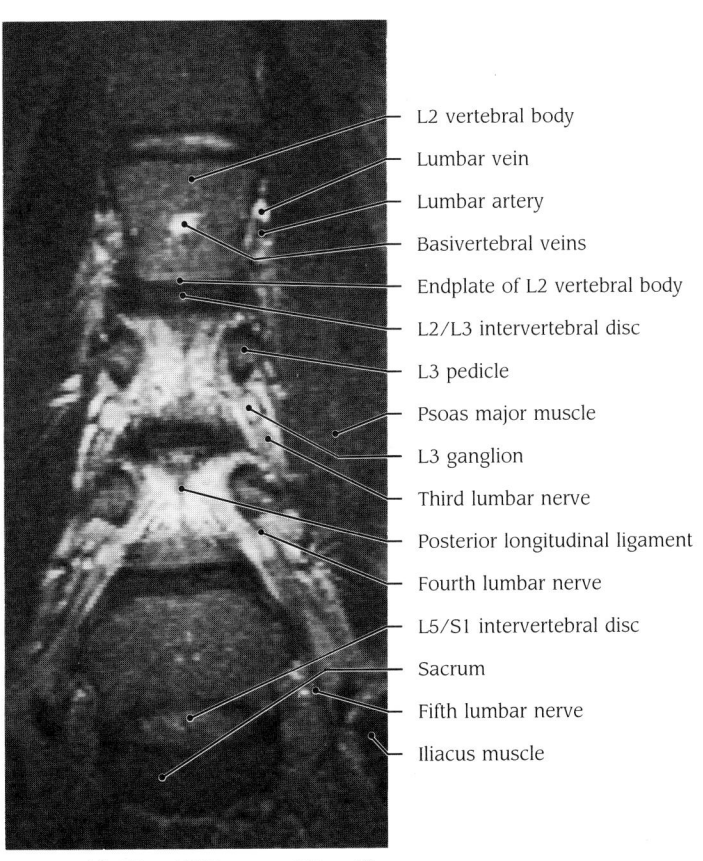

FIG. 11.44. TR = 5000 msec, TE = 64 msec.

263

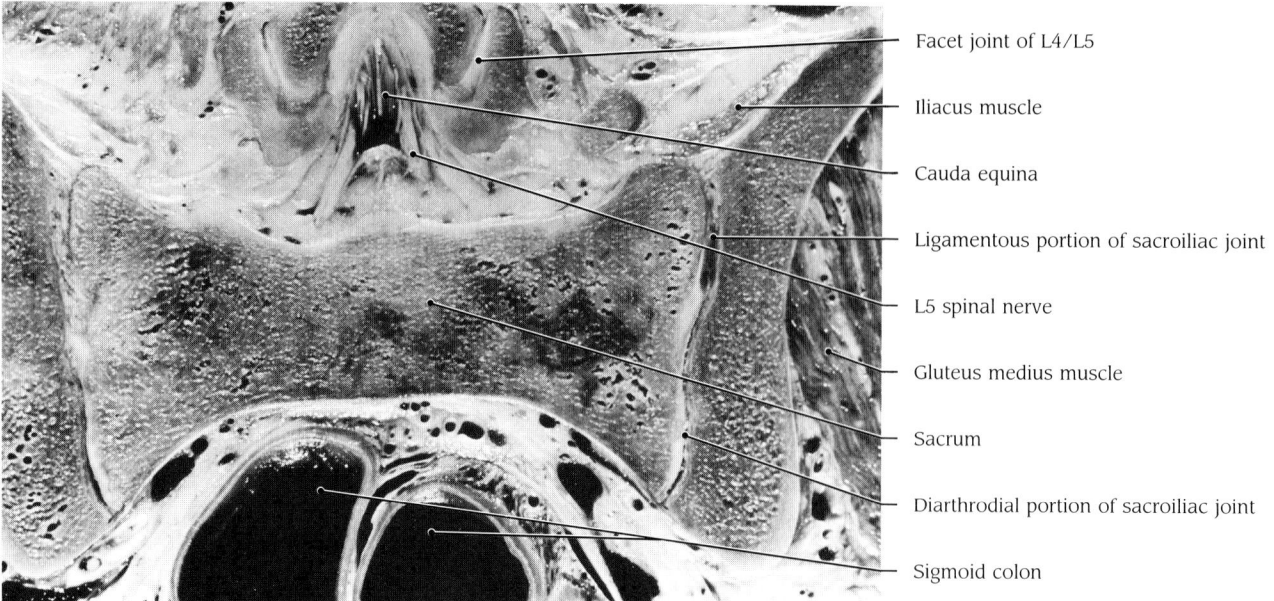

FIG. 11.45.

- The basivertebral veins are large, tortuous channels within the vertebral bodies. They emerge from foramina on the posterior aspect of the vertebral bodies and converge to form single or, occasionally, double veins that drain into the transverse branches connecting the anterior internal venous plexuses. The basivertebral veins additionally drain into the anterior external venous plexuses via foramina on the anterior and lateral surfaces of the vertebral bodies.

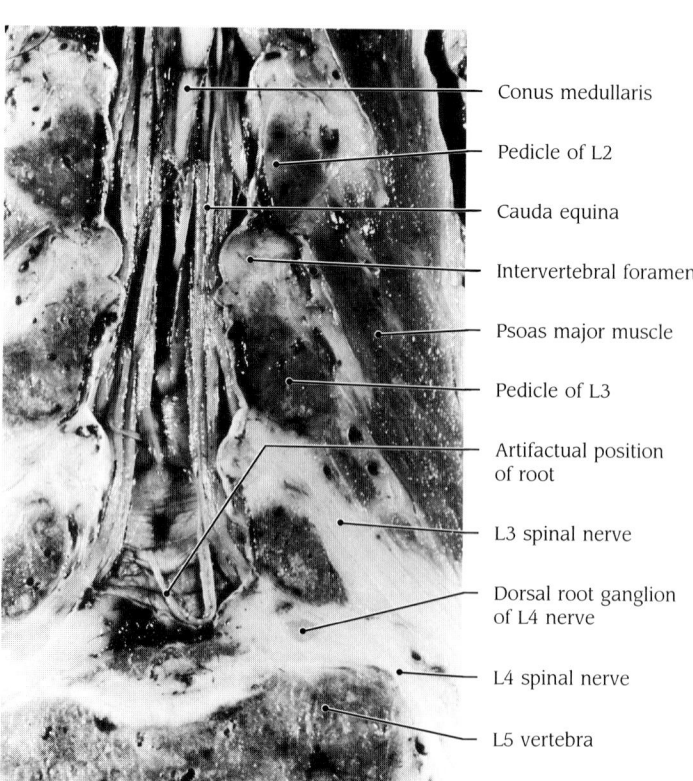

FIG. 11.46.

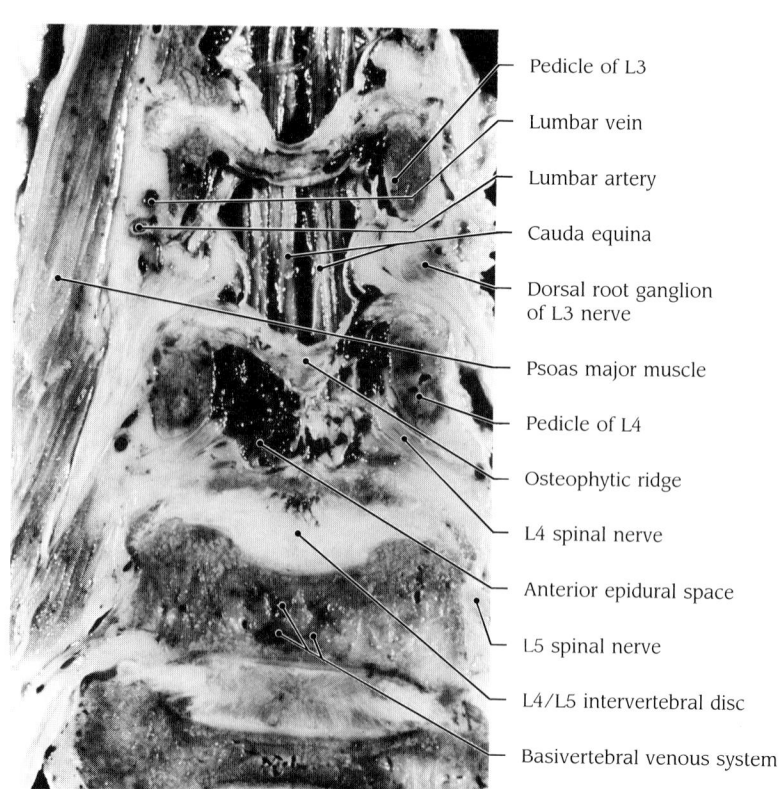

FIG. 11.47.

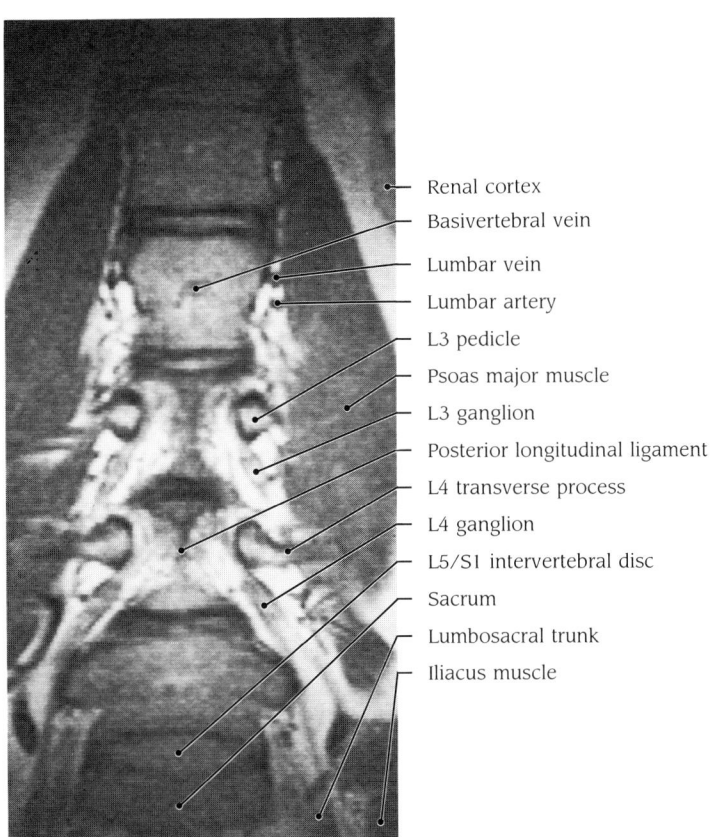

FIG. 11.48. TR = 837 msec, TE = 37 msec.

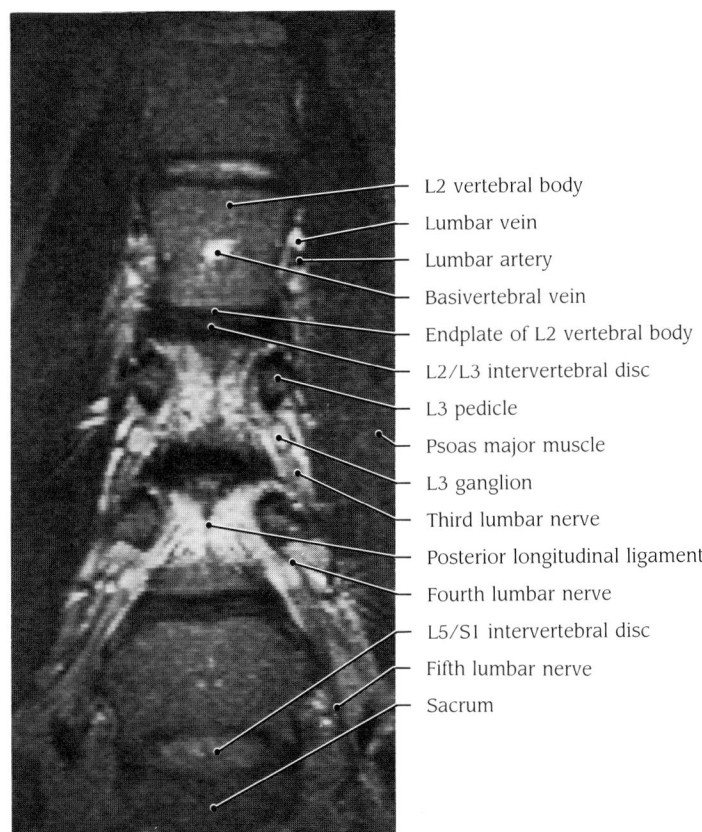

FIG. 11.49. TR = 5000 msec, TE = 64 msec.

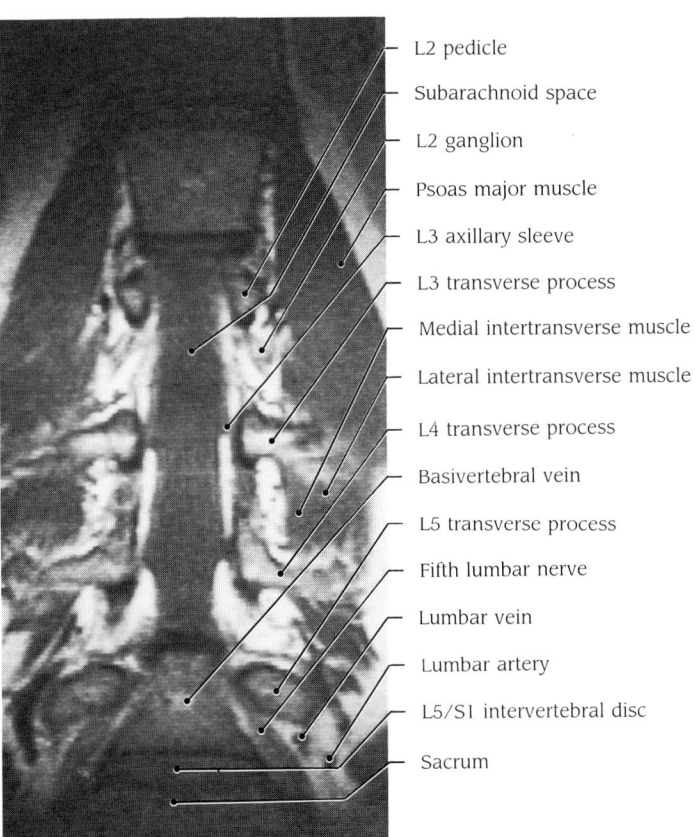

FIG. 11.50. TR = 837 msec, TE = 37 msec.

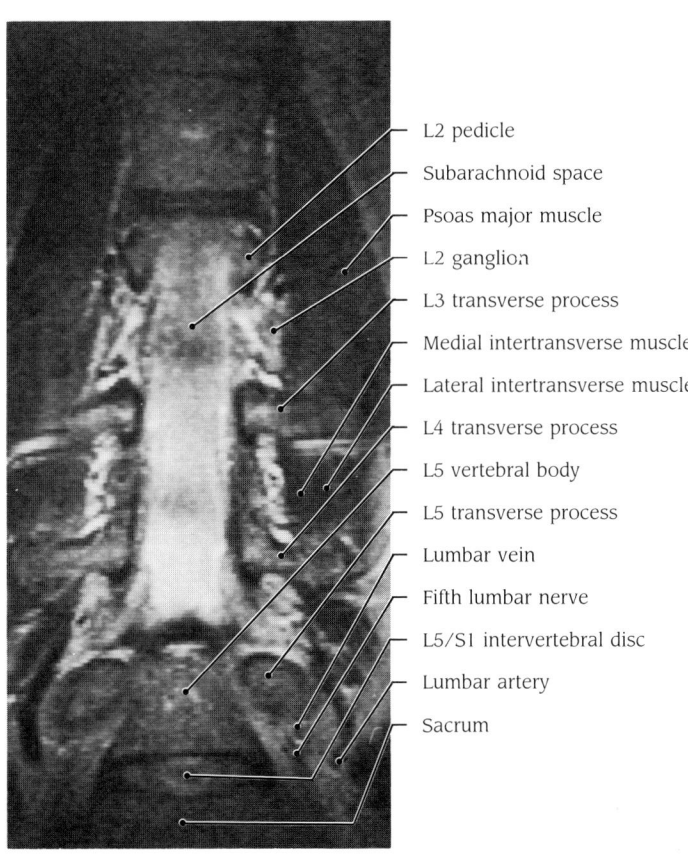

FIG. 11.51. TR = 5000 msec, TE = 64 msec.

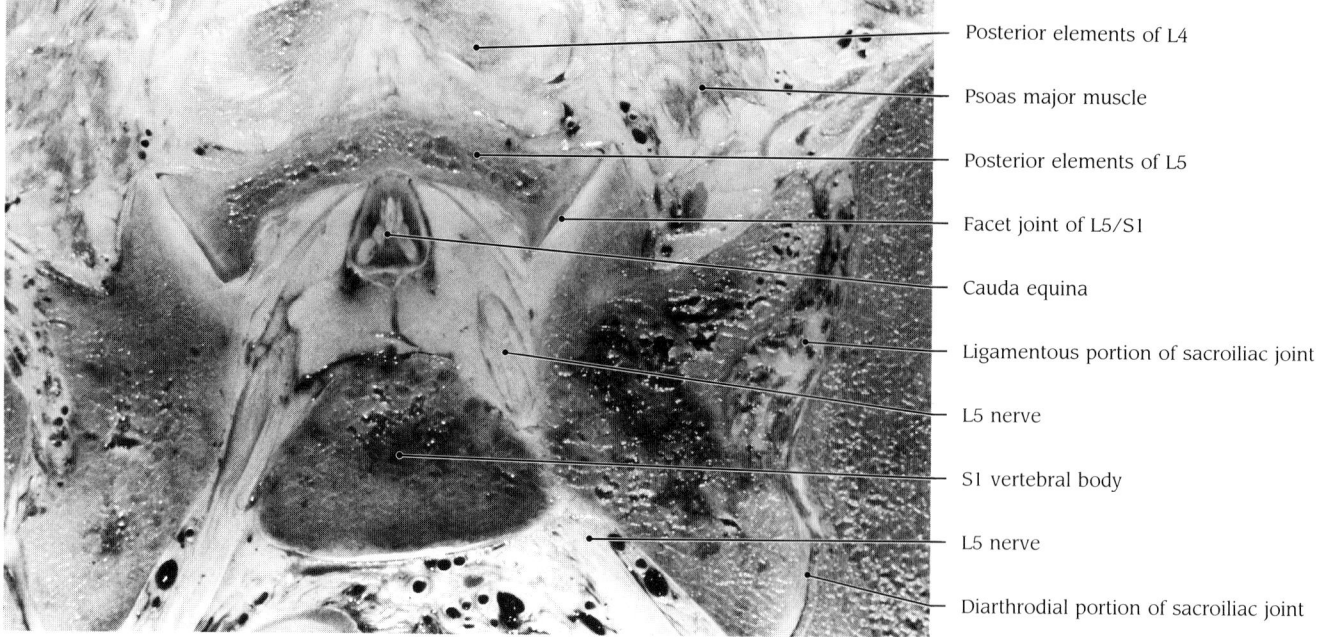

FIG. 11.52.

- A tubular prolongation of dura invests both the roots of the spinal nerves and the spinal nerves themselves as they pass through the intervertebral foramina. These dural sleeves are short in the upper part of the vertebral column, but gradually become longer more caudally because of the increasing obliquity of the nerve roots. The sacral and lower lumbar root sleeves may become wider and somewhat cystic in older individuals. These cystic dilations have been called Tarlov cysts or arachnoid diverticula.

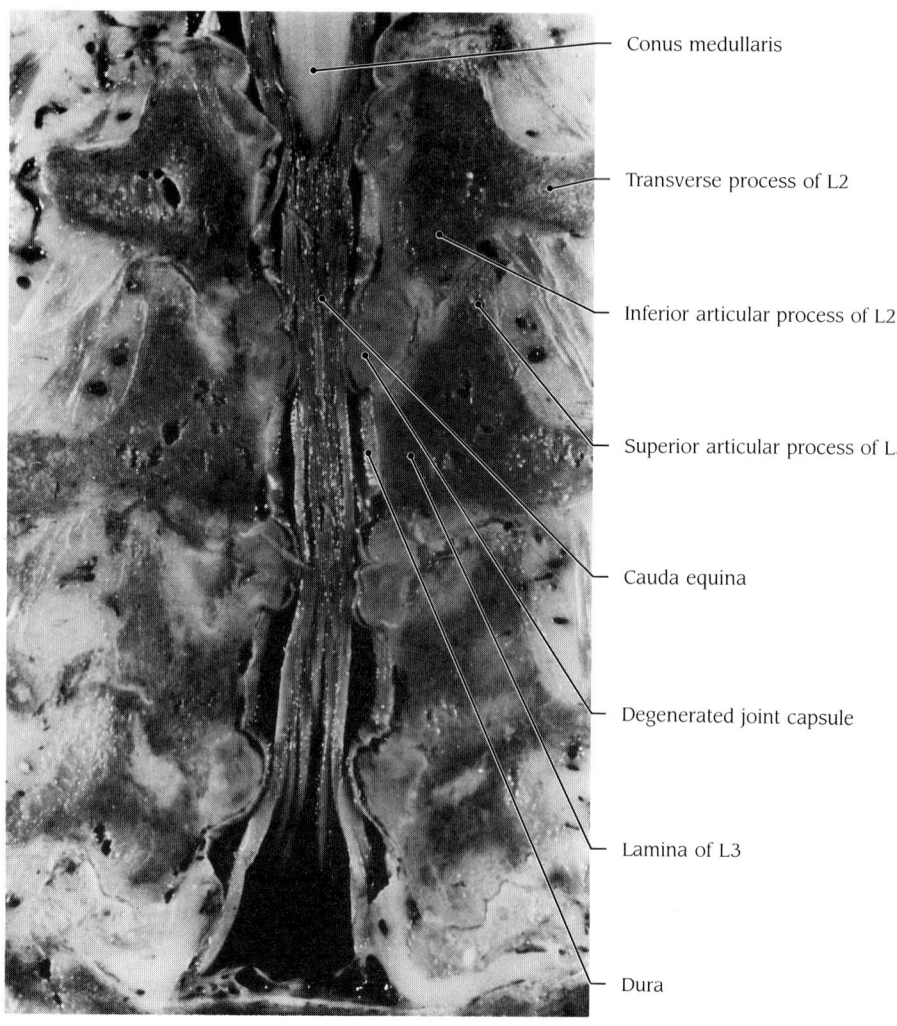

FIG. 11.53.

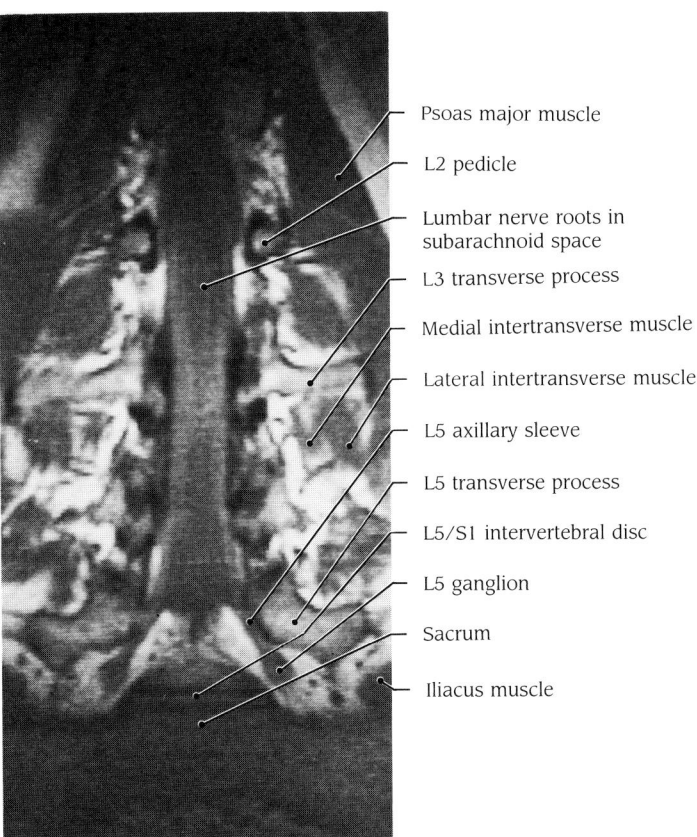

FIG. 11.54. TR = 837 msec, TE = 37 msec.

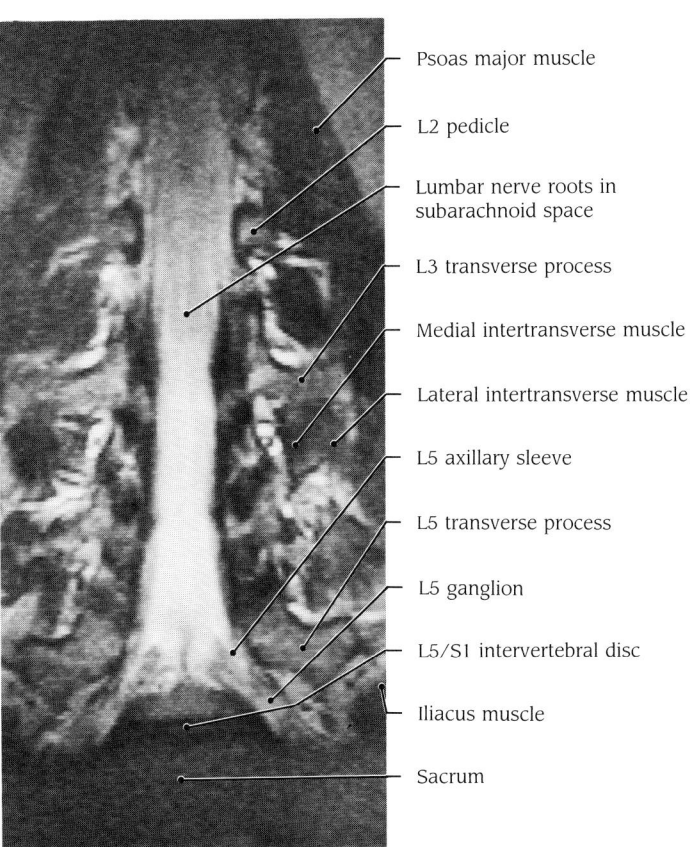

FIG. 11.55. TR = 5000 msec, TE = 64 msec.

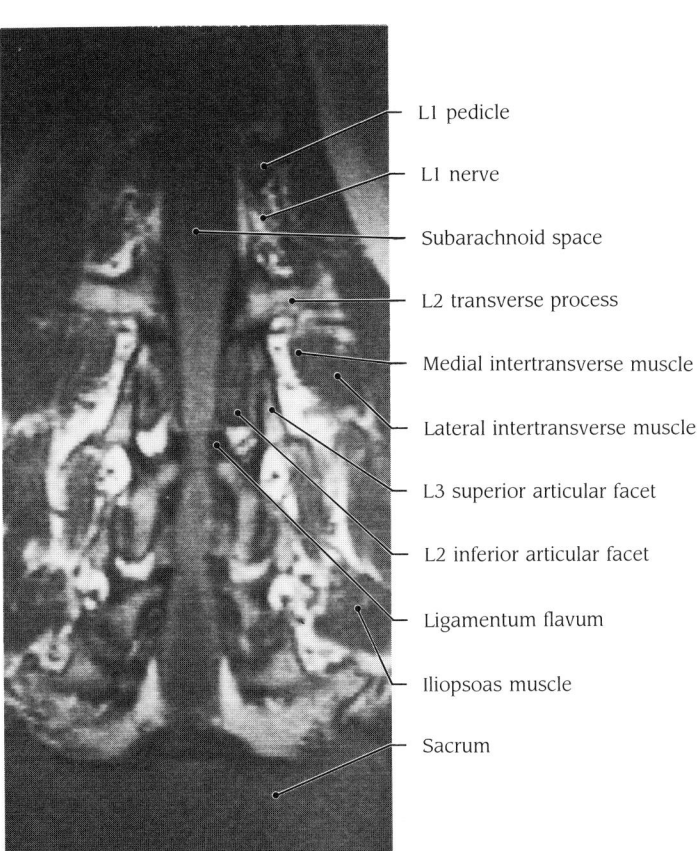

FIG. 11.56. TR = 837 msec, TE = 37 msec.

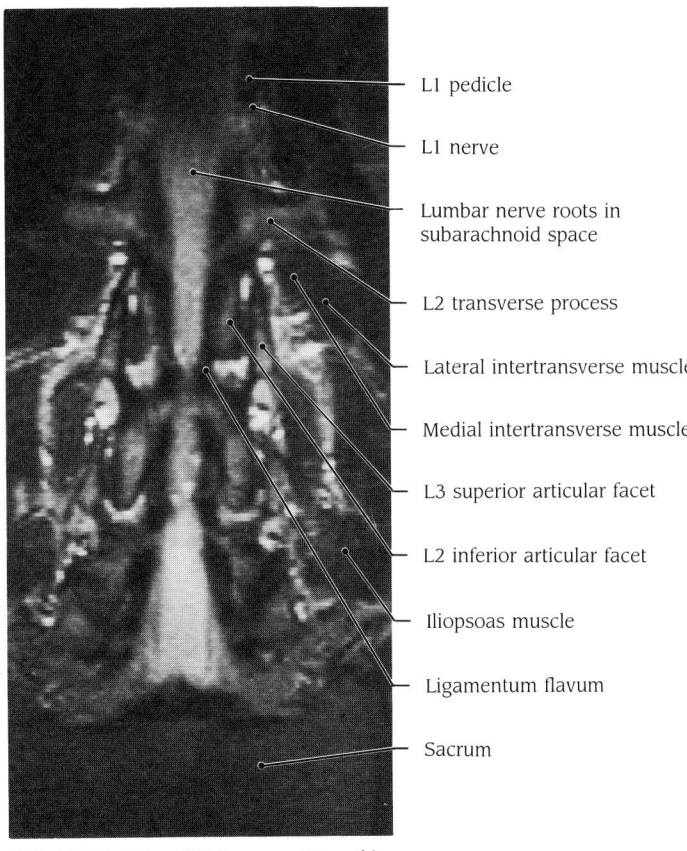

FIG. 11.57. TR = 5000 msec, TE = 64 msec.

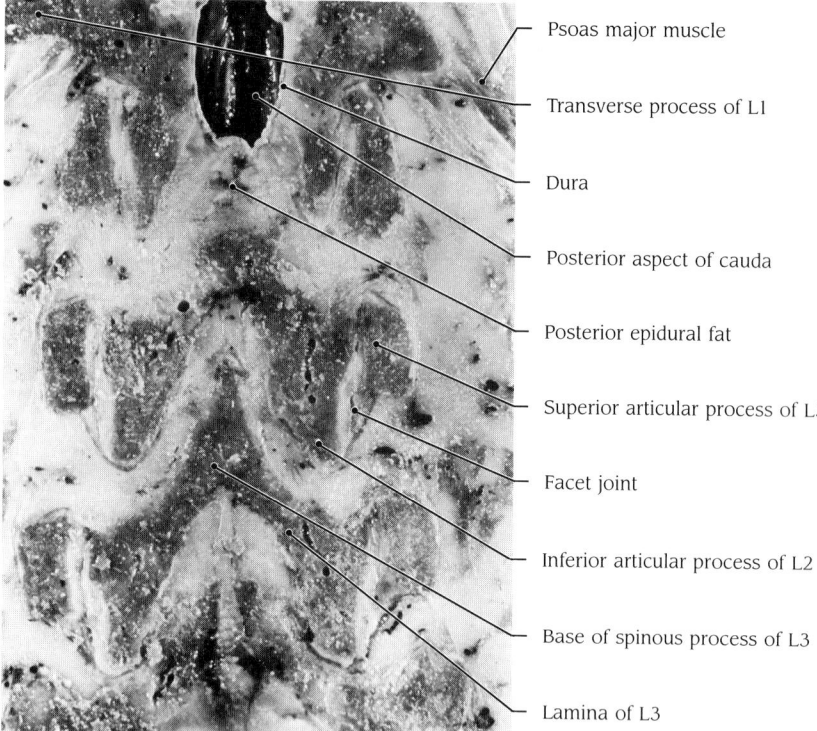

FIG. 11.58.

- Psoas major muscle
- Transverse process of L1
- Dura
- Posterior aspect of cauda
- Posterior epidural fat
- Superior articular process of L3
- Facet joint
- Inferior articular process of L2
- Base of spinous process of L3
- Lamina of L3

- The sacroiliac articulation may be divided into a diarthrodial synovial portion and a ligamentous portion. The articular surfaces exhibit irregular elevations and depressions that fit into one another, restrict movements, and contribute to the strength of the joint.

- The spinal portion of the arachnoid is continuous with the cerebral arachnoid superiorly. Inferiorly, it is broad, surrounds the cauda equina, and tapers off to end at the level of the second sacral vertebra in normal adults. Normal variations in the level of the end of the arachnoid and dural sac may range from the middle of the first sacral vertebra to the upper end of the third sacral vertebra.

- The sacrum articulates with the fifth lumbar vertebra by way of a large, anteriorly wide intervertebral disc, as well as by a coronally oriented facet joint. The distance between the superior articular processes of the first sacral vertebra is greater than at other levels in the vertebral column.

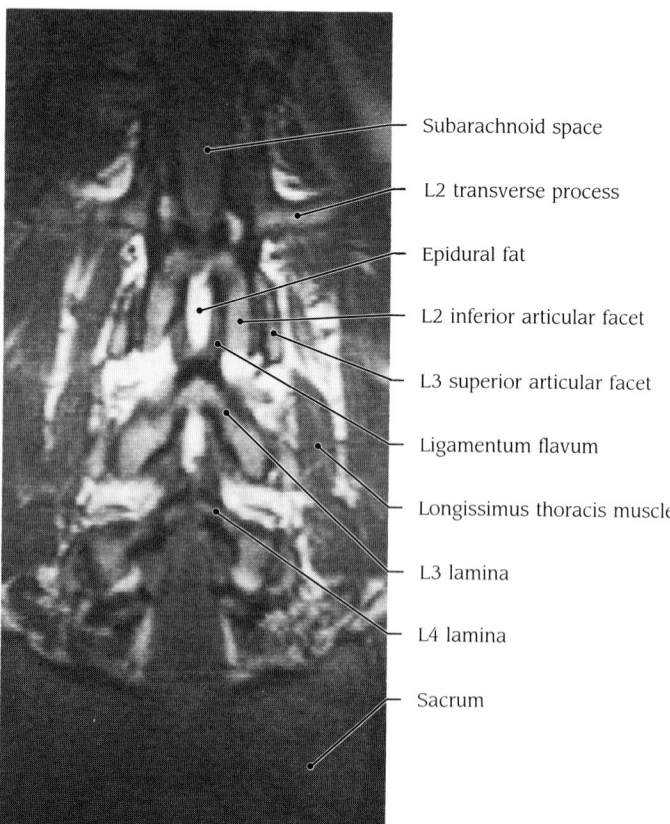

FIG. 11.59. TR = 837 msec, TE = 37 msec.

- Subarachnoid space
- L2 transverse process
- Epidural fat
- L2 inferior articular facet
- L3 superior articular facet
- Ligamentum flavum
- Longissimus thoracis muscle
- L3 lamina
- L4 lamina
- Sacrum

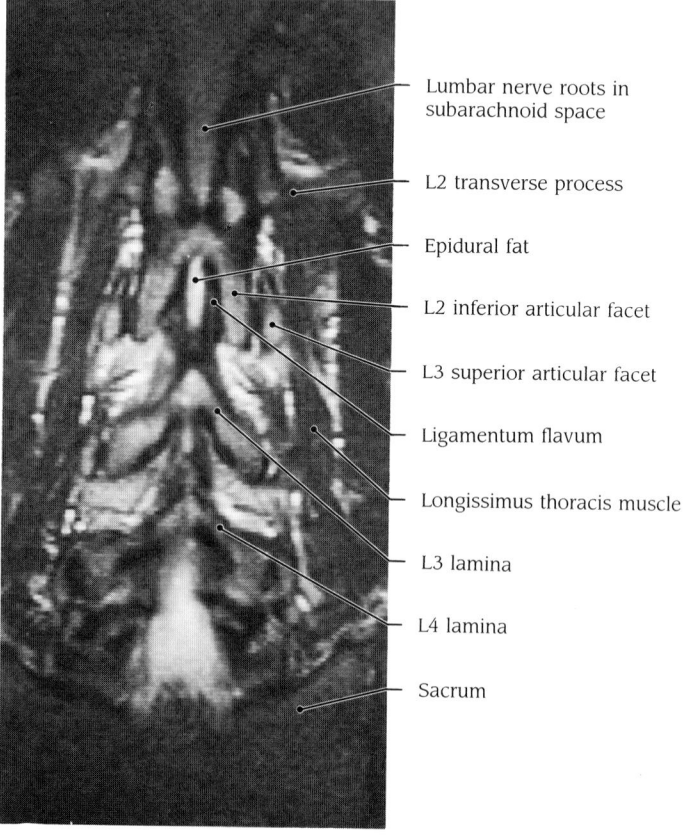

FIG. 11.60. TR = 5000 msec, TE = 64 msec.

- Lumbar nerve roots in subarachnoid space
- L2 transverse process
- Epidural fat
- L2 inferior articular facet
- L3 superior articular facet
- Ligamentum flavum
- Longissimus thoracis muscle
- L3 lamina
- L4 lamina
- Sacrum

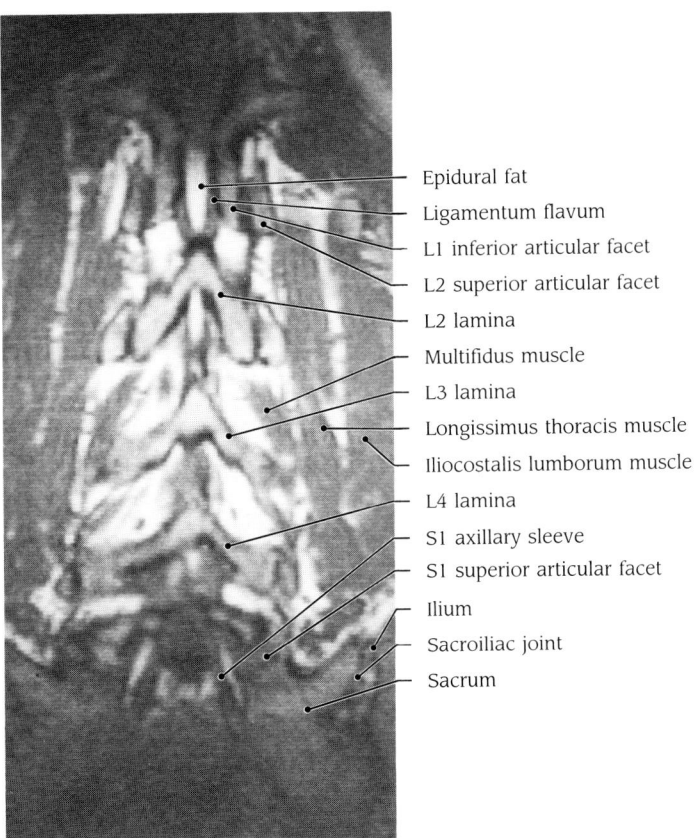

FIG. 11.61. TR = 837 msec, TE = 37 msec.

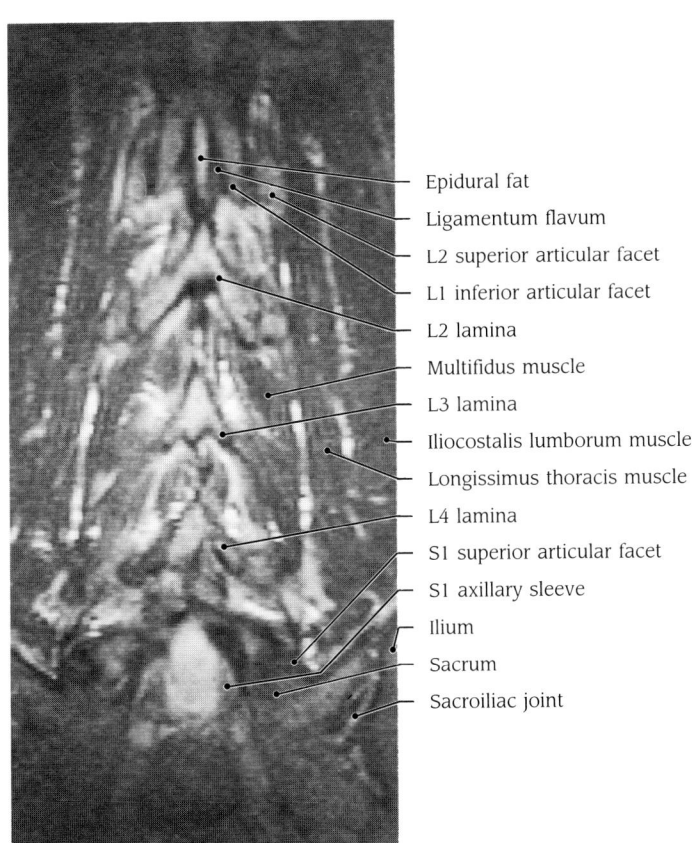

FIG. 11.62. TR = 5000 msec, TE = 64 msec.

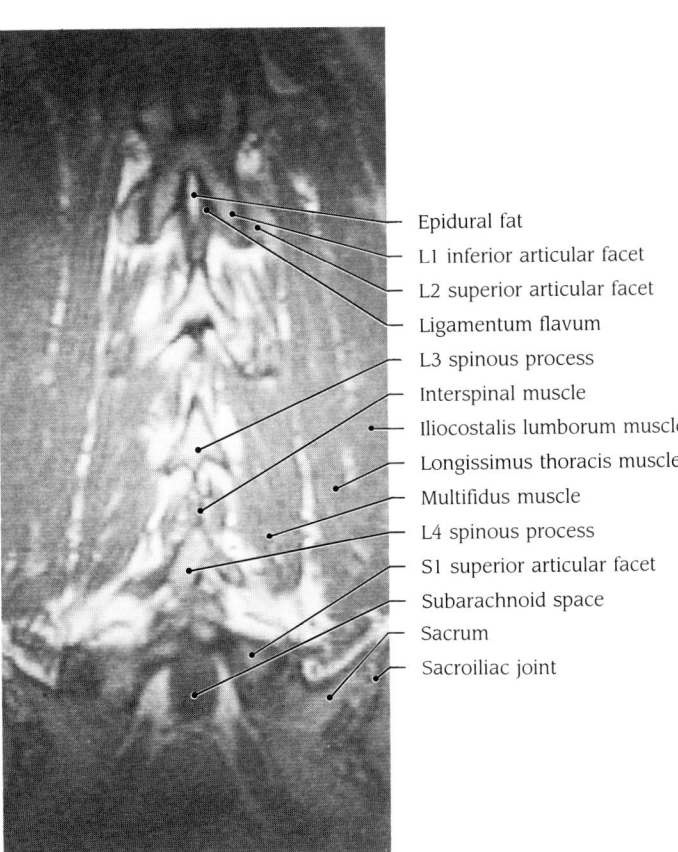

FIG. 11.63. TR = 837 msec, TE = 37 msec.

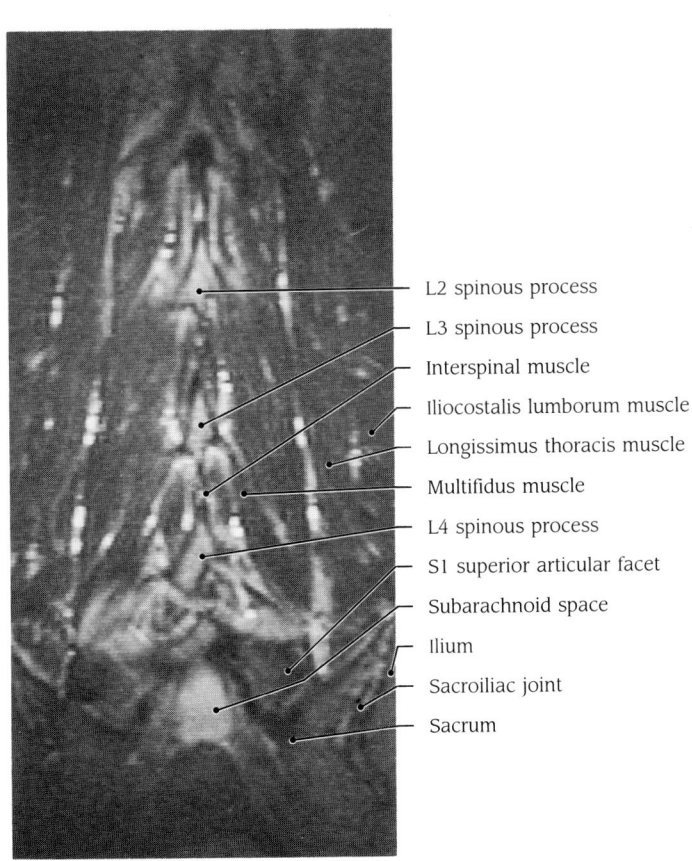

FIG. 11.64. TR = 5000 msec, TE = 64 msec.

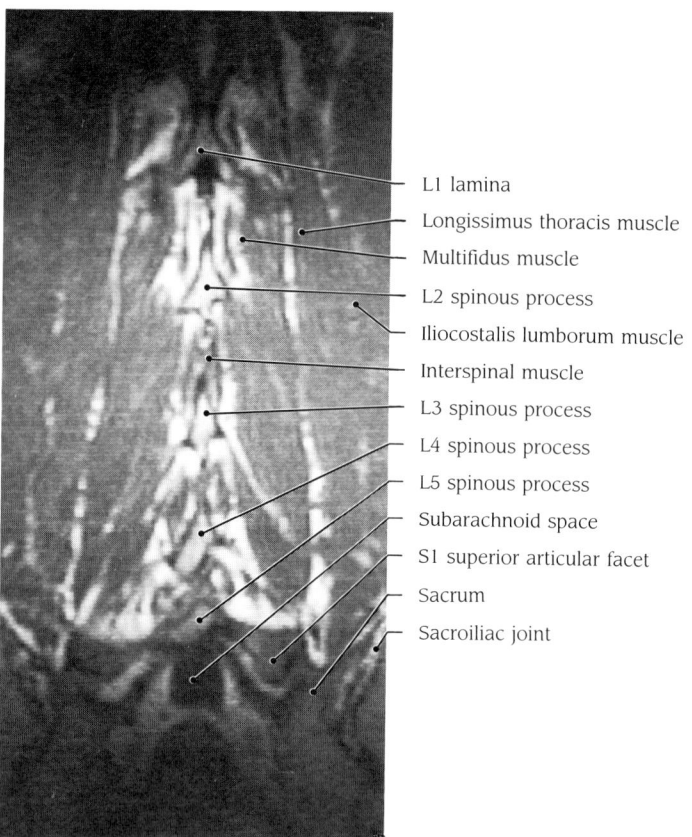

FIG. 11.65. TR = 837 msec, TE = 37 msec.

- The contents of the sacral canal include the cauda equina, filum terminale, and the spinal meninges. At the level of the middle of the sacrum, the subarachnoid and subdural spaces terminate, and the lower sacral nerve roots and filum terminale pierce the dura and arachnoid. The filum terminale continues inferiorly to reach the coccyx.

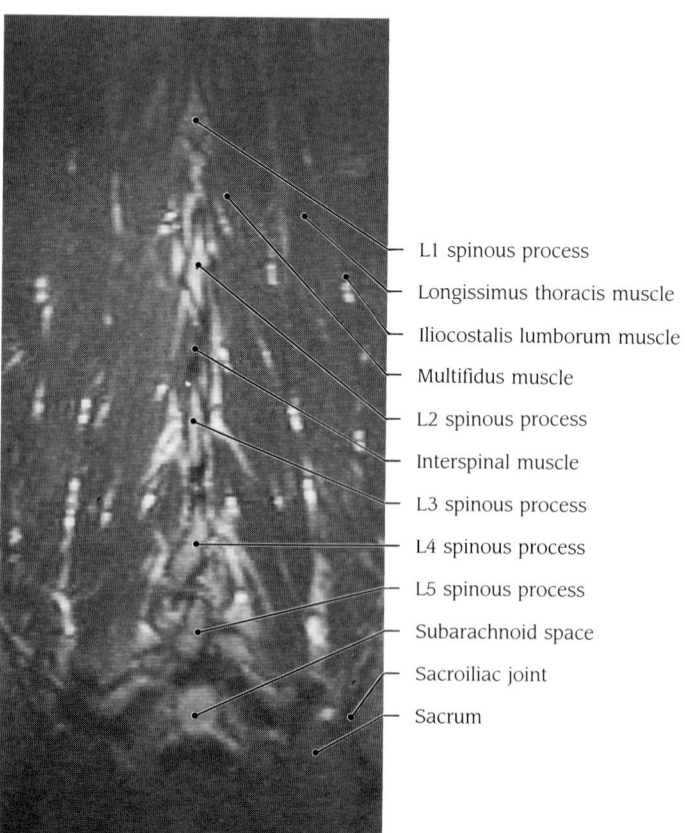

FIG. 11.66. TR = 5000 msec, TE = 64 msec.

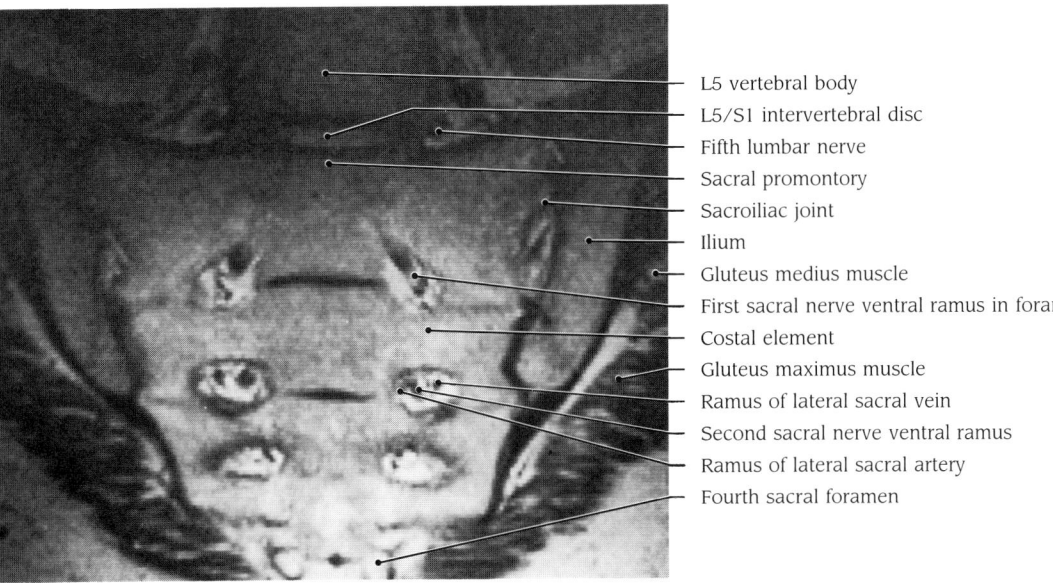

FIG. 11.67. TR = 739 msec, TE = 39 msec.

- L5 vertebral body
- L5/S1 intervertebral disc
- Fifth lumbar nerve
- Sacral promontory
- Sacroiliac joint
- Ilium
- Gluteus medius muscle
- First sacral nerve ventral ramus in foramen
- Costal element
- Gluteus maximus muscle
- Ramus of lateral sacral vein
- Second sacral nerve ventral ramus
- Ramus of lateral sacral artery
- Fourth sacral foramen

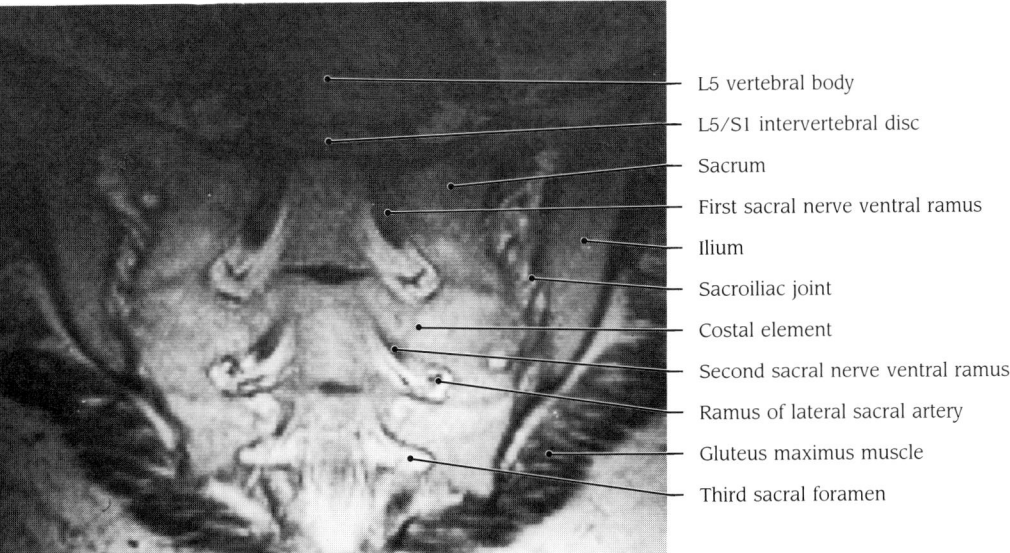

FIG. 11.68. TR = 739 msec, TE = 39 msec.

- L5 vertebral body
- L5/S1 intervertebral disc
- Sacrum
- First sacral nerve ventral ramus
- Ilium
- Sacroiliac joint
- Costal element
- Second sacral nerve ventral ramus
- Ramus of lateral sacral artery
- Gluteus maximus muscle
- Third sacral foramen

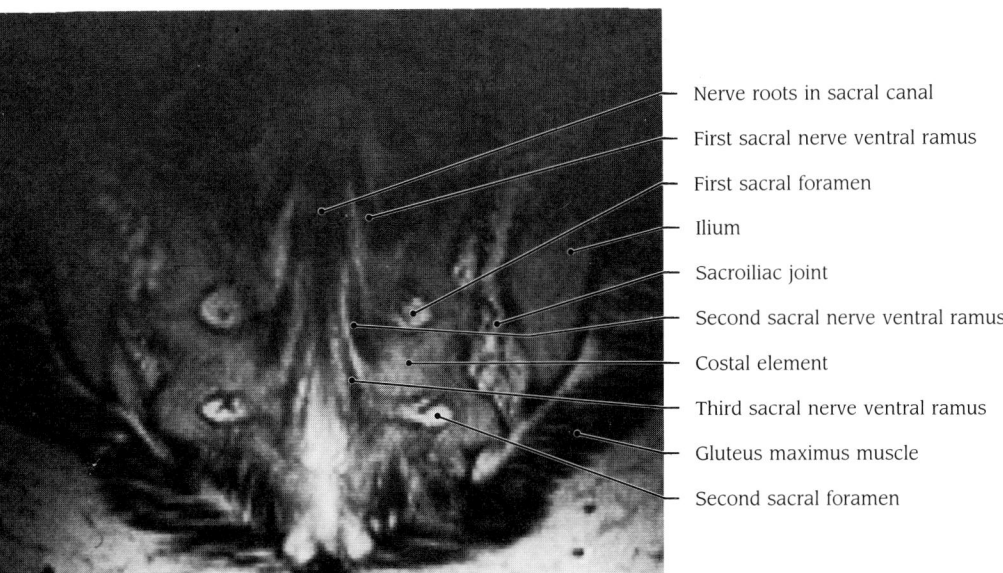

FIG. 11.69. TR = 739 msec, TE = 39 msec.

- Nerve roots in sacral canal
- First sacral nerve ventral ramus
- First sacral foramen
- Ilium
- Sacroiliac joint
- Second sacral nerve ventral ramus
- Costal element
- Third sacral nerve ventral ramus
- Gluteus maximus muscle
- Second sacral foramen

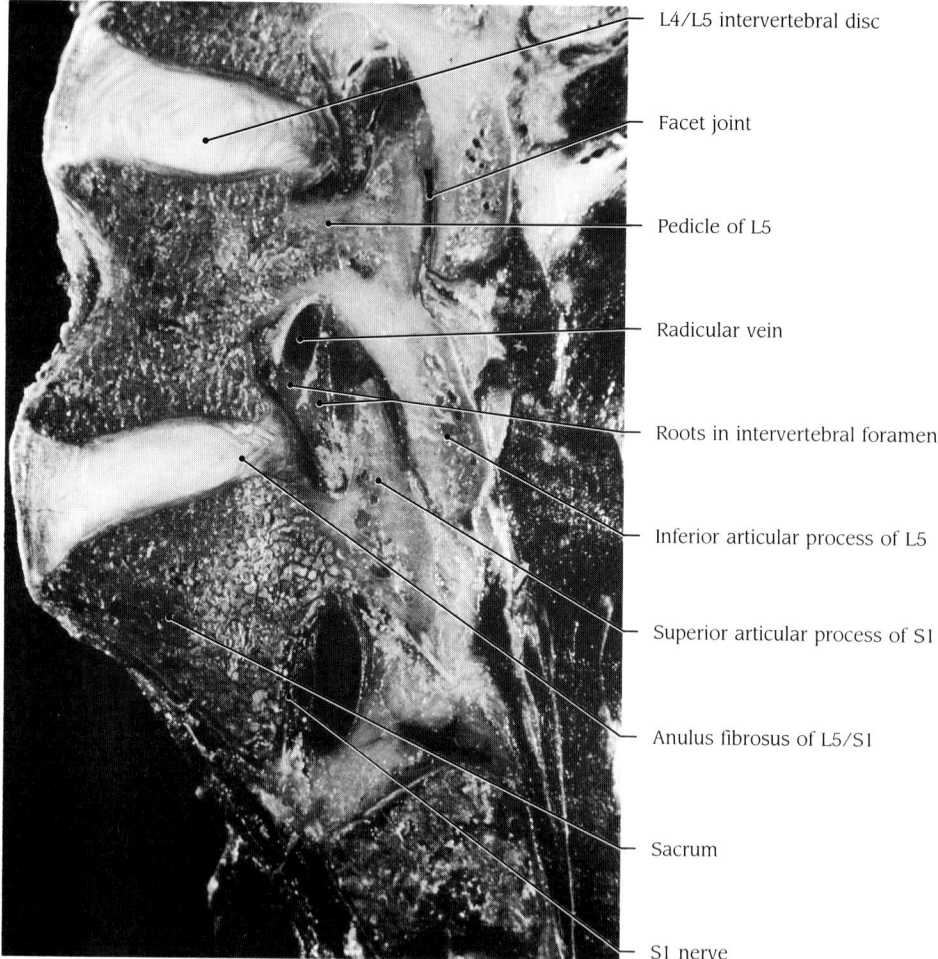

FIG. 11.70.

- The transverse processes of the lumbar vertebral bodies are thin and long, with the exception of the fifth lumbar transverse processes, which are more substantial. The length of the transverse processes progressively increases from the first lumbar to the third lumbar, which are the longest of all the transverse processes. The fourth and fifth lumbar transverse processes are shorter. The fibers of the longissimus thoracis muscles and the lateral intertransverse muscles are attached to the transverse processes.

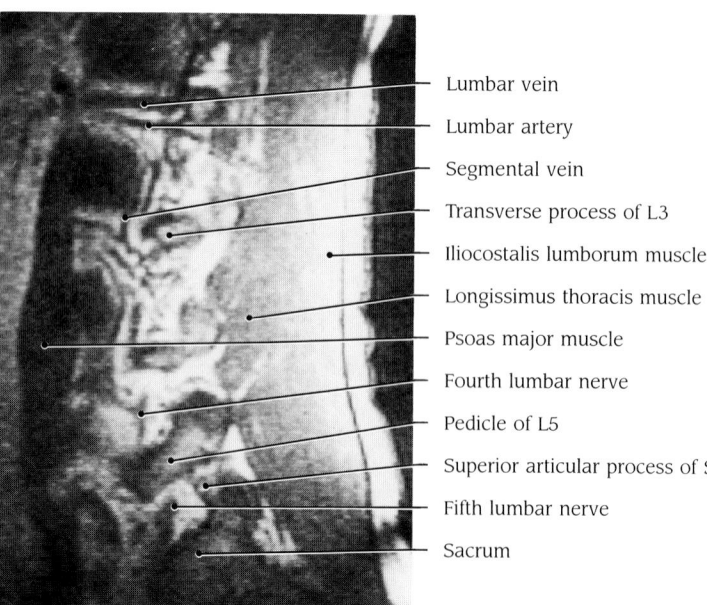

FIG. 11.71. TR = 837 msec, TE = 37 msec.

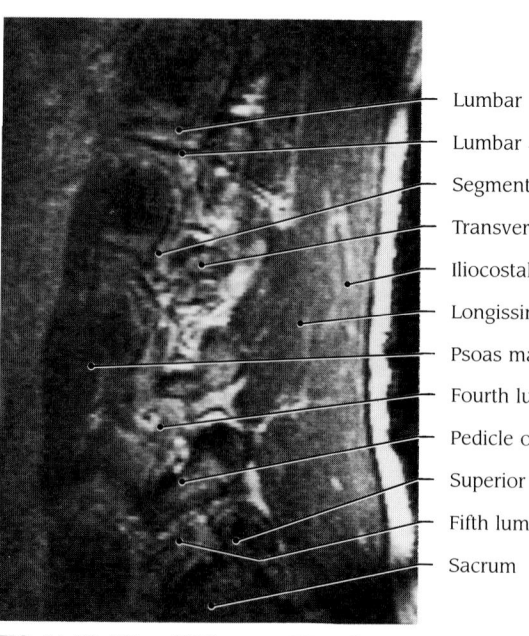

FIG. 11.72. TR = 5000 msec, TE = 60 msec.

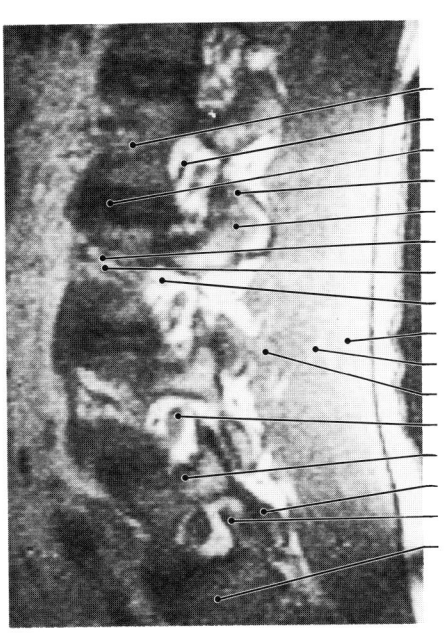

FIG. 11.73. TR = 837 msec, TE = 37 msec.

- L2 vertebral body
- Intervertebral vein
- L2/L3 intervertebral disc
- Mamillary process
- Superior articular process of L3
- Lumbar vein
- Lumbar artery
- Fat in intervertebral foramen
- Iliocostalis lumborum muscle
- Longissimus thoracis muscle
- Multifidus muscle
- Dorsal root ganglion of L4
- Pedicle of L5
- Inferior articular process of L5
- Superior articular process of S1
- Sacrum

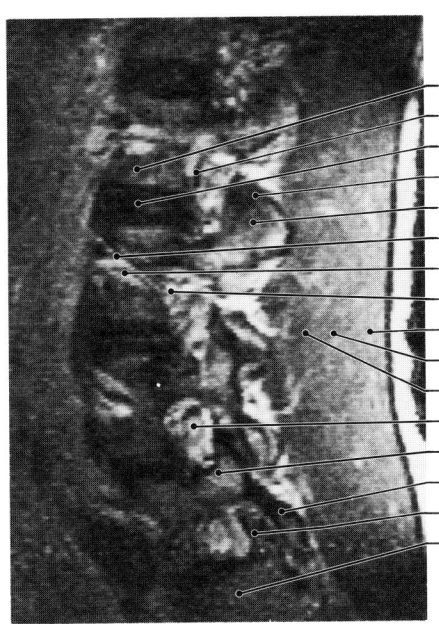

FIG. 11.74. TR = 5000 msec, TE = 60 msec.

- L2 vertebral body
- Intervertebral vein
- L2/L3 intervertebral disc
- Mamillary process
- Superior articular process of L3
- Lumbar vein
- Lumbar artery
- Fat in intervertebral foramen
- Iliocostalis lumborum muscle
- Longissimus thoracis muscle
- Multifidus muscle
- Dorsal root ganglion of L4
- Pedicle of L5
- Inferior articular process of L5
- Superior articular process of S1
- Sacrum

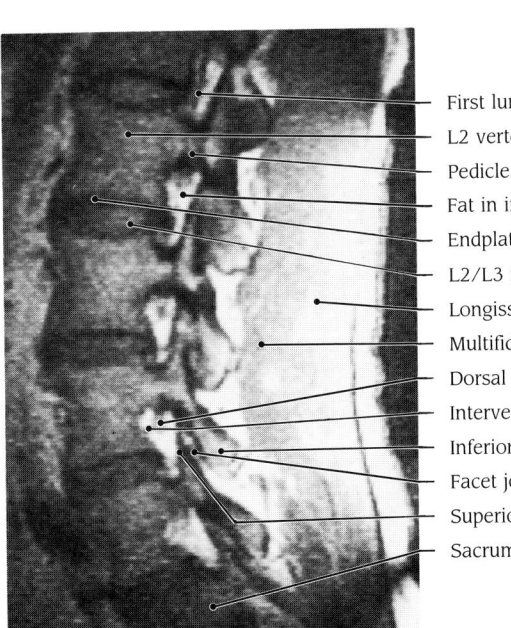

FIG. 11.75. TR = 837 msec, TE = 37 msec.

- First lumbar nerve
- L2 vertebral body
- Pedicle of L2
- Fat in intervertebral foramen
- Endplate of L2 vertebral body
- L2/L3 intervertebral disc
- Longissimus thoracis muscle
- Multifidus muscle
- Dorsal root ganglion of L4
- Intervertebral vein
- Inferior articular process of L4
- Facet joint
- Superior articular process of L5
- Sacrum

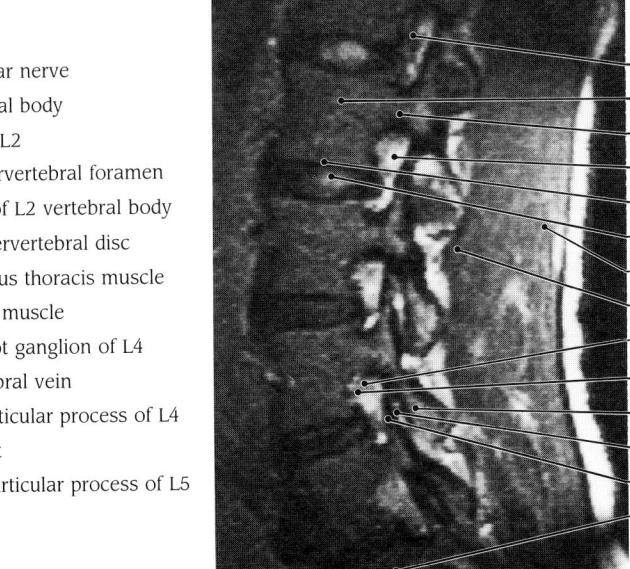

FIG. 11.76. TR = 5000 msec, TE = 60 msec.

- First lumbar nerve
- L2 vertebral body
- Pedicle of L2
- Fat in intervertebral foramen
- Endplate of L2 vertebral body
- L2/L3 intervertebral disc
- Longissimus thoracis muscle
- Multifidus muscle
- Dorsal root ganglion of L4
- Intervertebral vein
- Inferior articular process of L4
- Facet joint
- Superior articular process of L5
- Sacrum

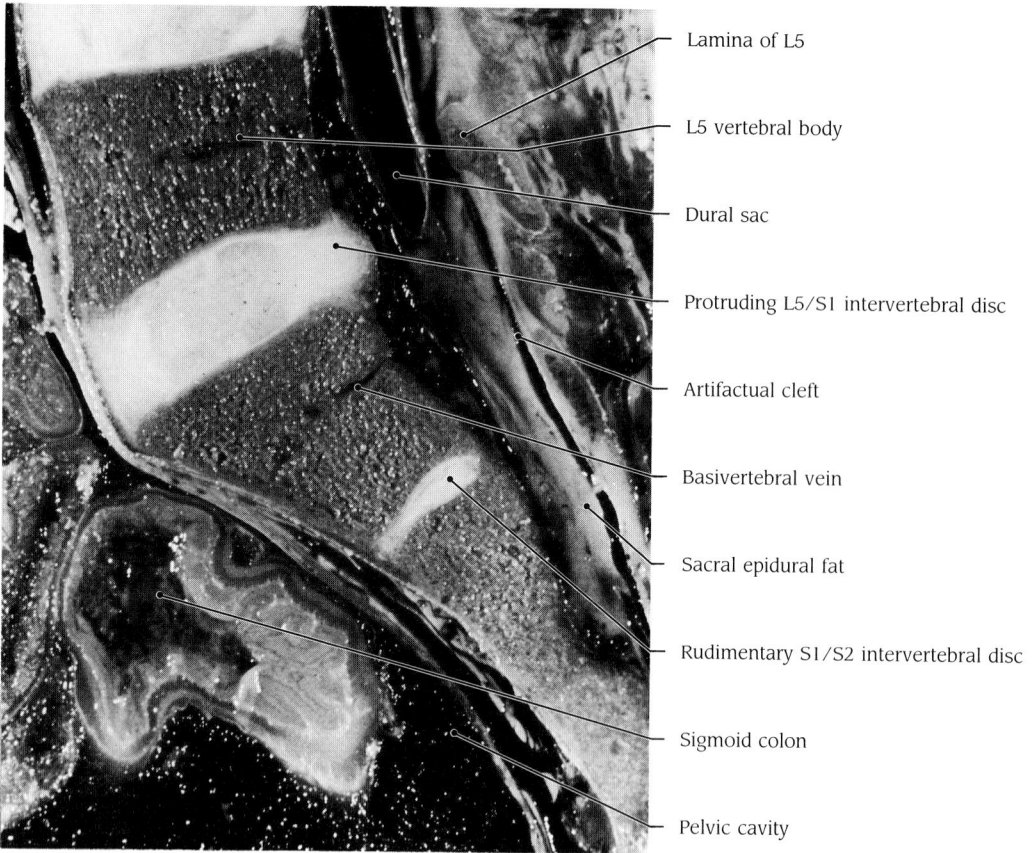

FIG. 11.77.

- The mamillary process is an irregular elevation on the posterior aspect of the superior articular process of each lumbar vertebral body. This process is homologous with the superior tubercle in the twelfth thoracic vertebra. It serves as the point of attachment for the multifidus and medial intertransverse muscles.

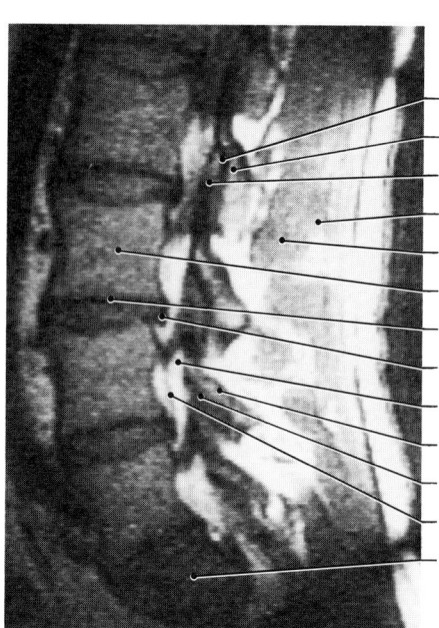

FIG. 11.78. TR = 837 msec, TE = 37 msec.

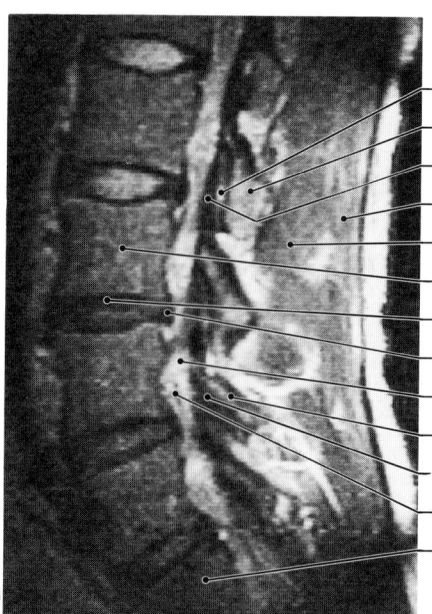

FIG. 11.79. TR = 5000 msec, TE = 60 msec.

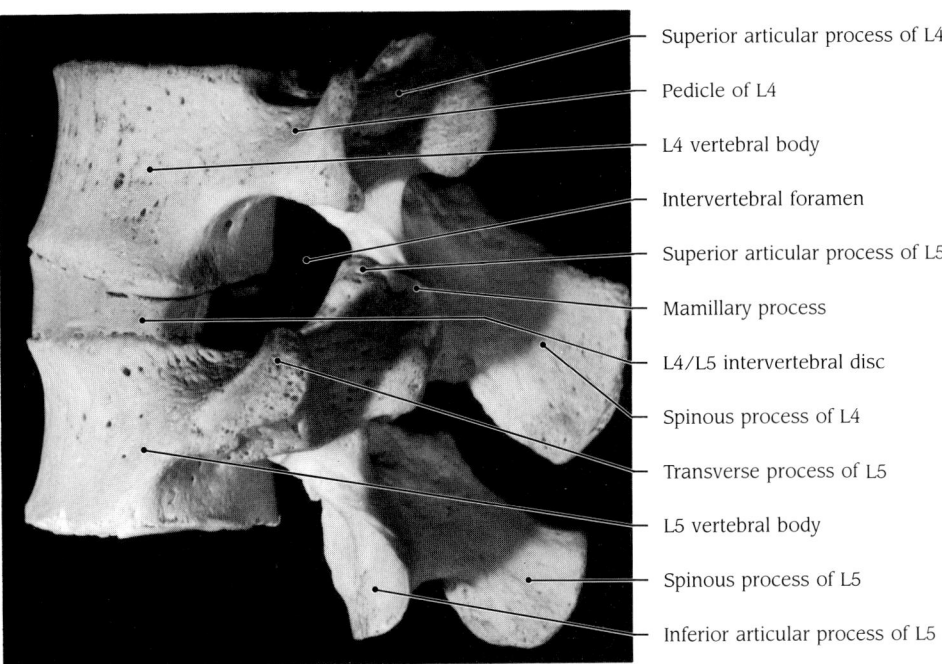

FIG. 11.80. (From de Groot, J: Correlative Neuroanatomy of Computed Tomography and Magnetic Resonance Imaging. Philadelphia, Lea & Febiger, 1984.)

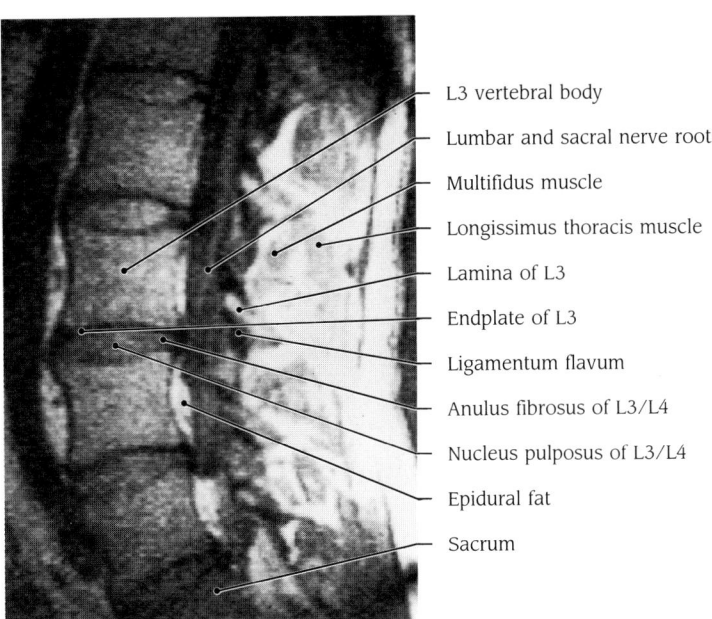

FIG. 11.81. TR = 837 msec, TE = 37 msec.

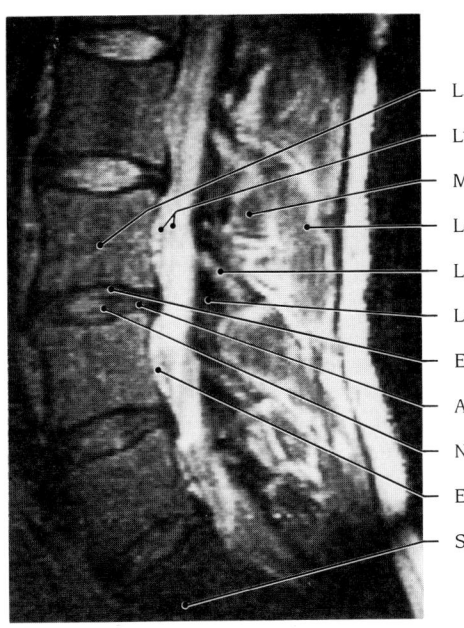

FIG. 11.82. TR = 5000 msec, TE = 60 msec.

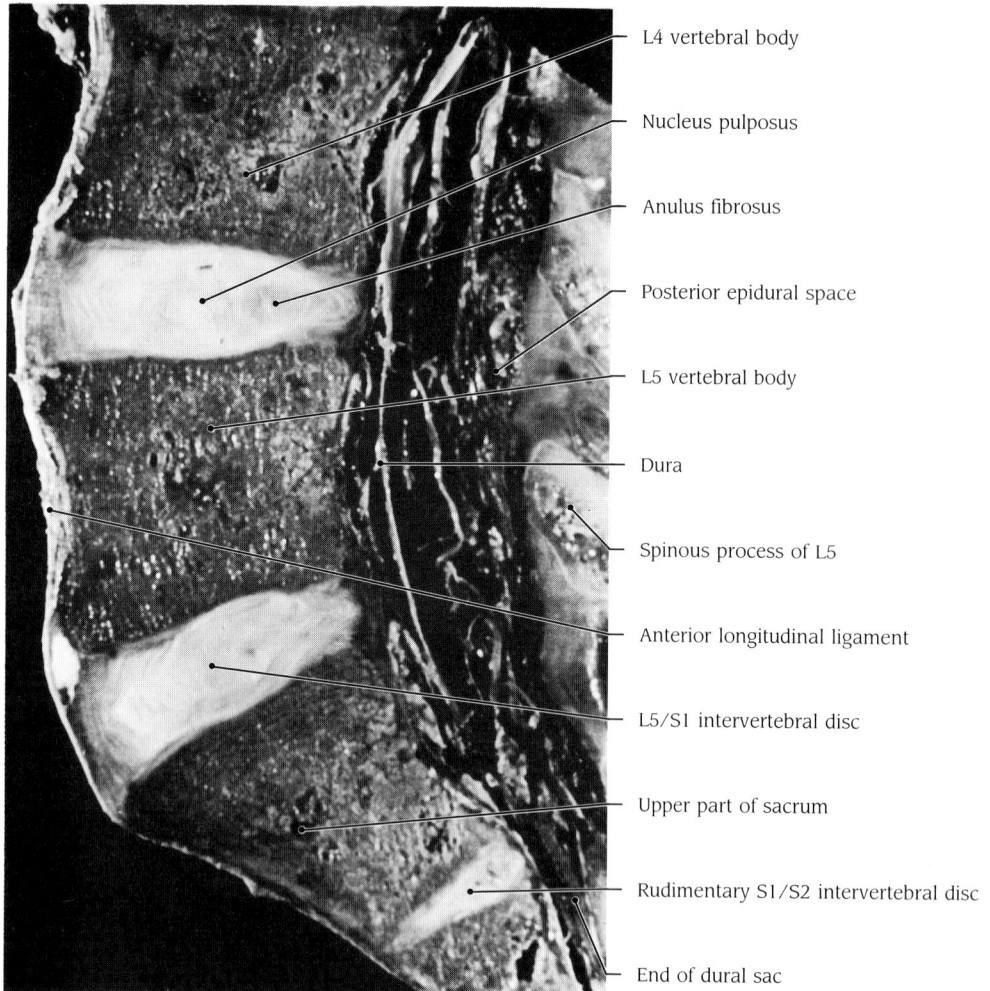

FIG. 11.83.

- The anterior longitudinal ligament attaches to the anterior margins of the vertebral bodies and the intervertebral discs. It originates at the basilar part of the occipital bone, extends to the anterior tubercle of the atlas, then continues to the anterior aspect of the body of the axis, and ends inferiorly at the superior portion of the sacrum. The anterior longitudinal ligament is composed of superficial fibers, which extend over three or four vertebrae, intermediate fibers, which extend between two or three vertebrae, and deep fibers, which attach to adjacent vertebrae.

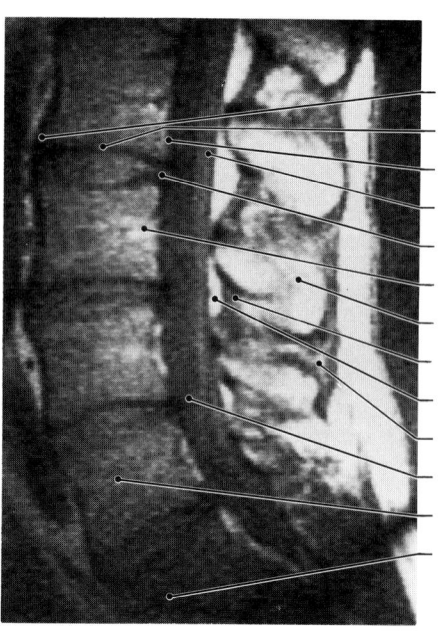

FIG. 11.84. TR = 837 msec, TE = 37 msec.

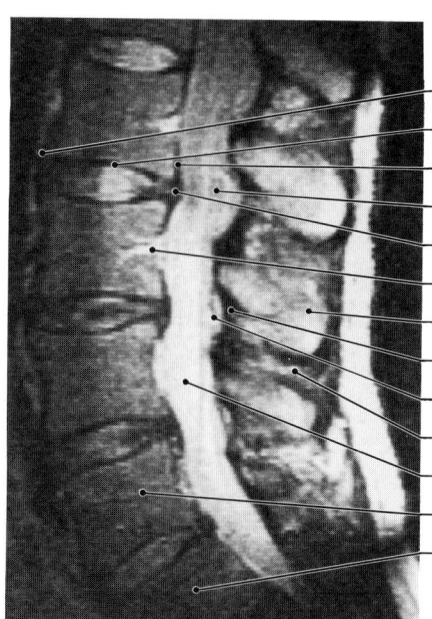

FIG. 11.85. TR = 5000 msec, TE = 60 msec.

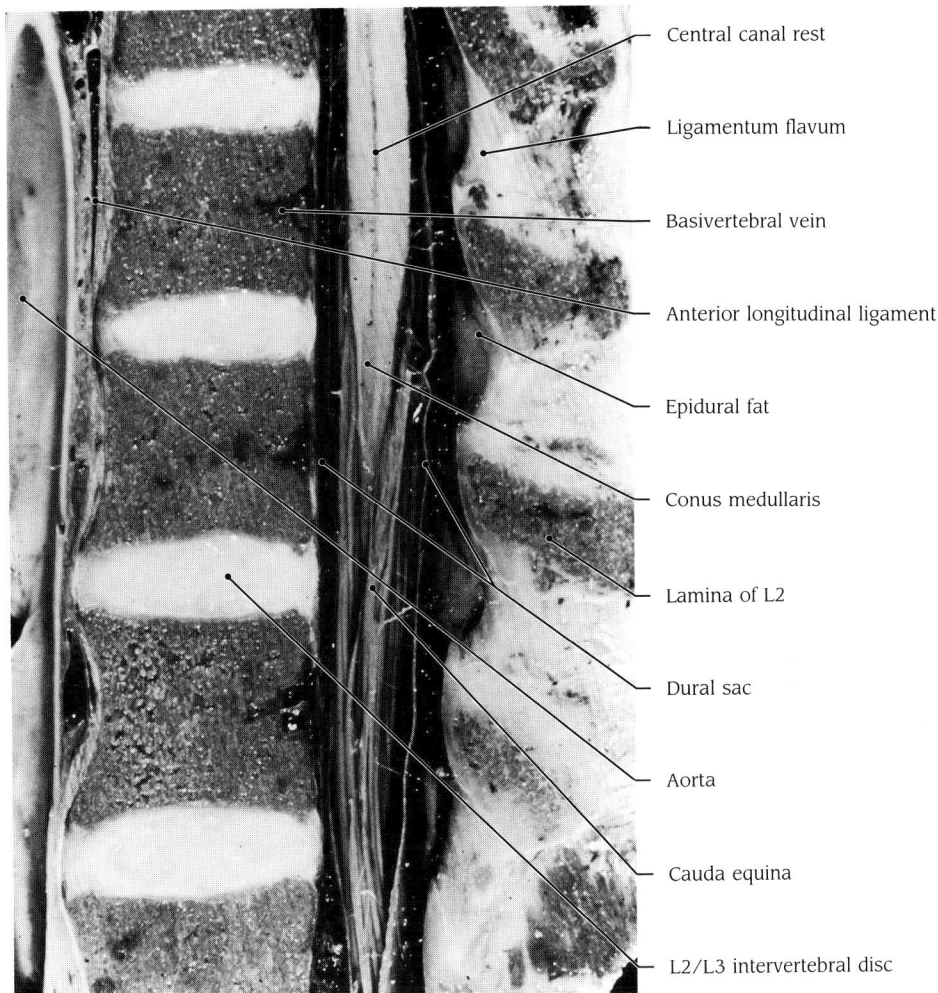

- Central canal rest
- Ligamentum flavum
- Basivertebral vein
- Anterior longitudinal ligament
- Epidural fat
- Conus medullaris
- Lamina of L2
- Dural sac
- Aorta
- Cauda equina
- L2/L3 intervertebral disc

FIG. 11.86.

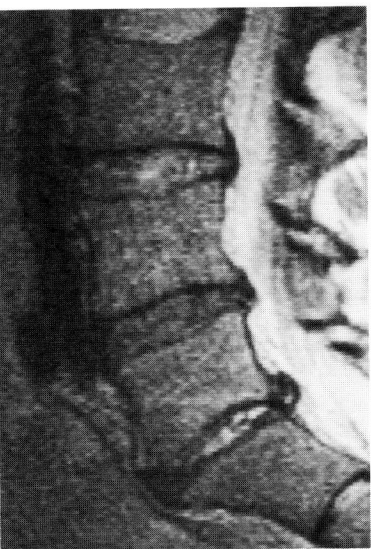

FIG. 11.87. TR = 5000 msec, TE = 60 msec. Desiccation of the lumbar intervertebral discs is present at the L3/L4, L4/L5 and L5/S1 levels. A disc herniation is evident at L5/S1, and disc protrusions are noted at L3/L4 and L4/L5.

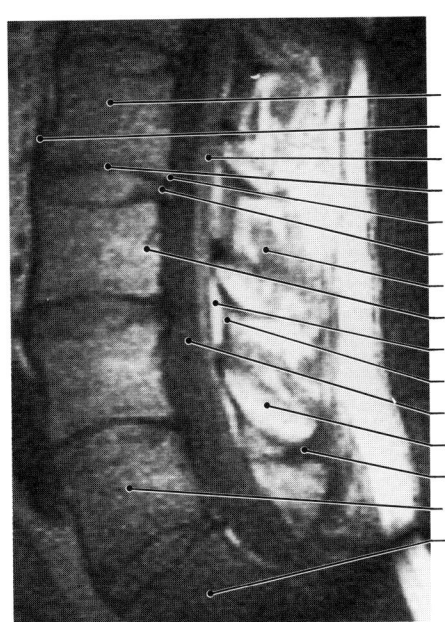

- L2 vertebral body
- Anterior longitudinal ligament
- Lumbar and sacral nerve roots
- Endplate of L2 vertebral body
- Posterior longitudinal ligament
- L2/L3 intervertebral disc bulge
- Multifidus muscle
- Basivertebral vein
- Epidural fat
- Ligamentum flavum
- Subarachnoid space
- Spinous process of L4
- Interspinal muscle
- L5 vertebral body
- Sacrum

FIG. 11.88. TR = 837 msec, TE = 37 msec.

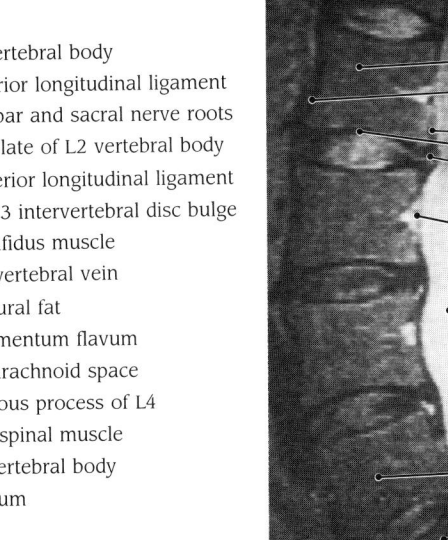

- L2 vertebral body
- Anterior longitudinal ligament
- Lumbar and sacral nerve roots
- Posterior longitudinal ligament
- Endplate of L2 vertebral body
- L2/L3 intervertebral disc bulge
- Multifidus muscle
- Basivertebral vein
- Epidural fat
- Ligamentum flavum
- Subarachnoid space
- Spinous process of L4
- Interspinal muscle
- L5 vertebral body
- Sacrum

FIG. 11.89. TR = 5000 msec, TE = 60 msec.

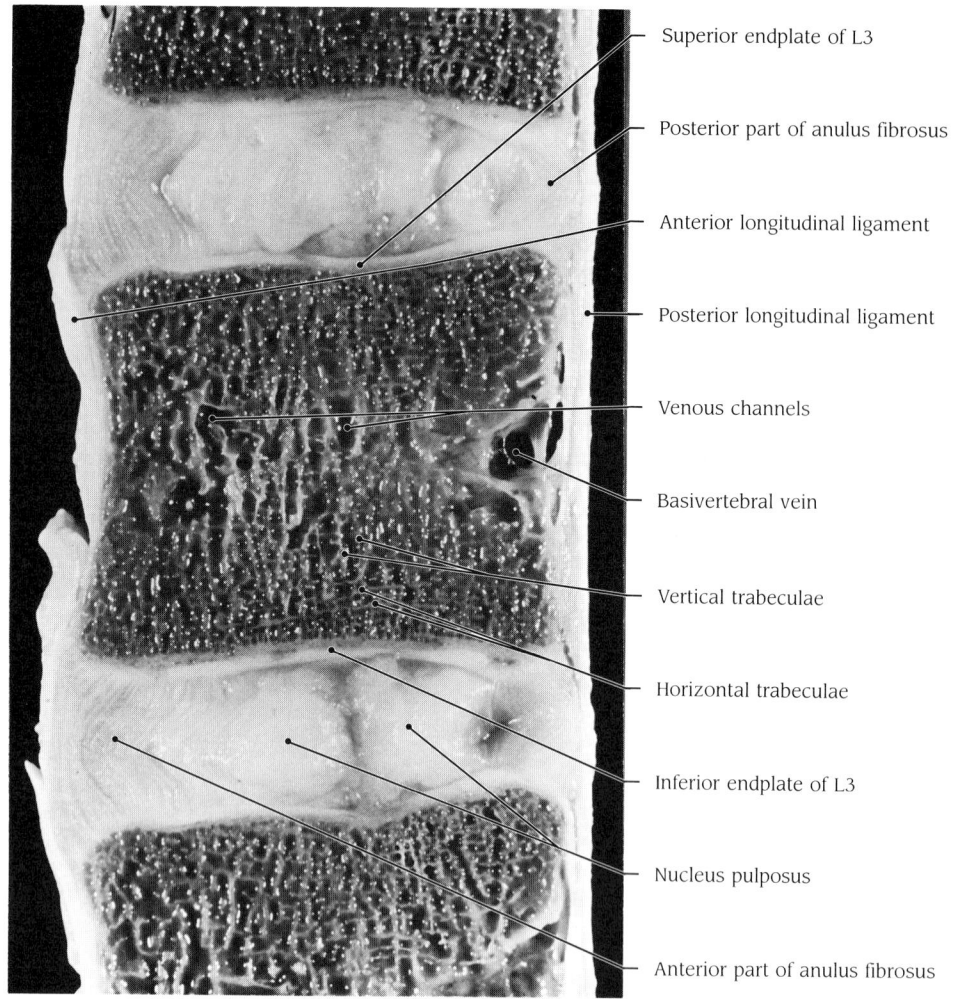

FIG. 11.90.

- The spinal nerves are formed by the union of the dorsal and ventral spinal nerve roots. The spinal nerves emerge through the intervertebral foramina, with the exception of the first cervical nerve, which exits the vertebral canal between the occipital bone and the atlas. The spinal ganglia are oval collections of nerve cells on the dorsal roots of the spinal nerves. The ganglia are usually in the intervertebral foramina, lateral to the point where the nerve roots perforate the dura mater. The exceptions are the first and second cervical ganglia, which are located on the vertebral arches of the atlas and axis, the sacral ganglia, which are inside the vertebral canal, and the coccygeal ganglion, which is usually within the dura.

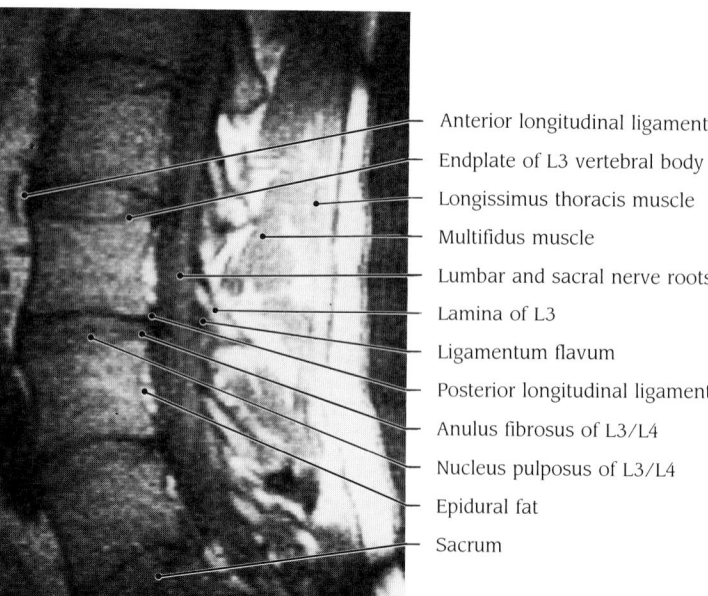

FIG. 11.91. TR = 837 msec, TE = 37 msec.

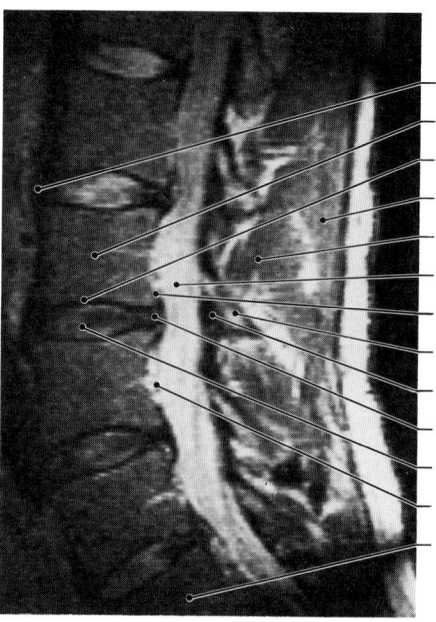

FIG. 11.92. TR = 5000 msec, TE = 60 msec.

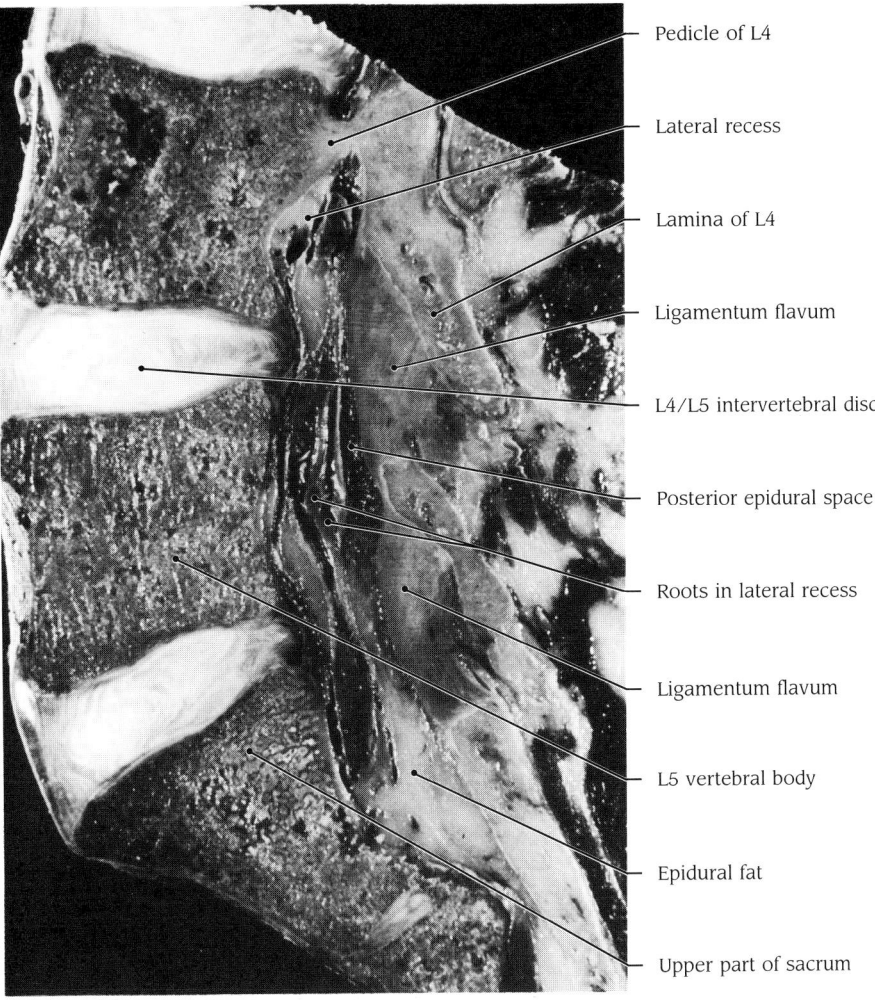

FIG. 11.93.

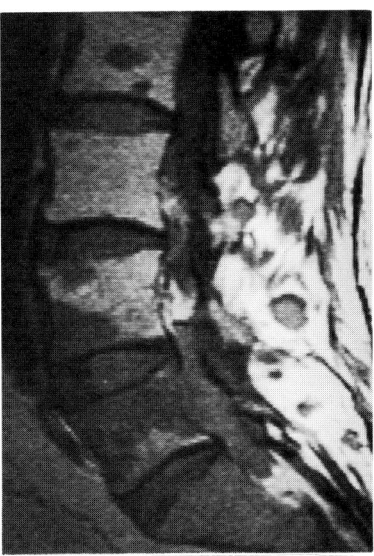

FIG. 11.94. TR = 739 msec, TE = 39 msec. Multiple low signal intensity foci of lymphoma replace the bone marrow of the L2, L4, and L5 vertebrae and of the sacrum. An epidural soft tissue mass extends from the lower border of L4 to S1. Multiple tumor nodules are noted in the soft tissues of the back.

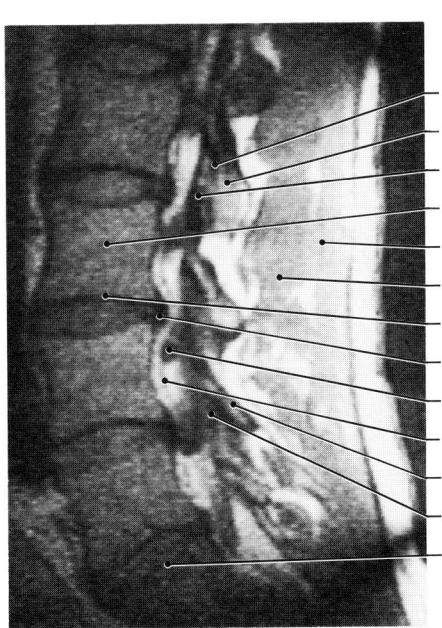

FIG. 11.95. TR = 837 msec, TE = 37 msec.

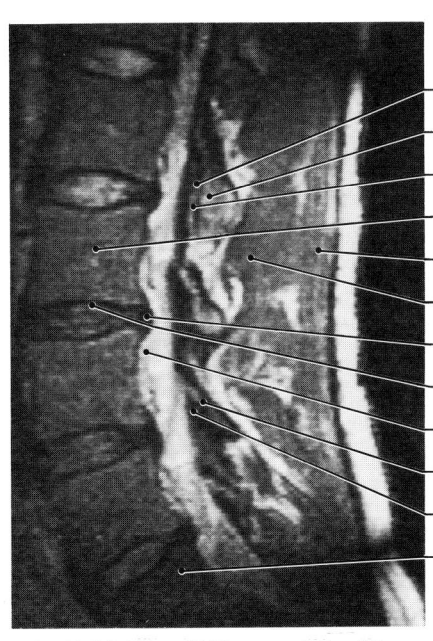

FIG. 11.96. TR = 5000 msec, TE = 60 msec.

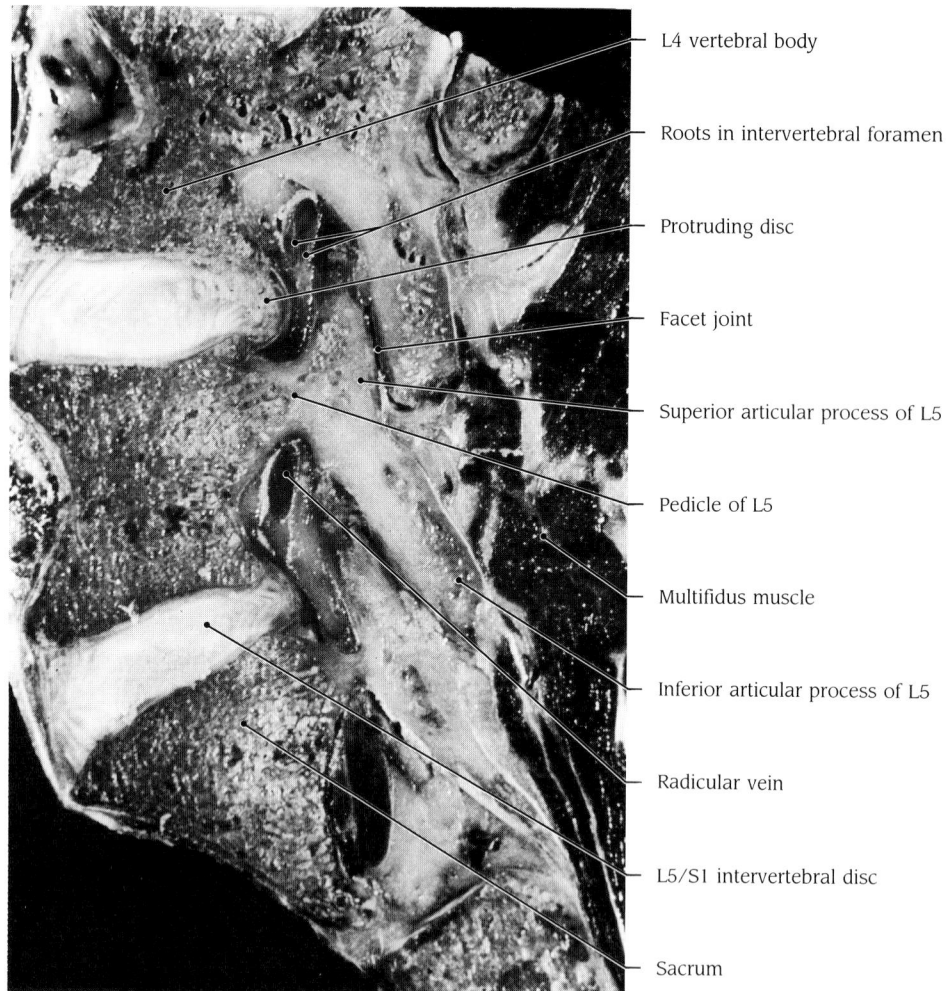

FIG. 11.97.

- The intervertebral veins pass through the intervertebral foramina and accompany the spinal nerves. They drain the veins from the spinal cord and from the internal and external vertebral plexuses. The intervertebral veins terminate in the vertebral, posterior intercostal, lumbar, and lateral sacral veins.

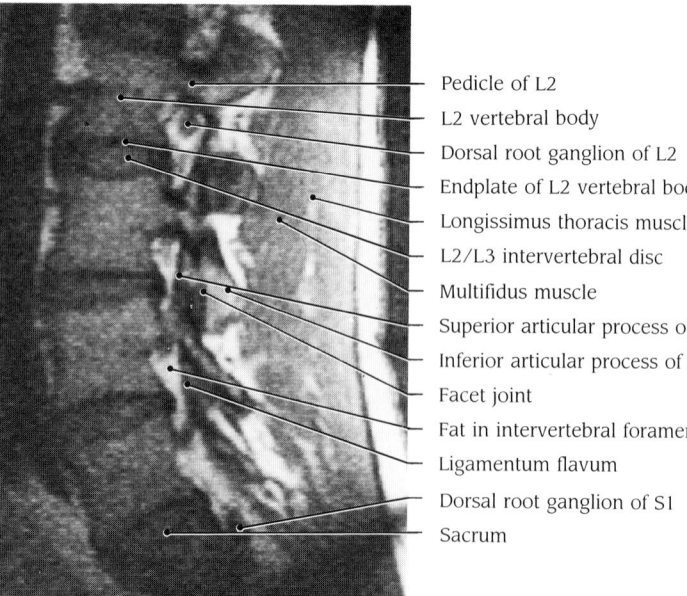

FIG. 11.98. TR = 837 msec, TE = 37 msec.

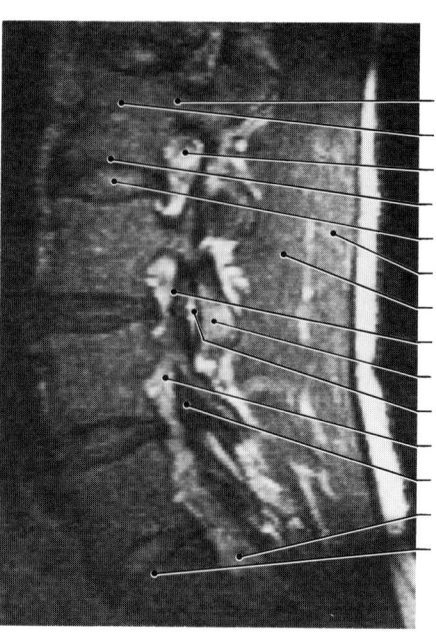

FIG. 11.99. TR = 5000 msec, TE = 60 msec.

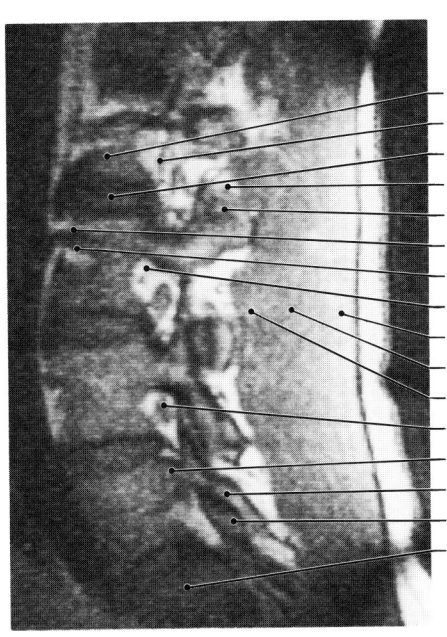

FIG. 11.100. TR = 837 msec, TE = 37 msec.

- L2 vertebral body
- Intervertebral vein
- L2/L3 intervertebral disc
- Mamillary process
- Superior articular process of L3
- Lumbar vein
- Lumbar artery
- Fat in intervertebral foramen
- Iliocostalis lumborum muscle
- Longissimus thoracis muscle
- Multifidus muscle
- Dorsal root ganglion of L4
- Pedicle of L5
- Inferior articular process of L5
- Superior articular process of S1
- Sacrum

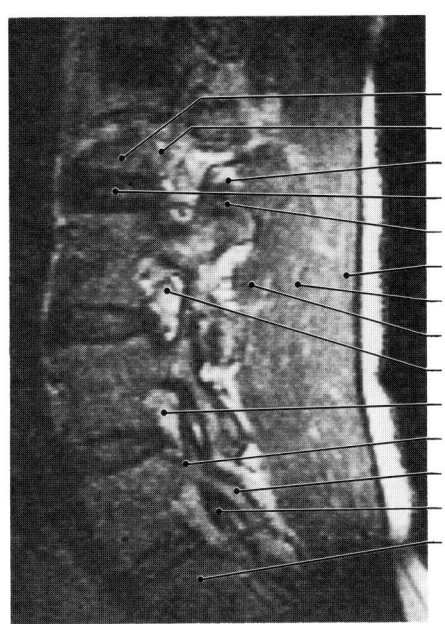

FIG. 11.101. TR = 5000 msec, TE = 60 msec.

- L2 vertebral body
- Intervertebral vein
- Mamillary process
- L2/L3 intervertebral disc
- Superior articular process of L3
- Iliocostalis lumborum muscle
- Longissimus thoracis muscle
- Multifidus muscle
- Fat in intervertebral foramen
- Dorsal root ganglion of L4
- Pedicle of L5
- Inferior articular process of L5
- Superior articular process of S1
- Sacrum

FIG. 11.102. TR = 837 msec, TE = 37 msec.

- Psoas major muscle
- Inferior vena cava
- Segmental vein
- Lumbar vein
- Transverse process of L3
- Lumbar artery
- Iliocostalis lumborum muscle
- Longissimus thoracis muscle
- Pedicle of L4
- Intervertebral vein
- Dorsal root ganglion of L4 in intervertebral foramen
- L4/L5 intervertebral disc
- Inferior articular process of L5
- Facet joint of L5/S1
- Superior articular process of S1
- Dorsal root ganglion of L5
- Sacrum

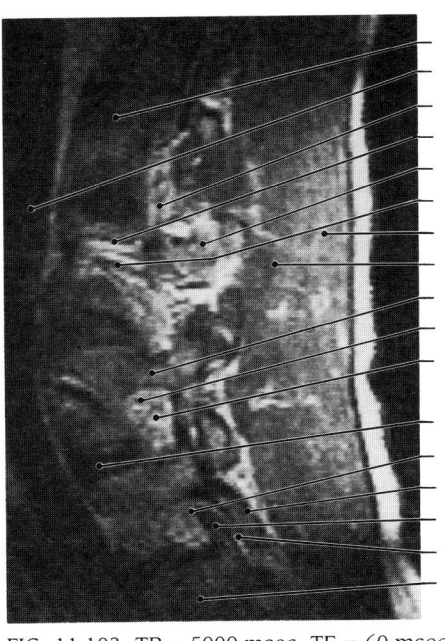

FIG. 11.103. TR = 5000 msec, TE = 60 msec.

- Psoas major muscle
- Inferior vena cava
- Segmental vein
- Lumbar vein
- Transverse process of L3
- Lumbar artery
- Iliocostalis lumborum muscle
- Longissimus thoracis muscle
- Pedicle of L4
- Intervertebral vein
- Dorsal root ganglion of L4 in intervertebral foramen
- L4/L5 intervertebral disc
- Dorsal root ganglion of L5
- Inferior articular process of L5
- Superior articular process of S1
- Facet joint of L5/S1
- Sacrum

Index

Adhesion, interthalamic, A 28, C 74
Aditus, of mastoid antrum, C 77
Amygdala, A 30, A 33–37, A 39, C 71–73, C 75, S 96, S 100–101, A 110, A 114, 156, S 157
Angle, iridocorneal, 118
Anulus fibrosus, S 204, S 240, S 242, A 248–250, A 252, A 254, S 272, S 275–276, S 278
Aorta, A 218–223, C 224–225, S 236–238, S 241, A 248–253, C 258, S 277
Aperture, pupillary, 118
Apex, of orbit, C 66
Apparatus, lacrimal, 112
Aqueduct, cerebral, A 32–35, S 88–89, C 77, A 110–112
Arch,
  of atlas,
    anterior, 56, S 88–90, S 205
    posterior, A 56, C 80, C 84, C 196–197, S 205, S 207
  zygomatic, A 49, C 64
Archicerebellum, 142, 152
Arcus parieto-occipitalis, 98, S 99
Area, Areas,
  cortical, of cerebrum,
    motor,
      speech of Broca, 158, S 159
      of Wernicke, 158, S 159
    numbered,
      areas,
        6, A 6
        8, 140
        17, 140, A 141, 154, A 155
    premotor, of cerebral cortex, A 6, 134
    prepiriform, 92
    pretectal, 140, A 141
    visual (calcarine), A 21, A 23–24, 140, A 141, 154, A 155
Arteries, named,
  alveolar,
    inferior, C 185
  angular, C 76
  aorta, see Aorta
  basilar, A 36–37, A 39, A 40–41, A 43–45, A 47, C 73, S 89, S 91, A 111–114, A 117, S 131
  calcarine, C 80
  callosomarginal, 16, A 17, A 19, A 21, A 23, C 66
  carotid,
    common, S 101, A 179, A 181, C 189, C 191, S 210–215
    external, A 46, A 54, A 56, S 105, A 167–171, A 173, A 177, C 190, S 212–213, S 215
    internal, A 35–55, A 57–59, C 68, C 70–73, 74, C 75, C 77–78, S 90–96, S 98–99, A 111–117, C 123, S 127, S 130–131, A 162–173, A 175, A 177–178, A 181, C 189–191, S 213–215
  cerebellar,
    inferior,
      anterior, A 37, A 41, A 45, C 77, C 79, S 93, S 95, S 97, S 99, S 101, S 103
      posterior, A 37, A 41, A 45, A 46, A 47, A 49, C 76,

Note: A, C, OR S REFERS TO AXIAL, CORONAL, OR SAGITTAL RESPECTIVELY

Arteries, named, cerebellar, posterior (*Continued*)
C 78–79, C 81, C 83, C 85, S 88–89, S 91, S 93, S 95, S 97, S 99, S 101, S 103, S 105, A 117
superior, A 29, A 33–34, A 37, A 41, C 77, C 79, C 81, C 83, C 85, S 89, S 91–93, S 95, S 97, S 99, S 101, S 103, S 105, A 111, A 114
cerebral,
anterior, A 5, A 7, A 9, A 13, 16, A 17, A 19, A 21, A 25, A 29, A 31–34, A 36–37, C 63, C 65, C 67–69, C 71, C 73, C 75, C 77, C 79, C 81, C 83, C 85, S 89, S 91, S 93, S 95, S 97, A 110–112, C 123
middle, A 7, A 9, A 13, A 17, A 21, A 25, A 29, A 33–35, A 37, A 41, A 45, C 63, C 65, C 67, C 69–71, C 73, C 75, C 77, C 79, C 81, C 83, C 85, S 93–101, S 103, S 105, S 107, A 111–112, C 123, S 124–125, S 127
posterior, A 13, A 17, A 21, A 25, A 29, A 33–34, A 37, A 41, A 45, C 73, C 75–77, C 79, C 81, C 83, C 85, S 89, S 91–93, S 95, S 97, S 99, S 101, S 103, A 110–112
choroidal,
anterior, A 29, A 33, A 37, A 41, C 71, C 73, C 75, C 77, S 93, S 95, S 97, S 99, A 110
communicating, of brain,
posterior, A 33, C 71
facial, C 184–188
frontopolar, S 88
iliac,
common, A 254–255, C 258–259
external, A 256–257
internal, A 256–257, C 258, C 262
iliolumbar, 254
intercostal, A 219–223, C 224–227, C 229–234, S 236–237, S 240, S 242–245
posterior, 236
superior, 230
lacrimal, A 111, 122
lenticulostriate, A 29, A 32, C 74
lateral, A 30, S 98, C 73
lingual, C 185, C 187
lumbar, 254, A 258, C 259, C 261, C 263–265, S 272–273, S 281
maxillary, A 48, C 72, S 96, S 102–103, S 105, C 122–123, 126, C 184–185, C 187, C 189
meningeal,
of lacrimal, 122
middle, C 71, 122
nasal, dorsal, 130
occipital, S 102, S 213
ophthalmic, A 39, A 41, S 95–96, A 110–114, 120, C 121–122, S 125–127, S 129–130
pericallosal, A 25, A 27, A 29, C 64, C 66–67, C 71, S 88–89, S 131
pulmonary, S 245
renal, C 224
sacral,
lateral, C 271
median, 254
spinal, S 239, S 244
subclavian, C 193
subcostal, 230
supratrochlear, 130
temporal,
superficial, A 17, A 31, C 70
vertebral, A 44, A 49, A 51–59, C 76–80, S 92, S 94–95, S 97, S 99, A 162, A 164–166, A 168–175, A 177–181, C 192–195, C 197, S 210–213, S 215
vidian, 44
Artifact, cerebrospinal fluid pulsation, A 218–223, S 241–242
Atlas, A 57, A 59, C 74
Auditory tube, see Tube, auditory

Basal ganglia, see Nuclei, basal
Basis pontis, see Pons, ventral (basilar part)
Body, Bodies,
amygdaloid, see Amygdala
ciliary, A 114–115, S 124–125, S 129–131
geniculate,
lateral, 32, 90, 94, 154, A 155
medial, 90, 150, A 151
mamillary, A 34–35, C 75, S 88–89, 90, A 110
pineal, see Pineal
pituitary, see Pituitary
vitreous, A 36, A 39, A 41, A 43, A 45, C 63, S 101, A 111–116, 118, C 119, 124, S 125–131
Bones, individual, see under individual names
Brachial plexus, see Plexuses of nerves, brachial
Bulb, olfactory, C 65, A 112–113, 156, S 157

Calcar avis, C 78, S 98
Calcarine cortex, see Area, Areas, cortical, of cerebrum, visual
Calvaria, 10
Canal,
abducent (Dorello's), S 92
alveolar, C 185–186
auditory,
external, A 42, A 44, C 77, C 191
internal, S 98, A 116
carotid, A 162
central, 194, S 241, S 277
hypoglossal, A 46, A 49-51, C 192, C 194
incisive, of maxilla, A 56
jugular, C 192
optic, A 112, 130
posterior condylar, A 162
pterygoid (vidian), A 44
sacral, 256, A 257
semicircular, C 77, 152
vertebral, see also Foramen, vertebral, S 208, 224, 250, A 251, 256
thoracic, C 224
vidian, see Canal, pterygoid
Canaliculus, lacrimal, 112
Capsule,
external, A 29, C 71, S 97
extreme, C 71
internal, 24, A 26, A 30, C 74–76, S 93–94, S 99, S 127, C 135, A 136–137, 150
anterior limb, 24, A 25–26, A 28–29, 70, C 71
genu, 24, A 29, A 31
posterior limb, A 24, A 27–31, C 73–75, S 97, 134, 144, A 146, 148
Cartilage,
arytenoid, A 172, A 176–179, C 186, C 188–189, 204, S 205–208, 210
of auricle, A 42, A 49, C 77, C 194
corniculate, 172, 204, S 205, 210
cricoid, 172, A 180–181, C 188–190, S 204–211, S 213
cuneiform, 172, 204, S 205, 210
epiglottic, S 88, S 90, A 168, A 170–171, 172, A 173, C 185, 186, C 187–189, 204, S 205–209, 210
nasal,
lateral (upper), A 114
septal, A 43, A 47, A 49
thyroid, A 172, A 174, A 176–178, A 180, C 184–190, S 204–211, S 213, S 215
Cauda equina, C 226, A 248–256, C 264, C 266, C 268, 270, S 277
Cava, vena, inferior or superior, see Veins, cava
Cave, Meckel's, A 40, A 115

Note: A, C, OR S REFERS TO AXIAL, CORONAL, OR SAGITTAL RESPECTIVELY

Cavity,
  abdominal, C 258
  middle ear, see Cavity, tympanic
  nasal, A 54, 64, 112, 126, C 184–185
  oral, 126, A 165–166, A 168
  pelvic, S 274
  tympanic, A 42, A 46, S 104
Cavum,
  septi, pellucidi, 24
  velum interpositum, see Cistern, subarachnoid, of velum interpositum
Centrum semiovale, A 12–13, A 15–17, A 19, C 64, S 98, S 100–103
Cerebellum, A 38, A 39, A 43, A 47, A 49, A 51–52, 78, 80, C 82, C 85, 88, S 96, S 98, S 102, S 105, 142, C 196, C 199–201
  corpus medullare, C 81, C 83–94, S 94, S 97, S 99–101, S 103
Chiasm, optic, 32, A 35–36, C 70–71, S 88–89, 90, S 91, A 110, A 112, 154
Choroid, of eye, 114
  plexus, see Plexus
Cingulum, A 16–17, C 73, S 93–95
Cistern,
  subarachnoid,
    ambient, A 32, A 34, S 94
    cerebellopontine, A 43, S 92, S 98, A 117
    crural, A 35
    interpeduncular, A 35, C 74–76, S 88
    magna, A 38, A 44, A 45, A 47, A 50–52, C 81–84, S 88–89, C 196, C 198, C 201
    medullary, see Cistern, premedullary
    pontine, 36, A 39, A 41, A 43, C 77, S 88, S 91, A 112, A 115
    premedullary, A 45, A 47, A 51, A 117
    prepontine, see Cistern, pontine
    quadrigeminal plate, A 26, A 28, A 30–32, A 34–35, A 44, C 78, S 90
    retropulvinar, A 25, A 27
    superior cerebellar, A 31, C 78, C 80–81, 84, S 88
    suprasellar, A 36, C 71–72
    sylvian, A 36
    of velum interpositum, A 22, S 88
Claustrum, A 24, A 29–30, C 71, C 75, 94, S 100, 138
Clivus, A 32, A 43, A 45, A 47, A 50, A 52, C 73–75, C 77, S 90–91, A 114–117, S 130–131, A 162, C 187, C 189–191
Coccyx, 270
Cochlea, A 42, A 177, 150, C 191
Colliculus, of midbrain,
  inferior, A 38, C 78, S 88, 150, A 151
  superior, A 29–30, 76, C 78, 88, 140, A 141
Colon,
  sigmoid, C 258, C 262, C 264, S 274
Column, Columns,
  of spinal cord,
    gray,
      anterior (ventral), 194, A 218, A 220–223
      lateral, 134, A 137, 194
      posterior (dorsal), 144, A 145, A 167, A 176, 194, A 218–223, C 230
    white,
      posterior (dorsal), A 54, A 56, A 59, A 165, A 175, A 177, C 230
Commissures,
  of brain,
    anterior, A 30, C 73, S 88, 156, S 157
    habenular, A 30, 90
    posterior, 90
  of spinal cord, 194, S 241
Concha, nasal,
  inferior, A 47, A 57, C 62–63, 64, C 65–67, C 69, S 90–93, C 118–122
  middle, A 51–53, C 62–67, A 117, C 119–122
  superior, A 49, 64
Condyle,
  occipital, A 48, A 53–55, C 76–77, C 79, A 162–164, C 192–193, S 209, S 211, S 213, S 215
Confluence of sinuses, A 33, C 85, S 91, S 97
Conus,
  medullaris, C 264, C 266, S 277
Cord, spinal, see Spinal cord
  vocal, see Fold, Folds, vocal
Cornea, A 115, S 124–125, S 129–131
Cornu ammonis, 96
Corona radiata, of brain, A 16, A 20, S 92, S 96–99, 134, C 135, A 136, 144, A 146
Corpus, Corpora,
  callosum, A 18–20, A 26, C 68, C 70, 72, C 76
    body, C 73–75, S 131, S 88–89, 92
    genu, A 22, A 24–25, A 29, C 66–69, C 71, S 91, 92, C 121–122, S 131
    rostrum, 68, 92, C 122
    splenium, A 21–23, A 27, A 32, C 77–79, S 88–89, S 91–92, S 129–131
  striatum, 70, 94, 138
Cortex, of cerebrum,
  calcarine, see Area, Areas, cortical, of cerebrum, visual
  prepiriform, see Area, Areas, cortical, of cerebrum, prepiriform
Crest or Crista,
  galli, A 34–35, A 40, C 62–63, 64, S 88, A 110–111, A 113, C 118–119
  lacrimal, 128
  occipital, external, A 162, A 164, 200
Cribriform plate, A 40
Crus, Crura,
  cerebri, C 75, 88
  of diaphragm, C 224–232, C 259, 260, C 261, C 263
Culmen, see Lobule, Lobules, of cerebellum
Cuneus, A 10, A 16–17, A 19, A 21, A 23, A 29, A 31, C 84–85, S 88–90, S 92–93
Cysts, Tarlov, see Diverticula, arachnoid

Declive, see Lobule, Lobules, of cerebellum
Dens, see Process, odontoid
Diaphragm, see Muscles, diaphragm
Diaphragma sellae, A 113
Diencephalon, 156
Diploë, A 5, A 10, A 17, A 19
Disc, see also Nucleus pulposus
  intervertebral,
    C2/C3, A 168, C 193
    C3/C4, A 170–171, C 191
    C4/C5, A 175, A 177, S 208
    C5/C6, A 179, C 192–193, S 205, S 208, S 236
    C6/C7, S 207
    C7/T1, S 244
    T2/T3, S 243
    T3/T4, S 241, S 244
    T4/T5, S 243
    T6/T7, A 220–221, S 240–244
    T7/T8, C 226–227, S 240–243
    T8/T9, C 225, S 239
    T9/T10, C 224–226, S 237, S 239
    T10/T11, C 224–225
    T11/T12, C 228, S 238, S 240
    L1/L2, C 260
    L2/L3, C 259, C 261, C 263, C 265, S 273, S 276–277, S 280–281
    L3/L4, C 258, S 274, S 279

Note: A, C, OR S REFERS TO AXIAL, CORONAL, OR SAGITTAL RESPECTIVELY

Disc, intervertebral (*Continued*)
    L4/L5, C 258, C 262, C 264, S 272, S 275, S 279, S 280
    L5/S1, A 255–257, C 258, C 263, C 265, C 267, C 271, S 274, S 276, S 280
    S1/S2, A 257, C 262, S 274, S 276
Diverticula, arachnoid, C 266
Dorsum sellae, A 32, A 36, A 113, A 115
Duct,
    nasolacrimal, A 44, A 46, A 50, C 63, S 92, 112, A 116–117, C 118–119
    parotid, 188
    submandibular, 212
Duodenum, C 226
Dura mater,
    cerebral, 4, C 75
    spinal,
        cervical, A 58, A 164, C 195, S 204
        lumbar, A 249–250, A 255–256, C 266, C 268, S 274, S 276–277
        thoracic, A 218, A 220, A 222, C 228–233, S 238, S 242–243

Ependyma, of third ventricle, 72
Epiglottis, see Cartilage, epiglottic
Epithalamus, 90
Esophagus, A 180, S 204–209, A 220–223, S 240, S 243
Eyelid, A 38, A 42, A 113

Facet, see Process, articular
Facet joint, see Joints, facet
Falx,
    cerebelli, A 36, C 200
    cerebri, 4, A 6–9, A 11, A 13–15, A 17, A 19–21, A 23, A 26, A 32–34, A 36, C 62–63, 64, C 65–66, C 69, C 77, C 82, C 85, C 118–119, S 130
Fascia,
    lacrimal, 116
    pharyngeal, A 162
    prevertebral, A 171, A 177
Fasciculus,
    arcuate, 158, S 159
    cuneatus, 176
    gracilis, 176, A 218–221, A 223
    longitudinal, medial, 140, A 141, 152, A 153
Fat,
    epidural,
        lumbar, C 230–231, A 248–257, C 268–269, S 275–278
        sacral, S 274, S 279
        thoracic, A 218–223, C 232–233, S 241–242
    epiglottal, see Fat, pre-epiglottal
    in intervertebral foramen, A 220–221, A 249, A 255, S 273–274, S 280–281
    orbital, A 45, A 110, A 115, A 117
    paraspinous, S 242–243
    pre-epiglottal, S 205–208
    retromandibular, A 44, A 52
Fiber, or Fibers,
    nerve, see also Tract
        corticobulbar, 76
        corticopontine, 24, 76
        corticospinal, 76
            in internal capsule, 24
        olivocerebellar, 142
        retrolenticular, A 31
        thalamocortical, 24
Field, cortical eye, A 140
Filum terminale, 270, C 271
    externa, 256
    interna, 256

Fissures, see also Sulcus, Sulci
    cerebellar,
        horizontal, C 79–80, C 82–84, S 100–103
        postpyramidal, S 89
        prepyramidal, S 89
        primary, S 89
    cerebral,
        calcarine, see Sulcus, Sulci, cerebral, calcarine
        choroid, C 76, S 96, S 98
        interhemispheric, A 6, A 8, A 14, A 18, A 27, A 31, C 63–64, C 66, C 70, C 120–121
        lateral, see Sulcus, Sulci, cerebral, lateral
        parieto-occipital, see Sulcus, Sulci, cerebral, parieto-occipital
    of skull,
        orbital, superior, A 40, C 68–69, A 114–115, 120, C 122
        pterygomaxillary, S 96
        tympanosquamosal, A 162
    of spinal cord,
        anterior median, A 218–223, C 228–229
        horizontal, C 227–228
Flocculus, A 41–43, A 46, S 96, A 116–117, 142
Floor, orbital, 64
Fold, Folds,
    aryepiglottic, A 175, C 187–189, 204
    glossoepiglottic,
        lateral, 204
        median, 204
    hyoepiglottic, A 173
    vestibular, A 174, 178, C 187, 206, S 207–208
    vocal, A 176–179, C 187, 206, S 207–208
Folium, see Lobule, Lobules, of cerebellum
Foramen, Foramina,
    caecum, of skull, 62
    emissary, A 162
    interventricular, A 29, C 72, C 75
    intervertebral, 280
        C7/T1, S 209
        T1/T2, S 209, S 244
        T4/T5, S 238
        T9/T10, S 239
        L2/L3, C 264
        L4/L5, S 275
    jugular, A 50–51
    lacerum, 44, A 162
    of Luschka, 82
    of Magendie, C 82
    magnum, 48, A 52, C 74, C 77, C 80, A 162, A 164, C 194–195, S 205, S 207
    mastoid, A 162
    Monro, see Foramen, Foramina, interventricular
    ovale, A 42, A 46
    sacral, C 271
        anterior, 256
        posterior, 256
    spinosum, A 162
    stylomastoid, A 162
    transversarium,
        accessory,
            C4, A 172
        C4, A 172–173, A 175
        C6, C 194
    vertebral, S 208, 224, 250, A 251, 256
Forceps,
    major, A 21, A 23, C 80, C 83, 92, S 93, S 95, S 97, S 99
    minor, A 20, A 29, C 65, 92, S 93, S 95
Formation,
    hippocampal, 96, 156
    reticular, paramedian pontine, 140, A 141
Fornix of brain, A 22, A 26, A 30, 72, C 74–75, S 88, S 92, 156, S 157

Note: A, C, OR S REFERS TO AXIAL, CORONAL, OR SAGITTAL RESPECTIVELY

body, C 72–73, S 88–91
columns,
  anterior, A 24–29
  posterior, A 22, A 24, A 28
crura, C 78
Fossa,
  cranial,
    middle, 122, 126
  glenoid, A 46, C 74, S 104, C 189
  hyaloid, 124
  infratemporal, 64
  jugular, A 162
  lacrimal, 112
  piriform, A 174–175, 188, C 189
  pterygopalatine, 44, A 116, S 125–127, S 129
  Rosenmüller, A 53, A 55, A 163, C 187
Frontal bone, A 4–7, A 13, A 15, A 17, A 19, S 107, C 119, 122
Funiculus of spinal cord,
  posterior, 176

Galea aponeurotica, A 8
Ganglion,
  basal, see Nuclei, basal
  pterygopalatine, 126
  spinal, 278
    C2, A 53, A 58, C 82, A 165
    C4, A 171
    C6, S 210
    C8, S 212, S 236
    T1, C 197
    T5, S 243
    T6, A 219–220
    T7, A 223, S 239, S 244
    T8, C 231–232, S 239, S 244
    T9, C 232
    T12, C 230
    L2, A 250, C 265, S 280
    L3, A 251, C 263–265
    L4, A 253, C 264–265, S 273, S 279, S 281
    L5, A 255, C 267, S 281
    S1, A 256–257, S 280
  trigeminal (fifth cranial nerve), A 38, 40, A 41, A 42, A 43, C 71–72, 74, C 75, S 94, A 114, A 116–117, A 148, C 187, C 189
Gland,
  adrenal, see Gland, suprarenal
  lacrimal, C 62–63, A 110–113, C 118
  lingual, anterior, 168
  parotid, A 52–57, A 59, C 70, C 72, C 75, C 77–78, S 105–106, 162, A 163, A 165, A 167, 168, 188, C 189, C 191, C 194
  pineal, see Pineal
  pituitary, see Pituitary
  salivary, 168, 212
  sublingual, 168, A 169, S 212
  submandibular, A 168, A 170–171, A 173, C 187–190, 212, S 213–215
  suprarenal, C 226, C 260
  thyroid, A 177–181, S 204, S 206–211, S 213, S 215
Globe, A 110, A 112, A 117, C 118
Globus pallidus, A 24, A 28–29, C 71, C 73, C 75–76, S 93–94, S 98, A 138, C 139
Granulations, arachnoid, A 4–5
Grooves,
  for digastric muscle, A 162, A 164
  for occipital artery, A 162, A 164
  for vertebral artery, A 164
Gyrus, Gyri,
  ambiens, 92, 156
  angular, A 14, A 17–19, A 21–24, C 79–81, C 83–84, S 98, S 102, 104, S 105, S 107, 158
  cingulate, A 10, A 12, A 14, A 16, A 18, A 20–24, C 66–68, C 70–72, C 75, C 77, S 88, S 90–91, 92, 156
  cuneate, 90
  dentate, 92, 96, 156
  fasciolaris (splenial), 96, S 97
  frontal,
    inferior, A 13–15, A 17, A 19–21, A 23, A 31–33, C 62–65, C 67, C 69, C 72, 100, S 102, S 105–106
    medial, S 88–92
    middle, A 9–19, A 21–23, A 28, A 33–34, A 36, C 62–67, C 69–70, C 72, S 100, S 102–103, S 105, 140
    superior, A 4–24, A 30, A 33, A 36, C 62–69, C 72, S 94–95, S 97–103, S 105
  fusiform, C 71
  intralimbic, 92
  lingual, C 81–83, 92, S 93–95
  long, of insula, S 101
  occipital,
    inferior, C 84–85, S 102, S 105
    superior, A 14, C 84–85, S 102
  occipitotemporal,
    lateral, A 32, C 77, C 79, C 82, S 102–103
    medial, S 96–101
  olfactory,
    lateral, 92
  orbital, 36, A 37, C 63–65, C 67, S 95–96, S 100–101, S 103, C 119–121, S 124–131
    anterior, A 110–111
    lateral, A 110–112
    medial, A 36, A 110–112
    posterior, A 110–111
  parahippocampal, A 24, A 36, A 41, A 43, C 73, 74, C 77, C 79, 92, S 94–95, 96, 156
  postcentral, A 4–11, A 13–19, A 21, A 23, C 74, C 76, S 94, S 97, 98, S 99, 102, S 106, 134, 144, A 146–147, 148, A 149, 152, A 153
  precentral, A 4–15, A 17, A 19–21, A 23, C 72, S 92, 102, S 106, 134
  premotor, see Area, Areas, premotor
  rectus, A 34–37, C 62–63, C 66–67, A 110–112, C 119–123
  retrosplenial, A 21, A 23, 156
  semilunaris, 92, 156
  short, of insula, S 101–103
  splenial, see Gyrus, Gyri, fasciolaris
  subcallosal, A 30, 156
  supracallosal, 96
  supramarginal, A 9, A 11–13, A 15, A 17, A 19–23, A 25, C 76–77, C 79, S 96, S 104–105, S 107
  temporal,
    inferior, A 38, A 40, A 45, C 73, C 77, C 79, C 81–82, S 105–107, A 114–117, C 122–123, C 125, S 128–129
    middle, A 37, A 39, C 68–71, C 73, C 77, C 79, C 81–84, S 104–107, C 122–123
    superior, A 25, A 31, A 33, A 35, C 68–71, C 73, C 77, C 82, 102, S 104–107, C 122–123, 150, A 151, 158
  transverse, 102, S 103

Hippocampus, see also Formation, hippocampal, A 30, A 32, A 34, 36, 72, C 73–76, C 78, S 94, S 96–100, 156, S 157
  fimbria, C 77
Humor,
  aqueous, A 114–115, 118, S 125, S 129–131
  vitreous, 114, 118
Hydromyelia, 194
Hyoepiglottic fold, see Fold, Folds, hyoepiglottic
Hyoid, A 171–173, C 184–188, C 190, S 204–210, S 213–215

Note: A, C, OR S REFERS TO AXIAL, CORONAL, OR SAGITTAL RESPECTIVELY

Hypopharynx, see Pharynx, cavity, laryngeal part
Hypothalamus, A 32, C 72, S 88–89, 90, 156, S 157

Ilium, A 256–257, C 269, C 271
Incus, C 77
Indusium griseum, S 89, 96
Infundibulum, of pituitary (hypophysis), A 35–38, C 70–71, S 88, 90, A 111–113
Insula, A 25, A 27–28, A 30, A 31, A 33–34, C 68–69, C 71–73, C 75–76, S 100, 102, A 110–111, S 128
Intestine,
   small, C 258, C 262
Iris, 114, 124
Isthmus,
   of parahippocampal gyrus, 92, S 94–95
   pharyngeal, 184, 186

Joints,
   atlantoaxial, A 53, 56, C 76, C 78, C 191–194, S 209–211, S 213, S 215
   atlanto-occipital, A 54, C 77, S 94–95, A 162–163, C 192–194, S 213, S 215
   capitular, S 210, C 228
   costotransverse, C 199, A 222, C 232–233, S 245
   costovertebral, C 195, A 218–219, A 221–222, C 229
   facet,
      C2/C3, S 96
      C3/C4, A 170–171, A 173
      C4/C5, A 174, A 177, C 192, S 213
      C5/C6, C 194, S 211
      C6/C7, S 210, S 236
      C7/T1, S 212
      T1/T2, S 244
      T6/T7, A 220, S 244
      T7/T8, S 239, S 244
      T8/T9, S 239
      T10/T11, C 232
      T11/T12, S 238, S 240
      T12/L1 C 230
      L1/L2, C 231
      L2/L3, A 249, C 268, S 274, S 279
      L3/L4, A 251, A 253, S 280
      L4/L5, A 253–255, C 264, S 272–273, A 280
      L5/S1, C 266, S 281
   sacroiliac, A 256–257, C 264, C 266, C 268–271
   temporomandibular, A 42
   uncovertebral, A 169, C 193
Jugular tubercle, see Tuber, Tubercle, or Tuberosity, jugular

Kidney, C 224–227, C 229, C 231–232, A 248–249, C 258–261, C 263, C 265

Labyrinth,
   vestibular, S 100, 152
Lacunae, venous of dura, C 80, 84
Lamina,
   cribrosa, 156
   papyracea, 62
   terminalis, A 31–32
   of vertebral arches,
      C1, A 163–164
      C2, A 166, C 194, C 197
      C3, A 168, C 195
      C4, A 172–174
      C5, A 173, A 176
      C7, C 198

T3, S 242–243
T4, S 239
T5, A 218
T6, A 219–222
T7, A 221, A 223, C 233, S 243
T8, C 233, S 240, S 243
T9, C 233, S 240
T11, C 232, S 238
T12, C 231
L1, C 231, C 270
L2, A 248–250, C 269, S 277
L3, A 251–253, C 266, C 268–269, S 275, S 278
L4, A 251, A 253–255, C 268–269, S 274, S 279
L5, A 255–256, S 274
Laryngopharynx, see Pharynx, cavity, laryngeal part
Larynx, 178, A 181, 188, 204, 206, S 208, S 212
   cavity, 178, C 189
   inlet, 178, 206
   saccule, 178
   sinus, 178, C 187
   vestibule, 178, 206
Lemniscus,
   lateral, 150, A 151
   medial, 144, A 145–146
      in pons, A 40–41, A 43, S 88–90
   trigeminal, A 148–149
Lens, C 62–63, S 98–100, A 114–115, C 119, S 124–126, S 129–131
Ligaments,
   apical, of dens, C 77
   arcuate,
      median, 260
   capsular, costovertebral, 228
   check, of eyeball,
      lateral, A 115
      medial, A 115
   costotransverse, 232, C 233
      lateral, 232
      superior, 232
   cricoarytenoid, 180
   cricothyroid, 180
   cricotracheal, 180
   flavum, A 177, C 197, S 204, A 218–223, C 230–233, S 238, S 240–243, A 248–256, 262, C 267–269, S 274–280
   hyoepiglottic, 172, C 187, 204
   iliolumbar, C 258
   interarticular, C 229–230
   interspinous, 200, S 204, 262
   intra-articular, costovertebral, 228
   longitudinal,
      anterior, A 57, C 190, S 204, S 242, A 251–255, 260, 262, S 276–278
      posterior, S 204, 226, C 227, C 229, S 242, A 248–256, 262, C 263, C 265, S 276–278
   nuchae, A 45, A 48, A 53–56, A 58–59, C 83–85, A 163–165, A 170, A 173, A 181, C 199–201, S 204–207, S 241
   palpebral,
      lateral, 128
      medial, C 63, 128
   petroclinoid, A 37, A 39, 74, S 92–93, A 114–115
   radiate,
      of rib, 228
   sacroiliac, C 258
   supraspinous, 200, 262
   suspensory, of lens, S 124
   thyroarytenoid, C 189
   thyroepiglottic, 188, 204
   transverse atlantal, A 53, A 56–57, A 59, S 88, A 164, C 192–193, S 205, S 207

Note: A, C, OR S REFERS TO AXIAL, CORONAL, OR SAGITTAL RESPECTIVELY

vestibular, 206
vocal, 206
Limen insulae, S 102
Lingula, see Lobule, Lobules, of cerebellum
Lip, A 166, A 168
Liver, C 224–226, C 228–232, S 240
Lobe, Lobes,
  flocculonodular, 142, A 143, 152, A 153
  frontal, 16, C 118, 156
  limbic, 156, S 157
  occipital, 80, S 96–97, S 99–100, 104
  piriform, 92
  temporal, 16, 36, A 44, C 66, 106
Lobule, Lobules,
  of cerebellum,
    central, C 79, S 89
    culmen, 28, A 29, A 31–32, A 34, C 80–81, S 89
    declive, A 36, C 80, C 82–83, S 89
    folium, C 84, S 89
    lingula, S 89
    nodule, A 38, A 42, C 80, S 89, A 116, 142
    pyramid, A 38, A 46, S 89
    tuber, A 42, C 84, S 88–89
    uvula, C 81, C 83, S 89, A 116, C 198
  paracentral, A 6–9, A 11, A 13, S 88–92
  parietal,
    inferior, A 7, A 9, A 11–13, A 15–17, A 19, A 34, C 78–79, C 81–85, S 100, 102, 104, S 105
    superior, A 5–8, A 12–16, C 74, C 78–85, S 96–97, 98, S 99–101
Locus ceruleus, A 36
Loop, of Meyer, 154
Lung, C 195, C 197, S 209, S 211, S 213–215, A 218–223, C 224–233, S 236, S 244–245
Lymph nodes, A 50
  lumbar, C 259, C 262

Malleus, C 191
Mandible, A 44, A 49–53, A 55, A 59, C 63, C 66, C 68–69, C 72, S 105, C 122–123, A 166–168, A 170–171, A 173, C 184–189, S 204–209, S 211–215
  condyle, A 47, C 72, S 102, S 105, C 189–190
  coronoid process, A 47, C 184–185
  neck, C 189, C 191
  ramus, A 54, A 56, C 66, C 70, C 74, A 164–165, C 187
Mass,
  lateral,
    C1, A 56, A 58, C 75, C 77, 94, A 164–165, C 190–193, 196, S 209, S 211, S 213, S 215
Massa intermedia, see Adhesion, interthalamic
Mastoid, see Temporal bone, mastoid portion
Matter, gray,
  periaqueductal, A 110, A 112
Maxilla, A 55–56, C 63–64, S 104, 128, A 164–165, S 215
Meatus, acoustic,
  external, A 41, A 46, S 106–107
  internal, A 42, C 77, S 96, S 101, S 103
Medulla, A 44–45, A 47, 48, A 49, A 51, 78, C 79, A 117, 134, 144, C 192, C 194–195
  closed, A 48, A 50
  open, A 46
Membrane,
  tectoria, of atlanto-occipital joint, 226
  thyrohyoid, 188
  tympanic, A 46, C 77
Metathalamus, 90
Midbrain (mesencephalon), A 32, S 88
Muscles,
  aryepiglotticus, S 208
  arytenoid,
    oblique, S 206, 208
    transverse, A 174, A 177, A 179–180, S 207–208
  buccinator, A 56, A 59, C 63–64, A 164–167, A 169, C 184–185, S 210, S 211, S 213
  cricoarytenoid,
    lateral, 208
    posterior, S 206, 208
  cricothyroid, S 208
  diaphragm, C 224, C 226, C 230–231, S 240
  digastric, A 54, A 56, A 59, C 76, C 79, A 162–166, A 170–171, C 185, C 190–191, C 193–195, S 212, S 214–215
  erector spinae, A 178, C 232, S 238, S 242
  genioglossus, C 68, S 88, S 90, S 92, A 168–169, C 184, C 187, C 189, S 204–207, S 209, S 212–213, S 215
  geniohyoid, C 74, A 171, A 173, S 205, S 206
  gluteus maximus, C 271
    medius, C 264, C 271
  hyoglossus, A 168–169, 171, A 175, C 184, C 186, S 208, S 214
  iliacus, C 258–259, C 263–265, C 267
  iliocostalis,
    cervicis, C 198
    lumborum, C 234–235, A 250–257, C 269–270, S 272–273, S 281
  iliopsoas, C 267
  intercostal,
    external, C 234–235
    internal, C 233–234
  interspinalis, C 197, C 269–270, S 276–277
  intertransverse, S 244
    lateral, C 265, C 267, S 272
    medial, C 265, C 267, 274
  intrinsic of tongue, see Tongue, muscles
  latissimus dorsi, A 250
  levator,
    palpebrae superioris, C 62–63, A 110–112, C 118–122, S 124–126, S 128–131
    scapulae, A 173, A 175, A 177, A 179–181, C 191, C 193–195, C 197–201, S 210, S 212, S 214–215
    veli palatini, A 48, A 53, A 57, C 71–72, S 98, A 163, 184, 186, C 187–188
  longissimus,
    capitis, A 173, A 175, C 195, C 201
    cervicis, A 173, A 175–177, A 181, C 194, C 196–197, S 210
    thoracis, A 218–223, C 233–235, S 236–237, S 244–245, A 248–255, C 268–270, S 272–275, S 278–281
  longitudinal,
    inferior, C 185
    superior, C 185
  longus,
    capitis, A 48, A 50–51, A 53–55, A 57, C 71–72, C 74, C 77, A 163, A 165–167, A 171, A 173, 174, A 177, C 187–191, S 208
    colli, 56, A 58, S 88, S 90, S 93, A 165–167, A 170–175, A 177, A 179–181, C 190–191, S 204–215
  masseter, A 47–49, A 51, A 53–57, A 59, C 64–70, C 72, C 74, S 98, S 102, S 105–107, C 122–123, A 163, A 165–169, C 184–185, C 187, C 189, S 214–215
  mentalis, S 204
  multifidus, A 171, A 177, A 179, A 181, C 196–201, S 205, S 207, A 218–223, C 232–234, S 237, S 239–245, A 248–257, C 269–270, S 273–275, S 277–281
  mylohyoid, C 72, A 168, A 171, C 184–186, S 204, S 209, S 211–215
  oblique capitis,
    inferior, A 56, C 78, C 80, C 84, S 100, S 102, A 164–167, C 194–198, S 207, S 209–211, S 213, S 215
    superior, A 52–53, C 78, C 197–198, S 209, S 211

Note: A, C, OR S REFERS TO AXIAL, CORONAL, OR SAGITTAL RESPECTIVELY

Muscles (*Continued*)
  oblique oculi,
    inferior, A 46, C 62–63, 110, A 116, C 118–119, S 124–126, S 129–131
    superior, A 35, A 40, C 62–64, 110, A 111–113, C 118–122, S 127, 130, S 131
  occipitofrontal, C 118
  omohyoid, A 177, A 179
  orbicularis,
    oculi, A 47, A 49, A 110–111, 116, A 117, S 124–131
    oris, C 66, S 90, A 165–167, A 169–170, S 208
  palatoglossus, 166, 168
  palatopharyngeus, 166, A 167
  pharyngeal constrictor, C 187–190, S 204, S 206, S 208–212, S 236
    inferior, 166, A 171, 172, A 173–178, A 181, S 206
    middle, A 164, A 166, A 170
    superior, A 53, A 58, A 165, 166, 170
  pharyngopalatinus, A 59, A 163–164, A 185, A 171
  platysma, C 70, A 170–171, A 175, C 185–186, S 213, S 215
  psoas,
    major, C 224, C 226, C 228, C 230, A 248–257, C 258–268, S 272, S 281
  pterygoid,
    lateral, A 47, A 49–51, A 53–54, A 56–57, C 68–70, C 73, S 96, S 98, S 100–104, A 177, C 122–123, S 124, S 128–129, A 162–164, 166, C 184–190
    medial, A 47–49, A 51–55, A 59, C 68, C 70–71, C 73, S 100–101, C 122–123, A 163–169, C 185–189, S 213–215
  quadratus,
    labii,
      inferior, A 169
      superior, A 48, A 52, A 54, A 56–57
    lumborum, A 248
  rectus capitis,
    anterior, A 48–49, A 163
    lateralis, A 53, A 55, A 163
    posterior,
      major, A 52, A 56, C 80, C 83, S 103, A 163–164, C 198–200, S 207, S 209, S 211
      minor, C 197–200, S 205, S 207, S 209, S 211, S 213, S 215
  rectus, of eye,
    inferior, A 42–43, A 46, C 62, C 64–65, S 95–97, 110, A 115–117, C 118–122, S 125–126, S 129–131
    lateral, A 38–41, C 62, C 64–65, S 94, 110, A 112–115, C 118, C 120–122, S 124–125, S 128–129
    medial, A 38–39, A 41, C 62–65, 110, A 113–115, C 118–122, S 126–127, 130, S 131
    superior, C 62–64, S 97–98, A 110–112, C 118–122, S 124–126, S 128–131
  risorius, C 66
  rotator, see Muscles, rotatores
  rotatores, C 196–198, C 231
    thoracis, C 233–234
  salpingopharyngeus, 166
  scalene,
    anterior, A 174, A 176–177, A 179, A 181, C 191, 196, S 214–215
    medius (middle), A 175, A 177, A 179, A 181, C 193, C 195–197, S 214–215
    posterior, A 177, A 179, A 181, C 193, C 195–197, S 214–215
  semispinalis,
    capitis, A 44, A 46, A 48–49, A 52–56, A 59, C 84, S 93–94, S 96, S 100–101, A 162–164, A 167–169, A 171, A 173, A 175, A 177, A 179, A 181, C 197–201, S 205, S 207–215
    cervicis, C 83, A 169–171, A 173, A 175, A 177, A 179, A 181, C 197, C 199–201, S 205, S 207–211, S 214
    thoracis, C 234–235
  serratus,
    anterior, C 193
    posterior, superior, C 199
  spinalis,
    cervicis, A 177, A 179, A 181
    thoracis, A 218–223, C 234–235, S 236–237, S 239–245
  splenius,
    capitis, A 49, C 80, C 82–83, S 93–94, S 96, S 100, S 102, S 105, A 162–164, A 166, A 169, A 171, A 173, A 175, A 177, A 179, A 181, C 194, C 196–201, S 205, S 207, S 209, S 211–215
    cervicis, C 195–196
  sternocleidomastoid, A 48, A 59, C 76, C 79, S 102, S 107, A 163, A 167, A 169–173, A 175, A 177, A 179–181, C 189–191, C 193–196, C 200, S 212–215
  sternohyoid, A 174, A 177, A 180–181, C 186, C 189, C 190, S 204–213
  sternothyroid, A 178–181, C 189, S 214
  strap, A 172, A 177, A 179
  styloglossus, S 98, 168, C 187–188, C 191, S 214
  stylohyoid, S 104, A 168, A 171, A 175, C 191, S 214
  stylopharyngeus, A 162, 166, A 167, A 171
  suboccipital, A 52, S 208
  subscapularis, C 193
  tarsal,
    inferior, A 115–117
    superior, 110, A 113–114
  temporalis, A 30–31, A 37–39, A 43, A 45–47, A 49, A 51–52, A 55, A 57, C 64–67, C 69, C 72, C 74, C 84, S 96, S 102–106, A 110–117, C 121–123, S 124, S 128, A 163–164, 166
  tensor tympani, A 42
  tensor veli palatini, A 48, A 54, A 57, C 72, C 123, A 163, C 185–186, C 188, C 190
  thyroarytenoid, C 186, 208
  thyroepiglotticus, S 208
  thyrohyoid, A 177, C 188, C 190, S 208
  tongue, see Tongue, muscles
  transverse, C 185
  trapezius, A 38, A 42, A 48, C 85, S 96, S 102, A 162–163, A 169–170, A 172–173, A 175, A 177, A 179, A 181, C 195, C 197, C 199, 200, C 201, S 205, S 207–209, S 211, S 213–215, A 222, S 236–237, S 239–240, S 242–245
  vocalis, A 174, A 176–179, C 188, S 208
  zygomatic, A 52, A 54–57, A 163

Nares, A 56
Nasal bone, A 112, C 118
Nasopharynx, see Pharynx, cavity, nasal part
Neocerebellum, 142, A 143
Neostriatum, 94
Nerve,
  abducens, A 36, A 38, 40, A 42, A 114, A 116, 122, 130, 140
  accessory, A 38, A 51, C 195
  auditory, see Nerve, vestibulocochlear
  facial, A 38, A 41–43, C 74, C 76–77, S 97, S 99, A 116–117, 148
  femoral, 262, C 263
  glossopharyngeal, A 38, A 44, C 76–77, 148
  hypoglossal, A 51, 168
  infraorbital, C 120–121
  intercostal, C 227, 230
  lumbar, C 265
  mandibular, C 73, C 187
  maxillary, 40, A 42, C 62, C 72, S 94, A 116–117, C 118, 126

Note: A, C, OR S REFERS TO AXIAL, CORONAL, OR SAGITTAL RESPECTIVELY

obturator, 262, C 263
oculomotor, A 36–38, A 40, A 43, C 71, C 73, A 113, 122, 130, 140
ophthalmic, 40, 122, S 127
optic, A 32, A 36–41, A 43, C 64–66, C 68, S 94, S 97–98, A 112–115, C 120–123, S 125–127, S 129–131, 154, A 155
plexuses, see Plexuses of nerves
spinal, 278, 280
  C1, C 194–195
  C2, C 194–195
  C3, A 169, C 195
  C4, A 174
  C5, A 174–177, C 194
  C6, A 176–177, A 179, S 210
  C7, A 178, S 210
  C8, A 181, S 212
  T12, C 230, 262
  L1, 262, C 267
  L2, 262, S 273
  L3, A 249, 262, C 263–265
  L4, 253, A 255, C 262–265, S 272, S 274, S 279
  L5, C 258, C 263–266, C 271–272
  S1, C 261, C 271, S 272
  S2, C 271
  S3, C 271
trigeminal, A 38, A 40, A 43, S 94, A 114–115, 122, 148
trochlear, A 36, A 38, 40, 122, 140
vagus, A 38, A 47, C 77, S 94, 148, 168, A 177, A 180, C 192
vestibulocochlear, A 38, A 41, A 42, C 74, C 76, S 97, S 99, A 116–117, 142, 150
Node, lymphatic, see Lymph nodes
Nodule,
of cerebellum, see Lobule, Lobules, of cerebellum
Schmorl's, C 224, S 242
Notch, cerebellar, posterior, C 84–85
Nuclei, of gray matter,
of abducent nerve, 140, 152
amygdaloid, 94
basal, A 28, C 73, 94, 138
caudate, A 18, 24, A 26, A 30, 70, C 74, C 76, S 92, S 94, S 127, S 129, A 138, C 139
  body, A 20–21, A 23, C 73, C 75
  head, A 20, A 22, A 24–25, A 27–29, A 30, C 67, C 69, C 70–72, S 93–95, C 122, S 126, S 130–131
  tail, A 25–27, A 30
claustrum, see Claustrum
of cochlear nerve, 150, A 151
cuneatus, 144
dentate, of cerebellum, A 36, A 38, A 40–43, C 78–80, S 93, S 95, A 116, C 195
dorsal column, A 51
facial, 134, 158
gracilis, 144
habenular, 90
of hypoglossal nerve, C 79, 134, 158
lentiform, 24, A 26, A 28, A 30, 76, 94, 138
of oculomotor nerve, 140, 152
olivary (inferior), C 76, 78
proprius, 194
red, A 32–34, C 75–76, S 88–89, 90, S 91, A 110–111, A 138–139, A 142–143
subthalamic, S 92, 138
of trigeminal nerve, 158
  motor, 148
  sensory, A 148
  spinal tract, A 148
of trochlear nerve, 140, 152
of vagus nerve, 158
of vestibular nerve, 78, 142, 152, A 153

  inferior, 152
  lateral, 138, 152
  medial, 152
  superior, 152
Nucleus pulposus, see also Disc, intervertebral, S 204, S 275–276, S 278
  C7/T1, S 242
  L2/L3, A 248
  L3/L4, A 252
  L4/L5, A 254

Obex, A 45, 48, C 78–79, 194, C 195
Occipital condyle, see Condyle, occipital
Opercula, of insula,
  frontal, S 102
  parietal, S 102
  precentral, S 102
  temporal, A 30, A 34, S 102
Optic chiasm, see Chiasm, optic
Optic radiation, see Radiation, optic
Ora serrata, 114
Orbit, A 34, A 44, A 46, 122, 126, 130
Oropharynx, see Pharynx, cavity, oral part
Ossicles, A 46

Palate,
  hard, C 62, 66, S 92, C 123, A 162–163, C 184–185
  soft, C 68–69, C 72, A 165, C 184–185, C 187, S 208–209, S 211
Palatine bone,
  plate, perpendicular, 126
  process,
    orbital, 126
    sphenoidal, 126
Paleocerebellum, A 142–143
Pancreas, C 225
Papilla,
  lacrimal, 116
  optic, S 126, S 130
Parietal bone, A 4–7, A 13, A 15, C 85, S 107
Pars or Part,
  opercularis, (posterior), 102
  triangularis, 102
Pedicle, of vertebra
  C5, A 175
  C6, S 236
  T1, S 209
  T2, S 209, S 244
  T5, S 238
  T6, A 218–219, S 239
  T7, A 222–223, C 232, S 243
  T8, C 231, S 239, S 244
  T9, C 229
  T10, C 229–230
  T11, C 227
  T12, C 229–230, S 238
  L1, C 267
  L2, C 264–265, C 267, S 273, S 280
  L3, A 249–251, C 263–265
  L4, A 251–253, C 264, S 275, S 279, S 281
  L5, A 254, S 272–273, S 280–281
  S1, A 256
Peduncles,
  cerebellar
    inferior, C 78, 142, A 143
    middle (brachium pontis), A 38, A 40–43, C 76–79, S 93, S 95, A 115–116, 142, A 143
    superior (brachium conjunctivum), A 36, C 78–79, 80, 142, A 143

Note: A, C, OR S REFERS TO AXIAL, CORONAL, OR SAGITTAL RESPECTIVELY

Peduncles (*Continued*)
  cerebral, A 31, A 33, A 35, C 74, C 76–77, 88, 134, C 135, A 137
  olfactory, A 38, C 120, 156, S 157
Pharynx, cavity,
  laryngeal part, A 171, 172, A 173–176, A 179, C 191, S 205–208, S 210
  nasal part, A 50, A 54–56, A 58, C 68, C 70–71, S 88, S 90–91, C 123, 162, A 163, C 185, 186, C 187, C 189, S 206
  oral part, A 59, A 164–169, A 171, C 186, S 205, S 207–209
Pineal, A 28, A 30–31, S 88–89, 90, C 76, C 78
Pituitary, A 36, A 39–41, A 43, C 70–71, S 88–89, A 114, A 131
  stalk, see Infundibulum, of pituitary (hypophysis)
Planum sphenoidale, see Sphenoid bone, planum
Plate,
  cribriform, of ethmoid bone, C 62, C 64, 66, C 121
  perpendicular, of ethmoid bone, C 63, C 65, 66, C 67, A 117, C 118–122
  pterygoid, see Sphenoid bone, pterygoid plates
Pleura, S 212, S 244
  parietal, C 227
Plexus,
  choroid,
    of fourth ventricle, C 78, S 91, C 195
    of lateral ventricle, A 22–23, A 25, A 27–28, A 31
    of third ventricle, C 78
Plexuses of nerves,
  brachial, A 178–181
  lumbar, 262
Plexuses of veins,
  vertebral,
    external, 240, 252, 280
      anterior, 252, 264
      posterior, 252
    internal, 240, 252, 280
      anterior, 226, A 248–257, 264
      posterior, 252
Pons, 24, A 42, A 44, C 76–77, 78, S 88–89, A 113–115, A 117, 134, 148, C 191
  tegmentum, see Tegmentum, of pons
  ventral (basilar) part, A 36, A 40–41, A 43
Precuneus, A 6, A 12–15, A 30, C 80–81, C 84–85, S 88–90, S 92
Process,
  alveolar, of maxilla, C 65–67
  articular,
    inferior,
      C1, A 164
      C4, A 173, A 175, C 195
      C5, A 174–175, S 211, S 213
      C7, S 209
      T1, S 209
      T3, S 224
      T5, A 218, S 238
      T6, A 220–221, S 244
      T7, C 233, S 239
      T8, S 244
      T9, S 239
      L1, C 269
      L2, A 249–250, C 266–268, S 274, S 279
      L3, A 251–253, C 268, S 280
      L4, A 251, A 253–255, S 273
      L5, A 255, S 272–273, S 275, S 280–281
    superior,
      C1, A 164
      C2, A 164
      C4, A 172, A 174–175
      C5, A 175, C 195, S 210–211, S 213, S 215
      C6, S 211
      T1, S 209
      T2, S 209
      T3, S 244
      T4, S 238–239
      T6, A 218
      T7, A 220–222, C 233, S 244
      T8, S 239, S 244
      T9, S 239
      T11, C 231
      L2, C 269
      L3, A 249–250, C 266–267, S 273–274, S 279, S 281
      L4, A 251–253, S 275, S 280
      L5, A 253–255, S 273, S 275, S 280
      S1, A 255–256, C 258, C 269–270, S 272–273, S 281
  ciliary, 118
  clinoid,
    anterior, A 20, 36, A 112–113, S 125, 130
  costal,
    cervical,
      C4, A 172, A 174
      C5, A 175, S 210
    sacral, C 271
  mamillary, A 162, S 273, 274, S 275, S 281
  mastoid, A 46, A 48, A 50, A 52–53, S 106–107, A 162, A 164, C 194, C 196
  odontoid (dens), A 52, A 56–59, C 74–75, C 77, S 88–89, A 164–165, C 191–193, S 205, S 207
  palatine, of maxilla, C 62, C 67
  pterygoid, see also Sphenoid bone, pterygoid plates, A 46, A 54, C 68–69, 126, C 186
  spinous, of vertebrae,
    C2, A 169, C 196, C 198
    C4, A 172–174, A 177
    C5, A 172–173
    C7, C 200–201, S 204–206, S 241
    T1, C 201, S 242
    T2, S 241
    T4, A 222, S 238–239
    T5, A 218–219, S 238–239
    T6, A 221–222, S 241
    T7, A 223, S 241–242
    T8, C 235
    T9, C 233–235
    T10, C 233
    T12, C 232
    L1, C 270
    L2, A 249–250, C 269–270
    L3, A 252–253, C 268–270, S 276
    L4, A 254–255, C 269–270, S 275, S 277
    L5, C 270, S 275–276
  styloid, A 48, A 52–53, A 162–164, C 191
  transverse,
    C1, A 58, A 164
    C2, A 164
    C3, A 171, C 193
    C4, A 174
    C6, A 178–179
    T1, C 197
    T2, C 201
    T3, S 245
    T5, A 222, S 239
    T6, A 218–219, S 236–237
    T7, A 223, C 233, S 236–237, S 245
    T8, C 233, S 245
    T9, C 232–234
    T11, C 231–232
    L1, C 231, C 268
    L2, C 266–268
    L3, A 250, C 265, C 267, S 272, S 281
    L4, A 251, A 253, C 265

Note: A, C, OR S REFERS TO AXIAL, CORONAL, OR SAGITTAL RESPECTIVELY

L5, A 254–255, C 265, C 267, S 275
uncinate, A 171–173, A 175–177, A 179, C 193
zygomatic, of frontal, 112
Promontory, sacral, C 271
Protuberance,
  mental, A 175
  occipital,
    external, 200
    internal, A 37, A 43–44, A 47, A 50–51, C 201
Pulvinar, A 25, A 27–28, C 77, S 92–95
Putamen, see also Nucleus, lentiform, A 24–25, A 27–29, A 31, C 68–69, 70, C 71–73, C 75–77, S 96–99, S 125–130, A 138, C 139
Pyramid, see also Lobule, Lobules, of cerebellum
  of medulla oblongata, A 31, A 44, A 47, A 52
    decussation, A 52

Radiation,
  acoustic, S 100–101, S 103
  optic, A 24–25, A 27–28, A 30–31, C 75, C 77–81, S 93, 94, S 95, S 97–99, 154, A 155
Raphe,
  lingual, A 170
Recess, Recesses,
  lateral,
    C5, S 208, S 279
    lateral dorsal of fourth ventricle, C 80–81
    median dorsal of fourth ventricle, C 80–81
  pharyngeal (fossa of Rosenmüller), A 48, A 163
  pineal (of third ventricle), C 76
  suprapineal (of third ventricle), C 76
  trigeminal, see Cave, Meckel's
Retinae, 154
Rhinencephalon, 156
Rib, A 181, C 195, C 197, C 199, C 201, S 214–215, A 218–223, C 224, C 226–235, S 236–237, S 244–245
Rima,
  glottidis, A 174, 178, A 179, C 185, C 187, 206, S 208
  vestibuli, 178, 206
Roots,
  of nerves,
    spinal, A 54, A 56, A 58, C 79, C 277, S 236, S 240, S 243–244, A 248–249, A 254–256, S 272, 278, S 279–280
      dorsal, C 230, C 232
      ventral, C 228–229

Sac, lacrimal, 112, 116, C 119
Sacculus, C 77
Sacrum, A 256–257, C 263–265, C 267–271, S 272–281
Scalp, A 4, A 8, A 10, A 19
Sclera, 114
Septum,
  nasal, A 48, A 50, A 52, A 54, A 56–57, C 63–64, C 66, C 122
  pellucidum, A 22, 24, A 25, A 27, C 68–71, 72, 156, S 157
  of spinal cord, posterior median, A 219, A 221–223
Sinus,
  of larynx, see Larynx, sinus
  paranasal,
    ethmoidal, A 39, A 45–46, C 62–63, C 65–66, S 90–92, A 112–116, C 118–121, S 127, S 131
    frontal, A 31–32, A 37, S 90–91, A 110–112, C 119, S 124–131
    maxillary, A 42, A 46–53, A 56–57, C 62, C 64–67, S 94–96, A 116–117, C 118–122, S 124–130, S 101, A 164
    sphenoidal, A 36, A 39–46, C 68–70, C 72, 74, S 89–90, S 92, A 114–117, C 122–123, S 126–127, S 130–131, C 184–186
  piriform, see Fossa, piriform
  venosus, sclerae, 118
  venous,
    cavernous, A 39, 40, A 41, A 43, C 70–71, 74, S 91, A 113–115, 120, C 123, S 127, S 130–131
    petrosal,
      inferior, A 43, A 45–47, C 75, A 117
    sagittal,
      inferior, 4, 82
      superior, A 4–11, A 13, A 15, A 17, A 19, A 21, A 32, A 35, 62, C 64, C 66–68, C 75, C 81–85, S 88–91
    sigmoid, A 37, A 42–43, A 46–47, 48, A 51, C 79–80, C 82, S 96, S 101–103
    straight, A 25, A 27, A 32, A 44, C 80–84
    transverse, A 37, C 81, C 83–85, S 99
Skull, A 4, A 8, A 10, A 19
Space,
  subarachnoid, thoracic, C 201
Sphenoid bone, 122
  planum, A 20, A 32, A 38, A 112, S 127, S 130–131
  pterygoid plates, see also Process, pterygoid, A 50, 126
    lateral, A 57
    medial, A 57
  rostrum, C 68, C 123, 184, C 185
  wings,
    greater, C 67–68, S 102
    lesser, S 124
Spinal cord,
  cervical, A 53, A 55, A 58, C 78, 134, A 162–164, A 168, A 172–173, A 177, A 194–197, S 204–205, S 207
  columns, see Column, Columns, of spinal cord
  lumbar, C 229
  thoracic, C 198–199, A 218–223, C 227–232, S 240–242
Spleen, C 224–227, C 229, C 231–233
Splenium of corpus callosum, see Corpus, Corpora, callosum, splenium
Stensen's duct, see Duct, parotid
Stomach, C 224–225
Stria, or Striae,
  longitudinal, of indusium griseum, S 89, 96
  terminalis, 156
Subiculum, 96
Substance,
  perforated, anterior, 100
Substantia,
  gelatinosa, of spinal cord, 194
  nigra, A 32–35, C 74–77, 88, S 90–91, A 110–111, A 138, C 139
Subthalamus, 90
Sulcus, Sulci, see also Fissures and Grooves
  cerebral,
    calcarine, A 20, A 22, A 28, A 30, A 32, A 34, C 82–84, S 90–92, S 94, 98
    callosal, S 90
    central, A 4–9, A 11–13, A 15–17, A 19, A 23, S 96–100, S 102, S 104, S 106, 134, C 135–136
      of insula, 102
    cingulate, A 12, 16, C 67, C 70, C 75–77, C 79, S 90
    circular, of insula, A 27, A 31, C 68, C 73–74, S 102
    collateral, C 70, C 78–79, C 81–83, 92, 96
    frontal,
      inferior, C 64
      superior, A 9, A 11, A 13, A 15, C 64
    intraparietal, C 82–85, 98, 104
    lateral, A 28, C 68–69, C 72, S 98, S 100–101, 102, S 103–107, S 124
    lunate, A 18
    occipital,
      lateral, C 85

Note: A, C, OR S REFERS TO AXIAL, CORONAL, OR SAGITTAL RESPECTIVELY

Sulcus, Sulci, cerebral (*Continued*)
    olfactory, C 66
    parieto-occipital, A 10, A 12–13, A 15–23, C 78, C 82, C 84–85, S 88–90, S 92, S 96, 98, 106
    postcentral, 104
    precentral, A 5–7, A 12
    rectus, A 110
    suprasplenial, 90
    temporal,
        inferior, 106, S 107
        superior, C 70, S 106–107
    median, posterior, A 222
Suture,
    coronal, A 4–5, S 96, S 100, S 106
    occipitomastoid, A 162, A 164
    petro-occipital, A 162
    sagittal, A 4–5, C 82
Syringomyelia, 194, A 223
Systems, nervous,
    acoustic, 150
    anterolateral (spinothalamic), 144
    extrapyramidal, 138
    lemniscal, 144
    limbic, 156
    oculomotor, 140
    olfactory, 156
    pyramidal, 134
    trigeminal, 148
    vestibular, 152
    visual, 154

Tapetum, 80, 92, 94
Tarsus, of eyelid,
    inferior, C 63, S 125–126, 128, S 129–131
    superior, C 63, 110, S 125–126, 128, S 129–131
Tectum, of midbrain, A 30, S 88
Teeth,
    mandible, A 59, C 63, A 166–168, S 209
    maxilla, A 55, C 63, A 165–166
Tegmentum,
    of mesencephelon, S 88
    of pons, A 37, A 39, A 41–43, A 116
Tela choroidea, of third ventricle, 72
Temporal bone,
    mastoid portion, A 42, A 45, A 47, A 49, C 74, C 76–77, C 79, S 106–107, A 115–117, C 195
    petrous portion, A 38, A 44, 48, C 74, S 102
    scutum, C 77
    zygomatic process, C 70
Tendon,
    of digastric muscle, C 187
    of rectus muscle
        inferior, C 63
        lateral, C 63
        medial, C 63, C 119
    of superior oblique muscle, A 36, A 41, A 110–111
    of temporalis muscle, C 66
    of tensor tympani, C 191
Tentorium cerebelli, 4, A 20, A 28–29, A 31–32, A 34, A 36, C 77–78, C 80–81, 82, C 83–84, S 92, S 96, S 100–101, A 112–114
Thalamus, A 20, A 22, A 24–27, A 30, A 32, C 73–77, S 90–91, S 94, S 129–131, 138, 152, A 153, 154
    nuclear groups,
        anterior, 156
        lateral, 144, A 146
        medial, 148, A 149
        ventral, A 138, C 139, A 142
Tongue, C 65, A 165, 168, C 184–185, S 206, S 210
    frenulum, C 184

muscles,
    extrinsic, 168
    intrinsic, C 66, C 70, 168, S 206, S 208, S 212
        longitudinal,
            inferior, C 185
            superior, C 185
        transverse, C 185
    septum linguae, (raphe), A 166, A 169, C 185–186
Tonsil,
    cerebellar, A 42, A 44–45, A 47–48, A 50–52, C 79–82, S 88–91, C 194–195, C 197, C 199
    lingual, 164
    palatine, 164, A 165–166, C 186
    pharyngeal, 164
Tooth, see Teeth
Torus,
    tubarius, A 51, A 53, A 55, A 163, C 187
Trabeculae, of bone, S 278
Trachea, C 187, C 189, C 190, C 193, S 205–208
    bifurcation, A 222
Tract(s) or Tractus, see also Fasciculus
    corticobulbar, 24, 134, 158
    corticorubral, 76
    corticospinal, A 52, C 76–77, 134, A 135, A 137, A 165
        anterior, A 220
        lateral, A 31, A 218, A 220–223
        olfactory, A 36
    cuneatus, 144
    gracilis, 144
    olfactory, C 64, A 110, C 120
    optic, 32, A 33–35, C 73–75, S 90, 154, A 155
    rubrospinal, 76
    spinocerebellar, 142
    spinoreticular, 144
    spinothalamic, 144, A 145–146
        anterior (ventral), A 218–221, A 223
        lateral, A 219–220
    thalamocortical, 76
    uveal, 114
Triangles,
    anterior, C 190, S 214
    carotid, S 214
    digastric, S 214
    muscular, S 214
    occipital, S 214
    posterior, C 190, S 214
    submental, S 214
    supraclavicular, S 214
Trochlea, of superior oblique, 120, S 127
Tube,
    auditory (eustachian), A 42, A 46, A 48, A 50–51, A 53, A 55, C 71–72, A 162–163, C 187, C 189–190
Tuber, Tubercle, or Tuberosity,
    of C1,
        anterior, C 190–191, 276
        posterior, C 83, A 164, C 199
    cinereum, A 33, A 110
    jugular, A 45, A 47, C 74, C 76, C 78, S 92, A 117, C 193–194
    pharyngeal, 56
    of vermis, see Lobule, Lobules, of cerebellum
Turbinate, see Concha, nasal

Uncus, 36, A 37, A 39, C 72, C 74–75, C 77, S 92, S 95, 96, A 111–114, 156
Ureter, C 258–259, C 261
Uvula,
    of palate, A 56, A 59, C 70, C 74, S 88, A 164–165, A 167, S 204–209
    of vermis, see Lobule, Lobules, of cerebellum

Note: A, C, OR S REFERS TO AXIAL, CORONAL, OR SAGITTAL RESPECTIVELY

Vallecula,
  of cerebellum, A 43, A 45–46, A 50–51
  of larynx, 172, A 173, C 187, 204, S 205
Veins,
  angular, C 63–64, S 94, A 112–113, 120, S 127, S 131, A 164–165
  azygos, A 218–223, 236, S 242–243
    lumbar, 218, 220
  basal, of Rosenthal, A 25, A 31, C 76, S 95
  basivertebral, A 173–174, S 204, A 219, A 223, C 225–227, S 241–242, A 250–253, A 255, C 260–261, C 263–265, S 274, S 276–278
  brachiocephalic, 236
  cava,
    inferior, S 240, A 248–255, C 258, S 281
    superior, 218
  cerebellar, superior, 82
  cerebral, internal, C 73, C 75–79, S 89, S 131
  cervical, A 48, A 52–53, A 58, A 82, A 164–165, A 169, A 172, A 177, A 179, 198, S 213
  ciliary, A 114, 118
  condylar,
    posterior emissary, A 52, C 193
  confluence, see Confluence of sinuses
  epidural, A 52, A 165, A 174, A 176, A 178–179, C 195, S 204, A 221–222, S 240, A 248–250, A 255, A 257
  facial, C 119, 120
    anterior, A 59, A 167–168, A 173, A 175
    common, 62, C 63, A 177
    posterior, A 52
  great cerebral, A 25, 82, S 88, S 91, S 130
  hemiazygos, 220, C 224–226, S 237, S 239–240
    accessory, A 218–223, C 226, 236, S 237
  iliac,
    common, A 255–257, C 259, C 261, C 263
    internal, C 258, C 262
  innominate, see Veins, brachiocephalic
  intercostal, A 222–223, C 224–234, S 236–237, S 244–245
    posterior, 236, 252, 280
    superior, 236
  intervertebral, S 239, S 244, 252, S 273, 280, S 281
  intravertebral, A 255
  jugular,
    anterior, A 179, A 181
    external, A 55, A 59, S 106–107, A 172–173, A 176, A 180, C 193
    internal, A 47–54, A 57–59, C 74, C 76–78, C 82, S 96, S 98, S 100–103, A 163–173, A 175–181, C 190–191, C 193, S 214–215
      bulb, 48
  lumbar, 252, C 258–259, C 261, C 263–265, S 272–273, 280, S 281
    ascending, 218, 220
  mastoid emissary, C 80
  occipital, C 201, S 215
  ophthalmic, 122
    inferior, A 115, C 120
    superior, A 36–37, C 65, A 110–113, 120, C 121, S 125, S 129–131
  pharyngeal, A 52, A 54, A 58, A 162–163
  pulmonary, S 245
  radicular, S 280
  renal, C 258
  retromandibular, A 54, A 163, A 165, A 167
  sacral,
    lateral, 252, C 271, 280
  segmental, S 272, S 281
  subcostal, 218, 220
  temporal,
    superficial, A 17, A 23
  thalamostriate, A 21–22, A 25, A 27, C 72–73, S 89, S 91–92
  vertebral, A 53, A 179, A 181, 236, 252, 280
Velum, medullary, superior, S 89
Ventricles, of brain,
  fourth, A 36–44, A 46–47, C 78–79, 82, S 88–90, A 113–116, 140, 152
  lateral, A 20, A 26, C 74, C 76, C 78–79
    anterior horn, A 25, A 27–28, A 30, C 66, C 68–72, S 90, S 94, C 122, S 126
    body, A 18–19, A 21, A 23, A 30, C 73, C 75, S 93–94
    inferior horn, A 26, A 30, A 32, A 35, A 37, 72, C 73–76, S 94, 97–98, S 100, 154
    posterior horn, A 31, C 78–82, S 96–98
    trigone (atrium), A 20, A 22, A 25–28, A 30, C 77, S 96, S 98–99
  third, A 20, A 27–29, A 30, A 31, A 32, A 33, C 72–75, C 77, A 110
Vermis, of cerebellum, see also Lobule, Lobules, of cerebellum, A 28, A 33, A 35, A 39, A 41, A 43, S 88–89, A 113, A 115
Vertebra,
  C1, A 52, A 163, C 195
  C2, C 84, A 164, A 167, C 191
  C3, C 82, A 171, C 192
  C4, A 172, A 174–175, S 204, S 206, S 208
  C5, A 174–175, A 177, C 196, S 215
  C6, A 178, A 181, C 194
  C7, A 181, C 193, S 206, S 209, S 212
  T1, C 195, S 207, S 242
  T2, C 197, S 209
  T3, S 243
  T4, C 228, S 239
  T5, A 222, S 238, S 244
  T6, A 218–221, S 241–244
  T7, A 222–223, C 227, C 229, S 239–243
  T8, C 226–227, S 241–243
  T9, C 224–225, S 237, S 239
  T10, C 225
  T11, C 224–225
  T12, C 226, C 228
  L1, C 224
  L2, C 259, C 261, C 263, C 265, S 273, S 276–277, S 279–281
  L3, A 249–251, C 258, C 260, S 274–275, S 278–279
  L4, A 251, A 253, S 275–276, S 280
  L5, A 254–256, C 261, C 264–265, C 271, S 274–277, S 279
  S1, A 257, C 266
Vertebral canal, S 208
Vestibular fold, see Fold, Folds, vestibular
Vestibule, of labyrinth of ear, A 42, A 117
Vitreous, see Body, Bodies, vitreous
Vocal cord, see Fold, Folds, vocal
Vocal folds, see Fold, Folds, vocal
Vomer, A 48, A 51, A 53, C 63, C 65–67, C 119–122, 184

Zygoma, S 100, S 105, S 128
Zygomatic bone, S 107, A 111–115, C 121, 128, C 185
  arch, C 68, C 70, A 116–117

Note: A, C, OR S REFERS TO AXIAL, CORONAL, OR SAGITTAL RESPECTIVELY

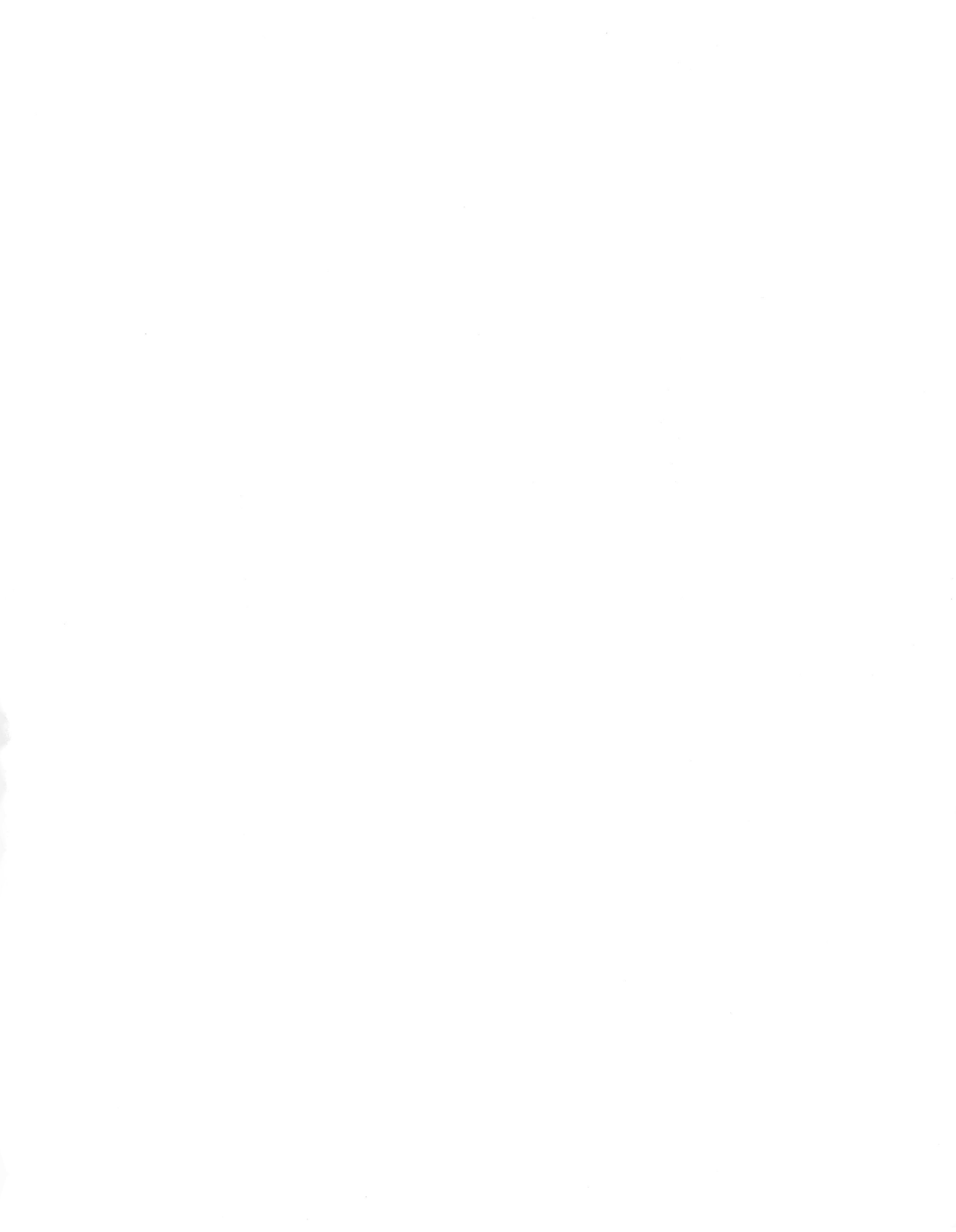

Discarded

University of Cincinnati
Blue Ash College Library